Intensive and Rehabilitative Respiratory Care

A Practical Approach to the Management of Acute and Chronic Respiratory Failure

Intensive and Rehabilitative Respiratory Care

THIRD EDITION

Thomas L. Petty, M.D.

Contributors:
Ernest K. Cotton, M.D.
Giles F. Filley, M.D.
J. Brevard Haynes
Louise M. Nett, R.N., R.R.T.
David J. Pierson, M.D.
Margo A. Pinney, M.S.N.
N. Balfour Slonim, M.D., Ph.D.
John L. Stauffer
Allan B. Wicks

University of Colorado Medical Center
Denver

LEA & FEBIGER • *1982* • *Philadelphia*

Lea & Febiger
600 Washington Square
Philadelphia, PA 19106
U.S.A.

Library of Congress Cataloging in Publication Data

Petty, Thomas L.
Intensive and rehabilitative respiratory care.

Bibliography: p.
Includes index.
1. Respiratory insufficiency—Treatment.
2. Respiratory insufficiency—Patients—Rehabilitation.
3. Critical care medicine. I. Title.
[DNLM: 1. Respiratory insufficiency—Therapy.
WF 140 P512i]
RC776.R4P47 1982 616.2'0046 81-23630
ISBN 0-8121-0764-0 AACR2

FIRST EDITION, 1971
Reprinted, April, 1973
SECOND EDITION, 1974
Reprinted, February, 1976
THIRD EDITION, 1982

PRINTED IN THE UNITED STATES OF AMERICA

Print No. 3 2 1

PREFACE

The practice and techniques of respiratory care continue to improve. Both intensive and rehabilitative respiratory care are now established services in most medical centers, and nearly every hospital has some means of caring for sudden unexpected acute respiratory failure. Blood gases are established in everyday practice, and the use of oxygen, mechanical ventilators, and hemodynamic monitoring along with other day-to-day respiratory care techniques serve millions of people each year.

Simultaneously our understanding of diseases characterized by chronic airflow limitation, bronchial asthma, interstitial lung disease, paralytic states, and the adult respiratory distress syndrome have improved, but much more progress is required in certain areas, particularly in the case of the adult respiratory distress syndrome, in order to begin to solve the basic problems of lung injury and repair.

This third edition emphasizes advances in respiratory care and includes a thorough review of both established and new techniques and concepts. New chapters have been added on Principles of Hemodynamic Monitoring and Ethical Considerations of Respiratory Care, which focuses on difficult human issues which are daily faced by those who care for patients with disordered breathing.

This edition is written for both beginning students and experts in modern respiratory care. Emphasis is placed on concepts and principles in greater detail than before. A systematic approach to management of the most pressing problems relevant to our field today is stressed throughout.

Denver, Colorado THOMAS L. PETTY, M.D.

ACKNOWLEDGMENTS

The assistance of the following current members of the respiratory care unit is gratefully acknowledged: Mrs. Jeanne Cleary, Mrs. Sandy Blegebron, Mrs. Patty Way, secretaries; Mr. B. Baidwan, technician; Miss Joan Balik, nurse; Mrs. Virginia Carpenter, social service worker; Mr. Alan Suzuki, statistician; Mr. Cleafe Best (deceased), consulting engineer; and Mr. G. Wayne Silvers, research associate.

The following contributors to the first and second editions are again acknowledged with great appreciation: Doctors David G. Ashbaugh, D. Boyd Bigelow; Nurse Martha L. Tyler, and Physical Therapist Georgia M. Foss.

CONTRIBUTORS

Ernest K. Cotton, M.D.
Professor of Pediatrics
University of Colorado Health Sciences Center
Denver, Colorado

Giles F. Filley, M.D.
Professor of Medicine, Emeritus
University of Colorado Health Sciences Center
Denver, Colorado

J. Brevard Haynes, M.D., Pulmonary Fellow 1977-1979
Pulmonary & Allergy Associates of Nashville, P.C.
Nashville, Tennessee

Louise M. Nett, R.N., R.R.T.
Associate Clinical Professor of Nursing
Instructor in Medicine
University of Colorado Health Sciences Center
Denver, Colorado

Thomas L. Petty, M.D.
Professor of Medicine
Head, Division of Pulmonary Sciences
University of Colorado Health Sciences Center
Denver, Colorado

David J. Pierson, M.D., Pulmonary Fellow 1972-1974
Associate Professor of Medicine
University of Washington
Seattle, Washington

Margo A. Pinney, M.S.N.
Pediatric Pulmonary Clinical Specialist
Instructor in Pediatrics
University of Colorado Health Sciences Center
Denver, Colorado

N. Balfour Slonim, M.D., Ph.D.
Director
Cardiopulmonary Diagnostic Laboratory
Denver, Colorado

John L. Stauffer, M.D., Pulmonary Fellow 1975-1977
Assistant Professor of Medicine, U.C.S.F.
Chief, Pulmonary Disease Section
Fresno Veterans Administration Hospital
Fresno, California

Allan B. Wicks, M.D., Pulmonary Fellow 1973-1974
Assistant Clinical Professor of Medicine
Pulmonary Physician Craig Rehabilitation Center
Denver, Colorado

CONTENTS

Section A
Acute Respiratory Failure—Methods of Care

Chapter 1

ACUTE RESPIRATORY FAILURE

(Manifestations, Clinical States, Arterial Puncture, Blood Gas and pH Analysis)

By Thomas L. Petty

DEFINITION

Acute respiratory failure occurs in many clinical situations and constitutes a medical emergency requiring prompt and exacting diagnosis, meticulous initial management, and effective follow-up care. It may be defined as the sudden inability of the respiratory apparatus and heart to maintain adequate arterial oxygenation and adequate carbon dioxide elimination. In the final sense, acute respiratory failure is present when tissue oxygen transport and carbon dioxide elimination are impaired; but because of the difficulties in estimating tissue gas tensions, arterial blood gas analysis is most commonly utilized to determine the presence and severity of acute respiratory failure. Arbitrarily, acute respiratory failure is defined as the sudden development of an arterial Po_2 of less than 55 mm Hg with or without CO_2 retention. An acute elevation of carbon dioxide tension to more than 50 mm Hg is called "acute ventilatory failure." The separation of hypoxemia from hypercapnia or so-called ventilatory failure has important therapeutic implications.

MANIFESTATIONS

Acute respiratory failure has become a frequently recognized clinical syndrome that can be encountered by physicians in the practice of any medical specialty, particularly internal medicine (e.g., emphysema due to chronic airflow obstruction, chronic bronchitis, and asthma). It can be associated with postoperative surgical states, trauma, neurologic emergencies, and accidental or self-induced poisonings. Table 1-1 lists the common disease states with which it may occur in adults; the table is organized according to the basic pathophysiologic process involved. (See also Chap. 16.)

Acute Respiratory Failure

A synopsis of the physiologic basis for the development of respiratory failure, including problems of ventilation and abnormalities of gas exchange (hypoxemia and hypercapnia), is given in Appendix A.

Various acute pulmonary insults are often precipitating factors in the development of acute respiratory failure, particularly when associated with underlying chronic airflow limitation (obstruction) or interstitial disease. These include pneumonia (Chap. 12), acute bron-

TABLE 1-1. Disease States Leading to Respiratory Failure

I. Impaired ventilation
   A. Chronic airflow obstruction
      Emphysema, chronic bronchitis, chronic asthma, cystic fibrosis
   B. Restrictive defects
      1. Decreased lung expansion
         Interstitial fibrosis, pleural effusion, pneumothorax, fibrothorax
      2. Limited thorax expansion
         Kyphoscoliosis, multiple rib fractures, thoracic surgery, ankylosing spondylitis
      3. Decreased diaphragmatic movement
         Abdominal surgery, ascites, peritonitis, severe obesity, diaphragmatic paralysis
   C. Neuromuscular defects
      Guillain-Barré syndrome, myasthenia gravis, multiple sclerosis, muscular dystrophy, botulism, tetanus, brain or spinal injuries, drugs or toxic agents (e.g., curare, acetylcholinesterase inhibitors, aminoglycosides), antibiotics, polio, porphyria
   D. Respiratory center damage or depression
      Narcotics, barbiturates, tranquilizers, anesthetics, cerebral infarction or trauma, uncontrolled high-flow oxygen therapy

II. Impaired diffusion and gas exchange
   A. Pulmonary fibrosis
      Interstitial fibrosis, sarcoidosis, pneumonoconiosis
   B. Pulmonary edema
      1. Cardiogenic
      2. Noncardiogenic
   C. Adult Respiratory Distress Syndrome
   D. Obliterative pulmonary vascular disease
      Thromboembolism with blood, fat, bone marrow, or amniotic fluid
   E. Anatomic loss of functioning lung tissue
      Pneumonectomy, tumor

III. Ventilation-perfusion abnormalities and venous admixture
   Asthma, emphysema, chronic bronchitis, bronchiolitis, atelectasis, pneumonia, thromboembolism, and respiratory distress syndromes

chial asthma (Chap. 9), and thromboembolism. These acute problems may also precipitate respiratory failure in patients with other chronic pulmonary conditions including restricted ventilation due to pulmonary fibrosis (Chap. 11). It is unusual for pneumothorax (unless accompanied by tension), small pleural effusions, and problems of impaired diaphragmatic excursion alone to cause respiratory failure in the absence of significant underlying lung disease, but these conditions may contribute to the development of acute respiratory failure when pulmonary reserve is impaired.

The clinical manifestations of acute respiratory failure are primarily those of the blood gas abnormalities involved. The major clinical signs are listed in Table 1-2. It is clear that these signs do not

TABLE 1-2. Clinical Manifestations of Acute Respiratory Failure

Manifestations of underlying disease plus:	
1. Restlessness	7. Hypotension
2. Confusion	8. Tremors—asterixis
3. Tachycardia	9. Poor chest expansion
4. Diaphoresis	10. Depressed respiration
5. Headache	11. Miosis, papilledema
6. Central cyanosis	12. Unconsciousness

necessarily direct one's attention to abnormalities of respiration. Hypoxemia and hypercapnia produce the signs of altered central nervous system function and impaired circulatory function.[1–5] This is the main reason that respiratory failure may be misdiagnosed. The most common misdiagnoses are (1) central nervous system catastrophe such as cerebral vascular accident, (2) congestive heart failure, and (3) pneumonia. One of the most common causes of impaired consciousness is acute respiratory failure.

The clinical signs observed in patients suffering from acute respiratory failure will be those of the underlying disease as well as the superimposed signs of hypoxemia or hypercapnia, or both. It is our experience that restlessness, headache, confusion, and tachycardia are the four most common signs encountered. It should be stressed that although the clinical features of acute respiratory failure may be obvious or dramatic at times (as in Adult Respiratory Distress Syndrome, unconsciousness due to drug ingestion, severe chest trauma, and status asthmaticus, or severe pneumonia), many patients, particularly those with chronic airway obstruction, become ill in so gradual and subtle a fashion that the attending physician, in making his rounds, may fail to spend time at their bedside lest he interfere with their "sleep." In some instances a sedative may be offered for bedtime restlessness.

DIAGNOSIS AND ASSESSMENT

Acute respiratory failure must be suspected by alert clinicians, nurses, and therapists who are aware of the clinical states in which respiratory failure is likely to occur. The diagnosis must be confirmed through laboratory study. Acute respiratory failure is most simply identified by means of arterial puncture and immediate analysis of a blood sample to determine the pH, Po_2, oxygen saturation, and Pco_2.[6] The safety and simplicity of arterial puncture have been established.[7] It is impossible to estimate the degree of hypoxemia from clinical signs alone, and cyanosis is a notoriously inadequate guide to determination of the degree of hypoxemia.[8]

Arterial Puncture

Figure 1-1 demonstrates the simple equipment needed for an arterial puncture (arterial stick)—a standard 10-ml glass syringe, disposable #20 needle, and dilute heparin (1000 units/ml). Disposable packages for this procedure have been marketed by several manufacturers.

The syringe is prepared by drawing sufficient heparin into it to wet the plunger and to fill the dead space of the syringe and the needle. The excess heparin is expelled with the syringe in the upright position. A palpable artery (radial or brachial) is selected. After skin preparation, the needle is directed into the artery as shown in Figure

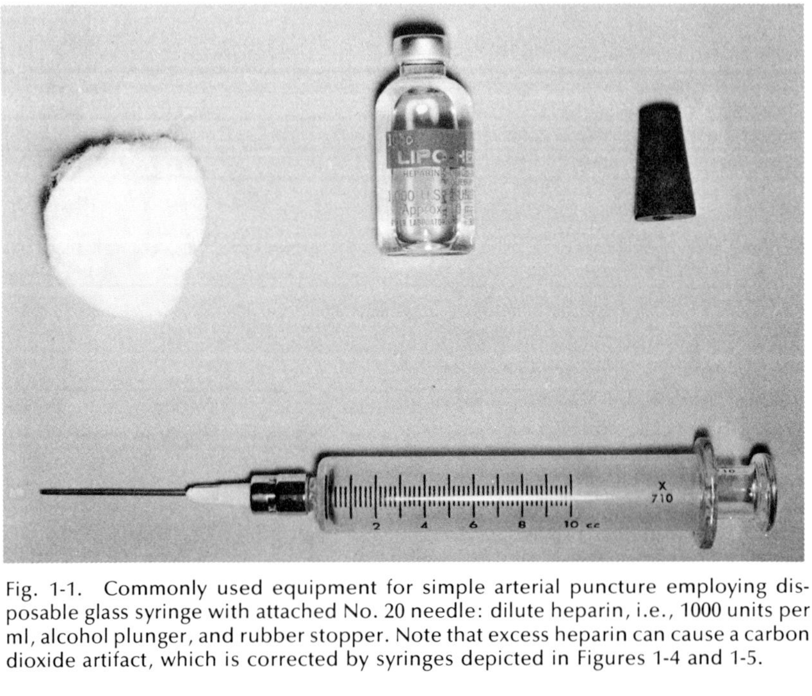

Fig. 1-1. Commonly used equipment for simple arterial puncture employing disposable glass syringe with attached No. 20 needle: dilute heparin, i.e., 1000 units per ml, alcohol plunger, and rubber stopper. Note that excess heparin can cause a carbon dioxide artifact, which is corrected by syringes depicted in Figures 1-4 and 1-5.

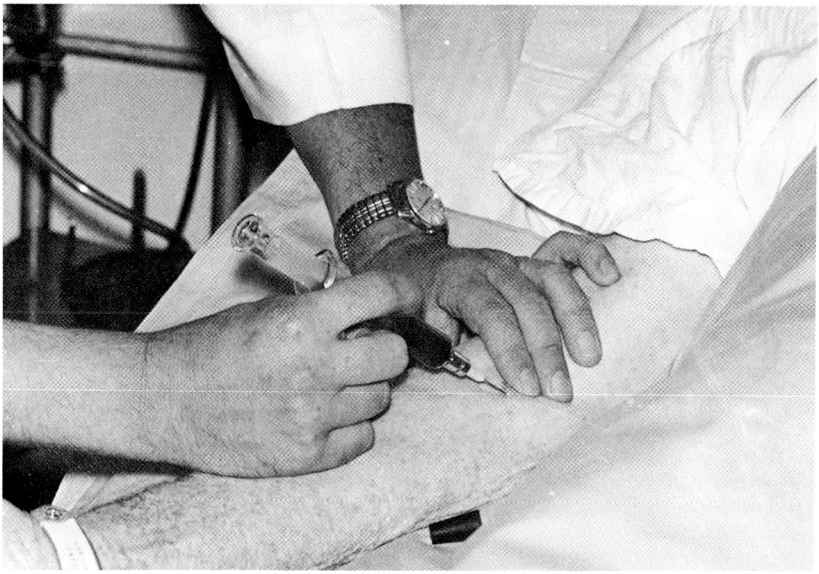

Fig. 1-2. Technique of arterial puncture, directing needle toward palpitating artery. The radial and brachial artery are most commonly used. Naturally, no tourniquet is used for arterial puncture.

1-2. Usually the initial thrust will bring a pulsating flow of blood into the syringe. It is not necessary to draw outward with the plunger; the spontaneous pulsating flow will be proof of entry into the artery. If the needle fails to enter the artery, simple redirection will usually result in its entry. Occasionally, the artery is pierced. When this happens, blood will flow when the needle is withdrawn slightly. After the blood sample has been obtained, the needle is plunged into a rubber stopper. The needle and syringe are then placed in a beaker of ice and taken to the blood gas laboratory for immediate analysis. Cooling reduces the metabolism of the cellular elements within the syringe (Fig. 1-3). The stability of a properly maintained "iced down" sample is revealed in Table 1-3.

This technique of arterial puncture has proved to be entirely satisfactory and safe with no identifiable complications in a large number of individuals followed for months after repeated arterial punctures.[7] The ease and relatively painless nature of the procedure make anesthesia and the use of indwelling needles and catheters unnecessary. Following these simple instructions, a clinician, nurse, or technician with no special background can learn to perform arterial punctures in a matter of two or three minutes.

Owing to the significant amount of dead space in large needles and the dead space of the 10-ml glass syringe in this illustration, significant errors can occur for P_{CO_2} when only small arterial blood samples are obtained.[9] The sample should be at least 5 ml and preferably more

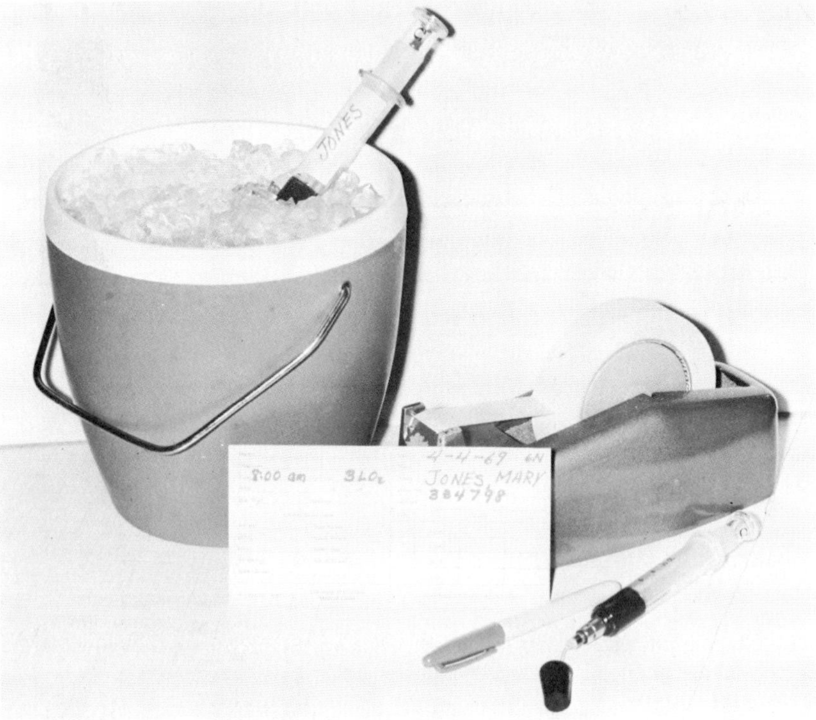

Fig. 1-3. Common method of placing syringe in ice for transport to laboratory. The sample should be determined directly, however. No icing is necessary if samples are analyzed within one hour.

when this technique is used. Arterial blood gas samples of less than 2 ml produce sufficiently large errors and are often misleading. Thus, all laboratories should refuse to perform determinations on inadequate samples.

New Blood Gas Samplers

Recently, a new device for arterial blood gas sampling that avoids this dead space problem has been evaluated and marketed.[9] Since

TABLE 1-3. Effects of Storage on Po_2 at Various Oxygen Tensions (8 to 10 ml Arterial Blood in Glass Syringe)

Duration of Storage (on-ice-hours)	Po_2	Po_2	Po_2	Po_2	Barometric Pressure (mm Hg)
0	116	216	290	520	636
1	113	212	290	512	636
2	112	211	285	500	635
3	111	214	290	510	635
24	111	189	275	350	634

resistance to filling is minimal, the device can be used with small-bore needles such as #23 to minimize trauma and hematoma formation. This is particularly important in patients who are receiving fibrinolytic therapy, with which hematoma and bleeding following arterial puncture are a problem.[10] Figure 1-4 diagrams the features of this new device.[9]

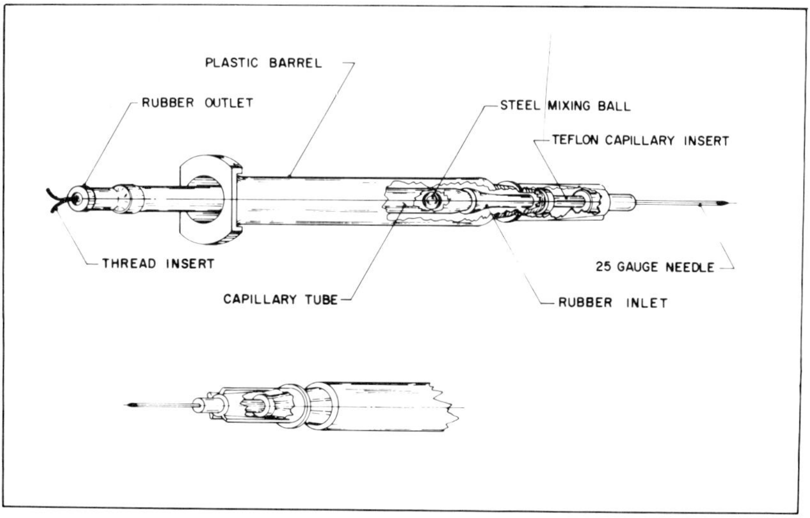

Fig. 1-4. Low-resistance arterial sampling device which avoids heparin artifact. Efficacy of device "mosquito" was previously reported.[9]

Figure 1-5 presents the features of the newest and most versatile device thus far available (Omnistik). The 2-ml glass syringe contains crystalline heparin. The plunger is set at the desired amount of arterial blood, such as 0.5 ml or more. When the artery is entered, blood can fill the preset volume, and air escapes via two vents in the plunger. These vents are retracted by simple rotation of the plunger handle to maintain an anaerobic sample. Small amounts of gas exchange at the filling blood-syringe air interface are negligible, and because only blood from the needle end of the syringe is introduced into the blood gas devices, no artifacts are encountered. This device has been recently evaluated in detail by the author and has been found very satisfactory in day-to-day use.

Blood Gas Instruments

Previous editions of this book presented pictures of the commonly used radiometer pH, P_{O_2}, and P_{CO_2} blood gas electrodes as well as the Astrup Tonometer for estimating P_{CO_2}. Blood gas technology has been refined although the electrode principles remain essentially unchanged. The design of blood gas systems has also changed considerably in recent years, and many other manufacturers have marketed

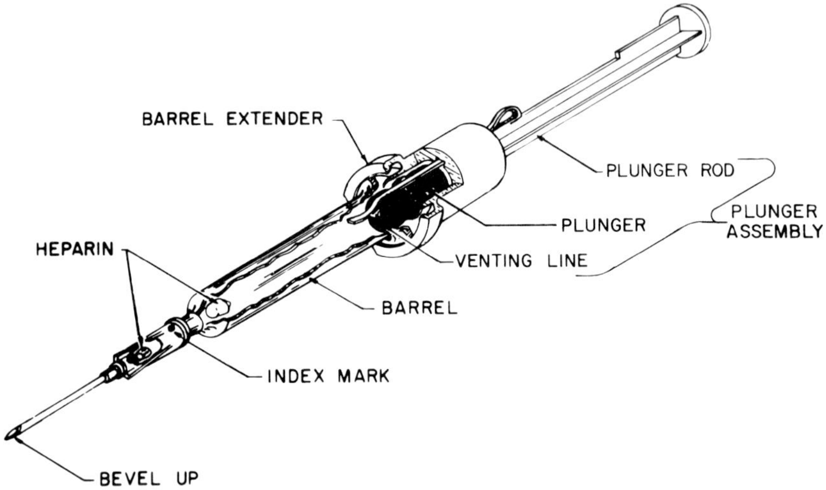

Fig. 1-5. A versatile blood gas sampler with 2-1/2 ml volume. Venting lines are retractable by twisting plunger rod. Lyopholized heparin is used to provide intimate contact between heparin and advancing blood sample. (Omnistik evaluated in laboratory of author.)

excellent automated devices. The automated radiometer device, used in our laboratory at the present time, is presented in Figure 1-6.

It is of more than passing interest to possess at least a casual knowledge of the principles of blood gas and pH analysis. For this

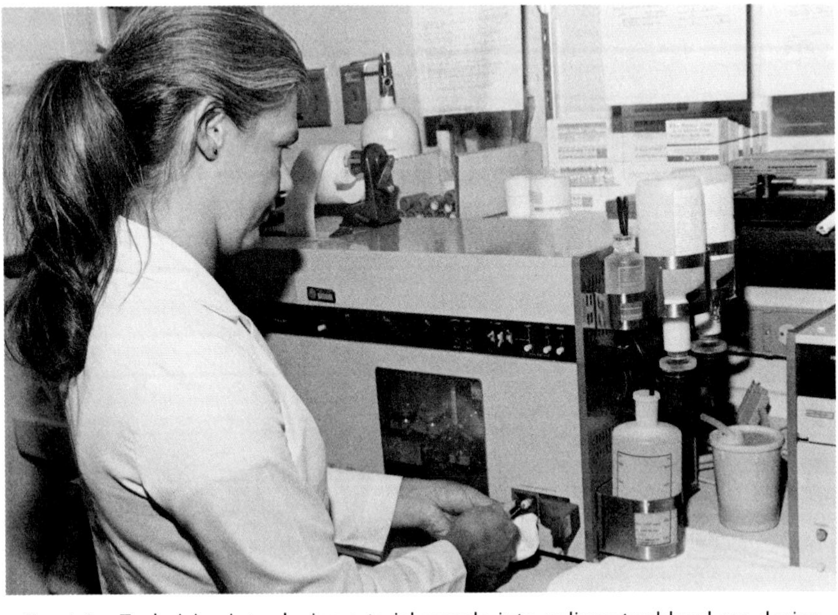

Fig. 1-6. Technician introducing arterial sample into radiometer blood gas device. This semi-automated machine gives both visual and paper printout.

reason Figures 1-7 and 1-8 are presented to diagram the construction and principles of P_{O_2}, P_{CO_2}, and pH analysis.[11,12] Figure 1-9 is the standard oxyhemoglobin dissociation relationship relating oxygen *amount*—a function of hemoglobin saturation on the vertical axis and oxygen tension on the horizontal axis—at three different pH values.[12]

Oximeters

Oxygen saturation can also be measured by a variety of oximeters that use reflected light at two wave lengths to reflect the reduced and oxygenated hemoglobin, expressed as a percentage. This directly measured oxygen saturation equals that calculated for pH and P_{O_2}.[12–14]

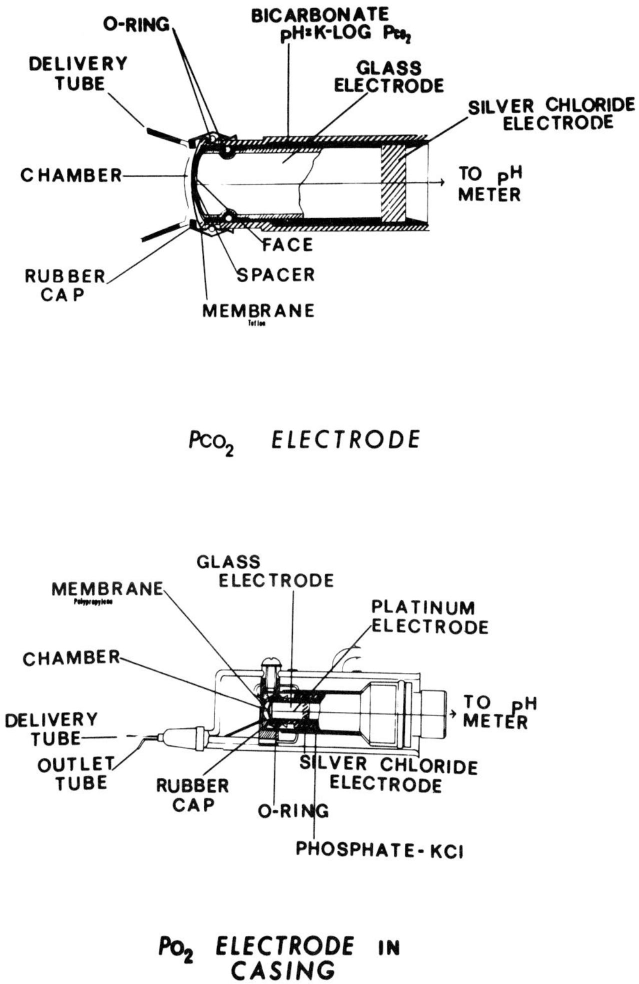

Fig. 1-7. Diagramatic representation of P_{O_2} and P_{CO_2} electrode. (Original radiometer used CO_2 and O_2 electrodes. New devices use the same principles.)

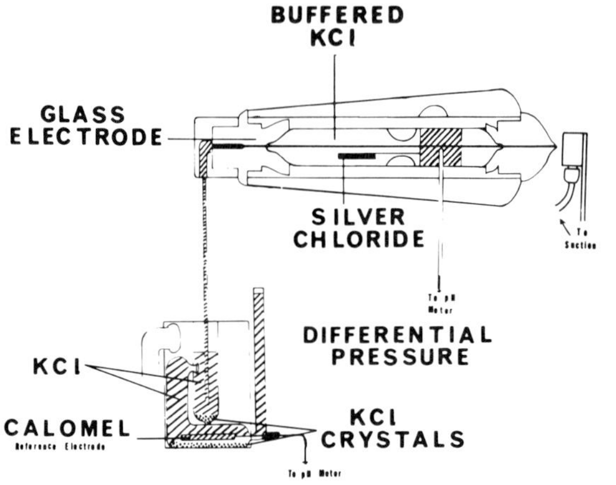

MICRO pH ELECTRODE UNIT

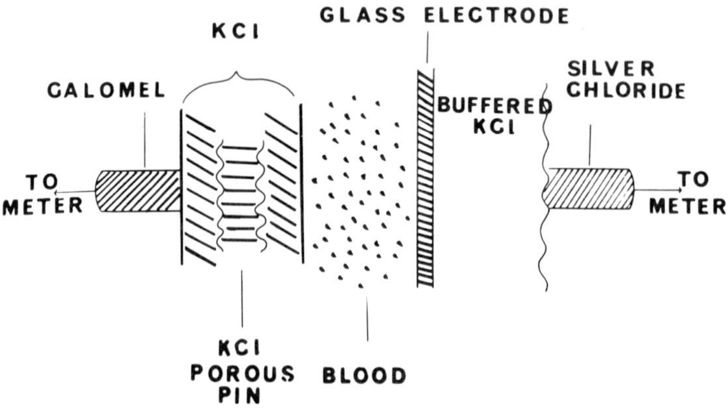

Fig. 1-8. Diagram of pH electrode. (Original radiometer electrode.)

A new ear oximeter has a similar accuracy.[15] The device uses the light transmission and in the case of normal ear perfusion gives a continuous record of oxygen saturation using a satisfactory ear probe (Fig. 1-10). A comparison of the accuracy of this device with that of the commonly used American Optical Oximeter or with calculated values from Po_2 and pH is shown in Figures 1-11 and 1-12. This device is particularly useful in making oxygen or ventilator adjustments when the main concern is adequacy of arterial oxygenation. When adjustments have been made at the bedside to satisfy the clinical situation, the full pattern of blood gas determinations can then be observed, with a final arterial puncture providing determinations of pH, Pco_2, and bicarbonate as well as oxygen saturation.

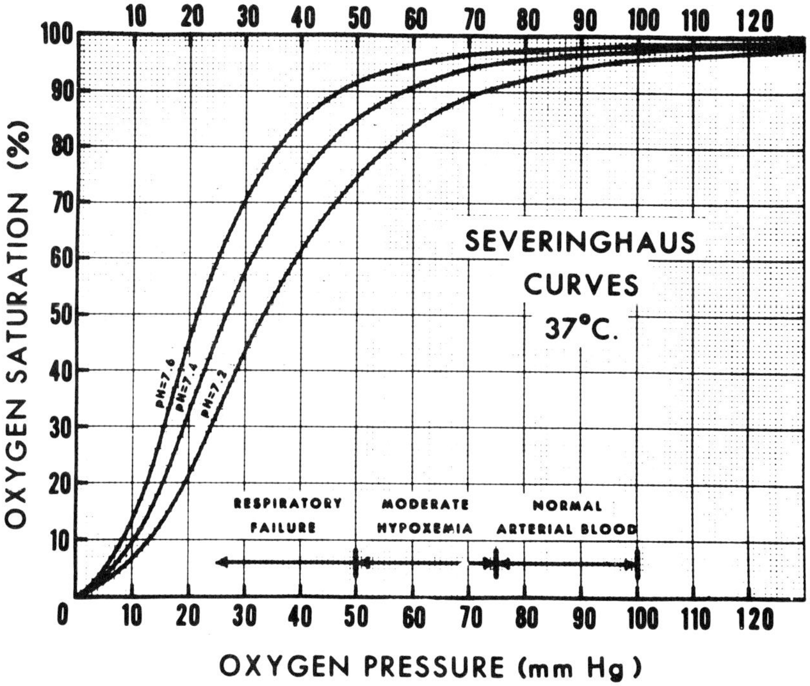

Fig. 1-9. Oxyhemoglobin dissociation curve showing relationship between oxygen tension (pressure) and oxygen saturation (%). Note shifts in curve due to pH changes.

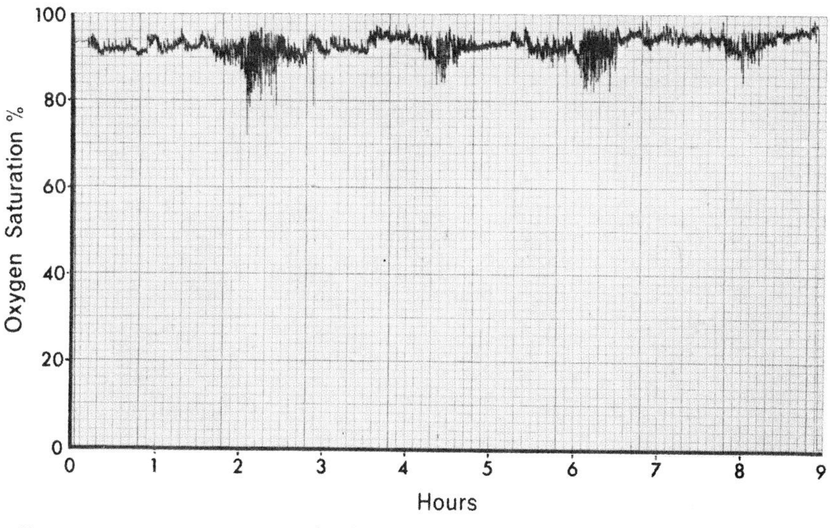

Fig. 1-10. Continuous record of oxygen saturation using Hewlett-Packard ear oximeter. (From Scoggin, C., Nett, L., and Petty, T.L.: Clinical evaluation of a new ear oximeter. Heart Lung, *6:*121, 1977.)

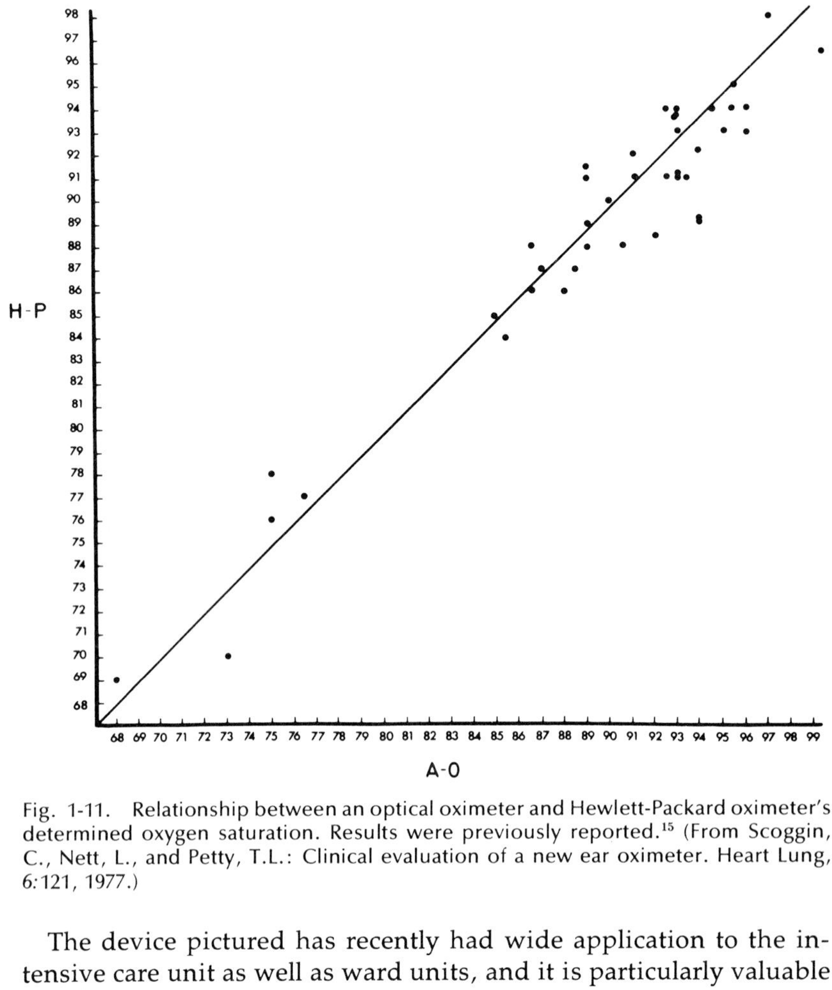

Fig. 1-11. Relationship between an optical oximeter and Hewlett-Packard oximeter's determined oxygen saturation. Results were previously reported.[15] (From Scoggin, C., Nett, L., and Petty, T.L.: Clinical evaluation of a new ear oximeter. Heart Lung, 6:121, 1977.)

The device pictured has recently had wide application to the intensive care unit as well as ward units, and it is particularly valuable when continuous noninvasive measurements of oxygen saturation are desirable.[15]

Arterial Blood Gas Diagram

A great amount of valuable clinical information is available from carefully performed and analyzed blood gas determinations. An arterial blood gas diagram suitable for clinical use has been offered to judge abnormalities of oxygen transfer and various levels of alveolar ventilation.[16] In brief, Figure 1-13 shows the normal relationship between arterial PO_2 and PCO_2 in normal subjects at rest as well as in subjects who performed breath-holding (for CO_2 retention) and voluntary hyperventilation. By contrast, Figure 1-14 shows the relationship between PO_2 and PCO_2 in subjects with various degrees of chronic obstructive pulmonary disease. There is a rough correlation between the expected and observed alveolar PO_2 for each increment of advancing chronic airflow obstruction (limitation). A similar rela-

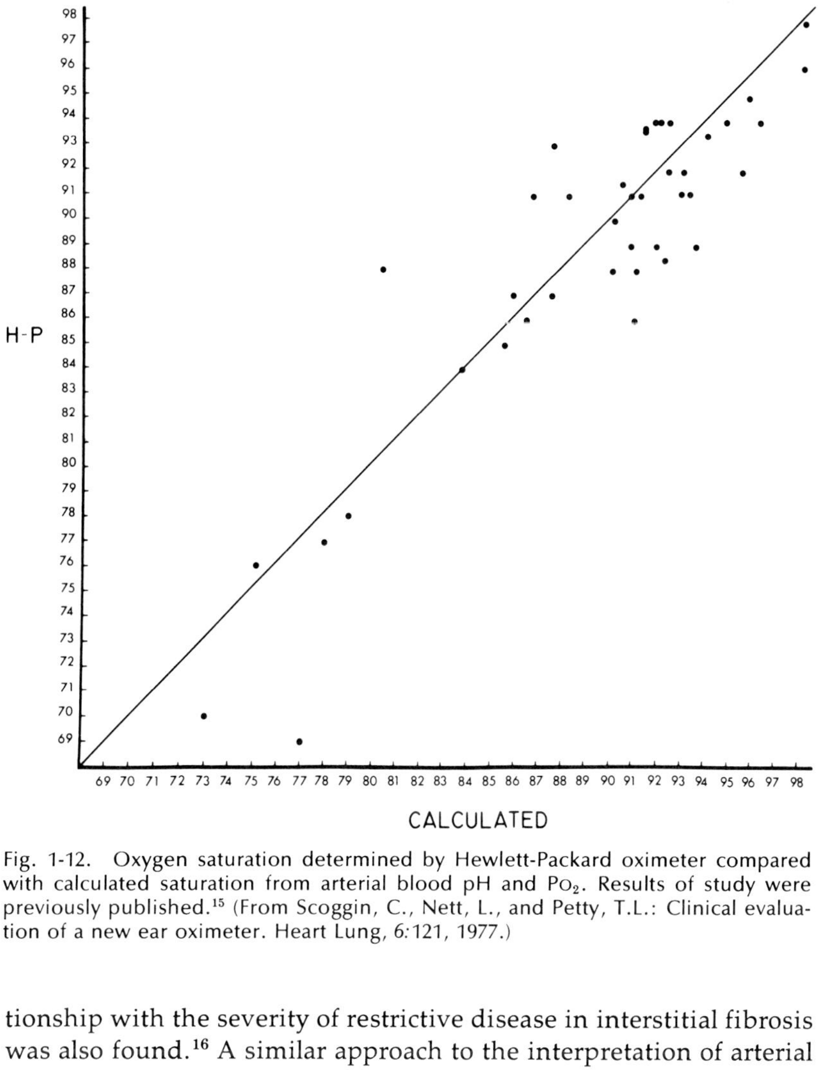

Fig. 1-12. Oxygen saturation determined by Hewlett-Packard oximeter compared with calculated saturation from arterial blood pH and Po_2. Results of study were previously published.[15] (From Scoggin, C., Nett, L., and Petty, T.L.: Clinical evaluation of a new ear oximeter. Heart Lung, *6:*121, 1977.)

tionship with the severity of restrictive disease in interstitial fibrosis was also found.[16] A similar approach to the interpretation of arterial oxygen–carbon dioxide partial pressures is offered in a companion article.[17] This offers a valuable approach to assessing the gas exchange function of the lungs.

Carbon Dioxide Homeostasis

In the normal individual, a delicate relationship exists between the metabolic production of carbon dioxide and its removal by alveolar ventilation so that there is a near-normal level of Pco_2—between 40 ± 4 mm Hg at sea level (36 ± 3 mm Hg Denver altitude). This results in a narrow pH range of 7.35 to 7.45. Pco_2 elimination has been compared with the renal clearance concept in the following relationship[18]:

$$\dot{V}_A \text{ (alveolar ventilation)} = \frac{\dot{V}co_2 \text{ (}CO_2\text{ production) in ml/mm} \times 0.863}{Pco_2}.$$

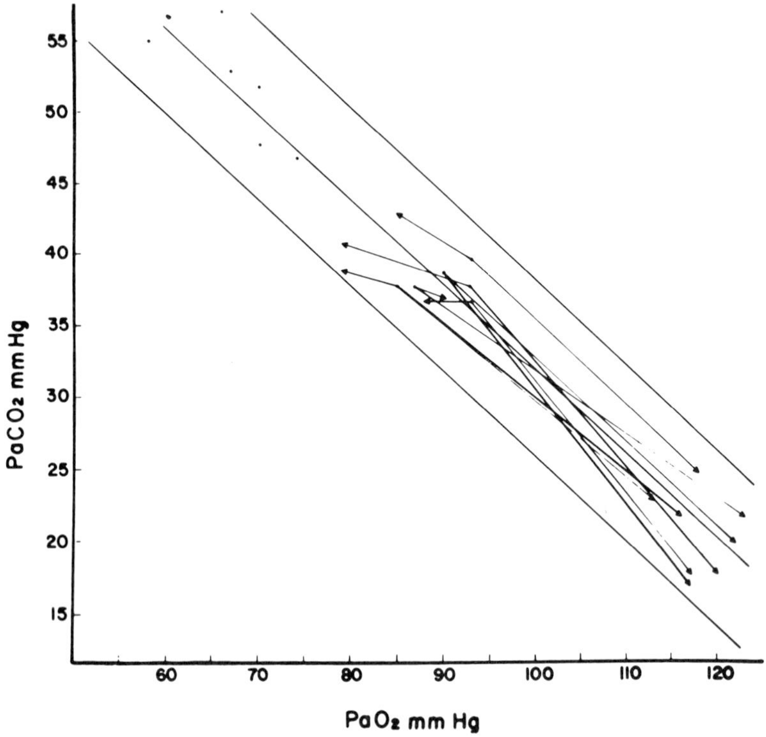

Fig. 1-13. Po_2, Pco_2 diagram for normal individuals. Solid dots are connected to arrows at rest. Arrows point to right during volunteer hyperventilation and to left during exhausting exercise. Discontinuous dots are a result of breath holding. This O_2-CO_2 diagram demonstrates the normal O_2-CO_2 relationship.

Others have preferred the simpler version[19]:

$$\text{arterial } P_{CO_2} \ \alpha \ \frac{CO_2 \text{ production}}{\text{alveolar ventilation}}.$$

Ventilation-Perfusion Abnormalities

The bedside measurement of ventilation-perfusion abnormalities, when possible, reveals these categories: low ventilation to perfusion, no ventilation to perfusion (shunting), high-ventilation perfusion or high ventilation-no perfusion dead space units, or "ideal units" when there is excellent matching of ventilation and perfusion.[20,21] The method of using gases of six different densities infused into an arm vein, with determinations made from expired gas and arterial blood has offered a research technique that estimates the full range of ventilation-perfusion distributions as well as the percentage of shunting in critically ill patients.[21] These elaborate techniques are not sufficiently well established for routine use but are promising from

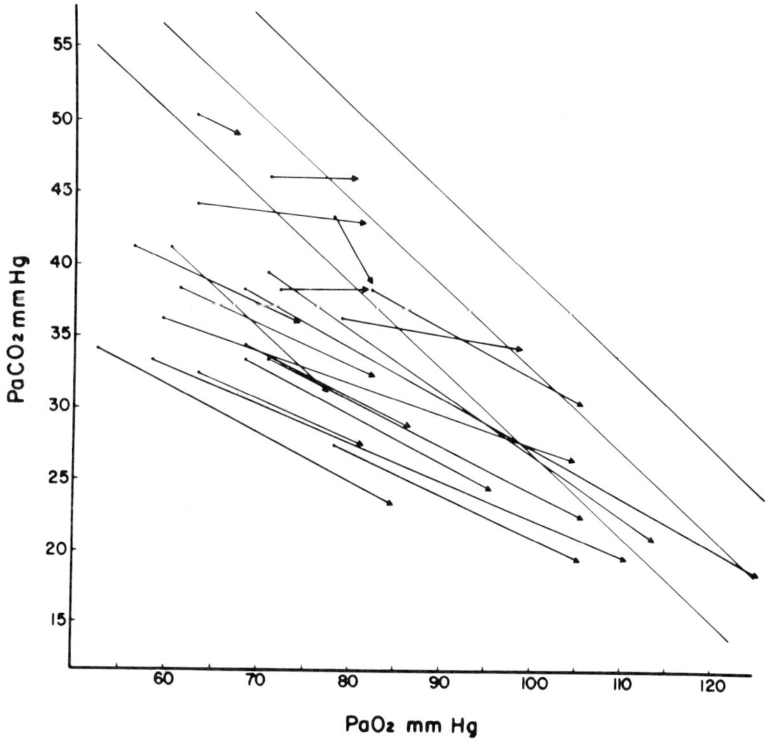

Fig. 1-14. Resting O_2-CO_2 diagram for patients with varying stages of COPD. Values are mostly outside normal range (*parallel lines*). Arrow results are a response to voluntary hyperventilation.

an investigational standpoint. Determinations using these techniques, however, have shown that the common technique of estimating shunting by measuring arterial oxygen tension after 100% oxygen breathing often increases the degree of shunting and is thus misleading. For this reason, we have always considered it best to measure the difference between inspired and arterial oxygen tension for an estimate of the efficacy of oxygen transfer across the lung.[22] This artifact on 100% oxygen breathing has also been established in recent clinical studies.[23]

Wasted Ventilation

It is also popular to estimate the ratio of dead-space ventilation to total ventilation by simultaneously measuring expired and arterial oxygen CO_2 tension in order to obtain the exact percentage of wasted ventilation according to the formula. Normal dead-space ventilation is only about 30% of minute ventilation and represents the ventilation of conducting airways and shunt units. Minute ventilation, of course, can be measured at the bedside with a Wright Respirometer attached to an endotracheal tube or a tracheostomy tube, or even used in conjunction with a mask. Normal anatomic dead space is approximately equal to the patient's weight in pounds; it is thus a simple matter to estimate alveolar ventilation from minute ventilation if one assumes that the anatomic dead space is normal. Of course, this is not normal in disease states. Therefore, it is best to judge alveolar ventilation by the P_{CO_2} as just indicated.

It would also be valuable to be able to measure respiratory work. This is not practical with present technology. It must be emphatically stated that bedside measurements of ventilation and blood gases tell what the patient has accomplished, but not how hard he has worked to accomplish it. Thus, in states of high work in near exhaustion, minute ventilation may be high and blood gases normal or near normal just before apnea occurs. In the final analysis, arterial blood gases are most useful in assessing respiratory failure and are particularly valuable if used in the context of the clinical state at hand. One must look at the oxygen tension, CO_2 tension, and pH and bicarbonate *together* within this clinical context. In so doing, valuable physiologic assessment can be made (see Chap. 6).

The delivery of oxygen to the tissues is another major consideration in the assessment of acute respiratory failure. It is particularly important in very critically ill patients with the adult respiratory distress syndrome (ARDS) who require mechanical ventilation in high tidal volumes and positive end-expiratory pressure (PEEP) along with high oxygen fractions (F_{IO_2}) (see Chaps. 5 and 8).

Oxygen delivery to the tissues is a product of cardiac output and the oxygen content of arterial blood. This is expressed in the formula $ST_{O_2} = CI \times Ca_{O_2}$ when CI = cardiac index or cardiac output/square meter body surface and Ca_{O_2} = oxygen content and thus is a product of oxygen saturation, dependent on P_{O_2} and pH, hemoglobin content and capacity for oxygen binding, and the trivial amount of oxygen physically dissolved in plasma.[12] Thus, oxygen content is $Hgb \times 1.34 \times Sa_{O_2} + 0.03\ P_{O_2}$ in ml/100 ml arterial blood. Cardiac output is conveniently and accurately measured by use of indicator dilution curves, usually using cold water (also see Chap. 5 on hemodynamic monitoring in ARDS).[24] Hemodynamic monitoring has therefore become commonplace in intensive care units and is particularly valuable, if not mandatory, in the most critically ill patients. Nonetheless, there are some pitfalls in these monitoring techniques which must be considered, particularly when observed measurements do not correlate with the clinical states of the patient (mental states, urine flow, blood pressure, arterial blood gas values, and skin temperature). These observations, carefully interpreted, often make direct hemodynamic monitoring unnecessary, particularly when experienced respiratory care workers are involved.

Additionally, calculation of systemic oxygen transfer still does not insure oxygen consumption in high-energy metabolism. Methods to measure oxygen consumption at the bedside have been introduced and may prove useful in daily practice.[25]

Oxygen delivery can be reflected by measurement of mixed venous oxygen tension or saturation, which are determinations that are eas-

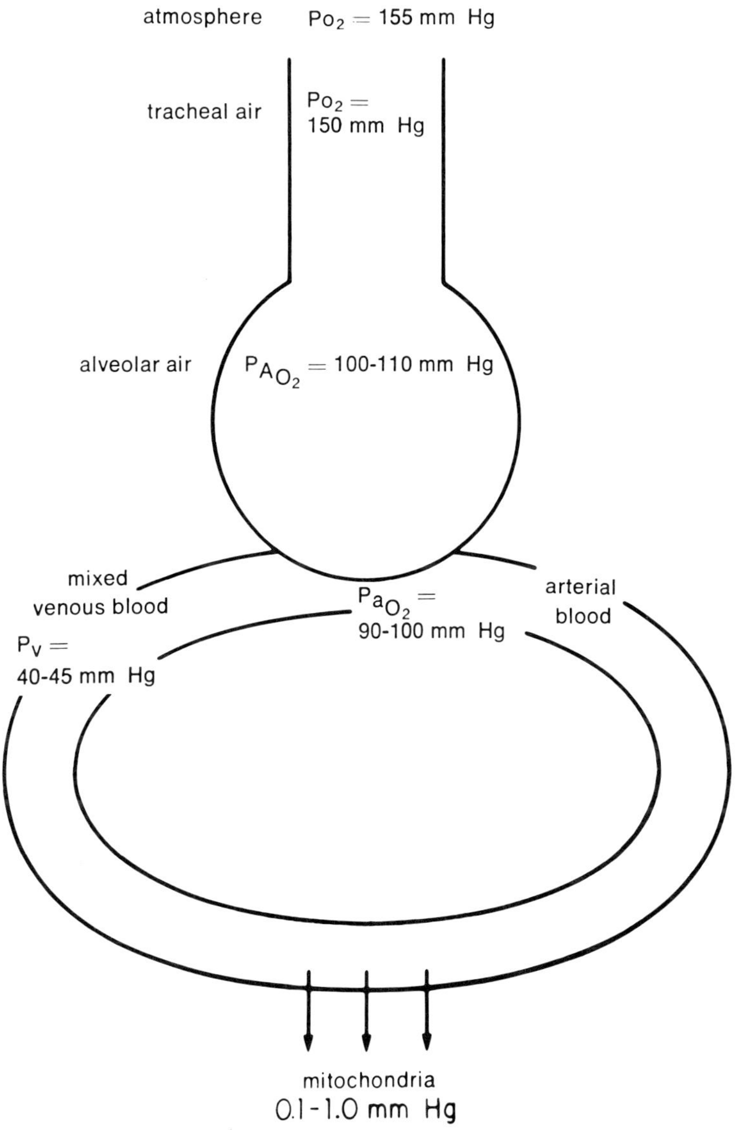

Fig. 1-15. Oxygen tensions and oxygen transport at sea level.

ily obtained with use of blood gas electrodes on blood drawn from Swan-Ganz catheters placed within the pulmonary artery.[25] Survival has been shown to correlate with these determinations.[26] A diagrammatic representation of arterial and mixed venous oxygen values is illustrated in Figure 1-15.

Shunt Fraction

Measurements of shunt fractions and dead-space ratios are fashionable, but they can hardly be considered as fundamental as arterial and mixed venous oxygen measurements, or direct measurements of cardiac output and systemic oxygen transport or of oxygen consumption in critically ill patients.[27]

SUMMARY

The diagnosis of acute respiratory failure must be based upon suspicion and identification of clinical states in which the condition can be expected, and it must be confirmed by immediate laboratory study. Identification thus becomes the first step in management.

Details of clinical management of patients with acute respiratory failure will be the subject of subsequent chapters. In brief, the principles involve clearing airways, maintaining adequate tissue oxygen transport by providing adequate arterial oxygenation and supporting cardiac output (tissue oxygen transport), controlling hydrogen ion concentration within narrow physiologic limits, and providing adequate CO_2 elimination commensurate with metabolic production. Management of acute respiratory failure can be divided into two phases: (1) support of respiration and circulation, and (2) treatment directed at prevention of precipitating and complicating features—such as infection, pulmonary embolus and pulmonary infarction, secretions, bronchospasm, and heart failure—leading to respiratory failure, and, when appropriate for the clinical situation, the management of trauma and poisonings. Artificial support of the patient's blood gases and circulation is provided in order to gain time for spontaneous recovery or improvement in response to management of the underlying problem. Since the individual details of care vary widely with each clinical situation, later chapters (Sections B and C) are devoted to each clinical type of respiratory failure commonly encountered today.

REFERENCES

1. Pitt, B., Alkaloy, I., Sweet, R., and Stein, M.: Respiratory failure with focal neurological signs. Ann. Intern. Med., *115:*714, 1965.
2. Cameron, A.S.: Marked papilledema in pulmonary emphysema. Br. J. Ophthalmol., *17:*167, 1933.
3. Miller, A., Bader, R.A., and Bader, M.E.: The neurologic syndrome due to marked hypercapnia with papilledema. Am. J. Med., *33:*309, 1962.

4. Refsum, H.E.: Relationship between state of consciousness and arterial hypoxemia and hypercapnia in patients with pulmonary insufficiency, breathing air. Clin. Sci., *25:*361, 1963.
5. Hamilton, J.N., and Gross, M.J.: Unusual neurological and cardiovascular complications of respiratory failure. Br. Med. J., *2:*1092, 1963.
6. Snider, G.L., and Maldonado, D.: Arterial blood gases in acutely ill patients. JAMA, *204:*133, 1968.
7. Petty, T.L., Bigelow, D.B., and Levine, B.E.: The simplicity and safety of arterial puncture. JAMA, *195:*693, 1966.
8. Comroe, J.H., Jr., and Butelho, S.: Unreliability of cyanosis in the recognition of arterial hypoxemia. Am. J. Med. Sci., *214:*1, 1947.
9. Petty, T.L., Bailey, D.B., and Best, C.: A new device for arterial blood gas sampling. JAMA, *239:*2016, 1978.
10. Urokinase Pulmonary Embolism Trial Study Group: Urokinase–Streptokinase Embolism Trial. JAMA, *229:*1606, 1974.
11. Severinghaus, J.W.: Electrodes for blood and gas P_{CO_2} and P_{O_2} and blood pH. Acta Anesth. Scand., *6*[Suppl. 11]:207, 1962.
12. Severinghaus, J.W.: Blood gas calculator. J. Appl. Physiol., *18:*1108, 1966.
13. Petty, T.L.: Acute Respiratory Failure. *In* Intensive and Rehabilitative Respiratory Care. 2nd Ed. Philadelphia, Lea & Febiger, 1974.
14. Oliva, J.V., Spellman, S., and Podgainy, M.: Ear lobe capillary blood for estimating arterial oxygen tension. JAMA, *223:*1388, 1973.
15. Scoggin, C.H., Nett, L.M., and Petty, T.L.: Clinical evaluation of a new ear oximeter. JAMA, *6:*121, 1977.
16. Mays, E.E.: An arterial blood gas diagram for clinical use. Chest, *63:*793, 1973.
17. Snider, G.L.: Interpretation of the arterial oxygen and carbon dioxide partial pressures. Chest, *63:*801, 1973.
18. Goldring, R.M., Heinemann, H.O., and Turino, G.M.: Regulation of alveolar ventilation in respiratory failure. Am. J. Med. Sci., *269:*160, 1975.
19. Fletcher, C.M.: Respiratory failure. Proc. R. Soc. Med., *55:*565, 1962.
20. Riley, R.L., and Cournand, A.: Analysis of factors affecting pressures of oxygen and carbon dioxide in gas and blood of lungs: Theory. J. Appl. Physiol, *4:*77, 1971.
21. West, J.B.: Pulmonary gas exchange in the critically ill patient. Crit. Care Med., *2:*171, 1974.
22. Harris, T.M., Gray, M., Petty, T.L., and Mueller, R.: Monitoring inspired oxygen pressures during mechanical ventilation. JAMA, *206:*2885, 1968.
23. Shapiro, B.A., Cane, R.D., Harrison, R.A., and Steiner, M.D.: Changes in intrapulmonary shunting with administration of 100% oxygen. Chest, *77:*142, 1980.
24. Swan, H.J.C.: The role of hemodynamic monitoring in the critically ill. Crit. Care Med., *3:*83, 1975.
25. Neukof, H., and Wolf, H.: Method for continuously measured oxygen consumption and cardiac output for use in critically ill patients. Crit. Care Med., *6:*155, 1978.
26. Kansnitz, P., Druger, G.L., Yorra, F., and Simmons, D.H.: Mixed venous oxygen tensions and hyperlactatemia. (Survival in severe cardiopulmonary disease.) JAMA, *236:*570, 1976.
27. Bageant, R.A.: Bedside techniques for calculating dead space/tidal volume ratio (V_D/V_T) and pulmonary shunt ($\dot{Q}_S/\dot{Q}_T$). Resp. Care, *22:*715, 1977.

Chapter 2

ESTABLISHMENT AND CARE OF THE AIRWAY

By John L. Stauffer

Management of the airway is one of the most fundamental aspects of critical care medicine and is perhaps the most vital aspect of treatment of patients with respiratory failure. Some patients with acute respiratory failure may be managed without an artificial airway, but most will require the insertion of a definitive airway into the trachea. Personnel caring for patients with acute or chronic respiratory diseases should be familiar with the principles and practical aspects of airway management including the use of artificial airways. Skill in establishing and maintaining a patent airway is based on an understanding of respiratory physiology and anatomy and is a prerequisite for all who provide intensive respiratory care, including internists, surgeons, anesthesiologists, nurses and respiratory therapists.

HISTORICAL PERSPECTIVE

Although tracheotomies may have been performed in ancient times, the first definite account of the use of tracheotomies did not appear until the sixteenth century.[1] However, tracheotomy was rarely performed before the nineteenth century, when it gained popularity in the emergency management of diphtheria. Credit for the first description of endotracheal intubation is usually given to Macewen, who in 1880 published a series about 4 patients intubated up to 36 hours with vulcanite tubes without any complications.[2]

Nevertheless, tracheotomy and endotracheal intubation had limited roles in the management of respiratory failure until the 1950s, when they were used in Scandinavian countries in the treatment of ventilatory failure accompanying poliomyelitis and drug overdose. During the last 3 decades, we have amassed extensive experience with artificial airways. In the last decade there have been major technical advances in the design of endotracheal and tracheostomy tubes and in the development of new methods of respiratory care. Disposable soft-cuff tubes of polyvinyl chloride or silicone composition have largely replaced the reusable rigid metal tracheostomy tubes and the hard red rubber endotracheal tubes with latex rubber cuffs that were popular in the 1950s and 1960s. Prestretching of cuffs in hot water has not been necessary since the introduction of high-volume, low-pressure cuffs in the early 1970s. Technical advances and improved respiratory care techniques have now made it possible to leave an artificial airway in place for extended periods with a low risk of complications. These developments have allowed the pendulum to swing toward endotracheal intubation as an alternative to tracheotomy in the management of most patients with acute respiratory failure. However, endotracheal intubation and tracheotomy are best considered as complementary procedures, since both have clear advantages and disadvantages.

ESTABLISHING A PATENT AIRWAY

The first step in the management of acute respiratory failure is establishment of a patent airway. Complete airway obstruction or apnea may lead to cyanosis within a minute, permanent brain injury within 4 to 5 minutes, and cardiac asystole within 5 to 10 minutes. In many cases of airway obstruction, patency may be re-established immediately without insertion of an intratracheal tube. Respiratory care personnel should be expert in this aspect of basic life support. The importance of the ability to provide relief of acute upper airway obstruction is underscored by the fact that 3000 Americans choke to death each year when nearly all these victims could have been saved.[3]

Airway obstruction may be caused by a variety of insults (Table 2-1), any one of which may cause life-threatening asphyxia. A common type of acute upper airway obstruction is that which is associated with loss of consciousness. In this setting, loss of muscle tone and gravity straighten the normal curvature of the cervical spine, angulating the pharynx and causing airway obstruction at the glottis. The tongue muscles also become flaccid, creating obstruction of the posterior oropharynx by the tongue. Immediate intervention by a person skilled in basic life support may relieve this type of airway obstruction and save the victim's life.

TABLE 2-1. Causes of Upper Airway Obstruction

Cause	*Example(s)*
1. Weakness or flaccidity of muscles maintaining patency of pharynx and glottis	Loss of consciousness Obstructive sleep apnea syndrome
2. Obstruction by foreign material	Gastric aspiration Foreign body
3. Trauma	Fracture of larynx
4. Retained secretions	Acute tracheobronchitis
5. Mucosal inflammation	Diphtheria Smoke inhalation
6. Neoplasm	Carcinoma of larynx
7. Chronic reaction to mucosal injury	Laryngeal granuloma Tracheal stenosis
8. Extrinsic compression	Aneurysm of aorta Retropharyngeal abscess
9. Laryngospasm	Post-extubation laryngospasm

The signs of airway obstruction are usually obvious. Partial airway obstruction is manifest by noisy respirations with or without retractions and signs of respiratory distress. Signs of complete airway obstruction include absence of airflow, intercostal and supraclavicular retractions, respiratory distress, and aphonia. Central cyanosis is a late manifestation of respiratory failure, and its absence should not preclude consideration of airway obstruction.

The sequence of methods to establish a patent airway in a patient with airway obstruction is outlined in Table 2-2. If a patient is found unconscious and the signs of airway obstruction are present, the following steps are useful either in the field or in the critical care unit before tracheal intubation is performed:

1. Positioning of the head and neck by the "head-tilt" method (the neck is flexed on the chest and the head is extended on the neck); an alternative method is the "jaw-thrust" maneuver.

TABLE 2-2. Sequence of Steps to Relieve Acute Airway Obstruction*

1. Proper positioning of head and neck (extend head, flex neck).
2. Positive pressure ventilation (mouth-to-mouth or bag-to-mouth).
3. Removal of any foreign material from the airway.
4. Jaw thrust maneuver.
5. Insertion of nasal or oral pharyngeal airway.
6. Endotracheal intubation (oral route usually attempted first).
7. Cricothyroidotomy.

* Modified from Young, J.A., and Crocker, D.[4]

2. Positive pressure ventilation by the mouth-to-mouth technique or with a self-inflating resuscitation bag.

3. Removal of any foreign bodies from the airway. If present, these may be detected because of increased airway resistance during assisted ventilation.*

4. Evacuation of secretions if suctioning is available.

5. Insertion of a nasal or oral pharyngeal airway if needed.

The "head-tilt" method is illustrated in Figure 2-1*A* and *B*. The patient is first rolled onto a hard, flat surface on his back. One hand is placed under the neck while the other tilts the head backward,

* The sequence recommended by the American Heart Association to remove an obstructing foreign body in an unconscious victim is four rapid back blows, four manual abdominal or chest thrusts, followed by a finger probe.

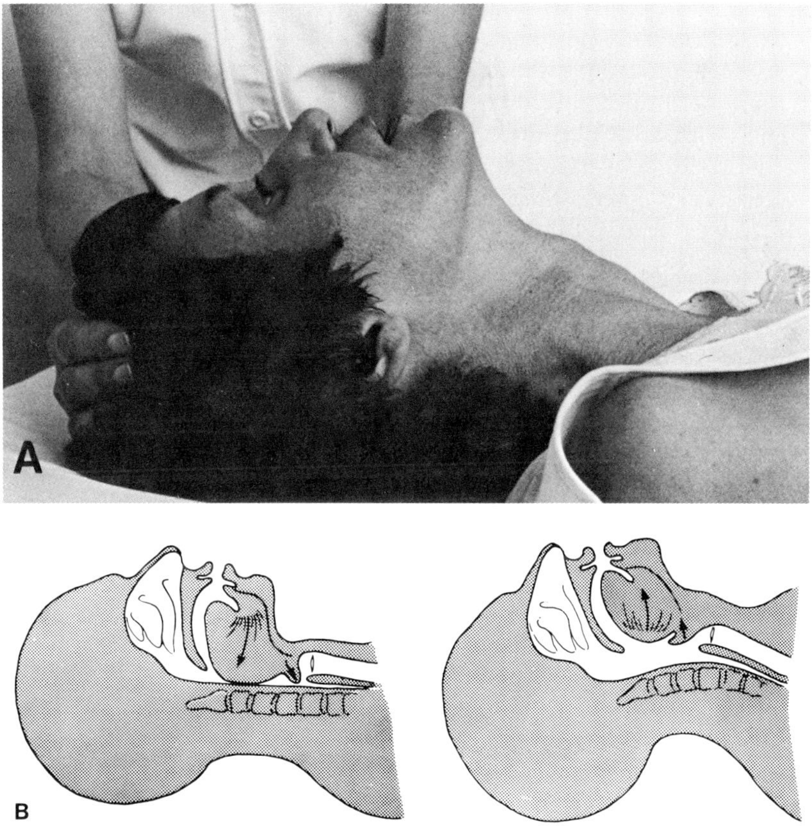

Fig. 2-1. *A*, The "head-tilt" method for relief of upper airway obstruction flexes the neck and extends the head.

B, Schematic diagrams illustrate obstruction of the airway at the level of the pharynx and glottis, and in an unconscious person (*left*), and relief by the "head-tilt" method (*right*).

restoring proper angulation of the head on the spine and relieving obstruction both at the level of the tongue and at the level of the glottis.[4–6] The alternative jaw-thrust maneuver is done either by displacing the mandible forward with the fingers behind the jaw while the head is tilted backward or by pulling the jaw forward with the thumb and index finger. After the head and neck are properly positioned, the patient may be able to breathe spontaneously, but if apnea persists assisted ventilation is begun.

Although it is possible to maintain a patent airway without intubation for many hours, the methods just outlined are usually temporary and are obviously not suited for long-term airway maintenance. The "head-tilt" method of airway maintenance does not protect against aspiration, and it is tiring for the rescuer to maintain. The jaw-thrust variation of this maneuver makes assisted ventilation by mouth-to-mouth (or nose) application very difficult. Furthermore, positioning methods do not provide a route for evacuation of tracheobronchial secretions. Thus, the "head-tilt" maneuver may be thought of as a temporary life-saving technique which most often is performed prior to the insertion of a definitive airway.

The esophageal obturator airway has gained some favor as an effective method for establishing ventilation during resuscitation. This alternative to the measures just discussed has some limitations, which are discussed in the section "Types of Artificial Airways."

ESTABLISHING A DEFINITIVE AIRWAY

A definitive airway is either an endotracheal tube or a tracheostomy tube inserted into the trachea. The decision to intubate the trachea either by the translaryngeal route or by tracheotomy is a clinical judgment which requires considerable wisdom and experience. The indications for tracheal intubation are as follows:

1. Relief of obstruction of the upper airway.
2. Stabilization and protection of the airway.
3. Facilitation of tracheobronchial suctioning.
4. Facilitation of assisted ventilation.

The patient with acute respiratory failure usually has several or all of these indications for intubation.

Relief of Obstruction of the Upper Airway

Translaryngeal endotracheal intubation relieves upper airway obstruction by bypassing obstruction in the pharynx or in the larynx. Acute obstruction of the upper airway resulting from conditions such as unconsciousness, laryngospasm, and diphtheria may be adequately managed with endotracheal intubation. Obviously, any foreign material in the upper airway should be removed before translaryngeal endotracheal intubation is attempted. Chronic disturbances such as carcinoma of the larynx and the obstructive type of sleep apnea syndrome may benefit from tracheotomy.

Stabilization and Protection of the Airway

Unconscious patients often require endotracheal intubation to protect their airways from aspiration. Patients with acute depression of consciousness caused by such conditions as head trauma, drug overdose, or stroke often need a definitive airway not only to maintain airway patency but also to prevent aspiration of upper airway secretions and gastric contents. Head positioning and pharyngeal airways may be used temporarily in the initial management of these patients, but to protect the airway from the possibility of aspiration, a cuffed endotracheal tube must be inserted until consciousness returns. Patients who remain comatose usually require tracheotomy.

Facilitation of Tracheobronchial Suctioning

A definitive airway is often inserted to facilitate clearance of tracheobronchial secretions. The normal person secretes 10 to 100 ml tracheobronchial secretions per day. Since the volume of the conducting airways in an adult is about 150 ml, ability to clear these secretions is obviously critical to maintenance of airway patency. Unless adequate tracheobronchial clearance is maintained, patients may literally drown in their own secretions. The volume of retained secretions depends upon a balance between production and clearance of mucus. Increased production of mucus occurs in chronic bronchitis, asthma, bronchiectasis, cystic fibrosis, thermal injuries, and inhalation injuries. Decreased clearance of mucus occurs in chronic obstructive pulmonary disease, upper airway obstruction, debility, depression of the central nervous system, muscle weakness, and chest trauma, and after thoracic and abdominal surgery. Certain drugs may also depress mucociliary clearance. When aerosol therapy and chest physiotherapy are not adequate to clear secretions in any of these settings, supervised coughing techniques and bronchial drainage with chest percussion are attempted. Pharmacologic measures such as inhalation of beta agonists, which increase mucociliary activity, and nasotracheal suction are often useful. If none of these measures prevents respiratory failure due to accumulation of retained secretions, the patient should be intubated. Transcutaneous cricothyroid catheters ("trach ticklers") are dangerous and should not be used to promote cough because of the risks of infection, bleeding, and subcutaneous emphysema.

Facilitation of Assisted Ventilation

The fourth indication for insertion of a definitive airway is facilitation of assisted ventilation in patients with alveolar hypoventilation or impaired oxygenation. Useful guidelines for use of assisted ventilation in adults with acute respiratory failure have been suggested by Pontoppidan.[7]

	Normal Range	Intubation and Ventilation Indicated
Mechanics		
Respiratory rate	12–20	>35
Vital capacity (ml/kg)	65–75	<15
FEV_1 (ml/kg)	50–60	<10
Inspiratory force (cm H_2O)	75–100	<25
Oxygenation		
Pa_{O_2} (mm Hg)	75–100 (air)	<70 (on Mask O_2)
$P(A\text{-}aD_{O_2})^{1.0}$ (mm Hg)	25–65	>450
Ventilation		
Pa_{CO_2} (mm Hg)	35–45	>55*
V_D/V_T	0.25–0.40	>0.60

The decision to intubate the trachea to provide assisted ventilation requires considerable judgment and is not based solely on "the numbers." There is, however, agreement that endotracheal intubation and mechanical ventilation are needed if apnea, severe hypoxemia, or hypercapnia is present that cannot be reversed within one to two minutes. When in doubt, the patient with ventilatory failure or hypoxemia should be intubated. Common disorders in which tracheal intubation and assisted ventilation are required include acute exacerbation of chronic obstructive pulmonary disease, adult respiratory distress syndrome (ARDS), pulmonary edema, central nervous system depression, severe chest trauma, and inadequate ventilation in the postoperative period.

The choice of the route of tracheal intubation (translaryngeal intubation vs tracheotomy) depends upon consideration of a number of factors. Some comparative advantages and disadvantages of endotracheal intubation and tracheotomy are listed in Table 2-3. During the last 3 decades—and with increasing experience with endotracheal intubation—the allowable period for "safe" translaryngeal intubation has steadily increased from as little as several hours in the early 1950s to 11 days in 1976.[8,9] There is, however, little evidence available establishing the duration of translaryngeal endotracheal intubation as a significant determinant of laryngeal complications. Nearly all patients who require a definitive airway may be managed initially with translaryngeal endotracheal intubation. We now feel

* Except in patients with chronic hypercapnia.

TABLE 2-3. Comparison of Advantages and Disadvantages of Endotracheal Intubation and Tracheotomy in Patients with Respiratory Failure

Advantages	*Disadvantages*
ENDOTRACHEAL INTUBATION	
Ease and speed of tube placement. Requires less experience than tracheotomy. Avoids many of the complications of tracheotomy. Less expensive than tracheotomy. Negligible mortality.	Numerous potential complications. Discomfort to patient. Difficulty with feeding. Difficulty evacuating tracheobronchial secretions. Possible laryngeal injury. Esthetically less pleasing. Not suitable for long-term airway maintenance. Bypasses upper respiratory tract defense mechanisms. Precludes effective cough.
TRACHEOTOMY	
Avoids upper airway complications of endotracheal intubation. Less discomfort in long-term use. Permits oral care, swallowing of secretions, feeding, and communication. Ease of evacuating tracheobronchial secretions.	3% mortality. Permanent scar. High incidence of tracheal stenosis. Numerous potential complications which tend to be more severe than those of endotracheal intubation. More expensive than endotracheal intubation. Bypasses upper respiratory tract defense mechanisms. Precludes effective cough.

that if indications for a definitive airway persist, the translaryngeal route may be used 2 to 3 weeks if necessary. If the patient requires an artificial airway for more than two weeks, tracheotomy should be strongly considered. However, a rote decision to perform tracheotomy because an arbitrary number of days of endotracheal intubation have elapsed should be avoided. The skilled clinician will consider a number of factors before proceeding with tracheotomy (Table 2-4).

TYPES OF ARTIFICIAL AIRWAYS

A large variety of artificial airways are available. Selection of the airway most appropriate for each patient depends upon a number of factors including the cause of respiratory failure, the patient's general condition, the presence or absence of airway obstruction, and the

TABLE 2-4. Factors to Consider Before Changing from Endotracheal Intubation to Tracheotomy

1. Estimated duration of need for artificial airway
2. Patient tolerance of endotracheal intubation—swallowing, discomfort, communication, nutrition, ease of suctioning, etc.
3. Complications of endotracheal intubation
4. Likelihood of improving patient's status with tracheotomy—nutrition, comfort, communication, ease of suctioning, etc.
5. Morbidity, mortality, expense of tracheotomy

anticipated duration of need for a definitive airway. Artificial airways may be classified in six broad categories: (1) pharyngeal airways, (2) endotracheal tubes, (3) tracheostomy tubes, (4) tracheostomy cannulas, (5) laryngectomy tubes, and (6) miscellaneous tubes.

Pharyngeal Airways

Oral or nasal pharyngeal airways are rubber or plastic tubes or struts which provide a patent airway down to the level of the larynx. These devices are particularly useful for temporary relief of airway obstruction at the level of the pharynx or hypopharynx, as in the unconscious patient, and for facilitation of suctioning of pharyngeal secretions. They are generally used only temporarily, often in conjunction with the "head-tilt" method of airway maintenance.

Oral pharyngeal airways are rigid or slightly flexible tubes with flange buttresses at the lips (Fig. 2-2*A*). They conform to the anatomy of the mouth and maintain patency of the oral portion of the airway by holding the base of the tongue away from the posterior pharyngeal wall (Fig. 2-2*B*). These devices permit evacuation of oral and pharyngeal secretions, facilitate mouth care, and, if properly used, prevent the patient from biting his tongue. They are also often used along with oral endotracheal tubes to prevent the patient from biting and occluding the endotracheal tube. The Guedel oral pharyngeal airway is a flexible rubber or polyvinyl chloride tube with a central channel for suctioning. The Berman oral airway is a rigid curved strut that lacks a central channel and is composed of polyethylene or ethylene vinyl acetate. A third type, the Safar "S" tube, is a modified Guedel type of oral pharyngeal airway with an extension adaptor for mouth-to-mouth or mouth-to-bag ventilation. The oral pharyngeal airway is inserted through the mouth after the lips are separated by means of the crossed-finger technique. The tongue is pulled forward or displaced forward with a wooden tongue blade. A rotation movement during placement permits atraumatic placement. It is desirable to use a topical anesthetic agent if time permits to suppress the gag reflex. The airway is then taped in place, if necessary, to prevent dislodgment by propulsive movements of the tongue. Frequent changing helps prevent infection and pressure ne-

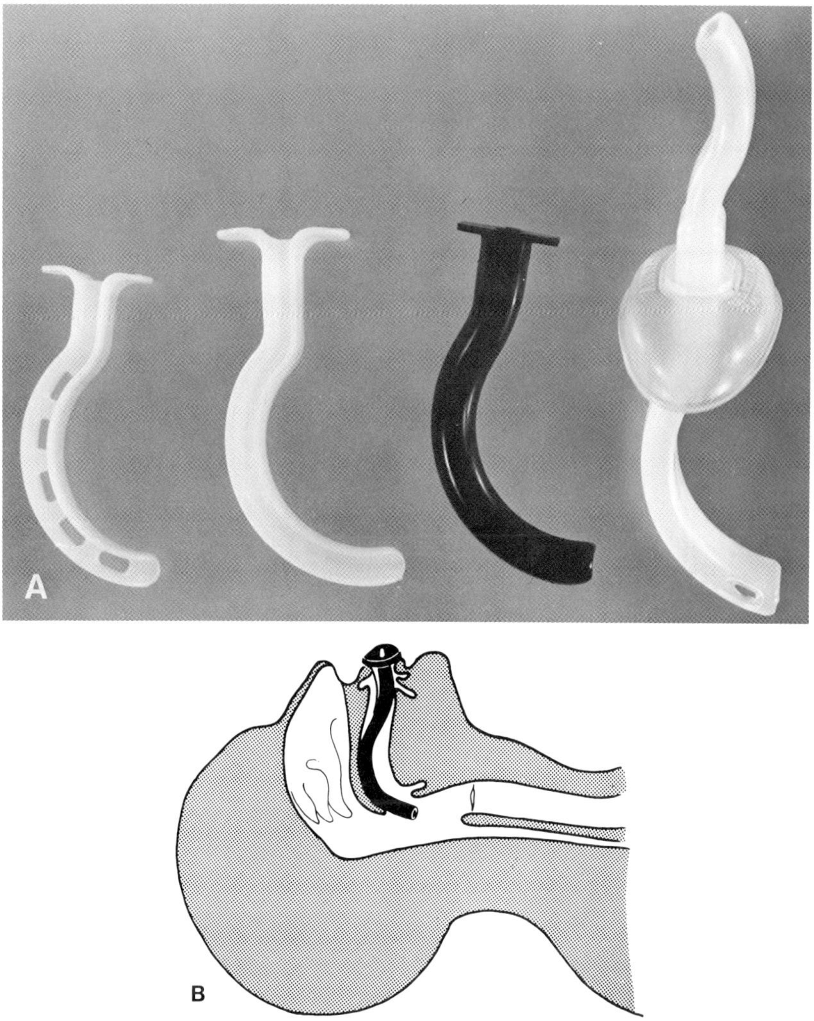

Fig. 2-2. *A*, Oral pharyngeal airways from left to right are (1) Berman with perforations, (2) plain Berman, (3) Guedel, and (4) Safar "S" tube.
B, Schematic diagram showing a Guedel oral pharyngeal airway in place maintaining patency of the airway to the hypopharynx.

crosis and ulceration of soft tissues. Limitations include patient discomfort, soft tissue injuries, and occasional gagging, retching, or vomiting.[10]

Nasal pharyngeal airways are curved, soft pliable tubes with a flange which are passed by way of the nose into the hypopharynx (Fig. 2-3*A*). Although less frequently used than oral airways, they also provide a patent airway down to the level of the larynx and aid evacuation of pharyngeal secretions. The nasal pharyngeal airway may also facilitate passage of the fiberoptic bronchoscope and bronchial catheters for suctioning or bronchography.[11] It may be used instead of the oral airway in a patient who clenches his jaw and will not permit passage of an oral airway. After topical anesthesia is given, the nasal pharyngeal airway is lubricated with a water-soluble jelly and is passed through the nostril so that the tip lies in the posterior pharynx just above the epiglottis (Fig. 2-3*B*). These tubes produce less gagging than oral airways and may be tolerated by unconscious patients for long periods of time. Limitations include

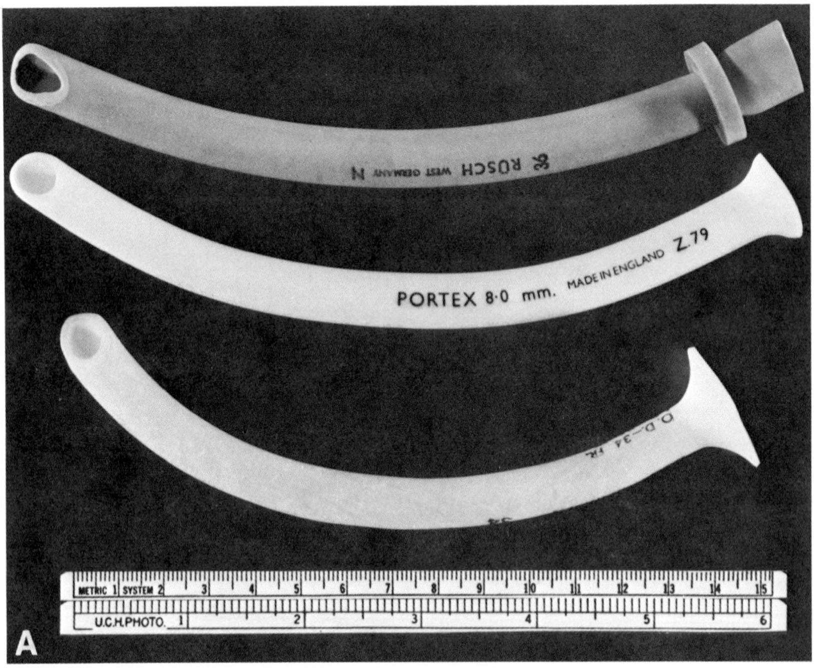

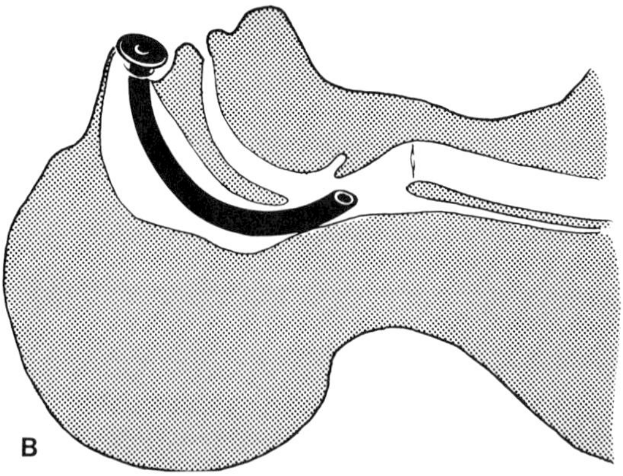

Fig. 2-3. *A*, Nasal pharyngeal airways are available in a variety of styles and sizes. *B*, The nasal pharyngeal airway provides patency of the airway to the glottis if properly positioned.

the presence of only a small channel for suctioning, occasional epistaxis, nasal mucosal ulceration, and sinusitis or otitis in long-term use. Inhalation of humidified air prevents crusting of secretions. These airways should be changed daily and should be shifted from one nostril to the other to avoid pressure necrosis.

The nasal pharyngeal airway is particularly useful in guiding a suction catheter into the trachea, with successful placement occurring in greater than 80% of attempts.[12] This may assist the sampling of tracheobronchial secretions for Gram staining and culturing, although the technique does not completely eliminate the possibility of contamination with pharyngeal organisms during insertion. Stimulation of the cough reflex and removal of tracheobronchial secretions in patients with retained secretions are additional advantages of this technique.

Endotracheal Tubes

Endotracheal tubes are definitive artificial airways inserted through the nose or the mouth into the trachea (Fig. 2-4). The typical features of a modern endotracheal tube are illustrated in Figures 2-5*A* and *B*. Most endotracheal tubes in use today are disposable tubes of polyvinyl chloride or silicone rubber (Silastic) composition. Red rubber tubes with latex cuffs and all reusable tubes are becoming less popular.

Recommended standards for endotracheal tubes have been provided by the Z-79 Committee of the American National Standards Institute (1430 Broadway, New York, NY 10018). Modern endotracheal tubes should be soft enough at body temperature to conform to the anatomy of the airway without kinking. The walls of the tube

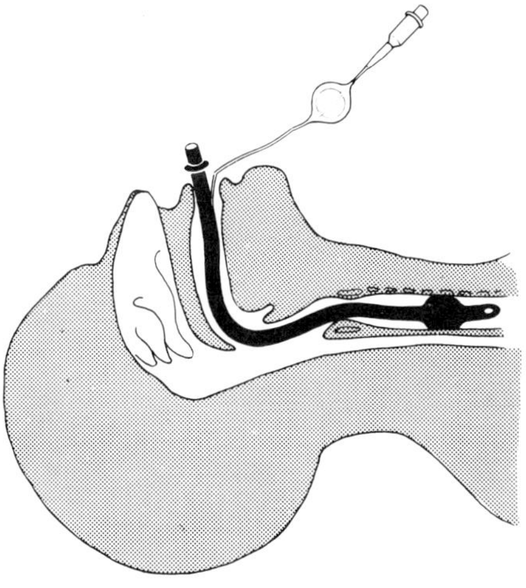

Fig. 2-4. A cuffed oral endotracheal tube is properly positioned in the trachea. Note that the distal tip of the tube is centrally located in the lumen of the trachea.

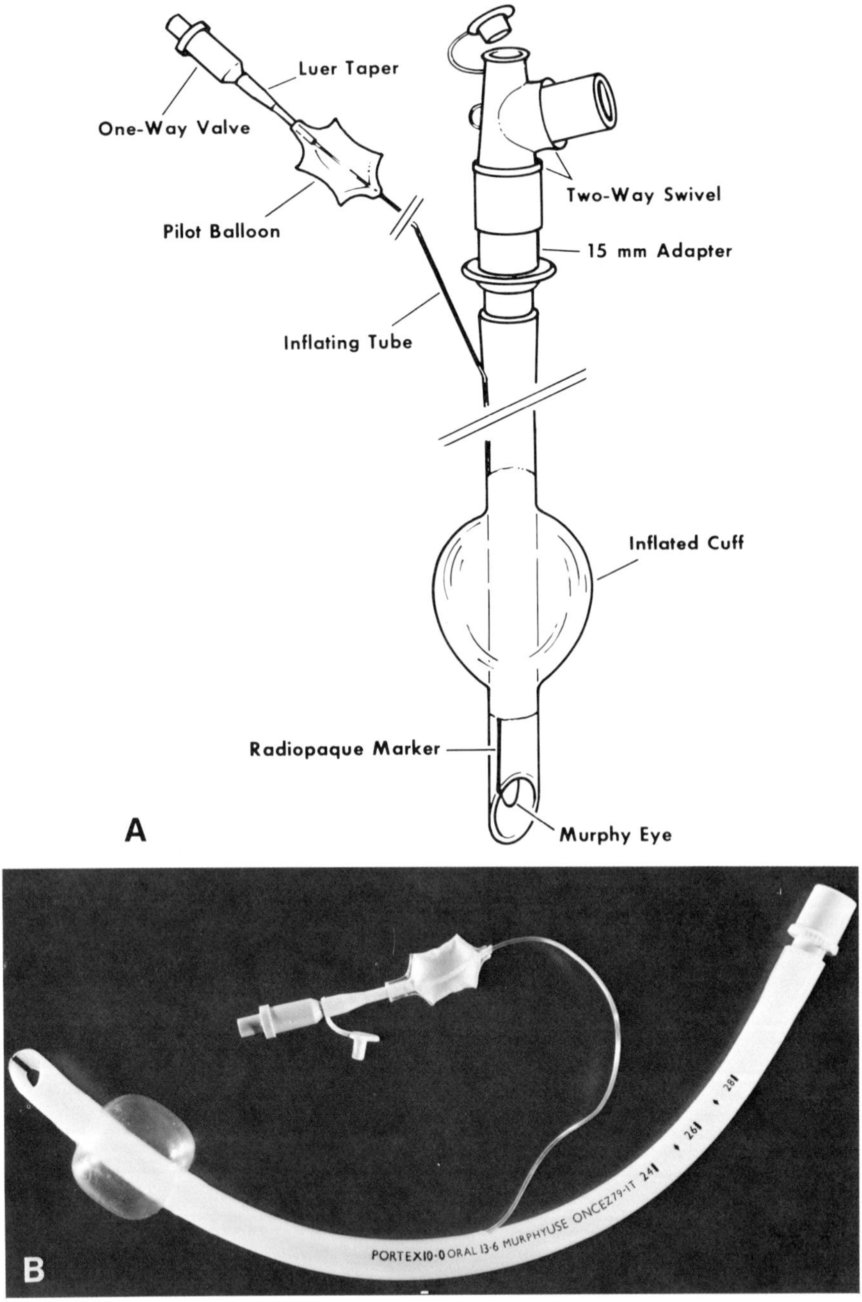

Fig. 2-5. *A*, Essential features of a modern endotracheal tube are illustrated. The shaft of the tube has been reduced in length for convenience of illustration.

B, A modern disposable Murphy-type oral endotracheal tube (Portex) with a soft cuff. Note the labeling of features along the shaft of the tube.

should be smooth and should offer little friction against suction catheters. Markings should be clear, indicating length, size, oral vs nasal tube, and so forth. Labeling of the package should clearly describe the type of tube enclosed. A radiopaque marker at the distal tip should be incorporated to aid localization by x-ray study. The pilot balloon attached to the inflating tube should reliably estimate the cuff pressure. A standard 15-mm adaptor should be attached for connection to ventilator tubing or resuscitation bag. Finally, the tube and cuff should be composed of materials proven to be nontoxic by implant testing ("IT" label).

A variety of sizes of endotracheal tubes is available. Sizes usually refer to the internal diameter in millimeters. Adult males generally require a size 8.5 to 9.0 tube, whereas adult females usually require one or one-half size smaller. Nasotracheal tubes are usually 1.0 mm smaller than orotracheal tubes. Oral tubes have a bevel angle of 45°, and adult size nasal tubes have a bevel angle of about 30°. The take-off point of the inflating tube may vary from oral to nasal tubes.

A few variations on the standard design are available. The Murphy-type endotracheal tube has an "eye" on one side at the distal tip, which is lacking on the Magill tube. This extra opening permits flow of air and secretions in the event of obstruction of the distal tip. Most endotracheal tubes have a bonded cuff ranging in length from 2.0 to 4.0 cm. Uncuffed tubes are also manufactured, but these do not prevent aspiration. Cuffs are generally not available on tubes smaller than size 5. Air-inflatable and polyurethane foam cuffs are available for larger tubes. Armored endotracheal tubes are available with a spring-like wire wall to prevent kinking and tube collapse. A double-lumen (Carlens) endotracheal tube is available to administer anesthesia gases and to suction secretions from each lung separately. The Robertshaw tube is another double-lumen tube which may be passed into either mainstem bronchus.

The endotracheal tube cuff has received great attention over the last two decades because of its potential for tracheal injury. Most respiratory care specialists prefer to intubate adults with tubes having a high-volume, low-pressure cuff, which is more compliant and less likely to produce injury than the older low-volume, high-pressure cuff (Fig. 2-6). The Portex Co. (Wilmington, MA) has introduced a low-pressure ("Profile") cuff which is designed to decrease cuff bulk, reduce contact area with the tracheal mucosa, and reduce "pistoning" motion of the endotracheal tube in the tracheal lumen (Fig. 2-7). The foam cuff, introduced by Kamen and Wilkinson, self-inflates to the contour of the trachea without air but is less popular than the air-inflatable cuff.[13] Foam cuffs exert low pressure (about 5 mm Hg) against the tracheal mucosa, but excess cuff bulk makes intubation or extubation potentially difficult. Foam-cuff tubes may

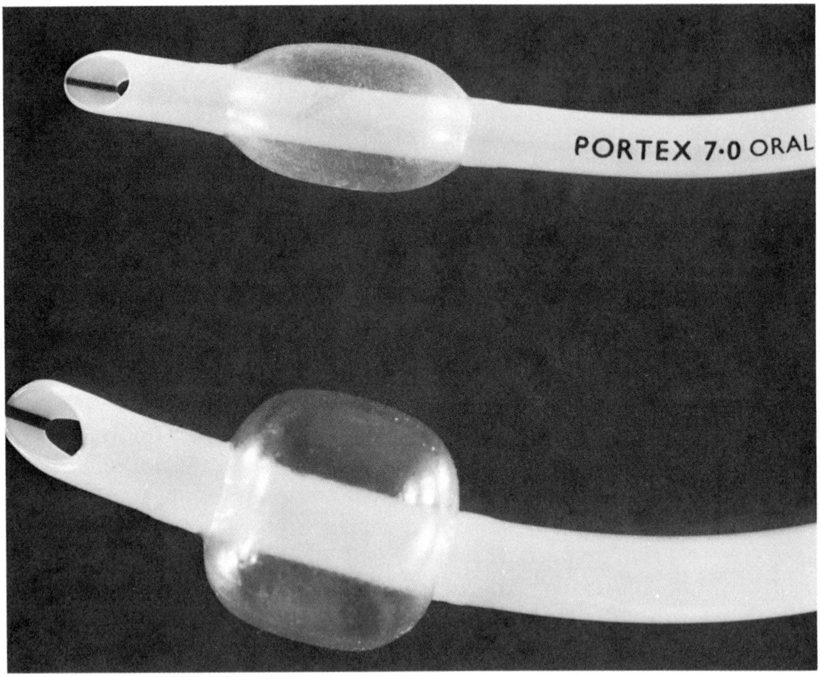

Fig. 2-6. Comparison of "hard" and "soft" cuffs on endotracheal tubes. The "hard" (low-volume, high-pressure) cuff (*top*) has a low contour but is less compliant than the "soft" (high-volume, low-pressure) cuff (*bottom*).

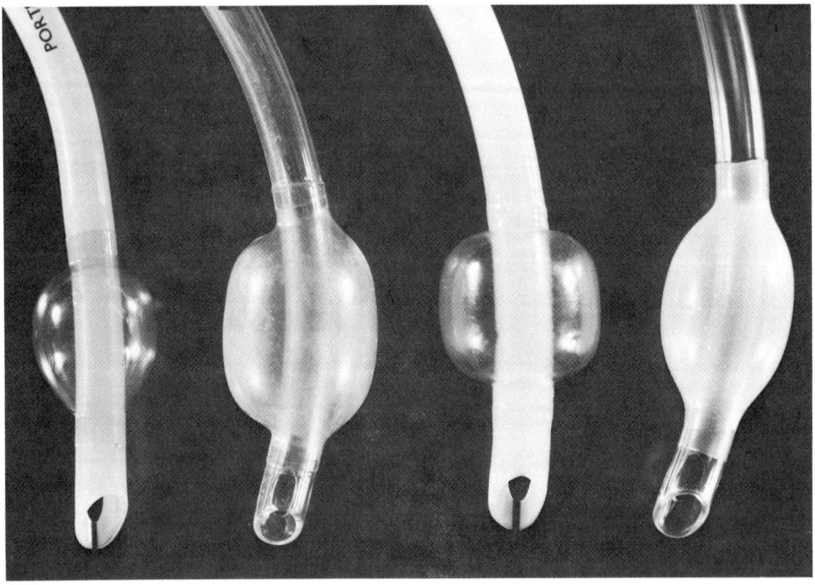

Fig. 2-7. Soft (high-volume, low-pressure) cuffs come in a variety of configurations. From left to right: (1) Portex "Profile" cuff, (2) National Catheter Corporation soft cuff, (3) Portex soft cuff, (4) Ohio soft cuff. The "Profile" cuff reduces contact area with the tracheal mucosa.

also fail to maintain airway pressure when high inspiratory pressures (>30 cm H_2O) are required.[13]

The pilot balloon connected to the inflating tube provides a very rough estimate of pressure in the cuff. The specialized pilot balloon system on the Lanz tube (Extracorporeal Medical Specialties, Inc., King of Prussia, PA) has an automatic device that controls pressure in the cuff, preventing possible overinflation and thereby reducing the risk of tracheal injury.[14–16] The pressure-regulating valve in this system automatically limits cuff pressure to 20 to 25 mm Hg.

Tracheostomy Tubes

Tracheostomy tubes are short curved tubes with a flange that helps anchor the tube on the neck. They may be passed either through a tracheostomy or, less frequently, through a cricothyroidostomy (Fig. 2-8*A*). A modern tracheostomy tube is illustrated in Figure 2-8*B*.

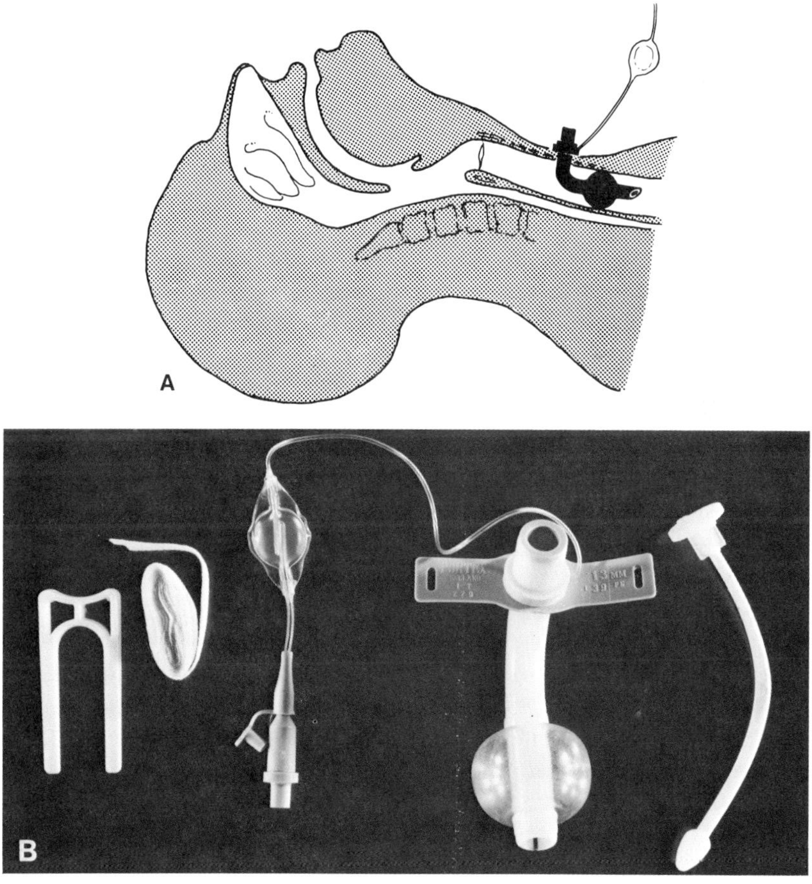

Fig. 2-8. *A*, A tracheostomy tube in proper position is illustrated. *B*, Soft-cuff tracheostomy tube (Portex) with plastic wedge and tape (*left*) and obturator (*right*).

These tubes should also meet the rigid standards of the Z-79 Committee for composition, shape, sizes, labeling, and toxicity. The cuff should be bonded to the shaft of the tube to decrease the risk of herniation over the distal end. Detachable balloon cuffs are dangerous and should not be used. The old standard double-cannula metal tracheostomy tube designed by Jackson is becoming less popular because of its rigid construction, lack of a standard 15-mm adaptor, and required cuff attachment.

Several accessory items are usually packaged along with modern disposable tracheostomy tubes. These include a disposable obturator for insertion, tape to hold the neck flange securely in place, and a two-way swivel adaptor. A plastic wedge to lift the tubing connector from the 15-mm adaptor is a helpful addition in some sets (Fig. 2-8*B*).

Several variations of the standard tracheostomy tube are available. Most disposable tracheostomy tubes have only an outer cannula, but an inner cannula is available with some to facilitate cleaning. Some tracheostomy tubes are fenestrated, allowing the patient to talk, to breathe through his upper airway as well as through the tracheostomy tube, and to cough up secretions on his own. Because fenestrated tracheostomy tubes allow the physician to monitor the function of the glottis in preventing aspiration, they may be useful for a short time prior to tracheal decannulation. Without an inner cannula, fenestrated tracheostomy tubes are, of course, not suitable for positive pressure ventilation and do not guard against aspiration. The Gabriel-Tucker metal tracheostomy tube has a flutter valve in the fenestration of the inner cannula, allowing the patient to talk without covering the tube with a finger (Narco Pilling Company, Fort Washington, PA). The Shiley fenestrated, cuffed tracheostomy tube set includes a cap to occlude the lumen of the outer cannula, thereby allowing the patient to breathe completely through the upper airway (Shiley Sales Corporation, Irvine, CA). The neck flange is usually fixed, but on the Shiley tracheostomy tube it may swivel and thus possibly reduce transmission of forces directly to the trachea.

Both cuffed and uncuffed tracheostomy tubes are available, the selection depending on the patient's needs. A double-cuff tracheostomy tube is available but has not been proven to decrease tracheal complications. Foam-cuff tracheostomy tubes are available but are sometimes difficult to insert or to remove because of the bulky cuff material (Fig. 2-9). Standard and pressure-regulating pilot balloon systems are available for tracheostomy tubes as well as for endotracheal tubes (Fig. 2-9). Soft, flexible Silastic tracheostomy tubes without cuffs are available for patients with chronic secretion problems or the obstructive type of sleep apnea syndrome (Fig. 2-10). Armored tracheostomy tubes are available to prevent tube compression and kinking.

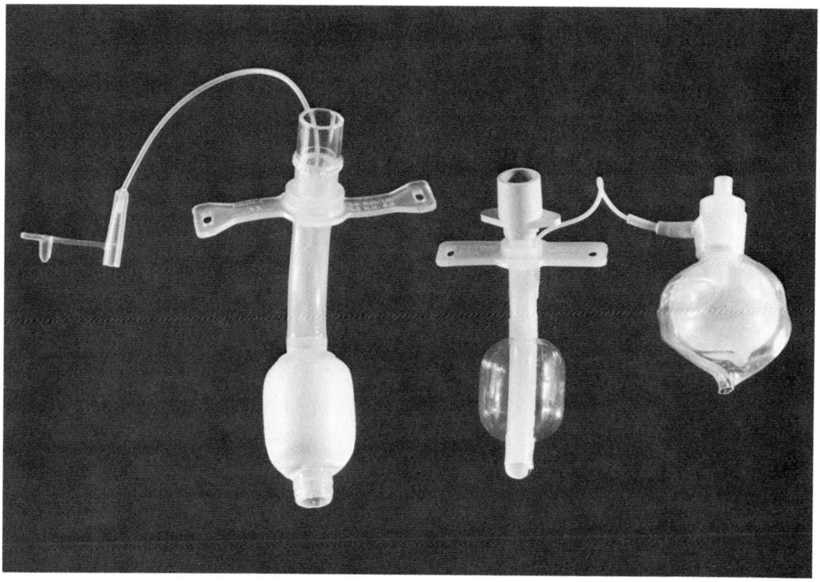

Fig. 2-9. *Left,* The foam cuff tracheostomy tube (Bivona Surgical Instruments, Inc., Chicago, IL).
Right, The Lanz pressure-regulating balloon system on a National Catheter Corporation soft-cuff tracheostomy tube (Extracorporeal Medical Specialties, Inc., King of Prussia, PA).

Tracheostomy Cannulas

Special tracheostomy tubes are available to provide a route for evacuation of secretions. The Kistner (Narco Pilling Company, Fort Washington, PA) and the Olympic (Olympic Medical Corporation, Seattle, WA) tracheostomy "buttons" are examples of this special-purpose tracheal cannula (Fig. 2-11). These are sometimes useful in the transition between prolonged use of a tracheostomy tube and decannulation. A cap is available on the Kistner button to close off the proximal end, allowing the patient to talk. The Olympic tracheostomy button has a series of "O"-rings to maintain proper placement of the tube against the anterior tracheal wall. The Olympic "Trach-Talk" is a one-way valve attachment to a standard tracheostomy tube that allows the patient to talk and cough (Fig. 2-12). The "Trach-Talk" should never be inserted if there is upper airway obstruction or if the patient has an inflated, cuffed tracheostomy tube in place, since there is no means of exhalation in these situations.

Laryngectomy Tubes

Laryngectomy tubes are available to provide a route for removal of secretions and to maintain patency of the airway after laryngectomy. Short metal tubes with an inner cannula and an obturator are commonly used for this purpose (Fig. 2-13). A nylon laryngectomy tube is also available (Narco Pilling Company, Fort Washington, PA).

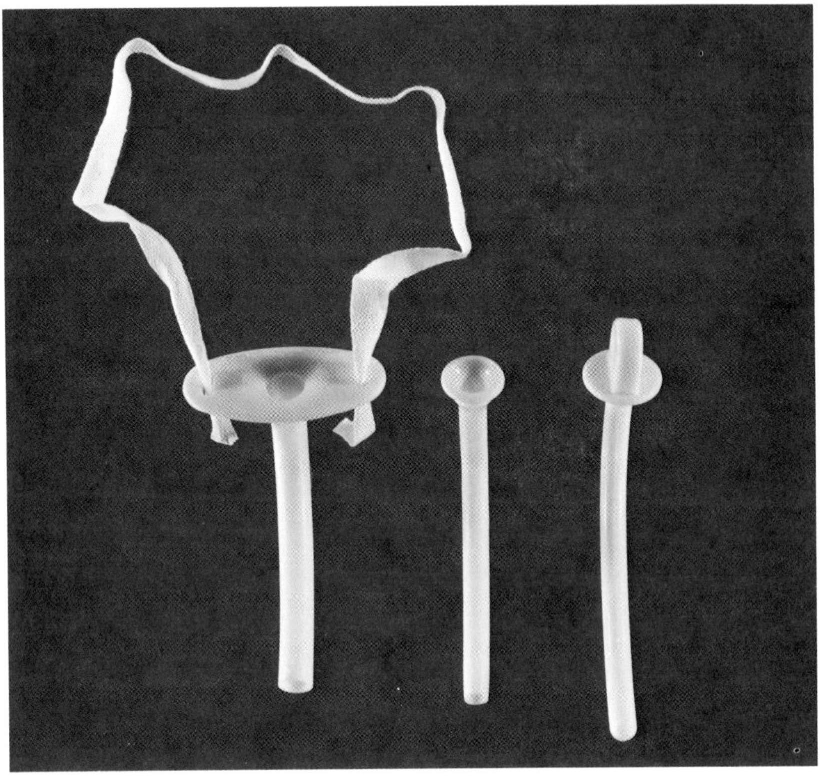

Fig. 2-10. Flexible Silastic Moore design tracheostomy tube with neck tape (*left*), inner cannula (*center*), and obturator (*right*) (Dow Corning Corporation, Midland, MI).

Miscellaneous Airways

The esophageal obturator airway, developed by Michael and associates, is available for emergency ventilation of unconscious adults by trained paramedical personnel (Brunswick Manufacturing Company, North Quincy, MA).[17] The advantage of this instrument is that it is easy to place by personnel not experienced in or authorized to do tracheal intubation during cardiopulmonary resuscitation. When this airway is placed into the esophagus, the esophageal cuff is filled with a set volume of air at a level just below the carina in order to prevent regurgitation of gastric contents. Ventilation is accomplished through perforations in the upper portion of the tube (Fig. 2-14). The esophageal obturator airway may be placed without extending the head, an advantage that may be useful in patients with possible cervical fractures. A semi-flexed head position facilitates insertion. When an endotracheal tube is subsequently inserted into the trachea, the esophageal obturator airway should be removed after intubation to prevent aspiration. The esophageal obturator airway is associated with a relatively low rate of complications; however, there are limita-

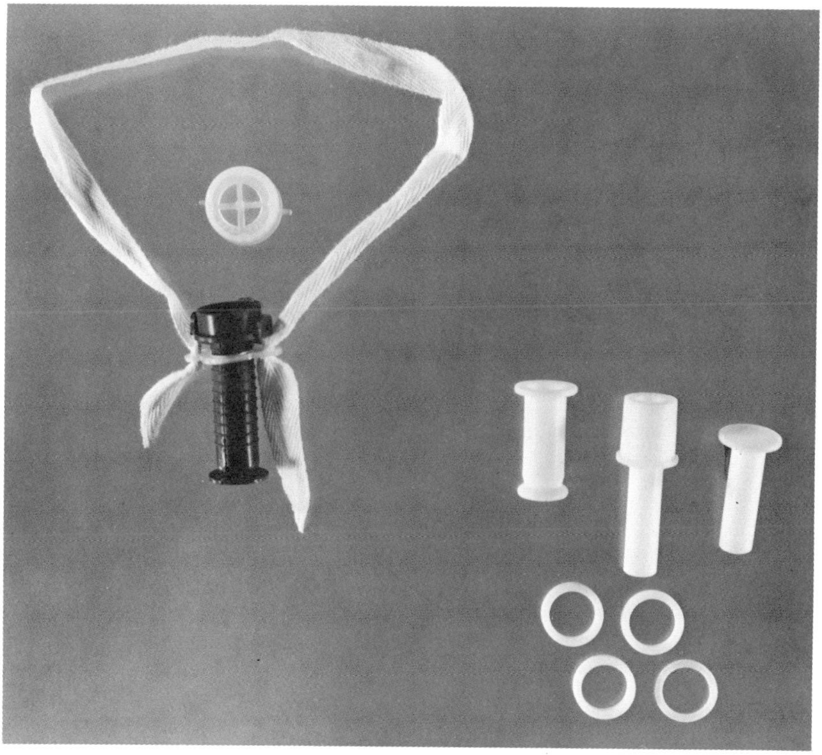

Fig. 2-11. Tracheostomy cannulas: The Kistner tracheostomy button *(left)* with neck tape attached has a detachable cap with a flutter valve, allowing the patient to talk. The Olympic tracheostomy button set *(right)* includes inner and outer cannulas, a cap, and "O"-rings for proper placement.

tions and complications, including the following: (1) No provision for suctioning of tracheobronchial secretions. (2) Occasional inability to intubate the esophagus. (3) Possibility of esophageal rupture from high cuff pressures in the esophageal balloon. (4) Inability to provide an airtight seal around the nose and the mouth. (5) Possibility of insertion into the trachea, thereby obstructing the airway. (6) Tracheal obstruction from placing the balloon too high in the esophagus. (7) Possibility of esophageal perforation caused either by the tip of the airway or by forceful retching.[18] A modification, called the "esophageal gastric tube airway" is now available and overcomes some of these limitations and risks.

Transtracheal catheters have been shown to be effective in providing adequate ventilation in selected patients during resuscitation and in animals, but the limitations of these devices are obvious.[19–22] A high-pressure source of air or oxygen is needed to overcome resistance in the catheter, and high-frequency respiration is also required. Experience with transtracheal catheter "jet" ventilation is limited, and this technique has limited clinical application at this time.

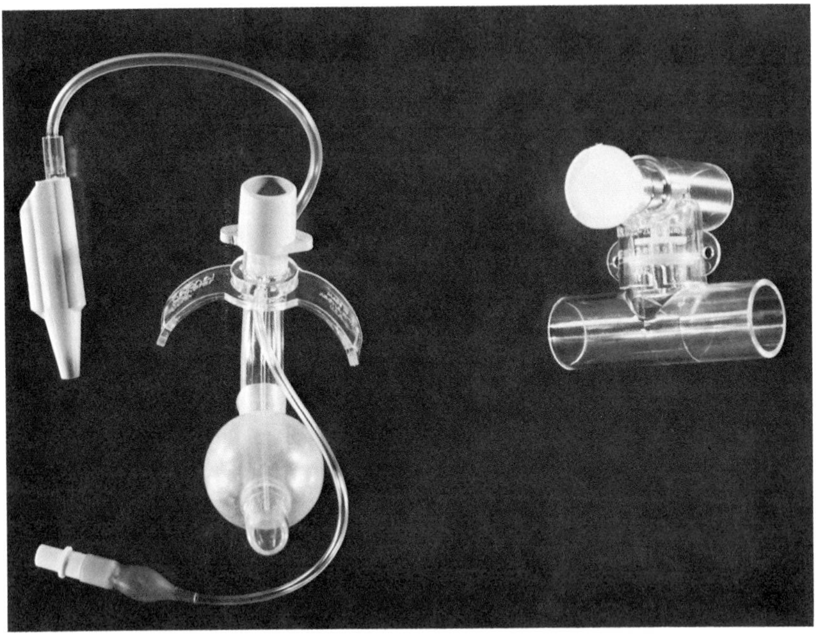

Fig. 2-12. Special tracheostomy tubes are available to allow the patient to talk. The National Catheter Corporation tracheostomy tube (*left*) has a "side-arm" which delivers air past the vocal cords through an opening above the cuff. The Olympic "Trach-Talk" (*right*) is a one-way valve which may be attached to a tracheostomy tube (see text for precautions).

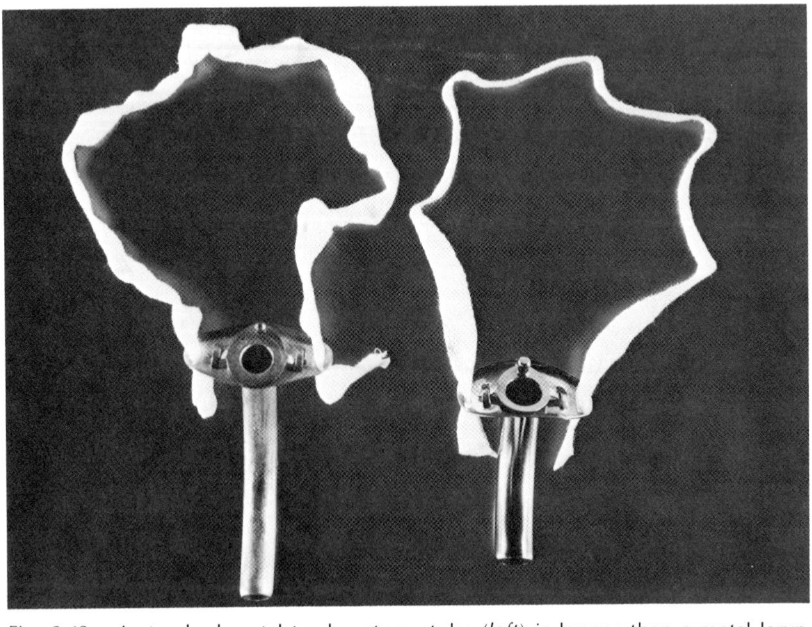

Fig. 2-13. A standard metal tracheostomy tube (*left*) is longer than a metal laryngectomy tube (*right*).

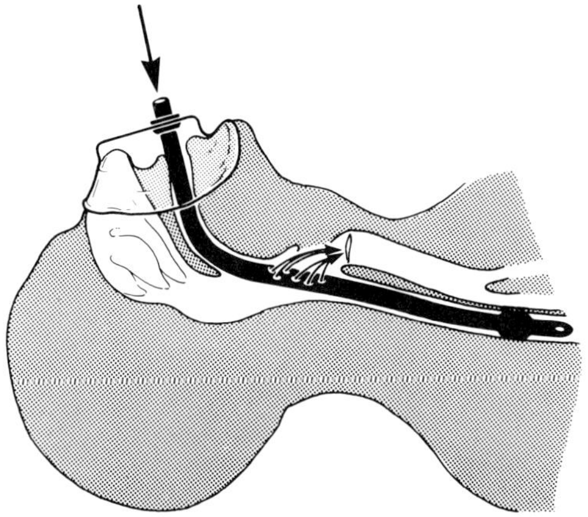

Fig. 2-14. The esophageal obturator airway is illustrated in proper position. Note that the cuff is inflated in the esophagus at a level below the carina. Airflow on inspiration is indicated by arrows.

ENDOTRACHEAL INTUBATION

Endotracheal intubation is the translaryngeal insertion of an airway into the trachea for one or more of the four indications previously listed. All respiratory care personnel should be able to perform endotracheal intubation, but this potentially difficult technique should always be attempted by the most experienced person immediately available, usually the physician. Whether elective or performed in an emergency, intubation should be attempted only after the patient is properly ventilated and oxygenated. Numerous studies and case reports attest to a higher complication rate when endotracheal intubation is performed in emergency settings.[23–25] Successful intubation depends in part upon a thorough understanding of the anatomy of the upper airway and, to a greater extent, upon experience acquired through practice in the operating room or on a deceased patient after unsuccessful cardiopulmonary resuscitation.

The route and type of definitive airway selected are matters of clinical judgment dependent upon many factors, including the duration of need for the airway. Endotracheal intubation by the oral route is the preferred method for immediate establishment of a definitive airway. We recommend oral endotracheal intubation for short-term airway management (up to 5 days) and nasal endotracheal intubation if an artificial airway is required for a longer time (5 to 14 $\pm$7 days). Some of the relative advantages of oral and of nasal intubation are listed in Table 2-5. Oral intubation is easier and quicker to perform and initially causes less discomfort for the patient. Emergency nasal intubation, without prior sedation and topical anesthesia, is a painful and harrowing experience for the patient and often results in

TABLE 2-5. Comparison of Advantages of Oral and Nasal Endotracheal Intubation

Advantages of Oral Endotracheal Intubation
Easier, faster, less painful procedure
Larger size tube tolerated
Easier suctioning
Less chance of tube kinking
Avoids nasal, paranasal complications
Advantages of Nasal Endotracheal Intubation
Allows patient to swallow oral secretions, communicate with lips
Permits oral care
Easier fixation and anchoring of tube at anterior nares
Less gagging
Prevents tube obstruction by biting
Less discomfort after tube placement
Laryngeal ulceration less common
Avoids oral complications

nasal hemorrhage. However, once the tube is in place, the nasal route is generally better tolerated than the oral route, and there is less gagging.

Our procedure for endotracheal intubation is outlined in Table 2-6. All intubation equipment should be assembled and checked for proper function before intubation is attempted. A tray or basket containing this equipment is immediately available in all critical care areas and on each hospital ward (Fig. 2-15). Ideally, two assistants should be available to help the intubator. A topical anesthetic applied to the oral or nasal mucosa before intubation is desired if the patient is conscious. Translaryngeal injection of topical anesthetic agents by way of the cricothryoid membrane is rarely necessary and should be attempted only by a skilled anesthesiologist. Prolonged attempts at endotracheal intubation are dangerous and unwarranted, and the unskilled person performing intubation is usually unaware of how much precious time has elapsed. If an endotracheal tube cannot be placed successfully in one minute, the attempt should be temporarily aborted, and ventilation and oxygenation should be resumed, utilizing the "head-tilt" method to maintain airway patency.

After intubation, it is usually desirable to obtain a chest roentgenogram to confirm proper positioning of the tube in the trachea. The radiopaque tip ideally should be located 5 ± 2 cm above the carina in an adult when the neck is in neutral position, which is about the level of the third or fourth thoracic vertebral body.[26] The shaft of the endotracheal tube should then be marked at the lip or nostril or should be trimmed for future reference to avoid slipping in or out. Special oral endotracheal tube holders are available to secure tube placement, but often these are not well tolerated because of

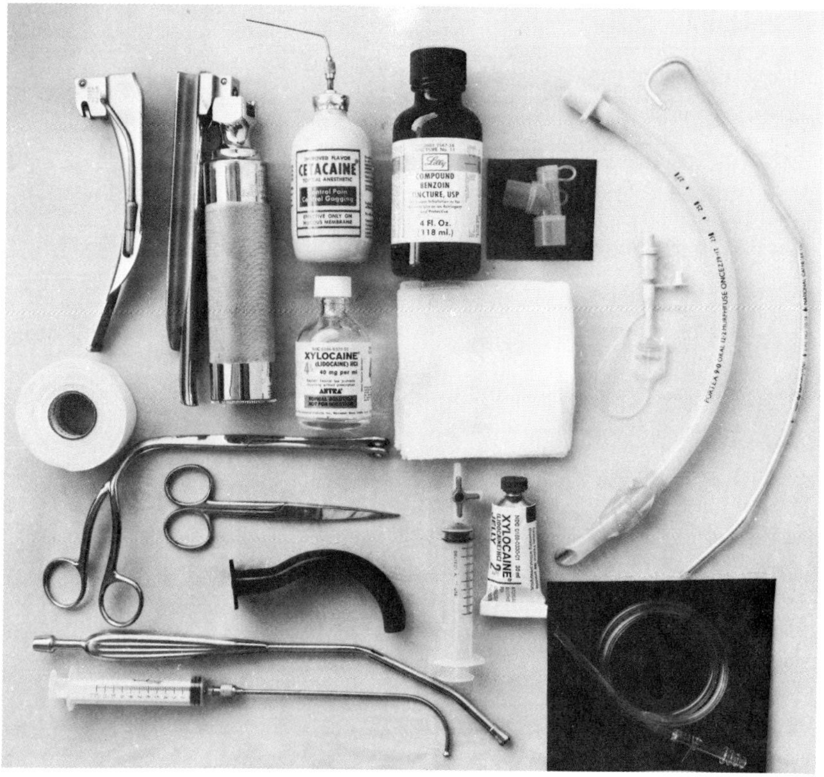

Fig. 2-15. All necessary equipment for endotracheal intubation is assembled in a tray or basket for convenience.

gagging or pressure necrosis of soft tissues. An oral pharyngeal airway should be used in conjunction with endotracheal intubation only if absolutely necessary to prevent biting and obstruction of the oral endotracheal tube, to permit evacuation of secretions, to prevent tongue biting, or to provide a buttress to stabilize tube placement in edentulous patients.

Endotracheal intubation is usually a simple task for the experienced clinician, but in some circumstances, it may be difficult and challenging to even the most experienced anesthesiologist. In certain unusual circumstances—i.e., ankylosis of the temporomandibular joint, flexion deformities of the cervical spine, mandibular fractures, ankylosing spondylitis, and cervical fractures—special techniques of intubation are usually necessary. For difficult intubation, we use a fiberoptic bronchoscope to visualize the vocal cords and to guide the endotracheal tube into place. A flexible intubation laryngoscope may also be used for this purpose.[27] Both the fiberoptic bronchoscope and the flexible intubation laryngoscope may be used to confirm proper placement of the tip of the endotracheal tube in the midportion of the trachea. Threading an endotracheal tube over an introducer or suc-

TABLE 2-6. Procedure for Oral and Nasal Endotracheal Intubation

EQUIPMENT

1. Endotracheal intubation tray or basket which includes:
   a. Soft-cuff endotracheal tubes of various sizes (nasal and oral)
   b. Stylet for endotracheal tube
   c. Water-soluble lubricant
   d. Syringe
   e. Four-way stopcock
   f. Two-way swivel adaptor for endotracheal tube
   g. Topical anesthetic and applicator
   h. Laryngoscope handle, curved and straight blades
   i. Magill forceps
   j. Adhesive tape
   k. Scissors
   l. Tincture of benzoin and 4 × 4 gauze
   m. Oral pharyngeal airway
   n. Yankauer pharyngeal suction tip
   o. Endotracheal suction kit with gloves, catheter, and water cup
2. Portable or wall suction apparatus, ready for use.
3. Self-inflating resuscitation bag with mask connected to high-flow oxygen source.

PROCEDURE FOR OROTRACHEAL INTUBATION

1. Keep patient NPO for at least six hours if intubation is elective.
2. Assemble the necessary equipment and check for proper function (laryngoscope blade and light, cuff of endotracheal tube, etc.).
3. Explain the procedure and provide reassurance if the patient is conscious.
4. Maintain adequate ventilation and oxygenation while intubation equipment is being assembled.
5. Remove any dental appliances and foreign bodies from the mouth. Suction any secretions from the mouth and pharynx.
6. Apply topical anesthetic to the mouth and posterior pharynx if time permits.
7. Remove headboard from patient's bed.
8. Lubricate tip of endotracheal tube with water-soluble anesthetic ointment. Evacuate all air from the cuff.
9. Place the patient in the supine position with neck flexed on the chest and head extended on the neck at the atlanto-occipital joint.
10. Administer a short-acting parenteral sedative drug only if necessary to calm the patient and only if ventilatory support is immediately available.
11. Open the lips with crossed-finger technique to protect the lips during insertion of the laryngoscope blade
12. Lubricate laryngoscope blade with sterile water.
13. Using the left hand, pass the laryngoscope blade gently into the mouth along the right side of the tongue and posteriorly into the midline of the hypopharynx. Be careful not to exert leverage on the teeth and jam the blade tip into the pharynx. A straight blade tip should pass the epiglottis. If a curved blade is used, pass the tip into the vallecula.
14. Visualize the vocal cords by using a steady upward lifting motion of the entire laryngoscope.
15. With the right hand on the shaft of the endotracheal tube, pass the tip of the tube gently along the right side of the laryngoscope blade into the glottis while the vocal cords are continually visualized. The stylet may be useful to mold the tube in some instances, but if inserted, it should be lubricated first and never allowed to pass the tip of the endotracheal tube. Gentle external pressure exerted by the assistant on the larynx occasionally facilitates visualization of the vocal cords. Avoid blind jamming of the tip of the endotracheal tube.

TABLE 2-6. (*continued*)

16. Pass the tip of the endotracheal tube 5 to 6 cm beyond the vocal cords in adults.
17. Inflate the cuff to the appropriate pressure.
18. Ventilate the patient with a resuscitation bag connected to the oxygen source.
19. Auscultate the chest and observe for symmetry of chest expansion to be certain that the tube has not entered the right mainstem bronchus.
20. Apply benzoin to the skin and secure the shaft of the tube at the corner of the mouth with adhesive tape, using an oral pharyngeal airway for support only if necessary.
21. Attach ventilator tubing to two-way swivel connected to the standard 15-mm adaptor. Support the weight of any tubing attached to the endotracheal tube.
22. Obtain "stat" chest roentgenogram for confirmation of tube placement.
23. Trim off excess length of the endotracheal tube so that the 15-mm adaptor is at the edge of the lip. This provides a reference point to ascertain proper tube placement.
24. Protect the endotracheal tube from dislodgment and self-extubation.

PROCEDURE FOR NASOTRACHEAL INTUBATION

1. Follow steps 1 to 5 and 7 to 10 under "Procedure for Orotracheal Intubation."
2. Determine which side of the nose appears more patent for passage of the endotracheal tube.
3. Apply topical anesthetic agent to the nasal mucosa on the side selected. An agent with vasoconstrictive properties such as cocaine or phenylephrine may be useful to shrink the mucosa and expand the nasal passage.
4. The nasal endotracheal tube selected should be 1 to 2 mm smaller in internal diameter than an oral endotracheal tube for the same patient.
5. Pass the lubricated tube gently through the nostril into the nasal cavity. Do not jam the tube further if firm resistance is met. Try the opposite side of the nose if this occurs.
6. Pass the tube slowly into the hypopharynx and blindly into the glottis during inspiration, listening for airflow. Entry into the glottis is indicated by cough and rapid expulsion of air.
7. If two or three attempts are not successful or if more than one minute has elapsed, ventilate and oxygenate the patient. If further attempts at blind nasal intubation fail, attempt to visualize the vocal cords with a laryngoscope in the left hand and pass the tip of the nasal endotracheal tube into the glottis under direct vision. A Magill forceps can be used to facilitate passage into the glottis, but care should be taken to avoid grasping the cuffed portion of the tube.
8. Follow steps 16 to 24 under "Procedure for Orotracheal Intubation," anchoring the shaft of the tube at the nostril with tape and trimming excess tubing at the edge of the nostril.

tion catheter is sometimes done in a difficult intubation. Further suggestions for the occasional difficult intubation have been published by Salem and colleagues.[28]

TRACHEOTOMY

Tracheotomy is defined as the surgical creation of an opening in the trachea. The term "tracheostomy" refers to the opening so created and is loosely used to refer to the standard tracheotomy operation. Cricothyroidotomy is the surgical creation of an opening in the cricothyroid membrane and thus is really a "laryngotomy" procedure. Cricothyroidotomy is usually regarded as an emergency procedure, but its use in elective tracheal intubation has been described.[29]

The major advantage of this procedure is that it is easier and quicker to perform than the standard tracheotomy. Both tracheotomy and cricothyroidotomy are surgical methods of establishing a definitive airway.

The general indications for tracheotomy are those previously discussed for establishing a definitive airway. There are some additional specific indications for tracheotomy (Table 2-7). Tracheotomy also decreases anatomic dead space and decreases the work of breathing, but this minimal physiologic benefit is rarely important to the patient.[30]

Tracheotomy is rarely necessary as an emergency procedure because of the widespread availablity of endotracheal intubation. Whenever tracheotomy is performed as an emergency procedure in poor conditions, greater morbidity and mortality can be expected. In the rare emergency situation in which endotracheal intubation has not been successful, cricothyroidotomy should be performed, since it is easier and quicker than a standard tracheotomy procedure. Thus, in reality, the standard tracheotomy operation should never be regarded as an emergency procedure. Tracheotomy is best performed by experienced surgeons in the operating room with controlled aseptic conditions, good lighting, and ready availability of equipment. Occasionally, when there is great risk in transporting a critically ill patient to the operating room, tracheotomy may be performed at the bedside. Contrary to the tradition in many large teaching hospitals, tracheotomy should not be considered a "minor" procedure delegated to the most junior surgical house officer. The high complication rate associated with tracheotomy will be reduced if these principles are followed.

TABLE 2-7. Specific Indications for Tracheotomy

1. Patients with respiratory failure with prolonged need for a definitive airway (i.e., more than 2–3 weeks).
2. Chronic obstruction of the upper airway, including obstructive type of sleep apnea syndrome.
3. Retained or excessive secretions which cannot be evacuated by suctioning through an endotracheal tube.
4. Inability of the patient to tolerate endotracheal intubation.
5. Immediate need for a definitive airway when endotracheal intubation is not successful (cricothyroidotomy preferred).
6. Prophylactically—e.g., prior to radical neck surgery, various neurosurgical operations, ventilator management of severe flail chest, radiation therapy to the larynx, etc.
7. Chronic neurologic disorders with glottic incompetence predisposing to chronic pulmonary aspiration.
8. Laryngectomy.
9. Severe facial, pharyngeal, or laryngeal injuries or burns.
10. Certain congenital malformations of the upper airway.

A thorough discussion of the technique of tracheotomy is beyond the scope of this chapter. Readers are referred to standard surgical textbooks for this technical information. However, a few principles are worth mentioning here. The operation is performed with the neck extended and landmarks identified, always over an indwelling endotracheal tube with the patient properly ventilated and oxygenated. A transverse skin incision at or 5 mm below the cricoid cartilage is traditional. The tracheal incision is usually a vertical incision at the level of the second or third tracheal ring. Some surgeons prefer to create a small window in the anterior tracheal wall, but large portions of tracheal cartilage should not be removed because of the greater risk of stenosis.[31] Incisions above the second ring or below the fourth ring invite complications. The tracheotomy incision should not be sutured tightly upon closure, and the neck flange of the tracheostomy tube should not be secured tightly over the incision, since these practices will increase the risk of subcutaneous emphysema and infection. A postoperative chest roentgenogram is usually obtained to rule out pneumothorax. Care of the patient after tracheotomy is discussed next.

CARE OF THE PATIENT WITH AN ARTIFICIAL AIRWAY

The patient with an endotracheal or a tracheostomy tube is dependent upon respiratory care personnel to meet both physical and psychologic needs. The goals of management of the patient with an artificial airway are: (1) to treat the respiratory failure and its underlying cause, (2) to maximize patient comfort, (3) to support emotional needs, and (4) to prevent iatrogenic complications. Meticulous patient evaluation, careful scrutiny of all tubes and mechanical devices, and empathy for the patient are fundamental to achieving these goals.

A number of general guidelines are recommended for care of the patient with an artificial airway (Table 2-8). The patient is usually managed in an intensive care unit where skilled personnel and equipment are readily available. Patients with endotracheal tubes should be managed only in the intensive care unit or in the postoperative recovery room, while those with long-term tracheostomies may be managed on a hospital ward or in chronic-care facilities if skilled respiratory care is available. Some patients are able to care for their own permanent tracheostomies at home.

Intensive care unit patients with cuffed intratracheal tubes in place are unable to speak, are often restrained, and frequently are unable to communicate. Moreover, they are typically apprehensive, often depressed, and fully dependent upon attending personnel. Respiratory care nurses and respiratory therapists should be at or near the bedside around the clock to anticipate and to meet the patient's needs. Frequent visits by the physician and a careful daily examina-

TABLE 2-8. General Guidelines for Care of the Patient with an Artificial Airway

1. Maximize the patient's comfort.
2. Support the emotional needs of the patient.
3. Examine the patient and the airway frequently.
4. Humidify and warm inspired gases.
5. Evacuate and control tracheobronchial secretions.
6. Prevent infection.
7. Prevent pulmonary aspiration.
8. Minimize leverage on the tube and motion between the tube and the patient.
9. Use the lowest effective cuff pressure.
10. Provide adequate nutrition.
11. Avoid, recognize, and treat any complications.
12. Extubate or decannulate as early as possible.

tion with direct patient contact are reassuring. Personnel at the bedside should create an impression of confidence and optimism. Quiet times for rest and sleep without interruption should be provided. The patient should be oriented frequently to the time, the date, and the day by use of a calendar at the bedside and a clock. Patients are reassured by learning that the inability to talk with an intratracheal tube in place is normal and only temporary. A call bell to summon nurses should be within reach. Use of a writing pad or a "magic slate" also helps facilitate communication with the staff.

Humidification and Warming of Inspired Gases

Humidification and warming of gases inspired through the artificial airway help in the control of tracheobronchial secretions and in the prevention of lower respiratory tract infections. Although there is no firm scientific evidence that humidification of inspired gases and adequate systemic hydration enhance mucociliary clearance in patients with artificial airways, there is practical clinical benefit from these measures.[32] A definitive artificial airway bypasses the normal upper airway and its air-conditioning functions (filtration, heating, and humidification). Respiratory gases should be delivered to the trachea at or near body temperature and humidity to prevent tracheal injury. Inhalation of cold or dry gases depresses mucociliary transport and increases the risks of infection and atelectasis due to retained secretions. Inhalation of dry air produces tracheitis sicca with demonstrable histologic changes.

Humidifiers and nebulizers are available to add moisture to inspired gases. Humidifiers deliver water vapor to the airway by converting water to water vapor in a temperature-dependent process. The most common type of humidifier in use for patients with artificial airways is the heated cascade humidifier attached to the respirator. A bottle humidifier with a heating element attached to the wall is suitable for patients breathing spontaneously. Nebulizers produce a visible aerosol in which particulate water is suspended in the inspired gas—a process not dependent upon temperature. Ultrasonic nebulizers provide water particles less than five microns in diameter to maximize deposition in small airways. These devices should be used only for short periods, since inhalation of very fine particles may cause bronchospasm or fluid overload through pulmonary absorption. In patients on mechanical ventilators, a thermometer placed in line along the wide-bore tubing near the artificial airway is monitored to keep the inspired gas temperature between 85° and 95° Fahrenheit. Wide-bore tubing running from the humidifier or nebulizer to the airway should be as short as possible to avoid excessive condensation and cooling. Each foot of wide-bore tubing reduces the temperature of the in-line gas about 2°C. In-line condensate collection bags are useful to avoid spillage of condensed water directly into the airway. In patients breathing spontaneously, a "T-piece" attachment may be used to deliver inspired gas to the endotracheal or tracheostomy tube. A tracheostomy cover provides a dome for warm humidified gas without putting leverage on the tracheostomy tube (Fig. 2-16).

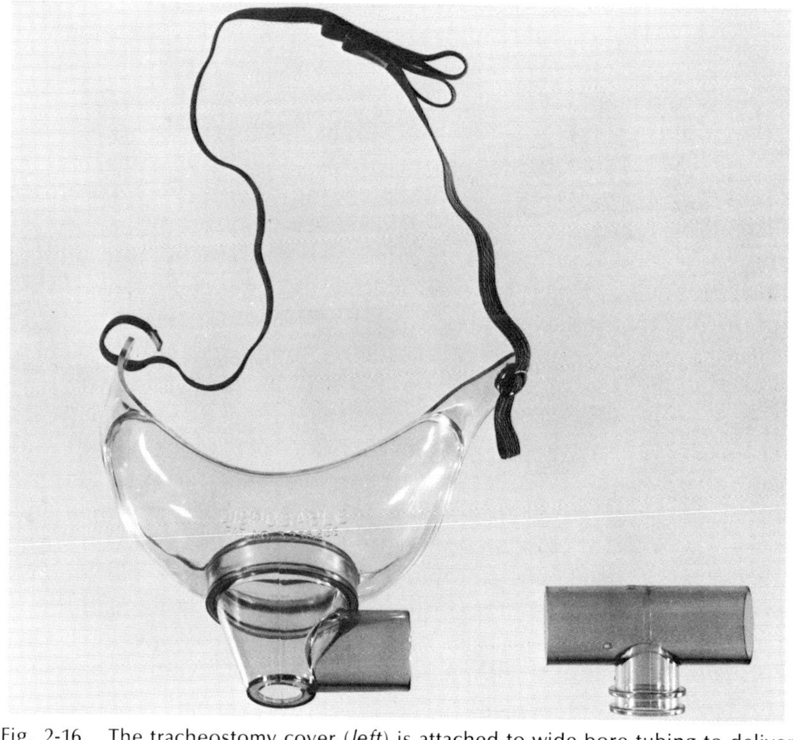

Fig. 2-16. The tracheostomy cover (*left*) is attached to wide-bore tubing to deliver inspired gas over the tracheostomy tube. The standard "T-piece" (*right*) delivers inspired gas to either an endotracheal or a tracheostomy tube.

Control of Tracheobronchial Secretions

The patient with a cuffed intratracheal tube usually has considerable difficulty in clearing tracheobronchial secretions for several reasons. First, cough is less effective since the vocal cords cannot close. Second, the cuffed tube produces a circumferential epithelial injury with loss of the ciliated columnar epithelium.[33,34] Interruption of the mucociliary escalator and obstruction by the cuff would be expected to block completely mucociliary transport at the cuff level. Finally, there is evidence that endotracheal tubes themselves with either high or low compliance cuffs suppress mucociliary clearance.[12,35]

Adequate control of tracheobronchial secretions requires attention to both decreasing the production of secretions and increasing their evacuation. This is usually accomplished by humidification and warming of inspired gases and skilled tracheobronchial suctioning, thereby reducing the risks of lower respiratory tract infection, atelectasis, and impaired gas exchange. Secretions should be kept thin and watery; the best agent for this purpose is water. Aerosolized water decreases sputum viscosity in chronic bronchitis patients.[36] Mucolytic agents should be avoided, since they may be irritating to the airway. The patient should be adequately hydrated systemically, since there is experimental evidence that water deprivation decreases tracheal mucous flow.[32,37] Agents that depress mucociliary transport such as anesthetic gases, high concentrations of inspired oxygen, atropine, acetylcysteine, and opiates should be avoided. Effective coughing and deep breathing may help raise sputum while the artificial airway is in place. Coughing should not be suppressed unless violent paroxysms of coughing produce complications. Beta-adrenergic agonists and methylxanthine agents may stimulate mucociliary clearance. Chest physiotherapy may be difficult to accomplish if the patient is intubated and on a respirator, but in selected patients it may be performed with beneficial results. Intermittent positive-pressure breathing (IPPB) has no proven value in clearing tracheobronchial secretions and should be avoided except to deliver aerosolized bronchodilator medications to distal airways.

Tracheobronchial suctioning is an efficient means to evacuate secretions in patients with artificial airways. Meticulous aseptic suctioning technique is necessary to avoid complications, some of which may be life threatening. Suctioning should be performed only by respiratory care personnel who are trained in this procedure and familiar with its complications. Deep suctioning is particularly hazardous. Our protocol for tracheobronchial suctioning is outlined in Table 2-9. The procedure is best performed by two persons. One ventilates the patient with a self-inflating resuscitation bag and stabilizes the endotracheal or tracheostomy tube with the opposite hand, while the other passes the suction catheter with sterile gloved

TABLE 2-9. Procedure for Endotracheal or Tracheostomy Tube Suctioning

EQUIPMENT

1. Portable or wall suctioning unit.
2. Connecting tube to suctioning unit.
3. Sterile suction catheters (size depends on diameter of endotracheal or tracheostomy tube). Avoid suction catheters with only one opening in the tip.
4. Sterile gloves.
5. Sterile cup containing 1 or 2 oz sterile water.
6. Sterile 10 ml syringe.
7. Normal saline, sterile, 5 ml.
8. Disposal bag for refuse.
9. Self-inflating resuscitation bag connected to a high-flow oxygen source.
10. Tracheostomy cleaning set with bowl, hydrogen peroxide, and pipe cleaners (for patients with a tracheostomy tube utilizing an inner cannula).

PROCEDURE

1. Wash hands.
2. Assemble necessary equipment.
3. Explain the procedure to the patient and provide reassurance.
4. Fill the sterile cup with 1 or 2 oz sterile water.
5. Open the disposable kit containing the catheter and gloves.
6. Put the sterile glove on the dominant hand and pick up the sterile catheter.
7. Using the ungloved hand, attach the catheter to the connecting tube.
8. Lubricate the suction catheter by suctioning a small amount of sterile water through it.
9. Estimate the length of suction catheter needed to enter the mainstem bronchi if deep suctioning is required.
10. Have the assistant ventilate the patient with the resuscitation bag connected to oxygen for 10 to 15 seconds. If possible, the patient should take 8 to 10 deep breaths while the assistant supplements ventilation with the resuscitation bag.
11. If the patient has a tracheostomy tube with an inner cannula, have the assistant remove the inner cannula and place it in the bowl of hydrogen peroxide for cleaning. The assistant cleans the inner cannula with a pipe cleaner and hydrogen peroxide and rinses it with sterile water.
12. With the gloved hand on the catheter tubing and the ungloved hand on the suction port, gently advance the catheter into the tube until resistance is met. Do *not* apply suction during introduction of the catheter. Angled (Coudé) catheters can be directed toward either the right or the left mainstem bronchus.
13. Withdraw the catheter slowly from the tube using intermittent suction and a gentle circular or twisting motion of the catheter. Each maneuver takes about five seconds and may be repeated once. The total period of suctioning should not exceed 10 to 15 seconds. Avoid vigorous suctioning and thrusting the catheter up and down the airway. Do not apply continuous suction. Remove thumb from the suction port if the catheter seems to be occluded because this may indicate grabbing of the mucosa by the catheter tip.
14. Rinse the catheter with sterile water.
15. Have the assistant repeat assisted ventilation with the resuscitation bag and oxygen before reconnecting ventilator or "T-piece" tubing.
16. After a 30-second rest, repeat suctioning only if necessary, since each time the catheter enters the trachea, the mucosa is abraded.
17. If the secretions are unusually thick and difficult to evacuate, instill 5 ml of sterile saline into the tube, ventilate and repeat Step 13. Remove needle from the syringe before use.

TABLE 2-9. (*continued*)

18. Auscultate both sides of the chest after suctioning to assess adequacy of the procedure.
19. The mouth and pharynx may be suctioned if necessary.
20. Discard used glove and catheter.

technique (Fig. 2-17). Suctioning should be performed whenever necessary to maintain patency of the airway. No rote schedule is appropriate for all patients, and those without secretions should not be routinely suctioned. A separate sterile catheter should be used to suction the artificial airway if the pharynx or mouth is suctioned beforehand. Sterile disposable suction catheters, gloves, and containers for sterile water are available in kits which facilitate the suctioning procedure.

Ideally, the patient should cough up secretions from deep in the lungs to the level of the artificial airway, where evacuation is then accomplished atraumatically with suction. Every time a suction catheter is introduced into the trachea, the mucosa is traumatized. A variety of suction catheters have been introduced in an attempt to reduce mucosal trauma, but trauma may be more dependent upon the suctioning technique than the design of the catheter.[38] However, suction catheters with multiple eyes at the tip are probably safer than those with single eyes.[39] In a study of dogs, Sackner and his col-

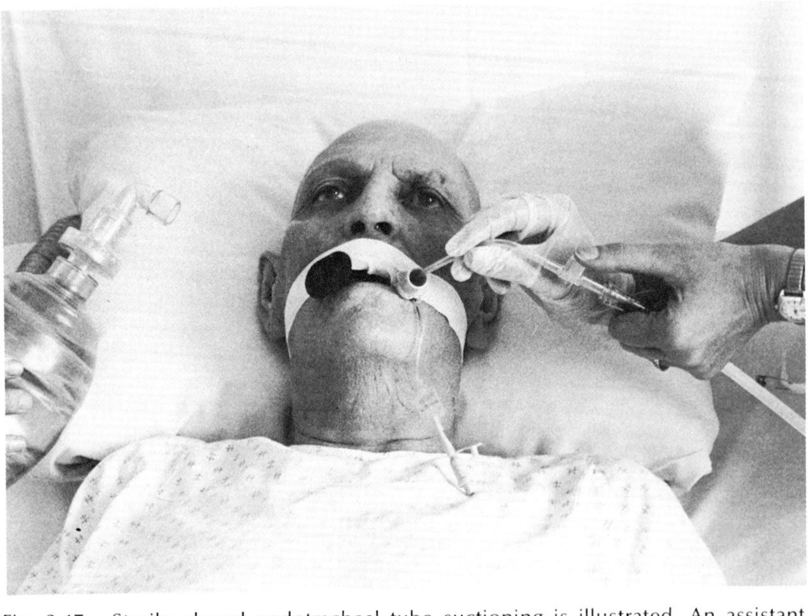

Fig. 2-17. Sterile gloved endotracheal tube suctioning is illustrated. An assistant (*left*) may stabilize the tube and provide ventilation with a self-inflating resuscitation bag connected to an oxygen source.

leagues demonstrated that use of an Argyle Aero-Flo catheter with several eyes above a beaded rim avoids invagination of the mucosa into the catheter during suctioning and decreases trauma.[12,40] Angled (coudé) catheters are available to help gain entry to the left or the right mainstem bronchus. The practice of turning the head to the left to enter the right mainstem bronchus with a suction catheter and vice versa is not effective and should be abandoned.[41]

Complications of tracheobronchial suctioning include patient discomfort and anxiety, mucosal trauma, hypoxemia in certain circumstances, cardiac arrhythmias in hypoxic patients breathing room air, and increase in resistance due to occlusion of the tube with too large a suction catheter.[42–44] Prolonged suctioning procedures are dangerous, particularly in patients who are hypoxemic.[12] One or 2 suctioning maneuvers lasting 10 to 15 seconds are usually well tolerated. In patients who require positive end-expiratory pressure (PEEP) on the respirator, an adaptor is available to maintain positive airway pressure during suctioning. Suctioning is performed only intermittently and with a traditional circular motion during withdrawal of the catheter to avoid stripping and tearing of the mucosa. Experimental studies reveal, however, that rotating the suction catheter does not cause the tip to rotate because of lack of torsional stiffness in suction catheters packaged in a coil.[39] The diameter of the suction catheter should be less than half the diameter of the endotracheal or tracheostomy tube. The catheter may be lubricated with sterile water or saline if dry insertion is difficult. In patients with unusually tenacious secretions, 5 ml of sterile saline solution may be injected directly into the lumen of the artificial airway, followed by ventilation with a resuscitation bag and repeat suctioning to attempt to break up thick secretions. This also stimulates cough. If the suction catheter meets a sudden resistance in the artificial airway, a kink in the tube should be suspected, and the tube should then be replaced.

Fiberoptic bronchoscopy is not a routine procedure in providing tracheobronchial toilet in patients with artificial airways because of expense and time commitments. Secretions can usually be controlled with suctioning through a plain catheter and with the measures just recommended. However, fiberoptic bronchoscopy may be useful in selected circumstances, including persistent atelectasis which is not responsive to simpler respiratory care measures and unexplained persistent lung infiltrates. Upper lobe or left lower lobe infiltrates or atelectasis due to retained secretions might benefit from fiberoptic bronchoscopy, since suction catheters are difficult to maneuver into these areas. Nevertheless, in one prospective study, fiberoptic bronchoscopy was shown to add nothing to respiratory therapy in the treatment of acute lobar atelectasis in critically ill patients.[45] Fiberoptic bronchoscopy used to evaluate the tracheobronchial tree to ascertain the safety of prolonged intubation has been advocated, but this practice should not be routine in our opinion.[46]

Prevention of Infection

Patients with artificial airways are particularly prone to developing respiratory tract infection because of impaired mucociliary transport, traumatic injury to the tracheobronchial mucosa caused by suctioning and intubation, and colonization of the airway with bacteria. Respiratory disease and tracheal intubation predispose intensive care unit patients to colonization of the airway with gram-negative bacilli, and colonization of the airway with gram-negative bacilli predisposes one to pneumonia.[47,48] The insertion of an artificial airway into the trachea introduces bacteria either through contamination of the endotracheal tube during its passage through the pharynx, through aspiration, or by direct extension of infection from a tracheostomy wound. A recent study has demonstrated an average of six bacterial isolates per aspirate from clinically stable patients with tracheostomy tubes.[49] Common organisms isolated from the respiratory tract in patients with artificial airways include gram-negative bacilli, especially *Pseudomonas* species, and *Staphylococcus aureus*.

Measures to combat infection in the patient with an artificial airway include humidification of inspired gases, aseptic suctioning technique, frequent changes of ventilator tubing and humidifiers, frequent changes of tracheotomy wound dressings, and hand-washing before and after patient contact. If lower respiratory tract infection due to the artificial airway is suspected, sputum should be aspirated into a sterile trap for Gram staining. In selected patients, obtaining of aerobic and anaerobic cultures may be helpful. A culture of sputum showing a potential bacterial pathogen should not be considered a sole indication for antibiotic therapy unless there is other evidence of nosocomial pneumonia such as fever, lung infiltrates, and leukocytosis. Patients with purulent tracheobronchitis may benefit from antibiotics in the absence of lung infiltrates. We rely on a daily Gram stain of sputum collected in a suction trap if infection is suspected, looking for a predominant organism.

Prevention of Pulmonary Aspiration

Pulmonary aspiration is a constant threat to patients with artificial airways and may be particularly difficult to diagnose.[50–53] Nasogastric tubes used concomitantly with artificial airways may impair the function of the lower and upper esophageal sphincters, increasing the predisposition for aspiration of gastric contents and infected pharyngeal secretions.[50,54] Depressed consciousness in critically ill intubated patients is also frequently associated with incompetence of the glottis, predisposing the patient to pulmonary aspiration. Furthermore, tracheotomy induces a functional incompetence of the glottis which lasts several days after the operation. Replacement of low-volume, high-pressure cuffs with high-volume, low-pressure cuffs on both tracheostomy tubes and endotracheal tubes has reduced the incidence of aspiration.[52,53] To reduce the risk of pulmonary aspiration in patients after tracheotomy, we keep a soft cuff inflated at all times at low ($\leq$20 mm Hg) pressure. Overinflation of the cuff puts pressure on the esophagus and prevents swallowing of pharyngeal secretions. For the first few days following tracheotomy, the patient is given no oral feedings. When oral feedings are initiated, the head of the bed is elevated. To test for possible pulmonary aspiration, the patient is given grape juice or a weak solution of methylene blue to drink, followed by aspiration of the trachea. Aspiration of secretions and water condensate in wide-bore tubing is avoided by frequent changing of these tubes and by the use of condensate collection bags.

Reduction in Leverage and Motion

Since artificial airways are levers as well as tubes, they transmit external forces directly to the patient. Motion of the artificial airway produces a raking action along the tracheal mucosa. Pressure points where contact of the artificial airway with soft tissues is the greatest include the lips (or anterior nares), the posterior pharynx, the posterior rim of the glottis, and the cuff site. Mucosal edema, inflammation, and ulceration are complications of excessive movement of the tube along these mucosal surfaces. Minimizing leverage on the endotracheal or tracheostomy tube and avoiding excessive motion between the tube and the patient should help reduce tracheal mucosal injury and other soft tissue complications. Particular care must be exercised to avoid direct transmission of forces to the tracheostomy tube, since the upper airway and glottis are not available to buttress the tube. The tracheostomy tube is anchored by a large neck flange and tape. Heavy tubing should not be allowed to hang from the patient's mouth or the tracheal stoma. Condensate should be emptied frequently to decrease the weight of wide-bore tubing. Wide-bore tubing is supported by a side arm of the ventilator or by a folded towel on the chest. Two-way swivel adaptors (Fig. 2-18) help reduce rotational forces. Corrugated elastic connectors between ventilator tubing and the artificial airway serve as a shock absorber to prevent transmission of various forces. The orotracheal tube should be taped securely at the lip to reduce motion. An oral airway is particularly helpful to buttress the orotracheal tube in edentulous patients. If the patient moves excessively, reassurance and sedation may be useful. Seizures, if present, should be controlled with anticonvulsants.

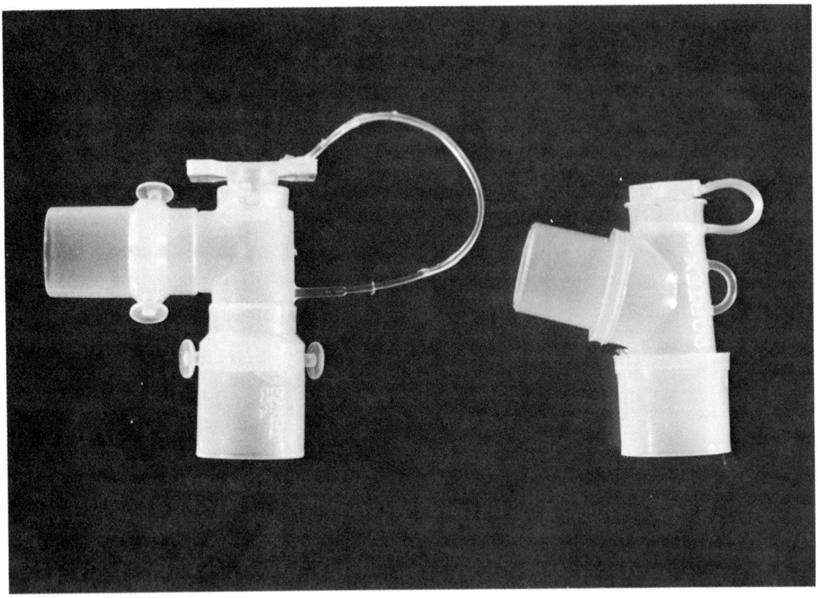

Fig. 2-18. Plastic two-way swivel adaptors help reduce rotational forces applied to the endotracheal or tracheostomy tube. Examples include the National Catheter Corporation adaptor (*left*) and the Portex adaptor (*right*).

Management of the Cuff

Attention to pressure in the cuff of the intratracheal tube is a vital aspect of modern respiratory care. Most definitive artificial airways now in use have air-inflatable cuffs to maintain positive airway pressure during mechanical ventilation and to reduce the risk of aspiration. An extensive experience and literature have developed during the last 15 years implicating cuff pressure as the single most important determinant of tracheal mucosal injury. Pressure necrosis of the tracheal mucosa at the cuff site may lead to tracheomalacia, tracheal dilatation, tracheal stenosis, tracheoesophageal fistula, and hemorrhage due to erosion into a major blood vessel. It is desirable to use the lowest effective pressure in the cuff that will maintain positive airway pressure during mechanical ventilation, reduce the risk of aspiration, provide the lowest lateral tracheal wall pressure, and keep the tip of the tube centrally located within the trachea. Because capillary perfusion pressure has been estimated to be about 30 mm Hg, cuff pressure should be kept well below this critical level to avoid necrosis.[55] Because of inherent compliance in the cuff material, the pressure exerted laterally against the tracheal wall is less than the pressure maintained within the air-inflated cuff. The pressure-volume relationship (compliance) of various cuffs is the major determinant of the pressure exerted upon the mucosa; it varies tremendously from one type of cuff to the next.[15] Compliant cuffs conform to the lumen of the trachea, while noncompliant cuffs distort the trachea before a seal is achieved.

Only sufficiently trained persons should manage the cuffed tube. The cuff pressure should be checked at least three times a day with a mercury or aneroid manometer open via a four-way stopcock to an air-filled 10-ml syringe (Fig. 2-19).[56] The cuff pressure recorded is written on a bedside chart or ventilator care sheet. This practice, although time-consuming, is more precise than the practice of relying on self-regulating cuff-pressure devices and provides assurance that a mechanical problem, such as rupture of the cuff, has not developed. Feeling the pilot balloon every so often is helpful, since the skilled clinician may be able to make a rough estimate of cuff pressure by noting the compliance or "give" of the pilot balloon. This practice takes considerable experience and is not foolproof.

Several different methods have been advocated to maintain inflation of the cuff. The "minimal leak" technique allows for a small rush of air upward past the cuff during the peak of the inspiratory cycle on

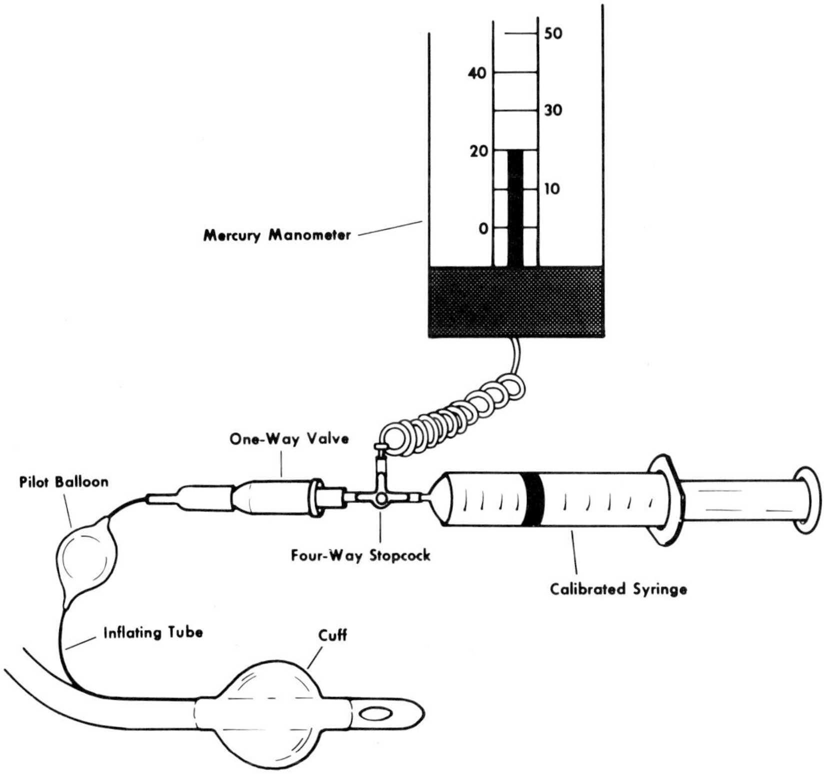

Fig. 2-19. Cuff pressure is measured on a manometer by way of an open four-way stopcock connected to an air-filled syringe and the luer adaptor on the inflating tube.

the mechanical ventilator. Advocates of this technique claim lesser tracheal mucosal injury because of the requirement for slightly less cuff pressure. When this technique is used, the tidal volume on the respirator must be increased to compensate for the leak and to maintain effective alveolar ventilation. Although the rush of air past the cuff may allow some patients to talk, this is a very brief benefit available only during inspiration. Furthermore, the rush of air into the pharynx is annoying to some patients, and the "leak" may allow for aspiration of infected secretions that have pooled above the cuff during exhalation. The "no leak" technique, sometimes called the "minimal occluding pressure" or "minimal occluding volume" technique, overcomes some of these objections. With this technique, the cuff is inflated just to that point at which the audible flow of air past the cuff during peak inspiration on the mechanical ventilator has ceased. The pressure at that level is measured and followed. Caution must be exercised that an excessive volume of air is not used to prevent the air leak, since the addition of only a few extra milliliters of air may create high cuff pressures, even in soft cuffs. Each of these two methods has specific advantages and disadvantages. Our preference is to use the minimal occluding pressure technique, which usually permits the use of less than 20 mm Hg of cuff pressure.

In our intensive care unit, we use only soft-cuff (high-volume, low-pressure) endotracheal and tracheostomy tubes. In patients who require positive pressure respiration and in those with a risk of pulmonary aspiration, the cuff is kept inflated all the time and the pressure is checked every nursing shift. The value of periodic deflation of soft-cuff tubes to reduce tracheal mucosal injury has not been established. In patients with artificial airways used only to bypass upper airway obstruction or to provide a route for evacuation of tracheobronchial secretions, the cuff may be kept deflated if aspiration is not a problem. Prior to tracheal decannulation, it is commonplace to leave the cuff deflated for short periods. Nevertheless, the patient must always be closely observed for the possibility of pulmonary aspiration. In patients breathing spontaneously, we set the cuff pressure at 20 mm Hg, an arbitrary level below capillary perfusion pressure. We avoid intratracheal tubes with excessively bulky cuff material because these permit a "pistoning" motion of the shaft of the tube inside the cuff and fail to keep the shaft of the tube within the center of the lumen. Redundant cuff material is also more likely to herniate over the tip and to cause pressure grooves in the mucosa.[57]

A few selected problems in cuff management are worthy of mention. First, the cuff pressure should be checked frequently after administration of a general anesthesia because of the possibility of diffusion of nitrous oxide into the cuff, resulting in high pressure.[58] Second, placing a hemostat clamp on the inflating tube of the pilot balloon should be avoided, since this may crimp the tube and prevent function of the inflating system. Third, whenever the cuff is deflated, aspiration of infected secretions which have pooled above the cuff may occur. Some tracheostomy tubes now have a side arm which allows aspiration of these secretions before the cuff is deflated. Whenever a cuff is deflated, the pharynx should be thoroughly suctioned beforehand, and the tracheostomy or endotracheal tube should be suctioned afterward. Finally, rupture of an inflated air-filled cuff is a common problem which may be identified by sudden inadequacy of ventilation, bubbling of frothy secretions in the mouth, ability of the patient to talk suddenly, and discrepancy between the selected tidal volume and the expired tidal volume. If the cuff will not hold air, the intratracheal tube should be replaced.

Nutrition

Nutrition is a vital yet often overlooked aspect of care of the intubated patient. Feeding should be initiated within 24 hours of intubation in order to prevent starvation and complications of negative nitrogen balance such as muscle wasting. There is no valid reason to starve the patient indefinitely while the intratracheal tube is in place. A nasogastric tube is often placed at the time of intubation and is an acceptable route for administration of liquid nourishment. However, because of long-term complications of nasogastric tubes such as otitis, sinusitis, nasal alar pressure necrosis, and increased risk of aspiration, a small pediatric-size feeding tube may be more suitable for long-term use.

We avoid the simultaneous use of nasogastric and nasotracheal tubes because of the risk of pressure necrosis of the thin, delicate nasal septum. Orogastric tubes are usually not well tolerated because of excessive gagging. Patients with orotracheal tubes are usually unable to swallow liquid nourishment, although in an exceptional patient, this is possible. Selected patients with nasotracheal tubes are able to swallow small amounts of liquids, but tube feeding is usually required to deliver adequate nutrition. After tracheotomy, patients are usually not given oral feedings for three or four days because of temporary glottic incompetence. After four days, however, liquid feedings may be initiated and may be quickly advanced to solids. The cuff on the tracheostomy tube should not be inflated with such a large volume that the esophagus is compressed. When prolonged use of an endotracheal or tracheostomy tube is necessary and enteral alimentation is not successful, intravenous hyperalimentation should be initiated.

Additional Aspects of Caring for the Artificial Airway

Personnel caring for patients with artificial airways should be able to respond immediately to airway emergencies, which are common in busy intensive care units. Common problems include self-extubation, accidental dislodgment of the tube, aspiration, rupture of the cuff, and disconnection from the respirator. Whenever an emergency occurs, the patient is taken off the respirator and is ventilated with a self-inflating resuscitation bag connected to oxygen. Patency of the airway is maintained, and a new artificial airway is inserted if necessary.

The artificial airway should be removed as soon as possible, consistent with optimal respiratory care. It is reasonable to suspect that the longer the duration of intubation, the greater the risk of complications. Every day, the physician should question the value of continuing the use of the artificial airway. Although most physicians are aware of the dangers of prolonged endotracheal intubation, there seems to be less enthusiasm for early removal of tracheostomy tubes. Again, the sooner the tracheostomy tube is removed, the lower the risk of complications.

Special Aspects of Endotracheal Tube Care

The patient with an oral or nasal endotracheal tube should be examined carefully every day for possible complications involving the mouth, nose, pharynx, sinuses, and ears. Otitis may result from prolonged use of nasogastric tubes, but it could also result from Eustachian tube obstruction accompanying the use of nasotracheal tubes.[59] Excessive taping of the orotracheal tube at the mouth should be avoided. The tube may be anchored at the lip without obscuring inspection of the oral cavity (Fig. 2-20). The orotracheal tube should be shifted in position every morning, and the tape should be replaced. This facilitates a thorough inspection and requires two personnel (Fig. 2-21).

Extubation requires considerable skill and should not be delegated to the most inexperienced member of the staff. The patient is adequately ventilated, oxygenated, and suctioned before the endotracheal tube is removed. After the cuff is deflated, the suctioning is repeated before the tube is actually removed. Supplemental oxygen is administered during and after extubation. A physician is always immediately available to reintubate the patient if necessary, and an intubation tray is kept nearby. The patient is observed carefully for labored breathing, retractions, and stridor, which may indicate upper airway obstruction due to laryngospasm or laryngeal edema. Inhalation of cool water aerosol after extubation by means of a face tent or mask is advised. Stridor following extubation often responds to parenteral corticosteroids (e.g., dexamethasone, 10 mg IM) and inhalation of a mist of racemic epinephrine.

The endotracheal tube is not changed routinely, but only if complications arise. Indeed, the same oral or nasal endotracheal tube may function perfectly well as long as three weeks according to our ex-

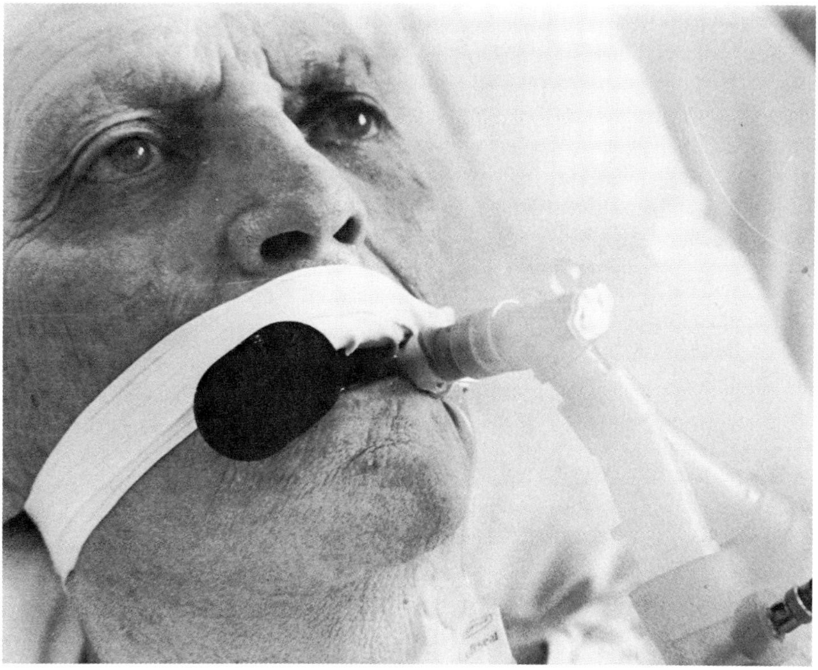

Fig. 2-20. An oral endotracheal tube may be anchored at the corner of the mouth with a minimum amount of adhesive tape so that the mouth is not covered. The oral pharyngeal airway is optional. Excess shaft of the endotracheal tube is trimmed at the corner to reduce leverage and to guarantee proper placement at the midlevel of the trachea. Use of the two-way swivel adaptor is shown.

perience. However, the physician may elect to convert from an oral to a nasal endotracheal tube after several days if long-term endotracheal intubation is indicated.

Special Aspects of Tracheostomy Care

In addition to the general recommendations for management of the artificial airway just mentioned, there are some specific aspects of tracheostomy care that deserve attention. The reader is referred to additional sources which review tracheotomy.[30,60,61] The tracheostomy is a surgical wound which requires aseptic care to combat the ever-present risk of wound infection. Sterile gloves should be used in handling this wound. After tracheotomy is performed, the staff should be alert for continued bleeding at the wound, which may indicate a nonligated wound vessel. A small amount of bleeding from skin vessels for the first three or four days after tracheotomy is considered normal. Tape securing the neck flange of the tracheostomy tube should be tied securely with a square knot. If the tape is tied too tightly, the neck flange will cover and compress the incision, increasing the risk of infection and subcutaneous emphysema. If the

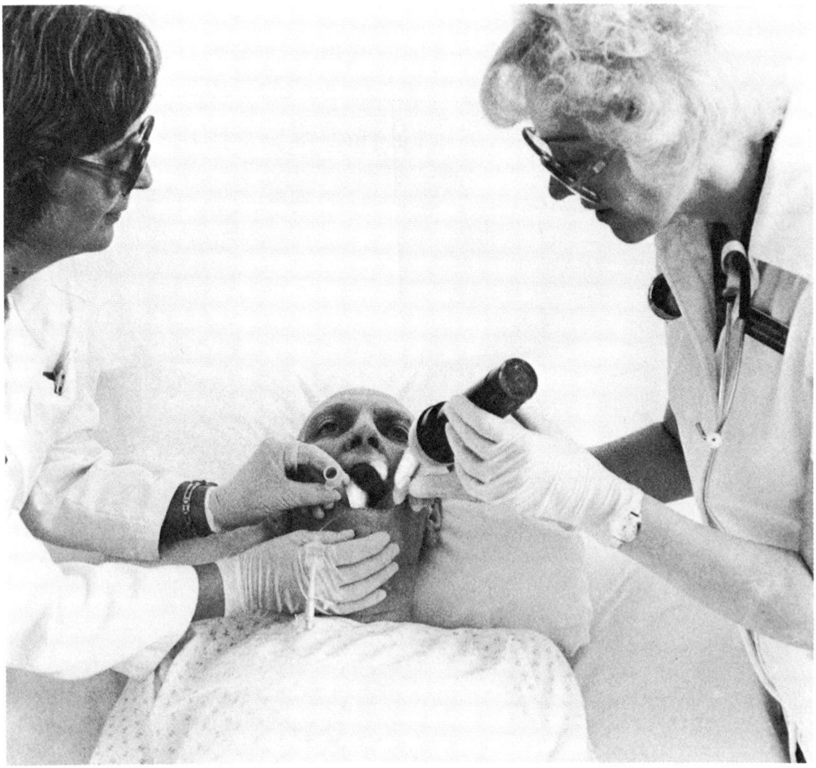

Fig. 2-21. The patient with an oral endotracheal tube is examined carefully every morning by trained respiratory therapists. (Ventilator tubing has been disconnected for the sake of illustration.) After the mouth is examined and oral care is given, the tube is retaped in the opposite corner of the mouth, as in Figure 2-20.

tape is tied too loosely, the tube will move excessively into and out of the stoma.

The tracheostomy tube is changed 48 hours after its placement by the same surgeon who performed the tracheotomy. Some surgeons prefer to use retention sutures to secure the trachea during the initial tube change. Others prefer to have a tracheal hook on hand in case the trachea slips away from view deep into the wound. A sterile catheter is sometimes used to guide the new tracheostomy tube into place the first time. Good lighting, suctioning equipment, and an assistant are important requisites for changing the tracheostomy tube. After one week, a tract develops which eases the placement of new tracheostomy tubes. Our practice is to change the tracheostomy tube every week. This may be performed by two trained respiratory nurses or therapists at the discretion of the surgeon. Whenever a tracheostomy tube is changed, intubation equipment should be immediately available to re-establish the airway. A tracheostomy change tray with all necessary equipment is helpful. If accidental dislodgment of the tracheostomy tube occurs, a physician should be called immediately, and patency of the airway must be reestablished. In an emergency setting, it is often easier to accomplish this with endotracheal intubation than with reinsertion of the tracheostomy tube. When the tracheostomy opening is reidentified, the tracheostomy tube may be reinserted under controlled conditions.

Care of the tracheostomy stoma includes frequent changing of tracheostomy dressings. We use precut Telfa or special gauze pads especially manufactured for this purpose. Cotton pads or gauze pads cut with scissors should not be used, since loose fragments of lint may lodge in the wound. The pads are changed every four hours or more frequently if excessive secretions accumulate. The skin around the stoma and neck is bathed with sterile water or hydrogen peroxide and is dried with sterile sponges. Encrusted secretions on the stoma may be loosened and removed with cotton-tipped applicators soaked in saline or hydrogen peroxide. Some surgeons prefer to use a small amount of antibiotic ointment on the stoma, applied with sterile applicators. When tracheostomy care is given, the wound is examined for infection or bleeding, and the tube is gently palpated for detection of pulsations, which might indicate impingement on the innominate artery. Tracheostomy tubes with an inner cannula should be cleaned every eight hours. The inner cannula is removed and is cleaned with hydrogen peroxide, then is rinsed with sterile water and reinserted.

The measures for tracheostomy care just given also apply to patients with prolonged or permanent need for a tracheostomy tube, such as those with severe brain injury. The tracheostomy tube is changed every week. Inflation of the cuff depends upon whether the patient aspirates and whether mechanical ventilation is needed. Uncuffed tracheostomy tubes may be used in selected patients, or the cuff may be periodically inflated, e.g., for one hour following meals. Permanent tracheotomies are sometimes performed, for example with laryngectomy or the obstructive type of sleep apnea syndrome. An uncuffed, pliable tracheostomy or laryngectomy tube is usually employed to facilitate control of secretions in these patients. These should be cleaned daily. The uncuffed Silastic tube used for patients with the obstructive type of sleep apnea syndrome should be changed every three to four months.

Decannulation or removal of a tracheostomy tube is performed when assisted ventilation is no longer required and when spontaneous ventilation has been proven to be adequate on a "T-tube." The patient must also be able to clear tracheobronchial secretions on his own and to protect his airway from aspiration. To perform decannulation, the physician reassures the patient and explains the procedure. The patient is ventilated and oxygenated, and tracheal and pharyngeal secretions are suctioned. The decannulation procedure then follows the same steps as just outlined for extubation. A moist gauze dressing is placed over the stoma and is kept in place until healing occurs, usually within four to five days. Delayed closure beyond one week may be caused by epithelialization of the stoma, which sometimes follows prolonged use of a tracheostomy tube. This may be treated surgically if it occurs. After decannulation, the patient is followed closely over the next two months for the possibility of tracheal stenosis. A tracheal tomogram is the best method to detect this cómplication.

COMPLICATIONS OF ARTIFICIAL AIRWAYS

Although endotracheal intubation and tracheotomy may save and sustain life, numerous and severe complications may accompany these procedures. The reader is referred to recent reviews on the subject.[9, 30, 31, 60, 62–72] Because most of the reports of complications of artificial airways are anecdotal or based on small series, the exact incidence of various complications is not known. Complications of artificial airways may occur during intubation or tracheotomy, while the artificial airway is in place; during extubation or decannulation; or after the tube has been removed. Although scores of different complications of artificial airways have been reported, some are rarely encountered. Selected complications which we often encounter in our hospitals are listed in Tables 2-10 and 2-11. Common postmortem lesions found in the larynx and trachea following prolonged endotracheal intubation are illustrated in Figure 2-22.

The determinants of injury from artificial airways are usually multiple, and it is often difficult to attribute complications to a single factor. Some of the many possible factors contributing to airway injury are listed in Table 2-12. With the exception of cuff pressure, few of these many possible determinants of airway injury have been studied in detail. Injury at the cuff site is, no doubt, multifactorial, but most of the attention has focused on cuff pressure as the single most important determinant of cuff site injury. Studies in both animals and man have proved beyond doubt that high lateral wall pressure exerted on the tracheal mucosa by high-pressure, low-volume cuffs injures the tracheal mucosa.[33, 55, 73–80] Epithelial injury at the cuff site is unavoidable, and mucosal erosion is possible with both high-pressure and low-pressure cuffs.[57] Cartilaginous necrosis occurs only with sustained or high lateral tracheal wall pressure and is less common with soft cuffs than hard cuffs.

A common injury due to endotracheal intubation is laryngeal ulceration.[59, 81–83] Laryngeal ulcers seen following endotracheal intubation are symmetric mucosal erosions on the posterior aspect of the true vocal cords or arytenoids, often as large as 1.5 cm in diameter. These "pressure sores" have been attributed to the mechanical force exerted by the endotracheal tube on the posterior rim of the glottis,

TABLE 2-10. Selected Complications of Endotracheal Intubation

1. *During Intubation:*
   - Pain, discomfort
   - Dental accidents
   - Soft tissue trauma to nose, mouth, pharynx, larynx
   - Retropharyngeal or hypopharyngeal perforation
   - Esophageal intubation
   - Aspiration
   - Laryngospasm
   - Right mainstem bronchus intubation
   - Cardiac/respiratory arrest
2. *While Endotracheal Tube is in Place:*
   - Pain, discomfort
   - Difficulty with feeding
   - Self-extubation
   - Ulceration of lips, mouth, nose, pharynx
   - Laryngeal injury—ulceration, motor dysfunction
   - Tracheal injury—ulceration, inflammation, tracheomalacia, dilatation
   - Mechanical problems: cuff rupture, inability to seal the airway, tube dislodgment, disconnection from respirator, etc.
3. *During Extubation:*
   - Laryngospasm or laryngeal edema
   - Bronchospasm
   - Aspiration
   - Adverse symptoms—hoarseness, sore throat, dysphagia
4. *After Extubation:*
   - Laryngeal motor dysfunction
   - Tracheal stenosis
   - Tracheal dilatation
   - Laryngeal or tracheal granuloma
   - Persistent adverse symptoms—hoarseness, sore throat, dysphagia

which serves as a fulcrum or pressure point.[82] Recent work indicates that laryngeal ulceration is twice as common with oral intubation as with nasal intubation, presumably because the mouth is less able to anchor an endotracheal tube than the nose.[83]

Tracheal stenosis is a common and dreaded complication of tracheotomy. This may occur at the level of either the stoma, the cuff, or the tube tip. Stoma site stenosis appears to be the most common and has been attributed to fibrous healing of the anterior tracheal wall defect with contracture.[31] Cuff site stenosis has been explained on the basis of fibrosis at the circumferential ring of mucosal ulceration and necrosis.[31] The role of infection in the pathogenesis of tracheal stenosis after either endotracheal intubation or tracheotomy is still unclear.

We recently concluded a prospective study of the complications of endotracheal intubation and tracheotomy in 150 critically ill adult patients in our medical and surgical intensive care units.[59] Sixty-two

TABLE 2-11. Selected Complications of Tracheotomy

1. *During the Operation:*
   - Hemorrhage
   - Subcutaneous emphysema
   - Pneumothorax, pneumomediastinum
   - Tracheostomy placed too low or too high
   - Mediastinitis
   - Placement of tip of tracheostomy tube in pretracheal space
   - Cuff laceration during tube placement
   - Cardiac/respiratory arrest
2. *While Tracheostomy Tube is in Place:*
   - Pain, discomfort
   - Wound infection, ulceration
   - Hemorrhage
   - Tracheal injury—ulceration, inflammation, tracheomalacia, dilatation
   - Aspiration
   - Sepsis
   - Mechanical problems: cuff rupture, inability to seal the airway, tube dislodgment, disconnection from respirator, etc.
   - Self-decannulation
3. *During Decannulation:*
   - Difficult decannulation
   - Patient discomfort
4. After Decannulation:
   - Scar
   - Tracheal stenosis
   - Tracheal dilatation
   - Tracheomalacia
   - Tracheal granuloma
   - Persistent open stoma
   - Persistent adverse symptoms—dysphagia

percent of 226 endotracheal intubations and 66% of 53 tracheotomies had one or more complications. We recorded one cardiorespiratory arrest in the endotracheal intubation group and 2 in the tracheotomy group as a direct result of these procedures. Early complications of endotracheal intubation included the requirement for excessive cuff pressure to seal the airway (19%), self-extubation (13%), inability to seal the airway (11%), right mainstem bronchus intubation (9%), aspiration (8%), and lip ulceration (7%). Difficulty in suctioning tracheobronchial secretions through the endotracheal tube was uncommon. Early complications of tracheotomy included serious stomal infection (36%), more than mild stomal hemorrhage (36%), assorted mechanical problems with the tracheostomy tube (31%), subcutaneous emphysema (9%), and aspiration (8%). The early complications of tracheotomy tended to be more severe than those of endotracheal intubation. Some patients appeared to tolerate endotracheal intubation well for as long as 3 weeks. An unexpected but

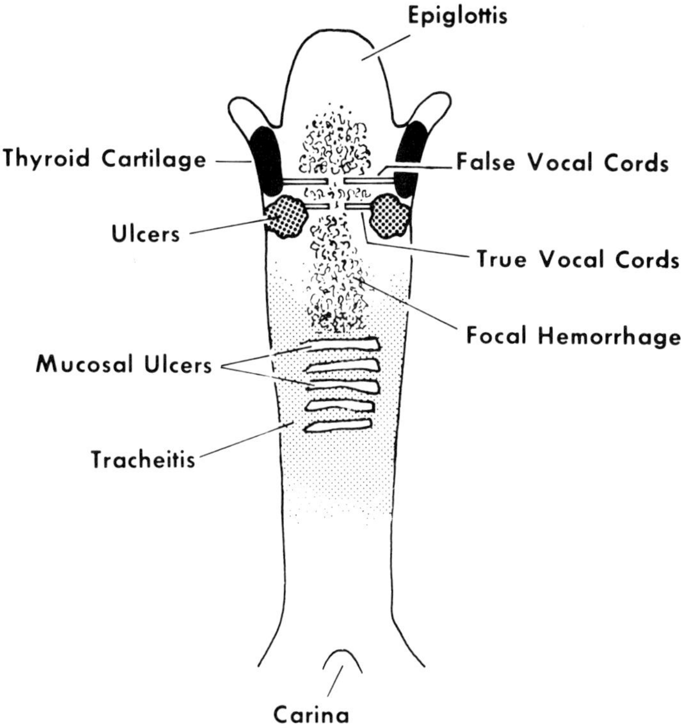

Fig. 2-22. Common laryngotracheal lesions following prolonged cuffed endotracheal intubation include mucosal ulcers on the posterior rim of the glottis, tracheal cuff site mucosal ulcers, tracheitis, and focal mucosal hemorrhage. The larynx and trachea are opened posteriorly to illustrate these lesions.

important observation was the finding of a 9% incidence of otitis in patients with artificial airways, which we related to concurrent prolonged use of nasogastric tubes. In survivors, tracheal stenosis was found in 19% of patients after endotracheal intubation and in 65% of patients after tracheotomy ($p < 0.01$). In nonsurvivors, ulcers on the posterior aspect of the true vocal cords were found in half the patients after endotracheal intubation. Tracheal injury found at autopsy was significantly more common following tracheotomy than following endotracheal intubation. Tracheal mucosal ulceration at the cuff site was the most frequent tracheal lesion. Laryngeal and tracheal granulomas and laryngeal synechiae were rarely seen, and tracheoesophageal fistula was not observed at all in this group of patients with soft-cuff tubes.

Members of a skilled respiratory care team should be able to avoid, recognize, and manage the common complications of artificial airways. A low rate of complications will be encountered if skilled respiratory care is practiced and a few principles are followed. Training, experience, and skill in intubation or performing the tracheot-

TABLE 2-12. Possible Determinants of Complications of Artificial Airways

General

1. Trauma during endotracheal intubation or tracheotomy
2. Duration of use of the artificial airway
3. Route of endotracheal intubation—oral or nasal
4. Pressure exerted on soft tissues
5. Size of tube relative to size of larynx, trachea
6. Motion between tube and patient
7. Compliance of tube at body temperature
8. Chemical irritants
9. Infection
10. Mechanical failure of tube
11. Suboptimal respiratory care

Cuff Site

1. Lateral wall pressure exerted by the cuff
2. Duration of cuff inflation
3. Sealing area
4. Redundancy of cuff material
5. Motion
6. Infection
7. Conformity of cuff to anatomy of trachea
8. Hypotension
9. Use of corticosteroids
10. Chemical irritants

omy are essential. These procedures should be performed in a controlled setting with all necessary equipment assembled beforehand. The bronchoscope should be used to facilitate difficult intubation. Only soft-cuff (high-volume, low-pressure), flexible, disposable endotracheal or tracheostomy tubes should be used in patients with respiratory failure. The guidelines previously outlined for care of artificial airways should be followed, and care should be taken to avoid self-extubation or decannulation. The artificial airway should be removed as soon as possible, and the patient should be followed closely with airway tomograms if necessary to look for late complications such as tracheal stenosis.

REFERENCES

1. Frost, E.A.M.: Tracing the tracheostomy. Ann. Otol. Rhinol. Laryngol., *85:*618, 1976.
2. Macewen, W.: Clinical observations on the introduction of tracheal tubes by the mouth instead of performing tracheotomy or laryngotomy. Br. Med. J., *2:*122, 163, 1880.
3. Heimlich, H.J., and Uhley, M.H.: The Heimlich maneuver. Clin. Symp., *31:*3, 1979.
4. Young, J.A., and Crocker, D.:Principles and Practice of Inhalation Therapy. Chicago, Year Book Medical Publishers, 1970, p. 118.

5. Shapter, R.K., Katz, H.J., Cobb, L.A., Grace, W.J., Nagel, E.L., Schwartz, M.L., Uhley, H.N., and Warren, J.V.: Cardiopulmonary resuscitation: basic life support. Clin. Symp., *26:*4, 1974.
6. National Conference on Cardiopulmonary Resuscitation (CPR) and Emergency Cardiac Care (ECC): Standards for cardiopulmonary resuscitation (CPR) and emergency cardiac care (ECC). JAMA, *244:*453, 1980.
7. Pontoppidan, H., Geffin, B., and Lowenstein E.: Acute respiratory failure in the adult. N. Engl. J. Med., *287:*690, 743, 799, 1972.
8. Lewy, R.B., and Sibbitt, J.W.: Tracheotomy in barbiturate poisoning. Am. Pract. Digest. Treat., *2:*527, 1951.
9. El-Naggar, M., Sadagopan, S., Levine, H., Kantor, H., and Collins, V.J.: Factors influencing choice between tracheostomy and prolonged translaryngeal intubation in acute respiratory failure: a prospective study. Anesth. Analg. (Cleve.), *55:*195, 1976.
10. Stauffer, J.L., and Petty, T.L.: Cleft tongue and ulceration of hard palate: complications of oral intubation. Chest, *74:*317, 1978.
11. Wanner, A., Zighelboim, A., and Sackner, M.A.: Nasopharyngeal airway: A facilitated access to the trachea for nasotracheal suction, bedside bronchofiberscopy, and selective bronchography. Ann. Intern. Med., *75:*593, 1971.
12. Sackner, M.A.: Tracheobronchial toilet. Weekly Update: Pulmonary Medicine. Princeton, NJ, Biomedia, Inc., 1978, pp. 2-7.
13. Kamen, J.M., Wilkinson, C.J., and Boon, J.: A new low-pressure cuff for endotracheal tubes. Anesthesiology, *34:*482, 1971.
14. Leigh, J.M., and Maynard, J.P.: Pressure on the tracheal mucosa from cuffed tubes. Br. Med. J., *1:*1173, 1979.
15. Lewis, F.R., Jr., Schlobohm, R.M., and Thomas, A.N.: Prevention of complications from prolonged tracheal intubation. Am. J. Surg., *135:*452, 1978.
16. McGinnis, G.E., Shively, J.G., Patterson, R.L., and Magovern, G.J.: An engineering analysis of intratracheal tube cuffs. Anesth. Analg. (Cleve.), *50:*557, 1971.
17. Don Michael, T.A., Lambert, E.H., and Mehran, A.: "Mouth-to-lung airway" for cardiac resuscitation. Lancet, *2:*1329, 1968.
18. Schofferman, J., Oill, P., and Lewis, A.J.: The esophageal obturator airway: a clinical evaluation. Chest, *69:*67, 1976.
19. Jacobs, H.B.: Needle catheter brings oxygen to the trachea. JAMA, *222:*1231, 1972.
20. Klain, M., and Smith, R.B.: High frequency percutaneous transtracheal jet ventilation. Crit. Care Med., *5:*280, 1977.
21. Rock, J.J., Pfaeffle, H., Smith, R.B., Mendelow, H., and Klain, M.: High pressure jet insufflation used to prevent aspiration and its effect on the tracheal mucosal wall. Crit. Care Med., *4:*135, 1976.
22. Smith, R.B., Schaer, W.B., and Pfaeffle, H.: Percutaneous transtracheal ventilation for anesthesia and resuscitation: a review and report of complications. Can. Anaesth. Soc. J., *22:*607, 1975.
23. Taryle, D.A., Chandler, J.E., Good, J.T., Jr., Potts, D.E., and Sahn, S.A.: Emergency room intubations—complications and survival. Chest, *75:*541, 1979.
24. Hawkins, D.B., Seltzer, D.C., Barnett, T.E., and Stoneman, G.B.: Endotracheal tube perforation of the hypopharynx. West. J. Med., *120:*282, 1974.
25. Stauffer, J.L., and Petty, T.L.: Accidental intubation of the pyriform sinus: a complication of "roadside" resuscitation. JAMA, *237:*2324, 1977.
26. Goodman, L.R., Conrardy, P.A., Laing, F., and Singer, M.M.: Radiographic evaluation of endotracheal tube position. Am. J. Roentgenol., *127:*433, 1976.
27. Whitehouse, A.C., and Klock, L.E.: Evaluation of endotracheal tube position with the fiberoptic intubation laryngoscope. Chest, *68:*848, 1975.
28. Salem, M.R., Mathrubhutham, M., and Bennett, E.J.: Difficult intubation. N. Engl. J. Med., *295:*879, 1976.
29. Brantigan, C.O., and Grow, J.B., Sr.:Cricothyroidotomy: elective use in respiratory problems requiring tracheotomy. J. Thorac. Cardiovasc. Surg., *71:*72, 1976.
30. Selecky, P.A.: Tracheostomy: a review of present day indications, complications, and care. Heart Lung, *3:*272, 1974.
31. Andrews, M.J., and Pearson, F.G.: Incidence and pathogenesis of tracheal injury following cuffed tube tracheostomy with assisted ventilation: analysis of a two-year prospective study. Ann. Surg., *173:*249, 1971.

32. Wanner, A.: Clinical aspects of mucociliary transport. Am. Rev. Respir. Dis., *116:*73, 1977.
33. Klainer, A.S., Turndorf, H., Wu, W.-H., Maewal, H., and Allender, P.: Surface alterations due to endotracheal intubation. Am. J. Med., *58:*674, 1975.
34. Paegle, R.D., Ayres, S.M., and Davis, S.: Rapid tracheal injury by cuffed airways and healing with loss of ciliated epithelium. Arch. Surg., *106:*31, 1973.
35. Sackner, M.A., Hirsch, J., and Epstein, S.: Effect of cuffed endotracheal tubes on tracheal mucous velocity. Chest, *68:*774, 1975.
36. Palmer, K.N.: Reduction of sputum viscosity by a water aerosol in chronic bronchitis. Lancet, *1:*91, 1960.
37. Yaeger, H.: Tracheobronchial secretions. Am. J. Med., *50:*501, 1971.
38. Jung, R.C., and Gottlieb, L.S.: Comparison of tracheobronchial suction catheters in humans: visualization by fiberoptic bronchoscopy. Chest, *69:*179, 1976.
39. Emergency Care Research Institute: Suction catheters. Health Devices, *6:*132, 1977.
40. Sackner, M.A., Landa, J.F., Greeneltch, N., and Robinson, M.J.: Pathogenesis and prevention of tracheobronchial damage with suction catheters. Chest, *64:*284, 1973.
41. Kirimli, B., King, J.E., and Pfaeffle, H.H.: Evaluation of tracheobronchial suction techniques. J. Thorac. Cardiovasc. Surg., *59:*340, 1970.
42. Boutros, A.R.: Arterial blood oxygenation during and after endotracheal suctioning in the apneic patient. Anesthesiology, *32:*114, 1970.
43. Naigow, D., and Powaser, M.M.: The effect of different endotracheal suction procedures on arterial blood gases in a controlled experimental model. Heart Lung, *6:*808, 1977.
44. Shim, C., Fine, N., Fernandez, R., and Williams, M.H.: Cardiac arrhythmias resulting from tracheal suctioning. Ann. Intern. Med., *71:*1149, 1969.
45. Marini, J.J., Pierson, D.J., and Hudson, L.D.: Acute lobar atelectasis: a prospective comparison of fiberoptic bronchoscopy and respiratory therapy. Am. Rev. Respir. Dis., *119:*971, 1979.
46. Amikam, B., Landa, J., West, J., and Sackner, M.A.: Bronchofiberscopic observations of the tracheobronchial tree during intubation. Am. Rev. Respir. Dis., *105:*747, 1972.
47. Johanson, W.G., Pierce, A.K., Sanford, J.P., and Thomas, G.D.: Nosocomial respiratory infections with gram-negative bacilli: the significance of colonization of the respiratory tract. Ann. Intern. Med., *77:*701, 1972.
48. Valenti, W.M., Trudell, R.G., and Bentley, D.W.: Factors predisposing to oropharyngeal colonization with gram-negative bacilli in the aged. N. Engl. J. Med., *298:*1108, 1978.
49. Bartlett, J.G., Faling, L.J., and Willey, S.: Quantitative tracheal bacteriologic and cytologic studies in patients with long-term tracheostomies. Chest, *74:*635, 1978.
50. Cameron, J.L., and Zuidema, G.D.: Aspiration pneumonia: magnitude and frequency of the problem. JAMA, *219:*1194, 1972.
51. Cameron, J.L., Reynolds, J., and Zuidema, G.D.: Aspiration in patients with tracheostomies. Surg. Gynecol. Obstet., *136:*68, 1973.
52. Spray, S.B., Zuidema, G.D., and Cameron, J.L.: Aspiration pneumonia: incidence of aspiration with endotracheal tubes. Am. J. Surg., *131:*701, 1976.
53. Bone, D.K., Davis, J.L., Zuidema, G.D., and Cameron, J.L.: Aspiration pneumonia: prevention of aspiration in patients with tracheostomies. Ann. Thorac. Surg., *18:*30, 1974.
54. Wynne, J.W., and Model, J.H.: Respiratory aspiration of stomach contents. Ann. Intern. Med., *87:*466, 1977.
55. Knowlson, G.T.G., and Bassett, H.F.M.: The pressures exerted on the trachea by endotracheal inflatable cuffs. Br. J. Anaesth., *42:*834, 1970.
56. Cox, P.M., and Schatz, M.E.: Pressure measurements in endotracheal cuffs: a common error. Chest, *65:*84, 1974.
57. Loeser, E.A., Hodges, M., Gliedman, J., Stanley, T.H., Johansen, R.K., and Yonetani, D.: Tracheal pathology following short-term intubation with low- and high-pressure endotracheal tube cuffs. Anesth. Analg. (Cleve.), *57:*577, 1978.
58. Stanley, T.H.: Nitrous oxide and pressures and volumes of high- and low-pressure endotracheal-tube cuffs in intubated patients. Anesthesiology, *42:*637, 1975.

59. Stauffer, J.L., Olson, D.E., and Petty, T.L.: Complications and consequences of endotracheal intubation and tracheotomy: a prospective study of 150 critically ill adult patients. Am. J. Med., *70:*65, 1981.
60. Timmis, H.H.: Tracheostomy: an overview of implications, management and morbidity. Adv. Surg., *7:*199, 1973.
61. Tracheostomy Care Handbook. Wilmington, MA, Portex Division, Smith Industries, Inc., 1976.
62. Blanc, V.F., and Tremblay, N.A.G.: The complications of tracheal intubation: a new classification with a review of the literature. Anesth. Analg., *53:*202, 1974.
63. Deane, R.S., and Mills, E.L.: Prolonged nasotracheal intubation in adults: a successor and adjunct to tracheostomy. Anesth. Analg., *49:*89, 1970.
64. Lindholm, C.-E.: Prolonged endotracheal intubation. Acta Anaesthiol. Scand. [Suppl.], *33:*1, 1969.
65. Tonkin, J.P., and Harrison, G.A.: The effect on the larynx of prolonged endotracheal intubation. Med. J. Aust., *2:*581, 1966.
66. Sellery, G.R., Worth, A., and Greenway, R.E.: Late complications of prolonged tracheal intubation. Can. Anaesth. Soc. J., *25:*140, 1978.
67. Dane, T.E.B., and King, E.G.: A prospective study of complications after tracheostomy for assisted ventilation. Chest, *67:*398, 1975.
68. Meade, J.W.: Tracheotomy—its complications and their management: a study of 212 cases. N. Engl. J. Med., *265:*519, 1961.
69. Stemmer, E.A., Oliver, C., Carey, J.P., and Connolly, J.E.: Fatal complications of tracheotomy. Am. J. Surg., *131:*288, 1976.
70. McClelland, R.M.A.: Complications of tracheostomy. Br. Med. J., *2:*567, 1965.
71. McGovern, F.H., Fitz-Hugh, G.S., and Edgemon, L.J.: The hazards of endotracheal intubation. Ann. Otol., *80:*556, 1971.
72. Davidson, I.A., Cruickshank, A.N., Duthie, W.H., Bargh, W., and Duncan, J.G.: Lesions of the trachea following tracheostomy and endotracheal intubation. Proc. R. Soc. Med., *64:*886, 1971.
73. Cooper, J.D., and Grillo, H.C.: The evolution of tracheal injury due to ventilatory assistance through cuffed tubes: a pathologic study. Ann. Surg., *169:*334, 1969.
74. Dunn, C.R., Dunn, D.L., and Moser, K.M.: Determinants of tracheal injury by cuffed tracheostomy tubes. Chest, *65:*128, 1974.
75. Grillo, H.C., Cooper, J.D., Geffin, B., and Pontoppidan, H.: A low-pressure cuff for tracheostomy tubes to minimize tracheal injury: a comparative clinical trial. J. Thorac. Cardiovasc. Surg., *62:*898, 1971.
76. Cooper, J.D., and Grillo, H.C.: Experimental production and prevention of injury due to cuffed tracheal tubes. Surg. Gynecol. Obstet., *129:*1235, 1969.
77. Shelly, W.M., Dawson, R.B., and May, I.A.: Cuffed tubes as a cause of tracheal stenosis. J. Thorac. Cardiovasc. Surg., *57:*623, 1969.
78. Mathias, D.B., and Wedley, J.R., Jr.: The effects of cuffed endotracheal tubes on the tracheal wall. Br. J. Anaesth., *46:*849, 1974.
79. Ching, N.P., Ayres, S.M., Paegle, R.P., Linden, J.M., and Nealon, T.F.: The contribution of cuff volume and pressure in tracheostomy tube damage. J. Thorac. Cardiovasc. Surg., *62:*402, 1971.
80. Dobrin, P., and Canfield, T.: Cuffed endotracheal tubes: mucosal pressures and tracheal wall blood flow. Am. J. Surg., *133:*562, 1977.
81. Burns, H.P., Dayal, V.S., Scott, A., Van Nostrand, A.W.P., and Bryce, D.P.: Laryngotracheal trauma: observations on its pathogenesis and its prevention following prolonged orotracheal intubation in the adult. Laryngoscope, *89:*1316, 1979.
82. Bergström, J., Moberg, A., and Orell, S.R.: On the pathogenesis of laryngeal injuries following prolonged intubation. Acta Otolaryngol. (Stockholm), *55:*342, 1962.
83. Dubick, M.N., and Wright, B.D: Comparison of laryngeal pathology following long-term oral and nasal endotracheal intubations. Anesth. Analg. (Cleve.), *57:*663, 1978.

Chapter 3

CLINICAL APPLICATIONS OF OXYGEN

By Thomas L. Petty

Oxygen is a fundamental drug in the management of patients with acute respiratory failure. Aerobic metabolism demands adequate tissue transport to provide a small O_2 tension at the tissue level, perhaps as low as 0.1 to 1 mm Hg for sustained aerobic, high-energy metabolism (see Fig. 1-5).[1] This requires an arterial P_{O_2} of at least 25 mm (saturation 40%), assuming normal hemoglobin content and cardiac output.[2] In most clinical situations with impaired circulation, anemia, or increased metabolic demands, higher oxygen saturations and tensions are required to support life.

By definition, hypoxemia is present in all states of acute respiratory failure (see Chap. 1). Mild degrees of hypoxemia do not necessarily indicate that tissue hypoxia is also present.[3] The adverse effects of hypoxemia on the circulatory and central nervous systems, and, indeed, on all cellular functions, demand correction far before the oxygen tension drops to 25 mm Hg; most would agree that adequate arterial oxygen tension must be greater than 50 mm Hg or an oxygen saturation of greater than 80% when circulation is adequate.[2,3] In states of circulatory collapse, higher arterial oxygen tensions are required.[1]

In poisonings, in paralytic states, and in respiratory depression in the postoperative period, the problem of hypoxemia is primarily one of hypoventilation and impaired ventilation-to-perfusion ratios. In these situations, support of ventilation corrects the hypoxemia (see Chap. 4). In chronic airflow obstruction (CAO-emphysema and chronic bronchitis), hypoxemia rarely results solely from hypoventilation.[4] The major reason for hypoxemia with chronic airflow obstruction is altered ventilation–perfusion (V/Q) matching (see Appendices A and B) superimposed upon some degree of underventilation and, often, abnormal reduced respiratory drives.

The rational use of oxygen in acute respiratory failure demands an understanding of tissue oxygen transport, which is a function of cardiac output and oxygen content. The proper use of oxygen in clinical medicine demands precision of administration and careful monitoring so that tissue oxygen transport is adequately maintained without harmful effects from imprecise and excessive use. The purpose of this chapter is to discuss practical means of oxygen administration in various common clinical situations.

OXYGEN ADMINISTRATION IN CHRONIC AIRFLOW OBSTRUCTION

Remaining controversies exist concerning the use of oxygen in patients with CAO in acute respiratory failure. The risk of carbon dioxide narcosis has been called to the attention of physicians for many years.[5–7] The development of precision in oxygen administration, however, has reduced the problem of CO_2 retention.[8–10] Also, the efficacy and safety of continuous oxygen therapy in acute respiratory failure in CAO are now established.

Oxygen can be administered by a variety of means to enrich the inspired air. A critical study of various means has been made by Kory, who found that adequate inspired concentrations of oxygen can be achieved by either the nasal cannula or catheter, and that suitable oxygen concentrations in the tracheal air can be maintained by either nose or mouth breathing.[11]

In acute respiratory failure in CAO, oxygen, when administered by controlled low flow utilizing nasal cannulae, has been highly effective in correcting hypoxemia without dangerous carbon dioxide retention.[10–12] Oxygen has also been effectively administered by means of the so-called Venturi mask discussed later.[2,13] Oxygen has thus become the basis of conservative treatment of acute respiratory failure in chronic obstructive lung disease.[14]

The oxygen delivery devices in most common use are the two-pronged nasal cannula and the nasal catheter (Fig. 3-1). Also, various masks have clinical application. Figure 3-2 shows a reservoir mask capable of delivering oxygen concentrations as high as 50 to 60%.

A single nasal prong with a retention rosette is as effective as the double nasal prongs in patients with chronic airflow obstruction (Fig. 3-3).[15] Table 3-1 compares the blood gas data for 10 random

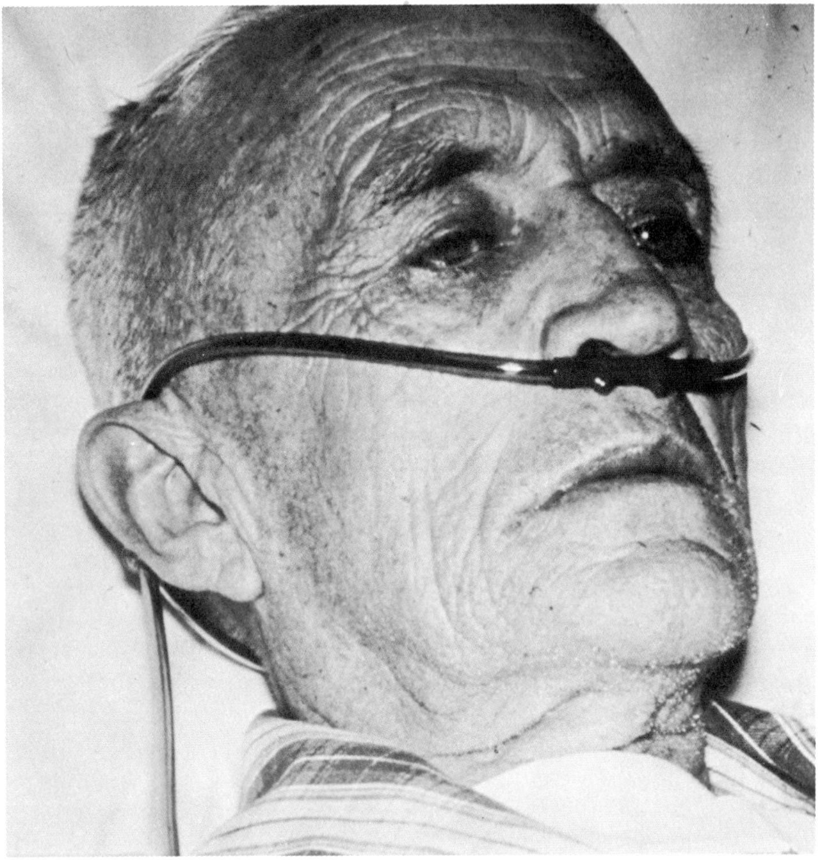

Fig. 3-1. The most common means of controlled low-flow oxygen administration via double nasal cannula. The advantages include comfort and ability to talk and eat. (From Rocky Mountain Med. J., *64*:66, 1967.)

patients hospitalized with various degrees of chronic airflow obstruction at various liter flows (range: 1 to 4 L/min) with double and single nasal prongs. Comparison data in 7 additional patients at both 1 and 3 L are presented in Table 3–2.

Much interest has been devoted to the Venturi mask because it is a means of controlling the inspired oxygen concentration accurately in spite of variable flows at the oxygen source (Fig. 3-4). This device will give fixed oxygen concentrations of 24%, 28%, or 35% or more as a fixed oxygen-to-air ratio and is controlled by the geometry of the Venturi apparatus.[13,16,17] The disadvantages of this device are that it is uncomfortable, it is unnecessarily expensive, and it must be removed during eating, a requirement which can be potentially disastrous in patients with profound hypoxemia. The cessation of oxygen administration even for a short period in severe airflow obstruction often causes the arterial oxygen tension to fall lower than it was

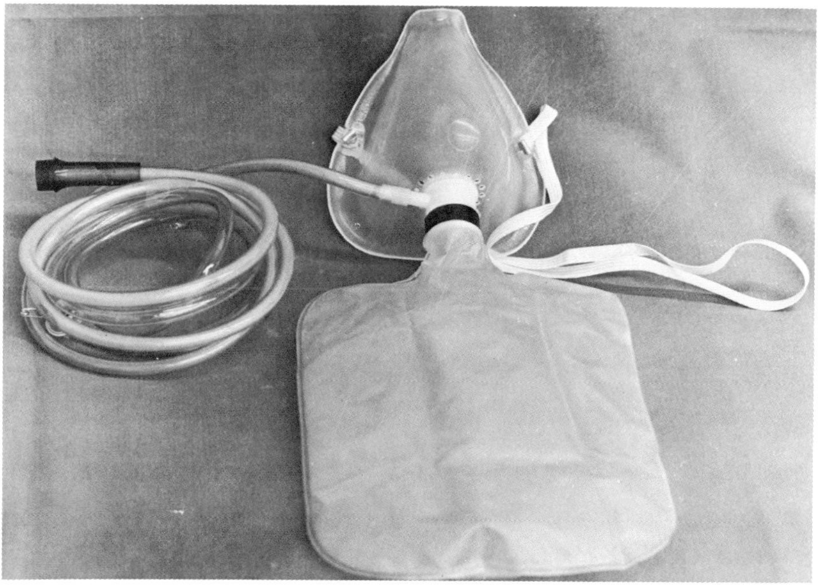

Fig. 3-2. Reservoir mask for higher oxygen fractions is achievable with use of double nasal cannulae. Masks and cannulae can be used together.

before the oxygen was given. If carbon dioxide retention occurs, the elevated CO_2 level further reduces alveolar oxygen tension when oxygen is discontinued. Profound hypoxemia and hypercapnia are potent respiratory stimulants, and the attempt at increased ventilation which results may increase oxygen consumption and carbon dioxide production, which further aggravate the situation in patients with severe CAO (see Chap. 10).

TABLE 3-1. Comparisons of Double vs Single Nasal Prongs (Group 1:10 Patients with CAO)

Patient	Double		Single	
	PO_2	PCO_2	PO_2	PCO_2
1	51	55	48	51
2	70	58	68	56
3	43	47	46	45
4	69	33	82	29
5	84	34	87	34
6	53	64	61	63
7	57	39	60	37
8	132	33	135	33
9	84	49	82	46
10	76	51	65	48

(Reproduced by permission from Chest, 64:146, 1973.)

TABLE 3-2. Comparisons of Double vs Single Nasal Prongs at 1 and 3 Liters/Minute Flow (Group 2:7 Patients with Severe CAO)

	Control		*1 L Double*		*1 L Single*		*3 L Double*		*1 L Single*	
Patient	PO_2	PCO_2	PO_2	PCO_2	PO_2	PCO_2	PO_2	PCO_2	PO_2	PCO_2
1	46	36	—	—	56	38	66	37	65	37
2	46	55	—	—	57	54	96	63	112	62
3	45	50	—	—	74	53	78	52	83	57
4	58	32	61	34	60	34	70	36	69	96
5	55	38	63	35	62	36	73	33	73	34
6	39	49	46	52	46	52	56	50	55	50
7	54	40	56	41	56	39	61	42	63	40

(Reproduced by permission from Chest 64:147, 1973.)

In addition, whereas the Venturi apparatus does provide for accurate control of the inspired oxygen fraction, the device does not guarantee sufficient arterial oxygen tension because the degree of lung disease and variable ventilatory response affect oxygen transport in the lung.[17] Moreover, in states of hypoventilation, it may not provide adequate oxygenation.[2]

Face masks with precise flow control are also effective, but their use must be accompanied by monitoring of arterial blood gas.[10,11,14] The nasal catheter is also an effective means of delivering oxygen, but it is uncomfortable.[10,11,14] Reservoir face masks (see Fig. 3-2) are of value when high oxygen fractions are needed, such as in shock states or severe interstitial disease with marked diffusion impair-

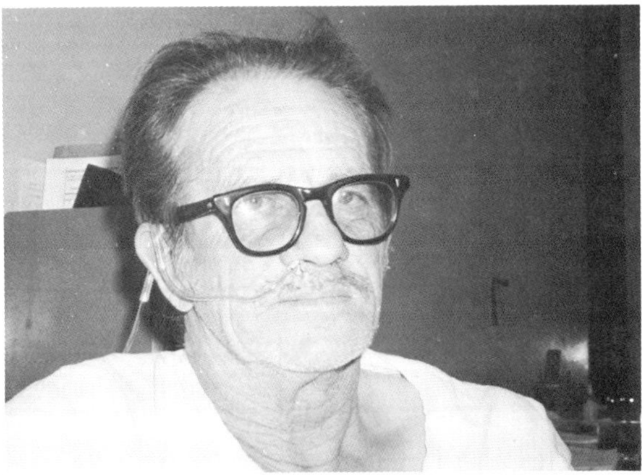

Fig. 3-3. Single nasal prong for oxygen administration. This is maintained in the nostril by a retention rosette. It is fitted to the ear with a valuable internal wire, or it can be fixed directly to the glasses frame. (Reproduced by permission from Petty, T.L., Nett, L.M., and Lakshminarayan, F.: A single nasal prong for continuous oxygen therapy. Chest, *64:*146, 1973.)

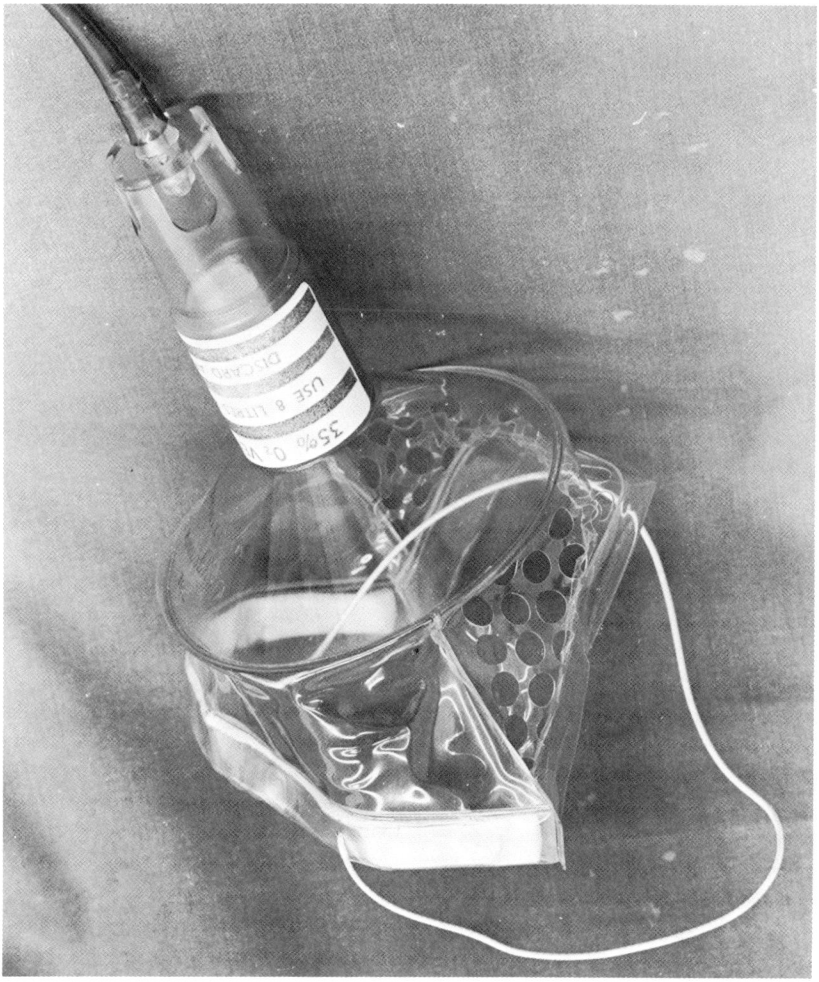

Fig. 3-4 Venturi mask employing high airflow oxygen-enrichment principles; flow at 6 L enters the Venturi tube. Entrainment of the atmospheric air controls oxygen fraction to 35% in this device. Other masks provide 24%, 28%, and 40% oxygen. Similar devices have a more continuous range of oxygen fraction.

ment (see Chap. 1). The exact concentration of oxygen achieved in the tracheal air via use of cannulae, masks, and face tents has been reported in normal volunteers.[18,19] The conclusions reached cannot necessarily be applied to the diverse clinical situations in which oxygen is required, however. In any case, all oxygen administration must be appropriately guided by arterial blood gas analysis (see Chap. 1). In long-term clinical practice, almost all patients with CAO can be well oxygenated via nasal prongs whether or not the patient's mouth is open. The nasopharynx is readily enriched by the nasal entraining mechanism, and, of course, the final tracheal oxygen con-

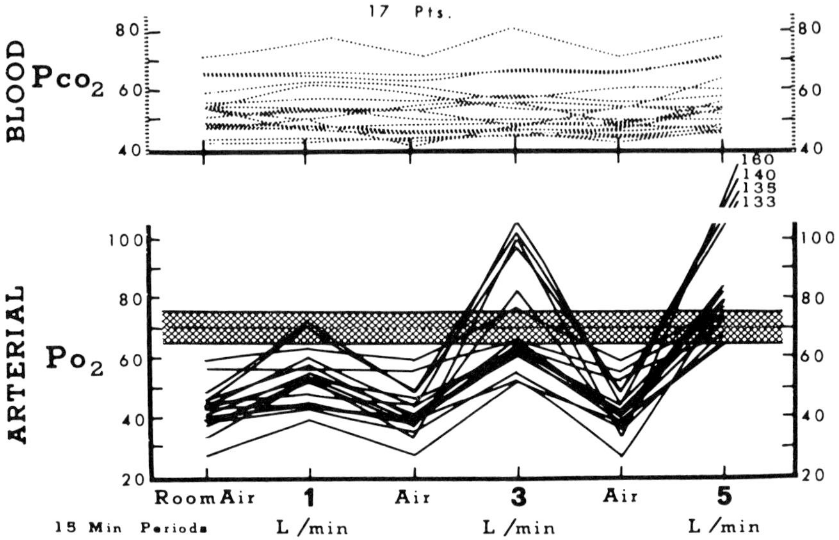

Fig. 3-5 Blood gas response to oxygen at 1, 3, and 5 L as compared with air breathing; 17 patients with CAO and acute respiratory failure had no other therapy during these steady states. Note wide range of blood gas values in response to oxygen breathing and lack of CO_2 elevation at 1 and 3 L, except in the patient with the lowest oxygen and highest carbon dioxide tension. Some CO_2 elevation is seen at 5 L, which is excessive oxygen flow for most. Cross-hatched area indicates normal oxygen tension for Denver—65 to 75 mm. (Reproduced with permission from Am. Rev. Resp. Dis., *96:*28, 1967.)

centration (fraction) will be a function of oxygen liter flow, minute ventilation, and the pattern of breathing.

Experience in our unit has repeatedly shown that a simple and comfortable device for delivery of oxygen is the two-pronged nasal cannula (see Fig. 3-1). It allows the patient to talk, cough, eat, and perform all necessary activities without interruption of oxygen flow. Use of this cannula has proved to be effective in providing adequate arterial oxygenation in patients with CAO studied over a 15-year period. The single prong, recently developed,* is equally comfortable. It may be particularly valuable in long-term home therapy, and it can be alternated from one nostril to the other.

Oxygen given into the nose is humidified by the normal nasal mechanism; it is doubtful that bubbling devices at the oxygen source, which are so popular, really add significant moisture to the oxygen.

The observations that originally established the effectiveness and safety of controlled low-flow oxygen at our center administered via double nasal prongs are illustrated in Figure 3-5. In brief, 17 patients

* Canulette.

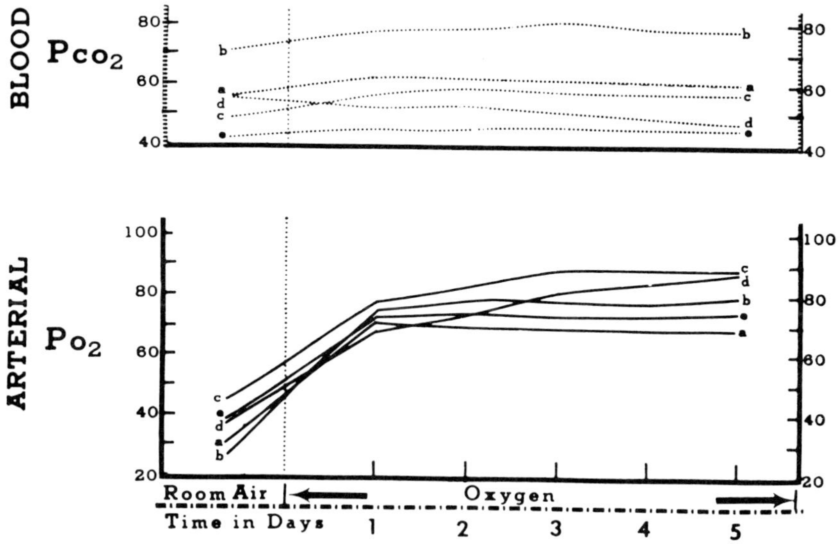

Fig. 3-6. Daily blood gas determinations and steady-state conditions for 5 of the 17 patients from Figure 3-5. Progressive carbon dioxide retention does not occur. (Reproduced with permission from Am. Rev. Resp. Dis., *96*:28, 1967.)

with acute respiratory failure associated with CAO were the subjects of this study.[20] Following placement of an intra-arterial cannula, these patients were allowed to breathe room air alternating with oxygen by graded flows for 15-minute steady-state periods. Blood gases were monitored throughout the study. Figure 3-6 reveals that 1-L flow improved the arterial oxygenation in all patients and in many was sufficient to elevate the oxygen tension to an acceptable level of approximately 50 mm Hg. The normal arterial P_{O_2} for Denver is indicated by the cross-hatched area (65 to 75 mm Hg). Three-liter flow provided adequate arterial oxygenation for all patients but excessive tension in some. Five liters elevated oxygen tensions in all patients at least to the normal range, but this flow produced excessive oxygen tensions in approximately 50% of the patients. During 1- and 3-L oxygen administration, carbon dioxide retention did not occur except in one patient who experienced modest elevations. This patient had the lowest initial oxygen tension and the highest carbon dioxide tension. Five-liter nasal oxygen flow did produce modest degrees of carbon dioxide retention in some patients, suggesting a threshold for oxygen-induced hypoventilation. We have further determined that after acute exposure, the continued use of precisely controlled oxygen caused no further CO_2 tension increase in patients for periods ranging up to 5 days (Fig. 3-6). Blood gas determinations were monitored in 5 patients for 5 days with no major change in their blood gas patterns. We do not wish to imply that carbon dioxide retention never occurs with continuous oxygen therapy. This has occasionally occurred in our institution as a result of *uncontrolled* oxygen therapy or sedation as well as in states of profound acute exacerbations of bronchitis leading to further ventilatory failure.

It should be stressed that the degree of hypoxemia in CAO and acute respiratory failure is quite variable and unpredictable and requires frequent laboratory analysis (Fig. 3–6).[9,10,12,20,21] It is rare for patients with even severe CAO to require more than 4 L/min to correct hypoxemia. Most patients are satisfactorily oxygenated with 1 to 3 L/min nasal flow.

Some patients with severe chronic airflow obstruction with hypoxemia require low oxygen flows for correction of the oxygen deficiency.[22] Flows as low as 0.25 to 0.5 L/min may be the desired amount. These patients have a low minute ventilation but little shunt-like effect or diffusion defect, and therefore small amounts of oxygen added to the small minute ventilation have a great effect on arterial oxygenation. A flowmeter* with 0.25 L/min accuracy has been developed for this purpose.[22]

OXYGEN IN OTHER PULMONARY DISEASES

Oxygen supplied by nasal cannula is also useful in the management of bronchial asthma (see Chap. 9). Often, higher flows than are commonly employed in CAO are required. Thus, 4 to 6 L or even more may be required, owing in part to severe ventilation–perfusion mismatching due to focal airflow abnormalities in asthma. Much higher flows per minute are also unlikely to improve oxygenation in asthma.

When severe oxygen transport problems occur, such as in overwhelming pneumonias (see Chap. 12), and in states of pulmonary edema including the early stages of adult respiratory distress syndrome (see Chap. 8), a higher oxygen concentration (fraction) may be required. Here is where oxygen masks are most useful, in addition to nasal cannulae or alone. Simple masks may also be sufficient or masks and nasal prongs can be used together (see Fig. 3-2).

Whenever tissue oxygen delivery is impaired owing to abnormal circulatory states, the highest possible oxygen concentrations are desired to help minimize tissue hypoxia. In these states, high-flow oxygen is used with no attempt to control exclusively the arterial oxygen tension. These high oxygen flows are used until circulation is restored. Thereafter, precise administration is again guided by blood gas analysis as necessary.

In general, sedatives should not be administered during oxygen therapy, and the patient's chart should be tagged to contraindicate sedation. Sedation will only cause CO_2 retention whenever this is a potential problem. When proper oxygen therapy principles are fol-

* Bethlehem Company, Bethlehem, PA.

lowed, oxygen has been effective in the so-called conservative management of a large number of patients with a variety of acute and chronic respiratory diseases, resulting in the control of hypoxemia without resorting to mechanical ventilation.

OXYGEN FOLLOWING SURGERY

It is well known that unpredictable hypoxemia may occur both during anesthesia and following surgery.[23,24] Monitoring for hypoxemia during anesthesia is beyond the context of this discussion but would be appropriate in borderline patients such as those with respiratory insufficiency. This can be done by means of intermittent blood gas analysis, ear oximetry in selected cases, or transcutaneous oxygen monitoring. Following surgical procedures, however, it is well known that significant hypoxemia is commonly present, probably owing to a combination of immobility, the reclining position, the effects of anesthetic agents, pooled secretions, and depressed respiratory drives as well as pain, which inhibits ventilatory responses in awake patients. It would be wise to perform arterial blood gas analysis in any patient at risk, and it would be prudent to give oxygen routinely in the postoperative period even in the absence of oxygen monitoring. Low-flow oxygen via nasal cannula would be satisfactory in most cases. Masks, including the Venturi device, would be acceptable alternatives but offer no advantages and great disadvantages compared with double nasal prongs or simple masks.

OXYGEN BY VENTILATOR

In paralyzed and postoperative patients, adequate arterial oxygenation will most likely be provided by ventilatory assistance with the ventilator functioning with room air (see Chap. 4). Patients with underlying pulmonary diseases will probably require an increased oxygen fraction. The details of oxygenation via a definitive airway (see Chap. 2) interfaced to a mechanical ventilator (closed system) are considered in detail in Chapter 4. Certain facts relevant to oxygenation are also considered in this chapter for the convenience of the reader. It should be stressed that when pressure-cycled ventilators (Bird and Bennett) are powered by an oxygen source, markedly elevated oxygen concentrations (60 to 80%) are often delivered in spite of a maximum air mix.[25] This subject is discussed in detail in Chapter 4. As in all forms of ventilatory support, the adequacy of arterial oxygenation and carbon dioxide elimination should be monitored with blood gas determinations. Patients should not receive prolonged oxygen concentrations higher than approximately 33% (inspired PO_2 of 235 at sea level) if possible; this may be the maximum tolerable inspired oxygen tension in normal man.[26] The inspired oxygen concentration from positive pressure respirators using oxygen should always be monitored frequently (see Chap. 4). Air-mix devices have recently become available to control oxygen concentrations.* Modern ventilators provide the means for effective control of the inspired oxygen fraction and tension.

LONG-TERM OUTPATIENT OXYGEN THERAPY IN ADVANCED CHRONIC OBSTRUCTIVE PULMONARY DISEASE

The use of long-term ambulatory oxygen therapy has been studied by many investigators, including the author and his associates, who recently summarized 13 years' experience in patients with advanced chronic obstructive pulmonary disease (COPD).[27] In these earlier studies, most patients were given oxygen because of severe hypoxemia, cor pulmonale, right heart failure, and associated exercise limitation. Hemodynamic benefit in terms of reduced pulmonary artery pressures and arteriolar resistance and reduction of an elevated red cell mass was found in some but not all patients in our original studies.[28] Our results have been confirmed by other investigators, and today, the overall clinical benefit of oxygen administration in selected patients with advanced COPD and demonstrable hypoxemia is no longer questioned.[29] Substantial neuropsychiatric benefit, reduced needs for hospitalization, and a return to gainful employment in a limited number of selected patients are additional major benefits of oxygen provided at home by both stationary and portable sources. The negative side of oxygen therapy, however, focuses on the substantial costs, often averaging $300 per month or more, and the question of possible tissue oxygen toxicity. There are cellular and fibrotic changes found in long-term COPD patients receiving oxygen that are not found in patients with similar degrees of illness who did not receive oxygen.[30] Thus, cost, inconvenience, and possible tissue oxygen toxicity must be considerations in continuous long-term oxygen therapy.

Studies from other centers have strongly suggested that less than 24 hours per day of oxygen may provide similar benefit, particularly from a hemodynamic standpoint.[31,32] If substantially less than 24-hour-per-day oxygen would provide not only physiologic benefit, but also improvement in neuropsychiatric function and quality of life, reduced hospitalization time, and overall improvement in functional capability, this would certainly be an advantage from the standpoint of logistics and cost. For this reason (following the NHLBI- and ATS/ACCP-sponsored Sugarloaf Conference to evaluate the scientific basis for respiratory therapy, focusing on the chronic stable outpatient with advanced COPD), studies were designed to evaluate the hypothesis that 12-hour oxygen might be equally as effective as and less toxic than 24-hour-per-day oxygen in patients with advanced COPD.[33]

* Veriflow Corporation, Richmond CA, and others.

Following a request for proposal, 6 centers were granted contracts (Chicago, Denver, Detroit, Los Angeles, San Diego, and Winnipeg), and a total of 203 patients were allocated at random to receive either 12- or 24-hour-per-day oxygen administration. Selection criteria for these patients included a clinical diagnosis of emphysema with or without chronic bronchitis fulfilling ATS definitions,[34] an arterial oxygen tension at rest breathing room air of 55 mm Hg or less during a 3-week steady-state period, or PO_2 of 59 mm Hg or less with ECG evidence of right ventricular hypertrophy, clinically determined right heart failure, or hematocrit of $>55\%$. Specific exclusions were designed to eliminate uncooperative patients and patients with other major organ system abnormalities, or any other clinical state that might alter the outcome parameters evaluated in the study. The study, just completed, was designed to evaluate the relative effectiveness of 12-hour versus 24-hour-per-day oxygen in terms of clinical, physiologic, and psychologic factors, quality of life, survival, and the possible presence of tissue oxygen toxicity in each therapy group.

The first report of major outcomes from this study has recently been revealed, showing a clear-cut benefit from 24-hour-per-day oxygen compared with 12-hour-per-day oxygen from the standpoint of survival at the 1- or 2-year evaluation point.[35] The relative benefits of oxygen in terms of neuropsychiatric function, quality of life, exercise parameters, and so forth are currently being analyzed, but continuous oxygen appears to be clearly advantageous in advanced patients compared with 12-hour-per-day oxygen. In another study conducted in the United Kingdom, a 15-hour-per-day oxygen group was compared with a control group receiving no oxygen. Again there was a clear-cut improvement in survival in the oxygen therapy group.[36] Thus, the immense value of controlled low-flow oxygen given on a continuous basis is now well established, and continuous or nearly continuous oxygen administration has been shown to be clearly more effective in advanced patients, at least compared with lesser periods of oxygen therapy. It must be pointed out, however, that oxygen administration is only one facet in the care of patients with advanced COPD, and its use must be integrated into an overall rehabilitation program, considered in further detail in Chapter 18.

In summary, the monitored use of oxygen is safe in CAO as well as other hypoxemic states and is effective in combating the profound hypoxemia that threatens life. In our experience, the precise use of oxygen has been safe, and fears of acute CO_2 retention and serious oxygen toxicity have not been realized. Oxygen is most easily administered via a nasal cannulae, but it can also be administered effectively by other devices, including mechanical ventilators. It is stressed, however, that oxygen, like any other drug, must be used with great precision. Lasting benefit from continuous oxygen use in advanced COPD with severe hypoxemia is now well established, but it must be integrated into a comprehensive care (rehabilitation) program. Thus, oxygen is life saving in both acute and chronic states of hypoxemia and is palliative therapy in advanced COPD.

REFERENCES

1. Flenley, D.C.: The rationale of oxygen therapy. Lancet, *1:*270, 1967.
2. Campbell, E.J.M.: The management of acute respiratory failure in chronic bronchitis and emphysema. Am. Rev. Resp. Dis., *96:*626, 1967.
3. Refsum, H.E.: Arterial hypoxemia, serum activities of GO-T, GP-T and LDH, and centrilobular liver cell necrosis in pulmonary insufficiency. Clin. Sci., *25:*369, 1963.
4. Sukumalchantra, Y., and Williams, M.H., Jr.: Pathophysiology of ventilatory failure. Am. Rev. Resp. Dis., *92:*428, 1965.
5. Bancroft, J.: Respiratory Functions of the Blood. Cambridge, England, University Press, 1914.
6. Comroe, J.H., Jr., Bolinson, E.R., and Coates, E.O.: Mental changes occurring in continually anoxic patients during oxygen therapy. JAMA, *143:*1044, 1950.
7. Westlake, E.R., Simpson, T., and Kaye, M.: Carbon dioxide necrosis in emphysema. Q. J. Med., *24:*155, 1955.
8. Campbell, E.J.M.: A method of controlled oxygen administration which reduced the risk of carbon dioxide retention. Lancet, *2:*12, 1960.
9. Hutchinson, D.C.S., Flenley, D.C., and Donald, K.W.: Controlled oxygen therapy: Respiratory failure. Br. Med. J., *2:*1159, 1964.
10. Cherniack, R.M., and Hakimpour, H.: The rational use of oxygen in respiratory insufficiency. JAMA, *199:*146, 1967.
11. Kory, T.C., Bergman, J.C., Sweet, R.P., and Smith, J.R.: Comparable evaluation of oxygen therapy techniques. JAMA, *179:*767, 1962.
12. Eldridge, F., and Gherman, C.: Studies of oxygen administration in respiratory failure. Ann. Intern. Med., *68:*569, 1968.
13. Smith, J.P., Stone, R.W., and Muschemheim, C.: Management of acute respiratory failure in bronchitis and emphysema with observations on controlled oxygen therapy. Ann. Intern. Med., *66:*1056, 1967.
14. Vendenbergh, E., Van de Woestijne, K.P., and Gyselen, P.: Conservative treatment of acute respiratory failure in patients with chronic obstructive lung diseases. Am. Rev. Resp. Dis., *98:*60, 1968.
15. Petty, T.L., Nett, L.M., and Lakshminarayan, S.: A single nasal prong for continuous oxygen therapy. Chest, *64:*146, 1973.
16. Campbell, E.J.M.: Respiratory failure: The relation between oxygen concentrations of inspired air and arterial blood. Lancet, *1:*10, 1960.
17. Schiff, M.M., and Massaro, D.: Effect of oxygen administration by a Venturi apparatus on arterial blood gas values: Patients with respiratory failure. N. Engl. J. Med., *277:*950, 1967.
18. Gibson, R.L., Comer, P.B., Beckman, R.W., and McGraw, C.P.: Actual tracheal oxygen concentrations with commonly used oxygen equipment. Anesthesiology, *44:*71, 1976.
19. Poulton, T.J., Comer, P.B., and Gibson, R.L.: Tracheal oxygen concentrations with a nasal cannula during oral and nasal breathing. Resp. Care, *25:*739, 1980.
20. Bigelow, D.B., Petty, T.L., Levine, B.E., Filley, G.F., and Finigan, M.M.: The effect of oxygen breathing on arterial blood gases in patients with chronic airway obstruction living at 5200 feet. Am. Rev. Resp. Dis., *96:*28, 1967.
21. McNicol, M.W., and Campbell, E.J.M.: Severity of respiratory failure (arterial blood gases: unsaturated patients). Lancet, *1:*336, 1965.
22. O'Donohue, W.J., and Baker, M.P.: Controlled low-flow oxygen in the management of acute respiratory failure. Chest, *63:*818, 1973.
23. Marshall, B.E., and Wyche, M.Q., Jr.: Hypoxemia during and after anesthesia. Anesthesiology, *37:*178, 1972.
24. Leigh, J.M.: Postoperative oxygen administration. Br. J. Anaesth., *47:*108, 1975.
25. Pontoppidan, H., and Berry, P.R.: Regulation of the inspired oxygen concentration during artificial ventilation. JAMA, *201:*11, 1967.

26. Roth, E.M.: Gas physiology in space operations. N. Engl. J. Med., *275:*255, 1966.
27. Petty, T.L., Neff, T.A., Creagh, C.E., Sutton, F.D., Nett, L.M., Bailey, D., and Fernandez, E.: Outpatient oxygen therapy in chronic obstructive pulmonary disease. Arch. Intern. Med., *139:*28, 1979.
28. Levine, B.E., Nett, L.M., Bigelow, D.B., Hamstra, R.A., Beckwitt, N.J., Mitchell, R.S., Stephen, T.A., and Petty, T.L.: The role of long-term continuous oxygen administration in patients with chronic airway obstruction with hypoxemia. Ann. Intern. Med., *66:*639, 1967.
29. Abraham, A.S., Cole, R.B., and Bishop, J.M.: Reversal of pulmonary hypertension by prolonged oxygen administration to patients with chronic bronchitis. Circ. Res., *23:*147, 1968.
30. Petty, T.L., Stanford, R.E., and Neff, T.A.: Continuous oxygen in chronic airway obstruction (observations on possible oxygen toxicity and survival). Ann. Intern. Med., *75:*361, 1971.
31. Stark, R.D., Finnegan, P., and Bishop, J.M.: Daily requirements of oxygen to reverse pulmonary hypertension in patients with chronic bronchitis. Br. Med. J., *3:*724, 1972.
32. Stark, R.D., Finnegan, P., and Bishop, J.M.: Long-term domicilliary oxygen in chronic bronchitis with pulmonary hypertension. Br. Med. J., *1:*467, 1973.
33. Oxygen Therapy (Recommendation Statement from the Conference). Am. Rev. Resp. Dis., *110:*4, 1974.
34. Definitions and Classification of Chronic Bronchitis, Asthma and Pulmonary Emphysema. Am. Rev. Resp. Dis., *85:*762, 1962.
35. Nocturnal Oxygen Therapy Trial Group: Continuous or Nocturnal Oxygen Therapy in Hypoxemic Chronic Obstructive Lung Disease. Ann. Intern. Med., *93:*391, 1980.
36. Long-term domicilliary oxygen therapy in chronic hypoxic cor pulmonale complicating chronic bronchitis and emphysema. Lancet, *1:*681, 1981.

Chapter 4

PRINCIPLES OF MECHANICAL VENTILATION

By Thomas L. Petty

A variety of mechanical ventilators, which are highly useful in providing the work to support ventilation, are now available. Although different capabilities were once represented by different devices, most modern volume-oriented ventilators used in supportive care possess similar capabilities which are adequate or even unnecessary in the care of most acutely ill patients. This chapter does not dwell on the engineering features of ventilators in common use today, and some currently available devices are not included for sake of brevity. The main purpose of this chapter is to consider principles of mechanical ventilation and weaning from mechanical ventilatory support.

All ventilators provide pressure to force gas into the lungs, so that in a sense, all machines are pressure oriented. Under given conditions, all machines deliver a certain volume of air depending upon the machine's capabilities and upon the clinical situation. Thus, all machines can be said to deliver a volume of air.

Today's ventilators are of several general types including simple pressure-cycled devices, time-cycled devices, and volume-cycled ventilators. Several new volume-limited ventilators have been introduced in recent years and enjoy great popularity, which is unjustified in certain instances.

The previously popular pressure-cycled machines—Bird and Bennett—have been relegated to a back-up role since other more versatile machines are available. Their main virtue is their relative simplicity. Most medical and paramedical personnel are generally familiar with their use.

A discussion of all the details of each ventilator's design is beyond the scope of this chapter, and the reader is referred to two complete texts which include functional schematic diagrams and define the various features of most ventilators currently available.[1,2] In brief, pressure-cycled devices allow inflow of air upon triggering of a valve by the patient's effort or by an automatic rate control; the flow continues until a preset pressure has been reached, whereupon the valve closes. The Bennett PR-1 and Bird Mark 7 ventilators, illustrated in Figure 4-1, are representative of this type of machine.

One of the greatest disadvantages of pressure-cycled respirators is that the varying resistance interferes with flow, since flow is a function of pressure and resistance. This resistance causes a change in tidal volume, since volume is a product of flow and time. Thus, the delivered volume varies as resistance varies. This may be a particular problem in patients with changing pulmonary resistance, such as in those in postoperative states (see Chap. 14) or in acute bronchospasm (see Chap. 9).

Another disadvantage of these devices is their low pressure capability (top effective peak pressure is 30 to 40 cm from a 50-lb-per-square-inch source). Moreover, these devices have poor control of the inspired oxygen concentration, unless powered by air-oxygen mixing devices (blenders).[3]

In contrast, so-called volume respirators deliver a metered amount of air at whatever delivery pressure is required, up to the peak pressure capability of the machine. Except for gas compression at high resistance and the compliance of the delivery system and machine bellows, these devices do deliver a fairly constant tidal volume. Small changes due to a high resistance are of little clinical importance.

A simple volume respirator still in common use in some centers is the Emerson device (Fig. 4-2). It is a motor-powered, piston-operated machine. It has a high pressure (approximately 100 cm H_2O) and flow capability and the ability to adjust inspiratory-expiratory ratios. This remains a reliable device that is often called into use because of its durability. It is less sophisticated than newer machines, but still useful in today's respiratory care. Newer modifications have also been introduced.

Two early popular volume-limited ventilators are the Bennett MA-1 (Fig. 4-3) and the Ohio 560. The Bennett MA-1 has a pressure capability of approximately 80 cm and various additional features, including the ability to vary the tidal volume periodically and provide a "sigh," which was originally designed to combat the microatelectasis and shunting that occurred with fixed low-tidal-volume

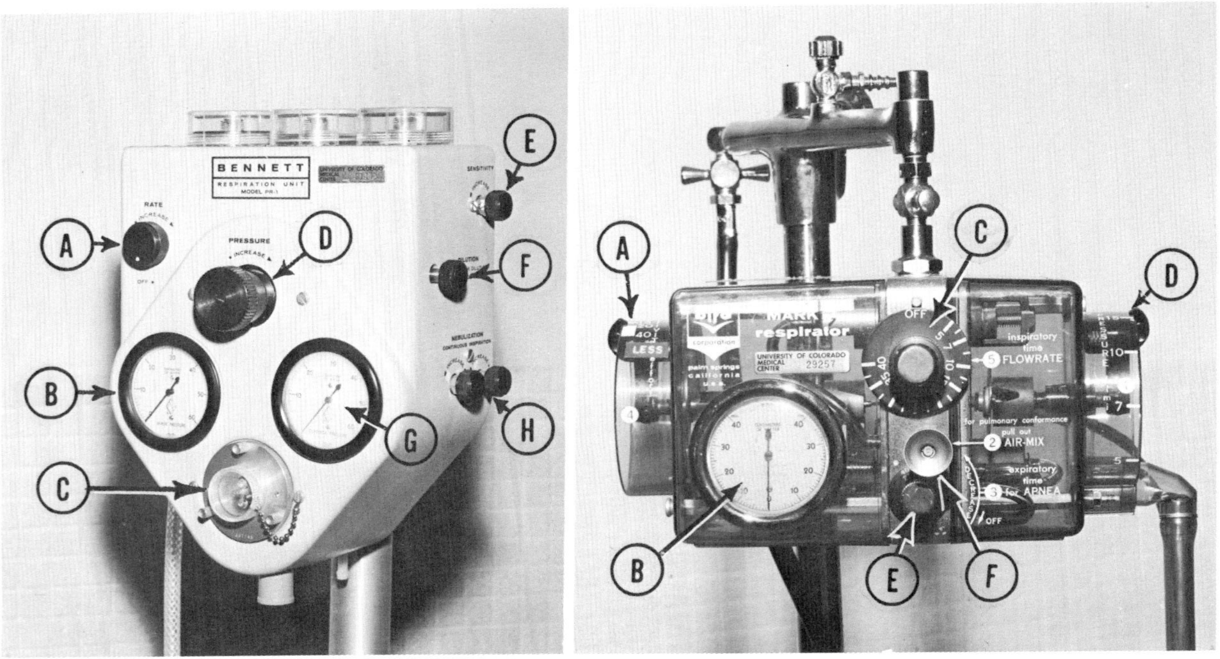

Fig. 4-1. Two pressure-cycled machines in common use. The Bennett PR-1 (*left*) has the following features: *A* = rate control; *B* = airway pressure indicator; *C* = flow-sensitive valve; *D* = pressure control; *E* = sensitivity control; *F* = oxygen diluter; *G* = machine pressure indicator; *H* = humidifier controls. The Bird Mark 7 (*right*) has: *A* = sensitivity control; *B* = airway pressure indicator; *C* = flow control; *D* = pressure control; *E* = rate control; *F* = oxygen diluter.

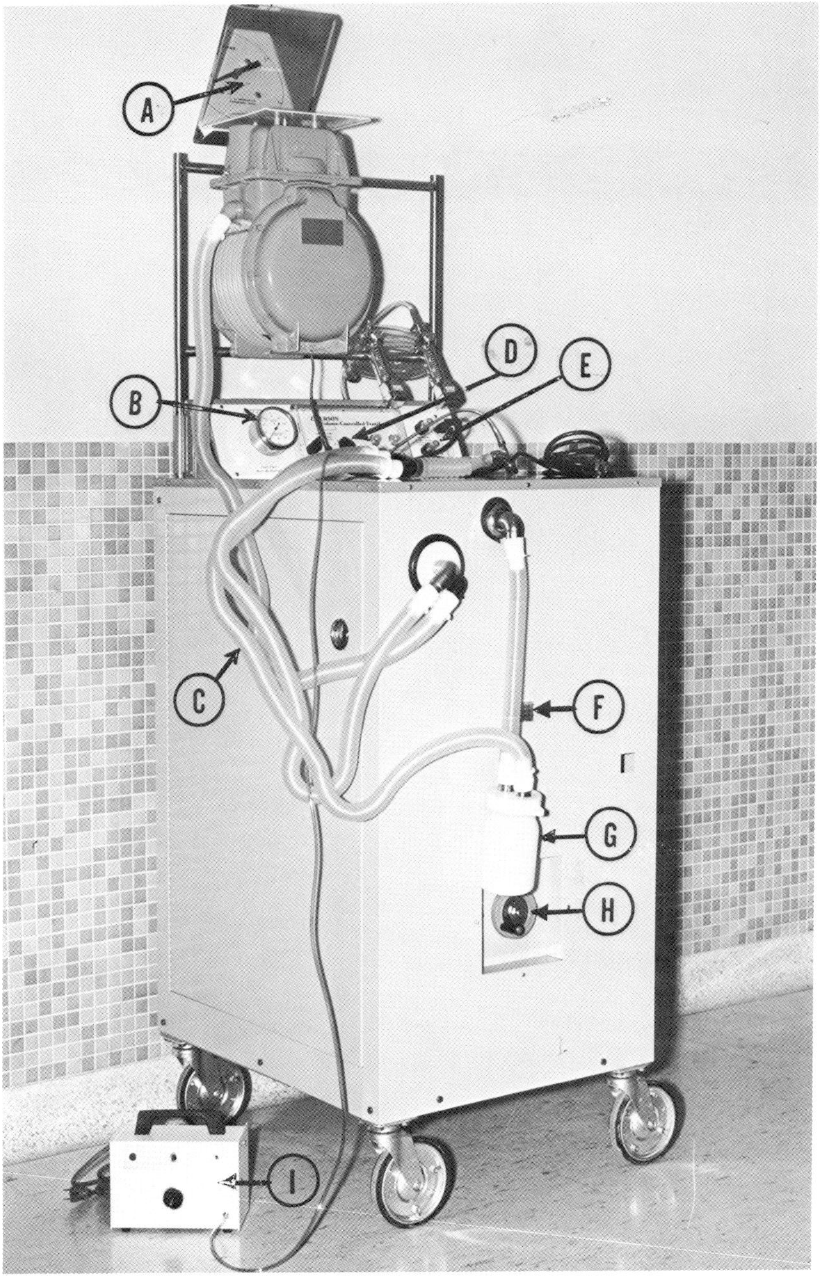

Fig. 4-2. Emerson volume-cycled respirator. *A* = volume indicator; *B* = delivery pressure gauge; *C* = hoses to airway; *D* = inspiration and expiration time controls; *E* = indicator lights; *F* = tidal volume setting; *G* = water trap; *H* = tidal volume control; *I* = accessory ventilator warning device.

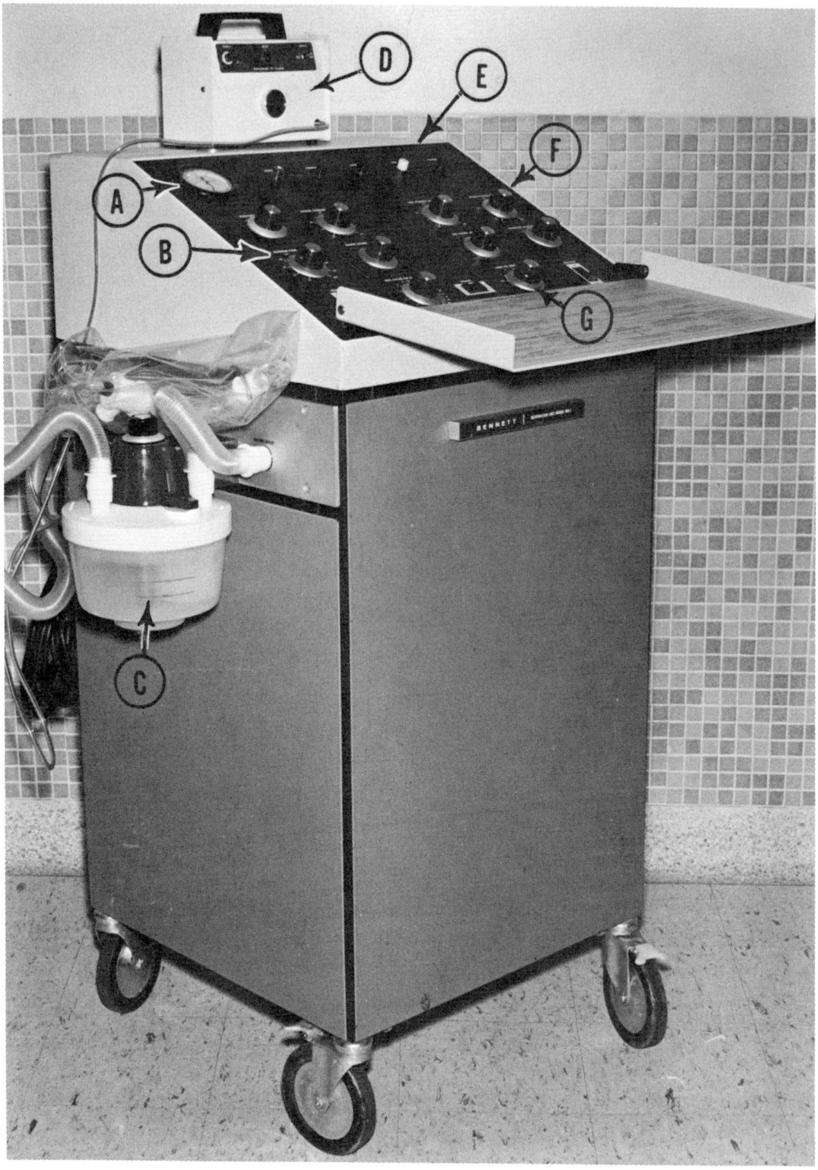

Fig. 4-3. Bennett MA-1 volume-cycled respirator. *A* = delivery pressure gauge; *B* = pressure, flow, and volume controls; C = Cascade humidifier; *D* = ventilator warning device; *E* = warning lights; *F* = oxygen control; *G* = sigh controls.

ventilation.[4] The MA-1 can also be cycled by the patient, and a wide range of flow rates is available. The oxygen fraction can be accurately controlled; a spirometer to monitor tidal volume and a warning device are available on this machine. The machines in Figures 4-2 and 4-3 are being used with a supplemental warning device.[5]

Recently, an MA-2 device has been introduced which offers more "capability." This is supported in part by the increased complexity of the device (Fig. 4-4). In many ways, its capabilities and design features are similar to the Bennett MA-1, and many feel that the MA-2 does not offer a significant advantage when cost is considered (MA-2, $11,110 vs MA-1, $9,440).

Figure 4-5 shows the original Ohio 560 device, which was introduced into respiratory care about the same time as the Bennett MA-1. This device is no longer being manufactured for the United States, but is still used in Europe under the label "Monaghan 250." This device, however, is still present in a number of intensive care units, primarily because of a high peak-pressure capability (approximately 100 cm H_2O), a wide range of flow capability, PEEP capability, and an excellent internal warning system.

Ohio Medical Products has their own critical care ventilator, shown in Figure 4-6, with capabilities summarized in Table 4-1.

Another device in common use offers the feature of fluidics control, thus minimizing the number of moving parts and eliminating electrical circuitry. The capabilities of this device, the Monaghan 225 (Fig. 4-6), and the 228, are listed in Table 4-1, along with the other volume-cycled respirators in common use in this country including the Bear 1, which enjoys considerable popularity today (Fig. 4-7).

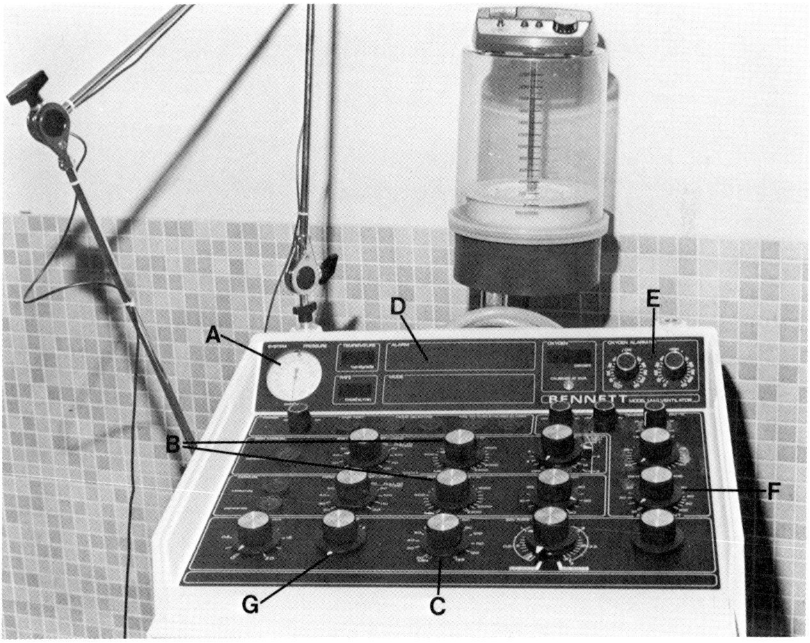

Fig. 4-4. Bennett MA-2 volume-cycled respirator. *A* = delivery pressure gauge; *B* = tidal volume and sigh volume controls; *C* = peak flow control; *D* = alarm displays; *E* = oxygen alarms; *F* = oxygen control; *G* = PEEP/CPAP control.

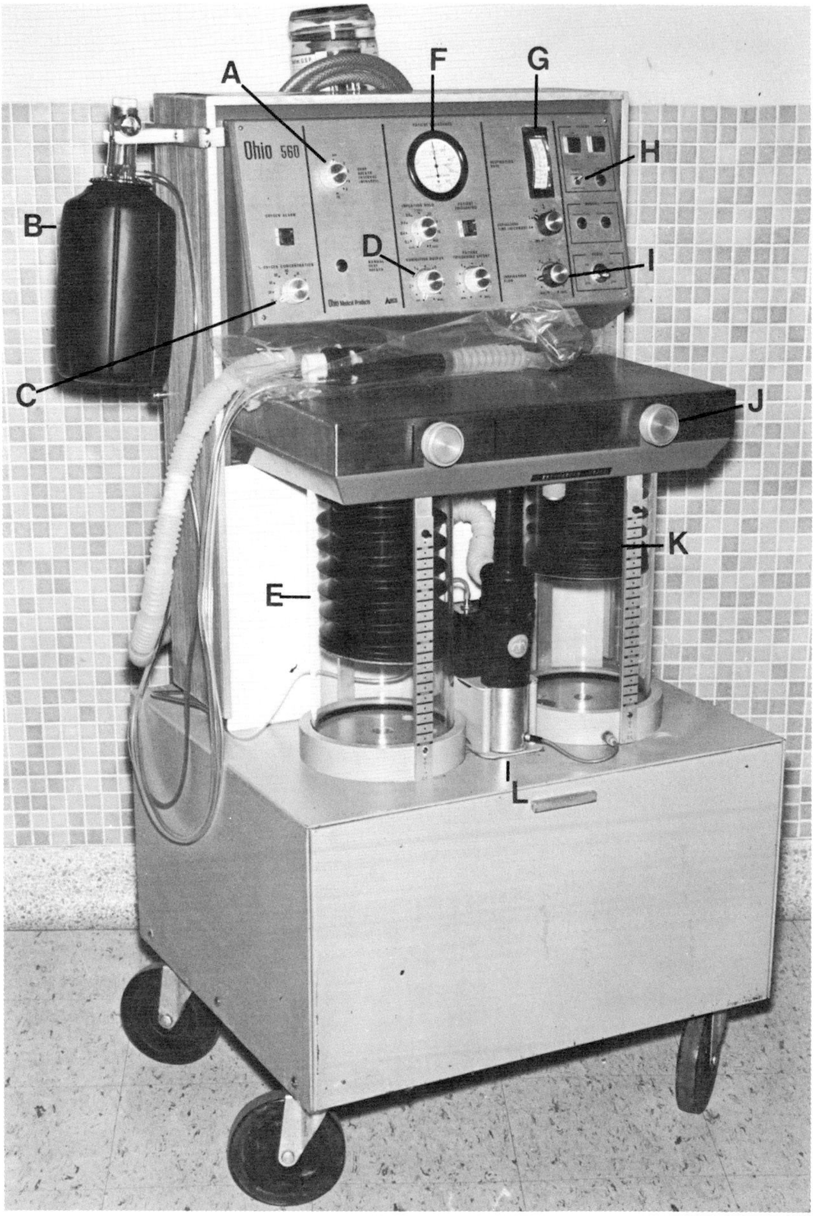

Fig. 4-5. Original Ohio 560 volume-cycled respirator. *A* = sigh timer; *B* = resuscitation bag; *C* = oxygen control; *D* = sensitivity control; *E* = sigh bellows; *F* = delivery pressure gauge; *G* = rate meter; *H* = warning lights and audible alarm; *I* = flow rate control; *J* = bellows control; *K* = tidal volume bellows; *L* = ultrasonic nebulizer.

INTERFACING THE VENTILATOR TO SERVE THE PATIENT

It must be emphasized that the purpose of mechanical ventilatory support is to serve the needs of the patient. Thus, the device must be adjusted to meet a wide variety of clinical situations, whereas certain

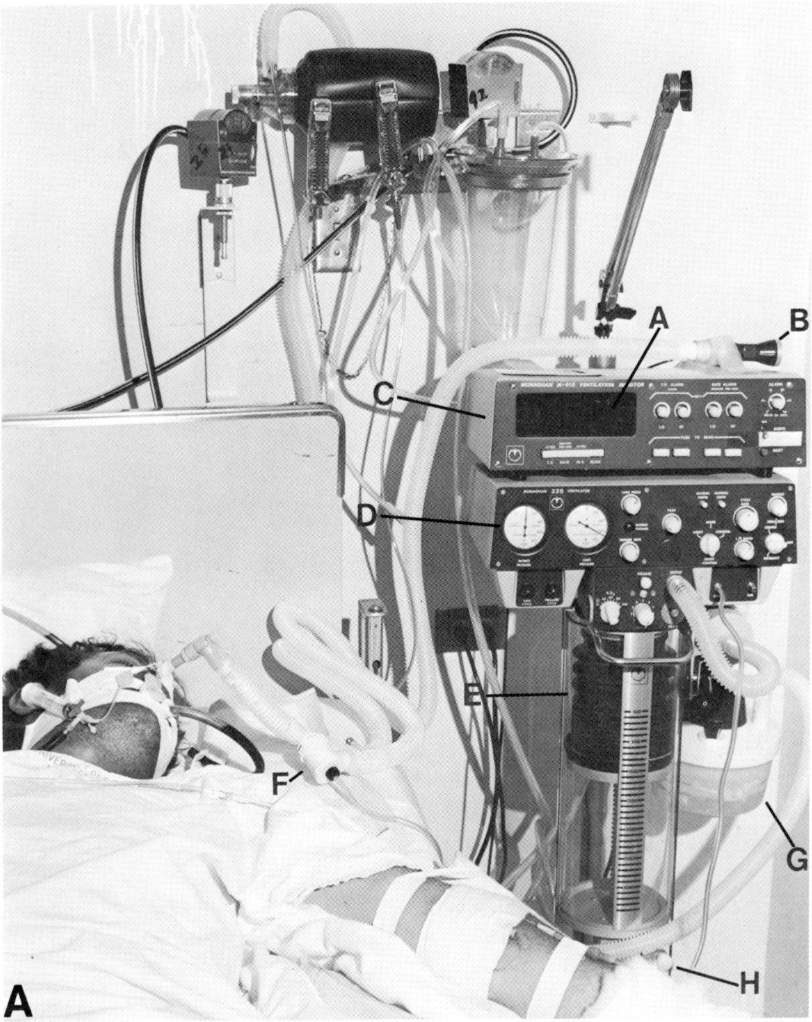

Fig. 4-6. Monaghan 225 volume-pressure and time-cycled respirator in clinical use (A); close-up of control panel (B) The device is being used with a prototype of the Monaghan 700 ventilator alarm system. *A* = digital monitor screen; *B* = thermistor for monitor; *C* = ventilation monitor; *D* = ventilator; *E* = tidal volume bellows; *F* = exhalation manifold; *G* = Cascade humidifier; *H* = crank to set tidal volume. (Continued on page 96.)

features of the machine can be set to meet the clinical situation at hand. The options that are available are considered in the following paragraphs.

Cycling Mode

This may be patient cycled (i.e., assist), control cycled wherein the machine picks a preset respiratory rate, or a combination of both so that the patient has the opportunity to select the respiratory rate according to his own respiratory drives. In case these respiratory

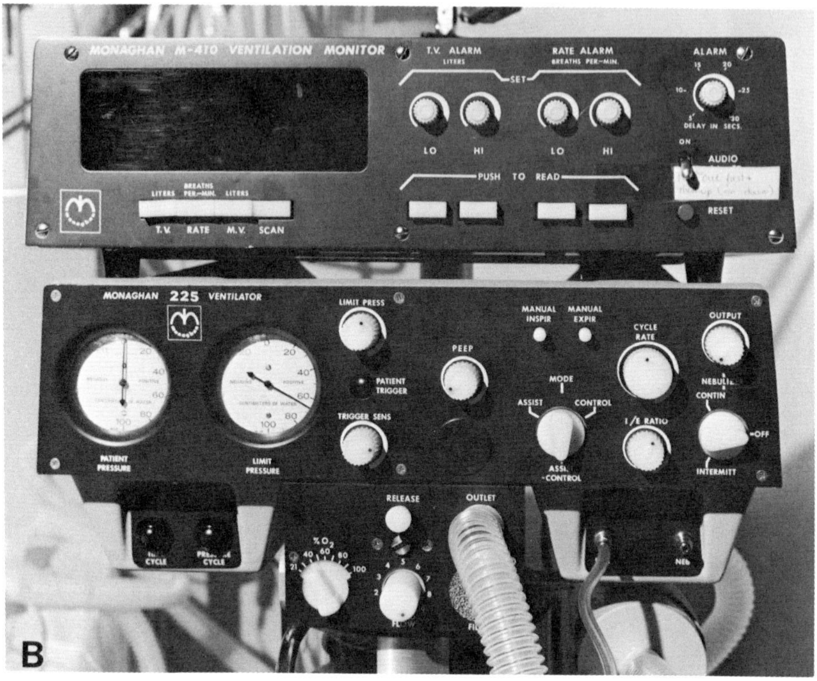

Fig. 4-6. (Continued.)

drives become diminished, a preset control rate, set at less than the patient's respiratory rate, cycles the machine (assist-control mode). This is the mode that is most commonly used, since it offers the advantage of allowing the patient to be in the "loop," i.e., to initiate an inspiratory breath whenever the urge to breathe occurs. The control rate will still cause the machine to cycle if the respiratory center fails, which is uncommon except in head trauma and poisoning.

Sensitivity

This determines the effort by the patient that is required to initiate assisted breathing. Generally, this should be set low, so that a small inspiratory effort will initiate machine cycling. The patient should not have to work to initiate the inspiratory cycle in most cases. Generally, 1 cm H_2O inspiratory effort or less should be the setting, but the setting should not be so exquisitely sensitive as to self-cycle or "chatter," meaning that any pressure transient will be sufficient to initiate the inspiratory cycle. A common respiratory rate setting is 12 to 14 breaths per minute in apneic individuals.

Tidal Volume

The usual necessary tidal volume is 10 to 15 ml/kg. Thus, an initial tidal volume setting of somewhere between 500 and 1000 at a slow rate, i.e., 10 to 14 per minute, is a starting point.

TABLE 4-1. Capabilities and Features of Volume Respirators in Common Use

	Bennett MA-1, MA-2	*Emerson*	*Original Ohio 560 Ohio CCV*	*Monaghan 225 and 228*	*Bourns Bear 1*
Cycling mechanisms	Rate control, patient cycled, volume cycled	Rate control, patient cycled	Rate control, patient cycled, volume cycled	Rate control, time, pressure, or volume cycled	Rate control, time, pressure, or volume cycled
Inspiratory-expiratory ratio	Variable	Variable	Variable	Variable	Variable
Peak pressure	80	100	100	100	100
Positive end-expiratory pressure	Yes	No	Yes	Yes	Yes
Inflation hold	No	No	Yes	No	Yes
Sigh feature	Yes	Yes	Yes	No	Yes
Moisture system	Humidifier	Humidifier	Ultrasonic nebulizer Ohio 560 Humidifier CCV	Humidifier	Humidifier
Alarm system	Yes	No	Yes	Optional	Yes
IMV	Yes	No*	Yes—Ohio CCV	Yes—M-228	Yes

* Emerson "IMV Ventilator" available.

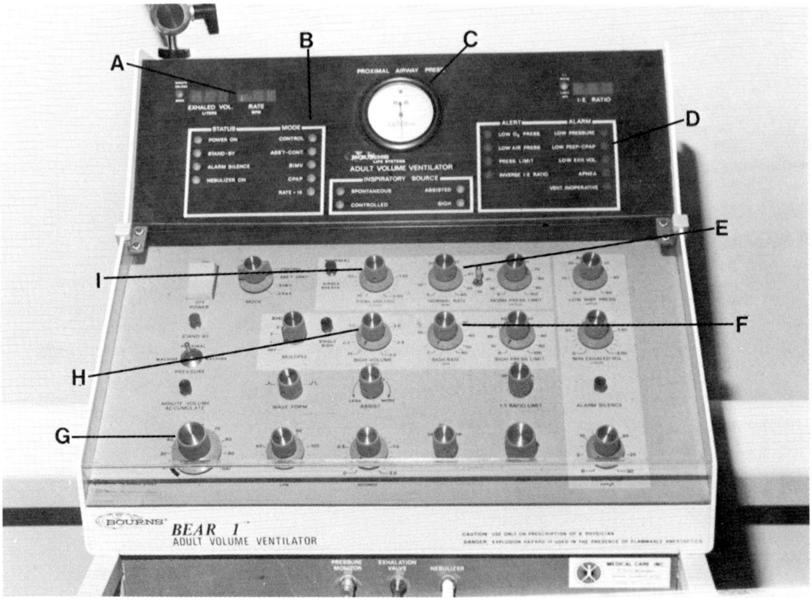

Fig. 4-7. Bear 1 adult volume ventilator. *A* = exhaled tidal volume digital display; *B* = rate display; *C* = airway pressure gauge; *D* = alarms; *E* = normal rate control; *F* = sigh rate control; *G* = oxygen fraction control; *H* = sigh volume; *I* = tidal volume.

Inspiratory-Expiratory Ratio

This can be set, but it is better to let the patient determine this himself. The respiratory rate will determine how many inspiratory cycles per minute are available to the patient, or the patient will choose the rate, which is based upon the urge to breathe. The inspiratory flow rate will control the inspiratory flow time, and the remainder of the time will be available for the expiratory time. (For example, 15 breaths per minute equals 4 seconds per breath for both inspiration and expiration; if inspiration takes 1 second, 3 seconds remain for expiration. Thus, assuming no pause at the end of inspiration, the I:E ration would be 1:3.) Therefore, an interrelationship between inspiratory and expiratory time will be determined by rate setting and inspiratory flow rate. Some machines have an override for expiratory time. Obviously, it is not possible to deliver a large tidal volume at a slow inspiratory rate with a fast overall respiratory rate, and so time becomes the "bottom line." Said another way, whatever rate and inspiratory time are required for delivery of the necessary tidal volume setting will determine the pattern.

F_{IO_2}

This controls the inspired oxygen fraction. It is extremely important to use the lowest possible inspired oxygen fraction that will provide adequate arterial oxygenation, i.e., an oxygen tension of 60 to 80 mm Hg. Oxygen tension may be improved by PEEP (see later). Problems of oxygen toxicity are considered in Chapter 8 on the Adult Respiratory Distress Syndrome.

PEEP

This useful technique is valuable in improving oxygen transfer across the lung in acute lung injury patterns termed the "Adult Respiratory Distress Syndrome." This is considered in detail in Chapters 5 and 8. Briefly, PEEP implies exhalation against a threshold resistor usually set a 5 to 15 cm H_2O. Exactly how PEEP works and its true value are considered in the commentary beginning on page 102.

Sigh

Sigh was originally added as a new feature to the Bennett MA-1 and the original Ohio 560 device. It was intended to combat the microatelectasis which was observed to occur in states of fixed low-tidal-volume ventilation.[4] Now that it has been established that high-tidal-volume ventilation, i.e., 10 to 15 ml/cm, is preferable and does not result in this problem of microatelectasis and shunting, sigh is considered essentially unimportant and a dead issue in the minds of many experts.[6]

Intermittent Mandatory Ventilation

The technique of intermittent mandatory ventilation (IMV) allows the patient to breathe in parallel with the machine spontaneously through the definitive airway, i.e., the endotracheal tube or tracheostomy, in between breaths selected by the rate setting on the respirator, which are mandatory breaths. This technique is also controversial, and the pros and cons of its use are considered in the following commentary.

First it must be pointed out that IMV is not new. Those who used older volume-oriented mechanical ventilators, including the 1952 model of the Engstrom or early Emerson volume-limited models—both of which had no capability for the patient to cycle the machine—will recall that the patient could still breathe at any time. With the Engstrom, the patient-initiated breath came from the balloon, which was charged according to the minute ventilation setting by an entraining system; in the Emerson, the patient could still breathe via the delivery system regardless of the cycle phase of the respirator itself. When the rate-controlled breath occurred, depending on the rate setting, the forced breath was delivered to the patient whether or not this coincided with the patient's urge to breathe. During this era, many patients would be seen to "fight the respirator," and for this reason the use of paralyzing and sedative drugs to gain control of the patient became commonplace. This mode of mechanical ventilation was indeed controlled in every sense of the word, and in fact these pharmacologic maneuvers really adjusted the patient to the respirator rather than vice versa. Those who witnessed these situations well remember the distress, anxiety, and, at times, anguish that this form of mechanical ventilatory support caused the patient, even though it was lifesaving at times.

The advent of a large number of newer mechanical ventilators, summarized previously and in Table 4-1, with the feature of patient cycling changed all this, so that in most cases it was possible for the patient to initiate an assisted breath with the slightest inspiratory effort adjusted by the sensitivity control of the machine. This feature, coupled with the high pressure and flow capabilities of most modern ventilators as well as the wide range of adjustable inspiratory-expiratory time capabilities (which give flexibility to the inspiratory-expiratory ratio), made it possible to do what one aims to do in modern respiratory care—adjust the respirator *to serve the needs of the patient.* Those experienced in respiratory care recognize the difference in terms of the comfort afforded the patient and the physiologic benefits of having the patient's respiratory center as an integral part of the relationship between patient and machine.

The technique of IMV allows the patient to breathe spontaneously and in parallel with the machine, which may be advantageous in certain clinical situations. One of these is when the patient is breathing irregularly or is driven to breathe by other than chemical drives, such as from reflexes, somatic sensations, anxiety, and so forth. When assisted mechanical ventilation, under these circumstances, leads to hypocarbia and respiratory alkalemia, allowing the patient to take over some of the work of breathing without assistance from IMV may lead to normalization of carbon dioxide homeostasis. This of course is advantageous. Other methods accomplish this same result, including adding mechanical dead space. Although writers also frequently comment upon using an increased $F_{I_{CO_2}}$ to correct hypocarbia, in fact this is not immediately practical in most hospitals. Thus, at this point we may score one advantage for IMV, although in a given patient the use of IMV may or may not provide better blood gas control than simple assisted mechanical ventilation.

The second situation in which intermittent mandatory ventilation is likely to be beneficial is when cardiac output and systemic oxygen transfer are reduced during PEEP (see Chap. 8). Interposing some spontaneous breaths will minimize the mean thoracic pressure over time, thus perhaps unburdening the circulatory system. A factor against this, however, is the work of breathing that the patient must perform during these intermittent breaths, which may be considerable in low compliance, high resistance states in which the work of breathing may account for as much as 30% of total oxygen consumption. Moreover, it must be emphatically stated that the most clinically useful levels of PEEP, i.e., 5 to 15 cm H_2O, are uncommonly associated with reduced tissue oxygen delivery.[7,8] Therefore, the use of PEEP to improve hemodynamics will be limited to a few patients in whom high levels of PEEP may, as a physiologic gamble, seem worthwhile. Against high levels of PEEP are many factors, including barotrauma, increased extravascular lung water, and initiation of cardiodepressor responses.[9,10] Thus, high PEEP levels, i.e., >15 cm, are not generally used, resulting in little need for IMV to reduce mean thoracic pressure. Since IMV may be beneficial in selected patients with PEEP, however, this is another point in favor of IMV.

The original reason for the popularity of IMV was to promote weaning from mechanical ventilation. Strategies for weaning are described later. Thus far, however, no controlled study has shown that mechanical ventilatory assistance can be shortened by use of IMV and, in fact, many including the author believe that IMV actually *delays* the decision to extubate by interposing an unnecessary period of intubation before the judgment is made to remove the tube. IMV requires considerable work and may result in chronic fatigue of the respiratory muscles, thus making extubation unlikely to succeed. Once the tube is out, airway resistance is lessened by the removal of the added resistance of the tube, which is in concert with the patient's own airway resistance. This offers the spontaneously breathing patient an advantage that is particularly important when pulmonary mechanics are severely impaired. Moreover, removing the endotracheal tube allows the patient to cough and thus clear secretions and use pursed lip-breathing if necessary. Finally, the undeniable advantage of the ability to communicate has a salutary effect on the critically ill.

When should the endotracheal tube be removed? Excellent criteria for judging when mechanical ventilatory assistance can be discontinued and extubation performed have been offered in at least one prospective study.[11,12] Techniques of weaning in diverse and sometimes difficult clinical states, including ARDS, advanced COPD, and neuromuscular disorders have been reported elsewhere, and these techniques are presented in greater detail later in this chapter.[11,12] Even some patients with poor ventilatory mechanics due to COPD or neuromuscular diseases can be successfully weaned and extubated. Selection of these patients and of strategies of weaning requires skill, of course. Therefore, since IMV has not been established to be advantageous in weaning, this is one point against IMV.

Finally, the additional circuitry required (valves with their inherent resistances), extra tubing connections, which can become disconnected or connected in an inappropriate fashion, and the increased expense of this technology added to the cost of the respirators should be considered. Since all these considerations are on the negative side of the ledger, they act as points against IMV.

Therefore, the tally rests: For IMV = 2; against IMV = 2. Evidently, the physician, nurse, or therapist will have to decide whether or not IMV will be useful based on the individual merits of the clinical situation encountered at the bedside.

CURRENT STATUS OF PEEP

The mechanism of improved arterial oxygenation by the mechanical ventilator technique, which causes expiration to take place against a threshold resistor, causing positive end-expiratory pressure (PEEP), has received extensive study since its introduction for management of the adult respiratory distress syndrome.[13,14] A reduction in intrapulmonary shunting, an increase in functional residual capacity and in lung compliance, and a reduction in the difference between inspired and arterial oxygen tension have been documented in both experimental animals and patients. *Exactly* how improved arterial oxygenation is accomplished, however, is not well understood, and how PEEP should best be applied in clinical situations is the subject of considerable debate.

What are the beneficial and the harmful effects of PEEP? Recently, an important question has been raised as to whether the use of PEEP really results in increased survival.[15] This study, however, suffers from its retrospective nature and from the fact that the selection of patients receiving PEEP and thus the clinical indications for its use were not well documented. It is therefore likely that PEEP was used in clinical states that were not likely to benefit from this ventilatory technique. Actually, patients receiving PEEP lived longer than those not receiving PEEP, but this is hardly the sole goal of therapy.

In another interesting study in a perfused excised lung model, various levels of PEEP were correlated with shunting, lung compliance, and extravascular lung water as judged by lung weight.[16] In this model, 5 and 10 cm of PEEP were clearly superior to 15 cm of PEEP from the standpoint of lung compliance and lung water, suggesting that there may be both good and bad effects of PEEP depending upon the level selected. The beneficial effects of 5 and 10 cm of PEEP were consistent with numerous clinical observations from this center and elsewhere, however.

That PEEP is not a panacea has been aptly pointed out in an editorial comment, and PEEP has not been shown in a controlled prospective clinical trial to reduce evidence of micro- or macroatelectasis in postoperative surgical patients.[17,18] Thus, we must continue to be critical about PEEP, its mechanisms, and its beneficial and harmful effects.

The purpose of PEEP is to improve arterial oxygenation *and* tissue oxygen delivery. That this can be accomplished in many patients is not in doubt.[19] PEEP generally reduces intrapulmonary shunting, but the mechanism of this shunt reduction is often a reduction of cardiac output.[8] If oxygen content is sufficiently increased by PEEP, however, even moderate reductions of cardiac output may result in increased net tissue oxygen transfer. However, in certain special cases, PEEP may even impair arterial oxygenation.[20] When PEEP allows the patients to be ventilated at a lower FIO_2 in acute lung injury states, such as the adult respiratory distress syndrome, it is likely that PEEP is beneficial. This should lead to improved survival if patients are properly selected and otherwise meticulously managed.

We should not, however, look upon PEEP as having a single mechanism, and, indeed, the effects of PEEP are many. Since these effects may be either beneficial or harmful, it is incumbent upon the physician, nurse, or therapist to judge whether or not PEEP should be instituted, at what level, and whether or not it is beneficial. Answers to these clinical challenges must be judged by the response of the individual patient. They should be based upon objective criteria for tissue oxygen transfer (see Chap. 8) and oxygen consumption whenever possible, or judged somewhat indirectly by studying a combination of arterial oxygenation, blood pressure, urine flow, state of consciousness, and temperature of the extremities as well as cardiac auscultation and chest examination. These are the things with which we should concern ourselves rather than isolated measurements of shunt, dead space ventilation, dead space ratio, ventilation-perfusion ratios, extravascular lung water, or any other single parameter that may alone be of trivial importance unless the tissues of the patient—indeed the intact human being—are served by this ventilatory technique.

CHOOSING THE VENTILATOR

Choosing the best ventilator for a particular clinical situation is considered a problem by some. It should be borne in mind that all available ventilators function by generating a transpulmonary pressure which inflates the lung. Each of the various ventilators just listed has individual special capabilities which must be appreciated by the physician, nurse, or technician involved in the use of the device. The pressure-cycled machines will suffice in most patients with chronic airflow obstruction, but their effective peak delivery pressure (about 30 cm H_2O) will not provide the necessary tidal volume in cases of high pulmonary resistance, and one will obtain little further output from this device at higher pressure settings. Volume devices have a far greater pressure capability. Moreover, it must be remembered that the inspired oxygen tension cannot be conveniently controlled unless newer mixing devices are used to power the pressure-cycled machine. On the Bird pressure-cycled device and the Bennett PR-2 pressure device, the ability to control the flow rate is a desirable feature that allows one to adjust the flow wave pattern and thus to improve patient comfort. Volume devices have features of high pressure capability and deliver a constant volume. Their additional capabilities of oxygen control are also desirable.

Adjustment of the machine-patient interface is an important matter. When patients fight the respirator, they usually (1) are hypoxemic, (2) are underventilated, (3) are uncomfortable because of an uncomfortable pressure wave form, or (4) suffer pain or anxiety. Blood gases will indicate abnormalities in ventilation and gas exchange. Adjusting the factors of ventilation (i.e., rate, speed of filling, and expiratory time) will allow one to judge the best inspiratory-expiratory ratio and the most beneficial pattern of ventilation by observing the patient's degree of comfort. Thereafter, adjustments made on the respirator should duplicate the required ventilator factors observed at the bedside. Simple reassurance will also help allay the inevitable anxiety the patient develops when placed on a respirator.

Pharmacologic adjuncts are rarely necessary. Small doses of intravenous morphine sulfate (i.e., 4 mg) are generally well tolerated by patients with chronic airflow obstruction and will quickly bring the patient into adjustment so long as shock is not present. Paralyzing doses of curare or, more recently, pancuronium are not desirable except in the most extreme situations, such as in the rare tetanus case requiring mechanical ventilation or in uncontrolled convulsive disorders, since the patient is thus entirely dependent upon the respirator and in a vulnerable position should a mechanical problem develop. A ventilator monitor is particularly necessary in these situations.

Ventilatory support is primarily used for patients with a profound derangement in their ability to ventilate and exchange oxygen. Once the patient is supported by the ventilator, definitive specific therapeutic efforts designed for each clinical situation must be directed at the underlying problem which precipitated the respiratory failure (see Chaps. 8 to 17).

PRINCIPLES OF WEANING FROM MECHANICAL VENTILATION

Periods of weaning from the respirator can be tried after the signs of disease (hypoventilation, hypoxemia, fever, congestive heart failure, weakness, and electrolyte abnormalities) are corrected, and it has become apparent that the patient's strength and vigor are improving. Measurements made with a hand spirometer will show whether or not the patient can maintain his necessary tidal volume. The Wright respirometer* (Fig. 4-8), a low-resistance hand spirometer, is accurate and can be attached to the tracheostomy tube with an adaptor. It is also useful in monitoring tidal volumes delivered by the various respirators. The forced vital capacity should be greater than 1L

* Harris Calorific, Cleveland, OH.

before attempts at removing the ventilator are made, but, in some patients with less ventilatory ability, "weaning" may still be tried with close observation.[21] Established criteria indicate that if the patient's spontaneous minute ventilation is less than 10 L, and if, on command, this can be doubled, and further, if an instantaneous negative pressure at the airway of 30 cm H_2O can be achieved, weaning will probably be successful.[11] The bedside systems used in these studies are simple. The method of measuring minute ventilation is illustrated in Figure 4-9, and that for measuring instantaneous negative pressure at the airway in Figure 4-10.

The respiratory care physician needs to be attuned to total care and to administer not only to the immediate medical problem but also to the nutritional and psychologic status of the patient. Successful weaning requires a systematic team approach by the physician, intensive care unit nurse, respiratory care specialist, and physical therapist. Some common conditions requiring ventilatory assistance may pose special problems in the weaning period. These are discussed under separate headings.

Chronic Obstructive Pulmonary Disease

The precipitating cause of acute respiratory failure (e.g., infection, heart failure, thromboembolism) should be treated while the patient's ventilation is mechanically supported. Minute ventilation should be adjusted to maintain the patient's "usual" P_{CO_2} levels. Often, this will be in the range of 60 to 70 mm Hg or higher. If the patient is hyperventilated on the respirator for 48 to 72 hours, renal bicarbonate excretion will occur to bring the pH into the normal range. When weaning is attempted, the patient will resume his "normal" alveolar ventilation, and the P_{CO_2} will rise toward its usual level. A dangerous respiratory acidosis may ensue, necessitating reinstitution of mechanical ventilation.

Prior to the start of weaning, maximum bronchodilatation should be achieved by administration of appropriate medication. In addition, the bronchial secretions should be cleared with adequate suctioning. At the time of weaning, the patient should be in an upright position and should be instructed to breathe in the most efficient manner (i.e., slow, controlled abdominal-diaphragmatic breathing). This results in a decreased respiratory rate, maximal tidal volumes, and relaxation of the accessory muscles of respiration. Owing to their severe ventilatory impairment, these patients frequently do not satisfy the proposed criteria for weaning. Therefore, when the patient appears to be clinically improved, attempts at weaning should be commenced. In many of these patients, early extubation will decrease the added resistance imposed by the narrow caliber of the endotracheal tube. Consequently, extubation should be performed after short T-tube trials. Certain patients require prolonged mechani-

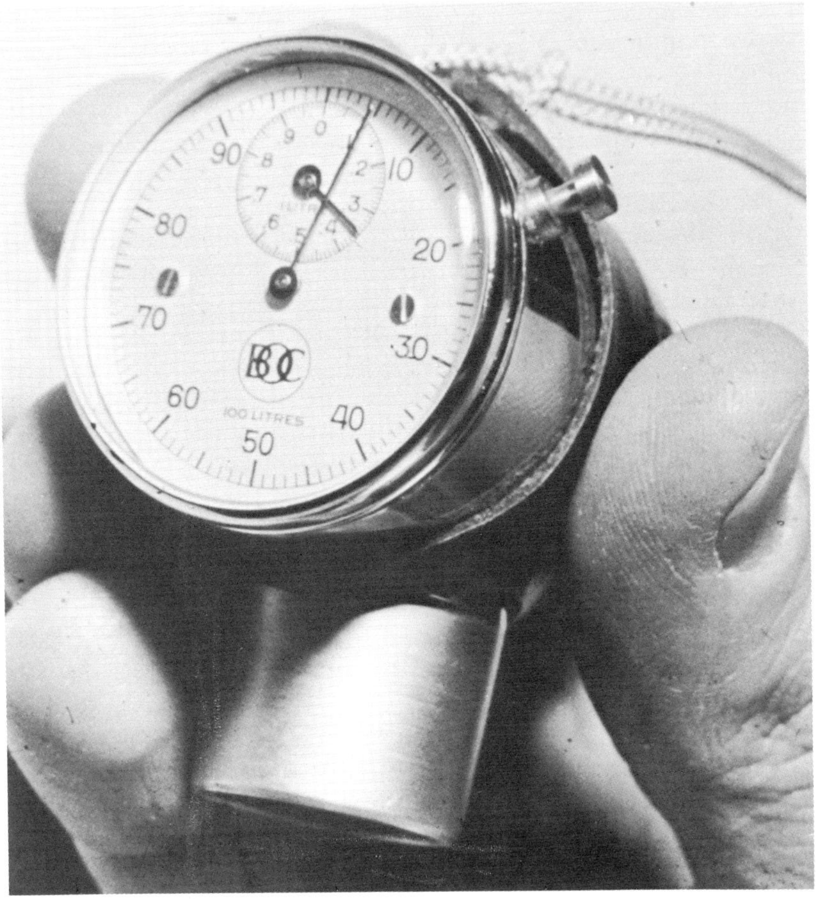

Fig. 4-8. Wright respirometer for monitoring tidal volume and minute ventilation.

cal support, and thus, the development of muscular weakness and poor nutrition complicate the situation. In these cases, special attention to nutrition, including eating full meals while being supported by mechanical ventilation, is essential. This is generally possible with a tracheostomy and is often not successful with an endotracheal tube. Ambulating the patient and walking with ventilation supported by a self-inflating bag are also useful in improving strength and coordination during the recovery phase.[21] These weaning techniques are considered further in Chapter 10.

Chest Trauma

With the increased incidence of motor vehicle accidents, chest trauma has become an important cause of respiratory failure.[22] A flail chest is frequently observed in the patient with multiple rib fractures. The current method of therapy for flail chest is internal stabili-

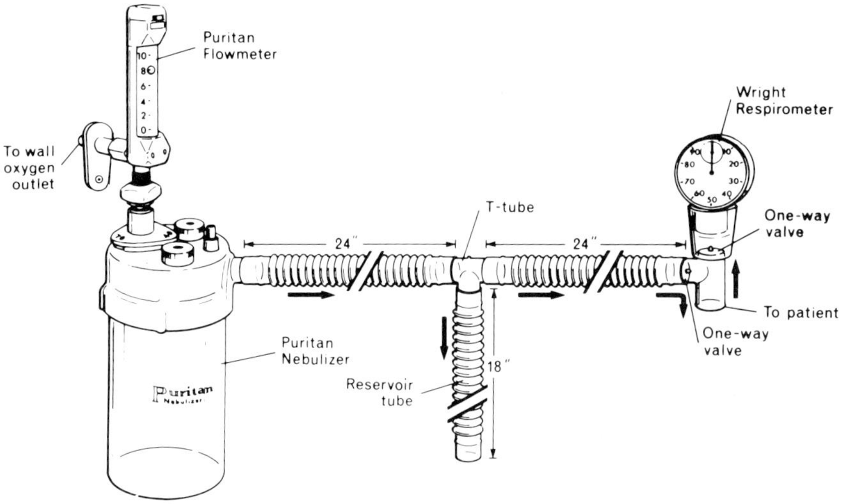

Fig. 4-9. System for bedside measurement of tidal volume and minute ventilation during weaning. (Reproduced with permission from Chest, *63:*1002, 1973.)

zation of the chest with the use of a mechanical ventilator. For adequate healing of the flail segment, the chest wall requires stability for approximately 10 to 21 days, necessitating the use of a tracheostomy. Weaning should not be attempted until there is no longer evidence of significant paradoxic motion of the chest wall during spontaneous breathing. Patients younger than the age of 30 usually require 7 to 10 days for chest wall stabilization. Older persons, those receiving corticosteroids, or patients with severe osteoporosis may take 3 to 4 weeks for stabilization to occur.

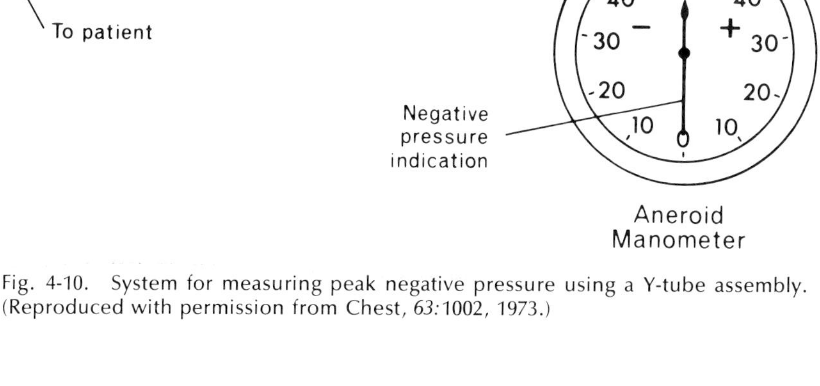

Fig. 4-10. System for measuring peak negative pressure using a Y-tube assembly. (Reproduced with permission from Chest, *63:*1002, 1973.)

Occasionally, when weaning a patient with flail chest from the ventilator, no paradoxic motion may be observed at first, but as respiration becomes more rapid (i.e., more than 35 to 40/min), paradoxic movement may occur. Therefore, it is important to observe the patient closely in the early weaning period, and if significant paradoxic motion occurs, mechanical ventilation should be reinstituted. When the flail segment is stable and the patient can maintain adequate ventilation, the use of the ventilator is discontinued and the tracheostomy tube is removed.

Head Injury

The respiratory consequences seen in association with acute brain injury are due to either the direct effect on the respiratory center or the changes in intracranial pressure, and respiratory complications are a significant cause of late mortality.[23] Depending on the location and severity of acute brain injury, different types of ventilatory disturbances, such as central hypoventilation and Cheyne-Stokes breathing, may occur.[24]

Often, the patient with acute brain injury is managed with an artificial airway (usually a tracheostomy) to aid in removal of bronchial secretions. However, the decision to use ventilatory assistance is based on the breathing pattern and arterial blood gas values. In some cases, mechanical hyperventilation may be employed to cause hypocapnic alkalosis and consequent cerebral vasoconstriction in an attempt to decrease intracranial pressure and perhaps aid in hemostasis in the contused brain.[25] In such circumstances, the decision to wean the patient should be made when the need for active cerebral vasoconstriction has passed.

In patients in whom arterial blood gas values indicate hypoventilation, mechanical ventilation is necessary until the patient's spontaneous minute ventilation becomes adequate. Patients with Cheyne-Stokes breathing or apneic spells require the use of either a ventilation monitor or mechanical ventilation, which should be continued until a regular respiratory pattern is established.[26] Pulmonary oxygen transport may be diminished as a result of associated causes, such as neurogenic pulmonary edema, pulmonary contusion, or aspiration requiring supplemental oxygen either with or without ventilatory assistance.

In the absence of pre-existing or complicating pulmonary disease, patients can be weaned rapidly once the underlying ventilatory disturbance is corrected. Once ventilatory assistance has been discontinued, the tracheostomy is often necessary in the obtunded patient to provide adequate bronchial hygiene.

Neuromuscular Diseases

The weaning from ventilatory support of patients with neuromuscular problems such as myasthenia gravis, poliomyelitis, Guillain-Barré syndrome, acute intermittent porphyria, and muscular dystrophy poses special problems owing to the prolonged duration of mechanical assistance.

As a consequence of prolonged ventilatory assistance, two physiologic features may occur: (1) a "resetting" of the patient's respiratory center to a lower Pa_{CO_2} level and (2) alterations in lung and chest-wall stretch receptors induced by large V_T.[27,28] During the weaning period, the patient may have to maintain a minute ventilation equivalent to that present during mechanical ventilation. This may, in turn, lead to early fatigue, requiring reinstitution of mechanical ventilation. In addition, the inability of the patient to achieve large V_T spontaneously could lead to dyspnea despite adequate arterial blood gas values.

The initial weaning attempt should commence when the patient can take reasonable tidal breaths (e.g., 5 ml/kg body weight). This criterion is obviously less stringent than those previously stated, but it is a useful guide for initiating weaning in this challenging group of patients. The first periods of weaning should be limited to three to five minutes each half hour, with gradual increments added as tolerated. At later stages, periodic large V_T should be provided, either by the ventilator or manually, if the patient is not capable of "sighing." In patients who experience excessive difficulty in the early phases of weaning, IMV may be beneficial. The tracheostomy should be maintained until the patient is capable of generating an effective cough, swallowing adequately, and maintaining normal arterial blood gas values over several days.

Adult Respiratory Distress Syndrome

The duration of weaning in the patient with the adult respiratory distress syndrome depends upon the severity of the acute lung injury, the presence of significant underlying lung disease, the age, and the general condition of the patient. If there are additional complications, such as oxygen toxicity or infection, long-term mechanical ventilation may be required and may interfere with weaning. The weaning period itself is usually prolonged during the slow healing process (see Chap. 8).

The patient with adult respiratory distress syndrome usually cannot be weaned if inspired oxygen fractions of greater than 0.4 or modifications of pressure wave forms such as positive end-expiratory pressure are required. A decrease in static recoil pressure indicates improved lung compliance and may be useful as a guideline to initiate weaning. In certain patients with diminished pulmonary oxygen transport, the transition to spontaneous ventilation may be expedited by the use of continuous positive-pressure breathing (CPPB), which provides positive end-expiratory pressure without a ventilator. This technique has also been called "continuous positive airway pressure." Continuous positive-pressure breathing may be achieved by use of a pressure source and reservoir on the inspiratory side and by immersing the expiratory line from the T-tube setup to the desired depth under water. As pulmonary oxygen transport improves, the F_{IO_2} can be reduced to 0.4; with an adequate arterial oxygen tension of more than 55 mm Hg, CPPB is discontinued, and the weaning process is continued in the conventional manner if oxygenation remains satisfactory.

Restrictive Pulmonary Disease

The necessity for ventilatory assistance is frequently due to an acute insult, such as pulmonary infection or a surgical procedure.

When the acute process has been resolved, weaning should be initiated. Since diminished pulmonary oxygen transport is the significant feature in patients with pulmonary fibrosis, supplemental oxygen should be used to achieve an adequate Pa_{O_2}. In contrast, the main problem of those with chest-wall restriction is alveolar hypoventilation during spontaneous breathing, and therefore a gradual weaning process is usually required.

USE OF VENTILATORS IN CARDIOPULMONARY ARREST

It must be emphatically stressed that the respirators described in this chapter are solely for the support of patients who require assis-

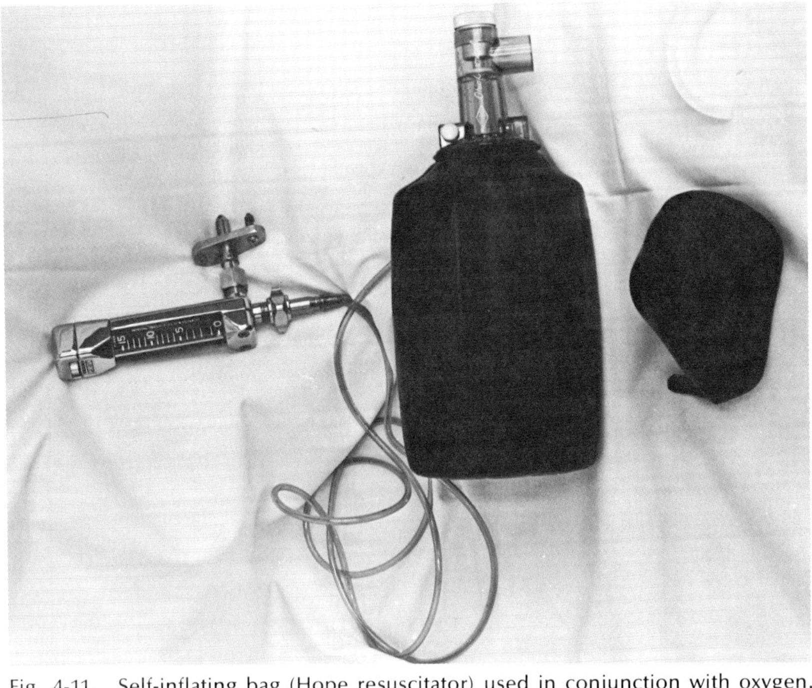

Fig. 4-11. Self-inflating bag (Hope resuscitator) used in conjunction with oxygen. May be attached directly to 15-mm connector of standard endotracheal or tracheostomy tubes or may be used with a face mask.

tance for ventilation and control of oxygen. The devices are not useful in resuscitation; in emergencies, the effective self-inflating bags such as the Hope resuscitator (Fig. 4-11), Ambu bag, and Air Viva are much more applicable to the situation at hand. All these devices have standardized 15-mm connectors to attach to the tracheostomy or endotracheal tube (see Chap. 2). They are simple to use and should be employed immediately for resuscitation in all forms of ventilatory failure. Their capabilities of oxygen delivery vary considerably, with the Ambu bag providing the highest oxygen concentrations.[29] They are often used with a simple face mask rather than a definitive airway. Once a definitive airway (endotracheal or tracheostomy tube) is in place, the device can still be used for situations in which ventilatory demands are changing. These situations may include the need to transport the patient or the discomfort of the patient when a pressure-cycled, volume-cycled, or time-cycled device is employed. Supplemental oxygen may be needed in shock states, but otherwise simple ventilation will provide adequate oxygenation.

Automatic ventilators are not found in our emergency room and are not available to the ward. They are used solely in the intensive care unit for the support phase of respiratory care while definitive therapy is being applied. The self-inflating bags are also valuable in the event of ventilator malfunction. They are delivered as standard equipment with each automatic ventilation device. One should not attempt to repair a malfunctioning ventilator while it is attached to the patient, but rather should use the simple self-inflating bag until the mechanical ventilator is replaced or appropriately repaired. The only possible disadvantage of self-inflating bags is the difficulty in achieving high oxygen fractions, through the side arm or terminal port for oxygen. Use of a reservoir tube or bag corrects this problem (Fig. 4-12).

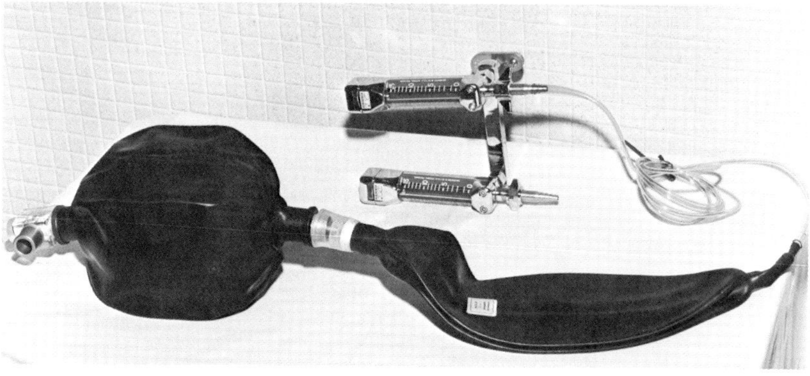

Fig. 4-12. Method of supplying 100% oxygen to self-inflating Ambu resuscitator. Oxygen from wall or portable source fills anesthesia bag, which serves as a reservoir for filling of Ambu bag.

In summary, industry has provided us with a variety of machines of varying capability, ranging from simple pressure-cycled devices to the more complex and excellently designed constant-volume ventilators. The choice of a ventilator depends upon the patient's individual needs, since all machines provide transpulmonary pressure and deliver airflow into the lungs. The abilities to control rate, volume, and inspiratory-expiratory ratio, to vary the tidal volume, and to control the inspiratory-expiratory pressure contour are desirable features of modern respirators.

REFERENCES

1. Heironimus, T.W.: Mechanical Artificial Ventilation: A Manual for Students and Practitioners. 2nd Ed. Springfield, IL, Charles C Thomas, 1971, p. 102.
2. Mushin, M.W., Baker, L.R., Thompson, P.W., and Mappleson, W.W.: Automatic Ventilation of the Lungs. 2nd Ed. Philadelphia, F.A. Davis, 1969, p. 841.
3. Harris, T.M., Gray, M., Petty, T.L., and Mueller, R.E.: Monitoring inspired oxygen pressure during mechanical ventilation. JAMA, *206:*2885, 1968.
4. Hedley-Whyte, J., Laver, M.B., and Bendixin, H.H.: Effect of changes in tidal ventilation on physiological shunting. Am. J. Physiol., *206:*891, 1964.
5. Petty, T.L., Nett, L.M., and Schmader, R.D.: A simple ventilator warning device. Inhal. Ther., *14:*67, 1969.
6. Fairley, H.B.: The mechanical ventilation sign is a dodo. Resp. Care, *21:*1127, 1976.
7. Nicrota, M.B., Stevens, P.M., Viroslav, J., and Alverez, A.A.: Physiologic evaluation of positive end expiratory pressure. Chest, *64:*10, 1973.
8. Dantzker, D.R., Lynch, J.P., and Weg, J.G.: Depression of cardiac output is a mechanism of shunt reduction in the therapy of acute respiratory failure. Chest, *77:*636, 1980.
9. Cassidy, S.S., Robertson, C.H., Pierce, A.K., and Johnson, R.L.: Positive end expiratory pressure in dogs. J. Appl. Physiol., *44:*31, 1978.
10. Manny, J., Grindlinger, G., Malke, A.A., and Hechman, H.B.: PEEP lung stretch and decreased myocardial contractility. Surgery, *84:*127, 1978.
11. Sahn, S.A., and Lakshminarayan, S.: Bedside criteria for discontinuation of mechanical ventilation. Chest, *63:*1002, 1973.
12. Sahn, S.A., Lakshminarayan, S., and Petty, T.L.: Weaning from mechanical ventilation. JAMA, *235:*2208, 1976.
13. Ashbaugh, D.G., Bigelow, D.B., Petty, T.L., and Levine, B.E.: Acute respiratory distress in adults. Lancet, *2:*319, 1967.
14. Petty, T.L., and Ashbaugh, D.G.: The adult respiratory distress syndrome—clinical features, factors influencing prognosis and principles of management. Chest, *70:*233, 1971.
15. Springer, R.R., and Stevens, P.M.: The influence of PEEP on survival in respiratory failure. Am. J. Med., *66:*196, 1979.
16. Toung, T.J.K., Paharia, P., Mitzner, W.A., Permutt, S., and Cameron, J.L.: The beneficial and harmful effect of positive end expiratory pressure. Surg. Gynecol. Obstet., *147:*518, 1978.
17. O'Donohue, W.J.: Positive end expiratory pressure is not a panacea. Chest, *76:*373, 1979.
18. Good, J.T., Wolz, J.F., Anderson, J.T., Dreisin, R.B., and Petty, T.L.: The routine use of positive end expiratory pressure after open heart surgery. Chest, *76:*397, 1979.
19. Peril, A., Olschvang, D., Eimeral, D., Kutzenelsm, R., and Coter, S.: The variable effect of PEEP in acute respiratory failure associated with multiple trauma. J. Trauma, *18:*218, 1978.
20. Kanarek, D.J., and Shanon, D.C.: Adverse effect of positive end expiratory pressure on pulmonary perfusion and arterial oxygenation. Am. Rev. Resp. Dis., *112:*457, 1975.

21. Petty, T.L., and Nett, L.M.: After-crisis care in chronic airway obstruction. Chest, *62:*58s, 1972.
22. Kemmerer, W.T., Eckert, W.G., Guithright, J.B., et al.: Patterns of thoracic injuries in fatal traffic accidents. J. Trauma, *1:*595, 1961.
23. Ulin, A.W., Rosomoff, H.L., Berkowitz, D., et al.: Acute head injury: A review of 1000 cases. Am. Surg., *19:*226, 1953.
24. Plum, F.: Neural mechanisms of abnormal respiration in humans. Arch. Neurol., *3:*484, 1960.
25. Gordon, E.: Controlled respiration in the management of patients with traumatic brain injuries. Acta Anaesthesiol. Scand., *15:*193, 1971.
26. Sutton, F.D., Nett, L.M., and Petty, T.L.: A new ventilation monitor for the intensive respiratory care unit. Resp. Care, *19:*196, 1974.
27. Smith, A.C., Spalding, J.M.K., and Watson, W.E.: CO_2 as a stimulus to spontaneous ventilation after prolonged artificial ventilation. J. Physiol. *160:*32, 1961.
28. Smith, A.C., Spalding, J.M.K., and Watson, W.E.: Ventilation volume as a stimulus to spontaneous ventilation after prolonged artificial ventilation. J. Physiol., *160:*20, 1961.
29. Carden, E.B., Chir, B., and Bernstein, M.: Investigation of the nine most commonly used resuscitator bags. JAMA, *212:*589, 1970.

Chapter 5

HEMODYNAMIC MONITORING DURING SUPPORTIVE MANAGEMENT

(With Reference to Adult Respiratory Distress Syndrome)

By J. Brevard Haynes

Since the introduction of the technique by Swan and associates in 1970, flow-directed, balloon-tipped catheterization of the pulmonary artery has become integral in the management of the critically ill patient. This technique has the advantage that the derived pressures provide a better index of overall cardiopulmonary function than do central venous pressures. The catheter has since been adapted to permit reliable, simple, serial determinations of cardiac output by means of the thermodilution technique. Percutaneous arterial catheterization has permitted continuous monitoring of systolic pressure and an easy access to arterial blood samples. Thus, the physician, nurse, or technician can measure numerous hemodynamic parameters at the bedside over a several-day period, which previously could be obtained only transiently in the cardiac catheterization laboratory. However, one should be thoroughly aware of the potential risks and sources of error inherent to these techniques. When one keeps this in mind, intelligent decisions can be made regarding the indications for these techniques and the utilization of these results to make appropriate changes in therapy.

The purpose of this chapter is to review cardiac performance and the bedside techniques that can be employed to assess this performance. The effects of positive end-expiratory pressure ventilation (PEEP) on the cardiopulmonary system are summarized. Finally, a practical approach to the patient with the adult respiratory distress syndrome (ARDS) that uses these techniques is presented (also see Chap. 8).

CARDIAC PERFORMANCE

Cardiac output is dependent upon heart rate and stroke volume. The three determinants of stroke volume are left ventricular end-diastolic volume (LVEDV), afterload, and contractility. In the intact heart, these factors are complexly interrelated, but they can be considered separately for purposes of discussion.

The Frank-Starling Law states that the amount of energy released during contraction depends upon the length of the muscle fiber prior to contraction. As the muscle fiber is progressively stretched during diastole, there is a progressive increase in the tension developed during systole. In the whole heart, this diastolic muscle-fiber stretch is proportional to LVEDV: The greater the LVEDV, the greater the average muscle-fiber stretch and, hence, the greater the stroke volume. This LVEDV is affected by total blood volume, distribution of that blood volume, the duration of diastole, and atrial systole. For a given state of left ventricular compliance, this LVEDV correlates with a given left ventricular end-diastolic pressure (LVEDP), a pressure that in general can be equated with left atrial and pulmonary wedge pressure (PWP). Thus, therapeutic manipulation of the LVEDV is an important means of altering stroke volume, and PWP may be used as an index of this LVEDV.

Ventricular afterload may be defined as the ventricular wall tension that develops during systole. According to the LaPlace Law, this tension is proportional to the systolic ventricular pressure and the ventricular radius. Thus, increases in afterload may occur with elevation of ventricular pressure resulting from an increase in aortic pressure or from aortic stenosis, or with increase in ventricular size. Increase in afterload causes a reduction in stroke volume. In the absence of valvular obstruction, mean systolic pressure is a rough index of left ventricular afterload, as mean pulmonary artery pressure is an index of right ventricular afterload.

Ventricular contractility is a measure of ventricular performance for a given LVEDV and afterload. Thus, if these latter two determinants of stroke volume are held constant, a factor that increases contractility will increase stroke volume. Many factors, both intrinsic and extrinsic, affect contractility, including sympathomimetic agents, neural impulses, and cardiac glycosides. Contractility is difficult to assess at the bedside in that it is difficult to separate the changes resulting from an increase in contractility from those resulting from an alteration of LVEDV and afterload. However, the use of a thermodilution Swan-Ganz catheter may permit a rough assessment of changes in contractility. For example, computation of cardiac output and heart rate permits calculation of stroke volume. An intervention that increases stroke volume without altering mean systolic pressure or pulmonary wedge pressure does so by increasing contractility.

PULMONARY WEDGE PRESSURE

Pulmonary wedge pressure (PWP) is measured through a catheter that has been inserted or wedged distally into a small branch of the pulmonary artery. If there is no flow around the catheter, the static column of blood distal to it will transmit impulses from the pressure source through the catheter to the transducer. If this column of blood is continuous from the catheter tip to the left atrium, the PWP will closely approximate left atrial pressure. Although pulmonary capillary pressure is difficult to measure directly, the PWP probably approximates the pressure of the pulmonary capillary bed. Thus, the PWP is used as (1) an index of LVEDV and (2) an index of pulmonary capillary hydrostatic pressure, an important Starling factor influencing fluid flux between the capillary and the interstitium. Two criteria are used to distinguish PWP: As the catheter tip becomes wedged by either inflation of the balloon or manual advancement of the catheter, (1) the phasic contour changes from pulmonary artery tracing to one resembling a left atrial tracing, and (2) mean PWP becomes less than mean pulmonary pressure (Fig. 5-1). However, even if both criteria are achieved, PWP is an index of LVEDV only if the following correlations are maintained:

1. Transmural LVEDP is an index of LVEDV.
2. LVEDP referenced against atmospheric pressure is an index of transmural LVEDP.
3. Atrial pressure is an index of LVEDP.
4. PWP is an index of left atrial pressure.
5. PWP is being accurately recorded.

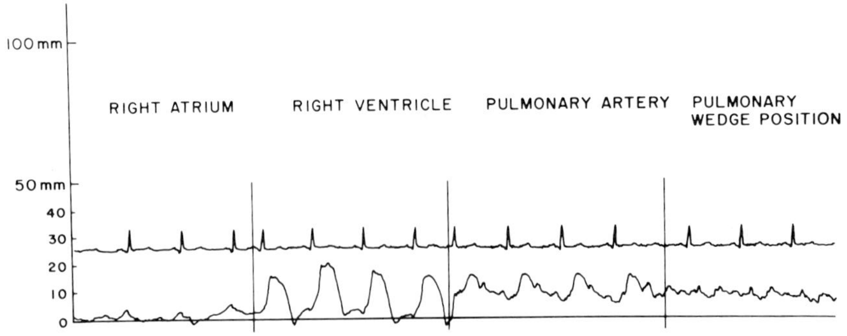

Fig. 5-1. Representative pressure wave forms recorded during advancement of a pulmonary artery catheter.

First, LVEDP may not be a valid index of LVEDV. The diastolic pressure–volume relationship may be altered in certain disease states in such a way that a given LVEDV is associated with either a higher or a lower LVEDP. For example, ventricular hypertrophy may stiffen the ventricle during diastole such that a higher pressure is associated with a given LVEDV; however, for a given state of hypertrophy, increases in LVEDV will be reflected in increases in LVEDP. In this situation, PWP may still be interpreted. Other situations, such as left ventricular ischemia or mechanical ventilation with PEEP, may alter the diastolic pressure–volume relationship only

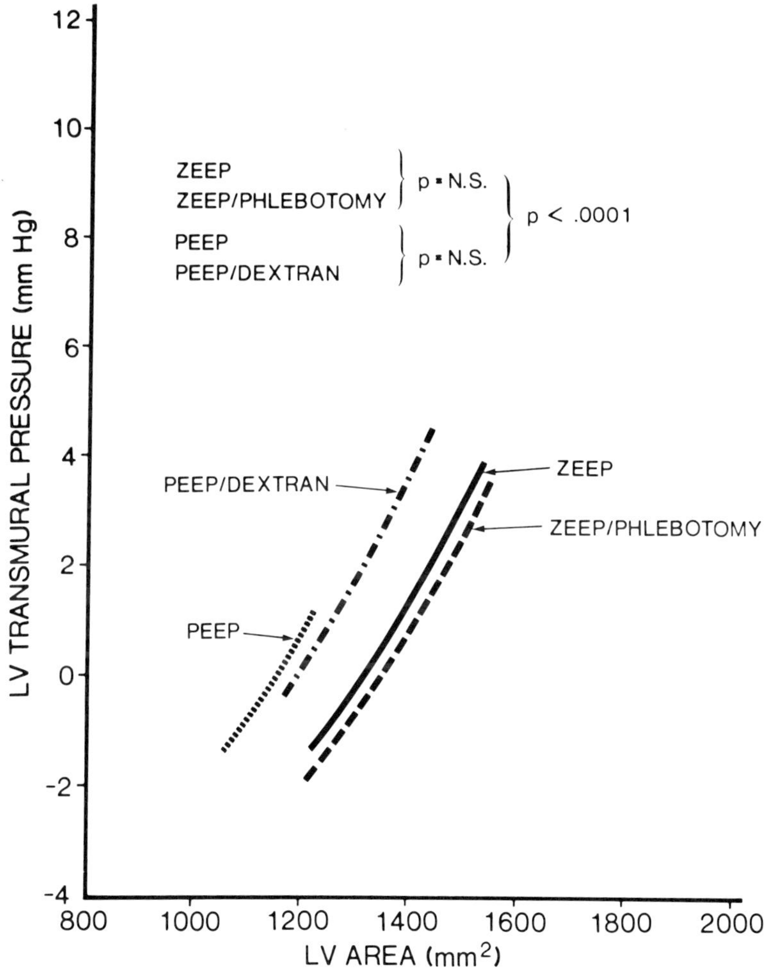

Fig. 5-2. Mean left ventricular pressure-area curves for four study conditions. Curves are drawn from the mean area at onset of diastole to mean area at end-diastole. Note that the PEEP-related conditions are shifted upward, consistent with PEEP-induced stiffening of the left ventricle.

transiently, making changes in PWP more difficult to interpret. PEEP transiently stiffens the left ventricle during diastole such that a given LVEDV is associated with a higher transmural LVEDP or PWP (Fig. 5-2).[1] These PEEP-induced alterations in diastolic pressure–volume relationships make interpretation of PWP difficult; one cannot be certain which component of an increase in "transmural" PWP is due to PEEP and which is due to a real increase in LVEDV. Indeed, these alterations may explain previous studies which conclude that PEEP depresses left ventricular contractility. The reduction in stroke volume, which may occur with PEEP when transmural LVEDP is maintained constant, has been interpreted as a PEEP-induced reduction in contractility when indeed the reduction in stroke volume is due to a reduction in LVEDV that is not reflected by a reduction in transmural LVEDP.

In all clinical situations, intracardiac pressures are referenced to atmospheric pressure because of the complexities of measuring pericardial or pleural pressure. This atmospheric referencing is satisfactory if intrathoracic pressure does not fluctuate widely. However, if intrathoracic pressure changes, the net diastolic filling of the ventricle is dependent upon the transmural pressure between the ventricle and pericardium (Fig. 5-3). Mechanical ventilation with PEEP results in an increase in alveolar pressure which, in turn, causes

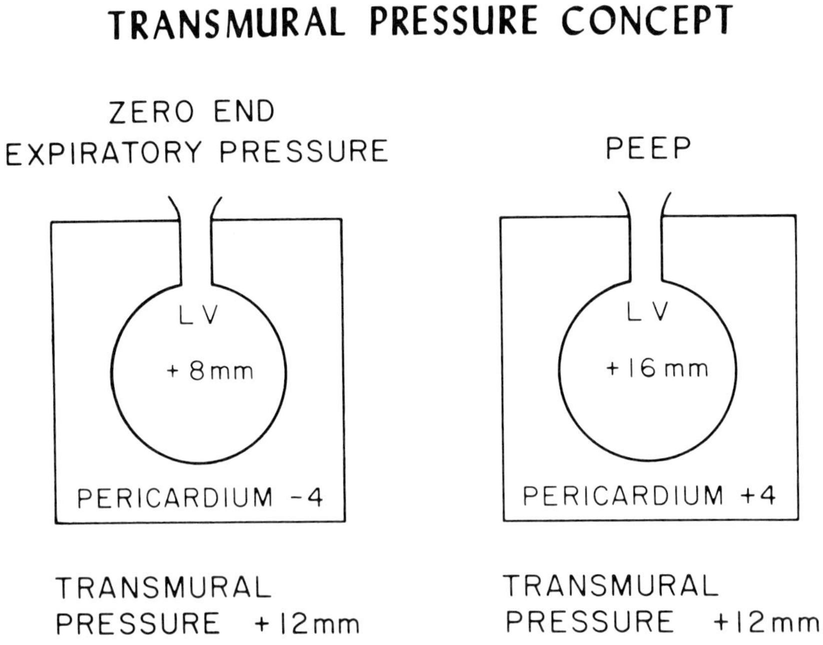

Fig. 5-3. Changes in pericardial pressure with use of PEEP necessitate the concept of a transmural pressure. See text for discussion.

pleural and pericardial pressures to increase. In animals, the increase in pleural or pericardial pressure is approximately 50 percent of the increase in end-expiratory airway pressure.[1,2] For example, if LVEDP and pleural pressure measured relative to atmospheric pressure are +8 mm Hg and −4 mm Hg respectively, the transmural LVEDP is +12 mm Hg. Ventilation with 15 mm Hg (20 cm H_2O) of PEEP would cause pleural pressure to increase approximately 8 mm Hg, from −4 to +4 mm Hg. If transmural LVEDP remains constant, mechanical ventilation with 15 mm Hg PEEP should cause LVEDP relative to atmospheric pressure to increase to 16 mm (12 mm + 4 mm) Hg. If the clinician interpreting PWP fails to consider these changes, he may falsely interpret the increase in PWP or LVEDP measured relative to atmospheric pressure as being consistent with increased LVEDV when, indeed, there has been no change.

The third assumption one must make in order to use PWP as an index of LVEDV is that left atrial pressure approximates LVEDP. This assumption is generally true unless mitral stenosis is present.

Pulmonary wedge pressure will approximate left atrial pressure if there is a static, continuous column of blood between the atrium and the catheter tip. West et al. have demonstrated that the distribution of blood flow throughout the pulmonary capillary bed is dependent upon mechanical forces, both inside and outside the pulmonary bed

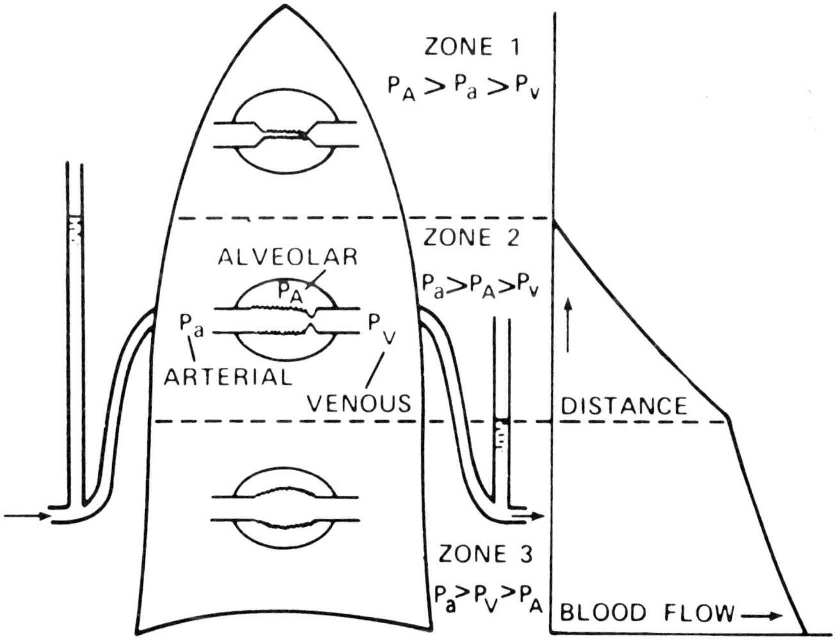

Fig. 5-4. Model to explain pressure-induced alterations in the distribution of pulmonary blood flow. (Reproduced with the permission of J.B. West.)

(Fig. 5-4).[3] Three zones have been described: In Zone I, alveolar pressure (P_A) is greater than both left atrial pressure (P_{LA}) reflected by P_V and pulmonary arterial pressure (P_{Pa}). In Zone II, P_{Pa} is greater than P_A, which is greater than P_{LA}. In Zone III, P_{Pa} is greater than P_{LA}, which is greater than P_A. If the catheter tip is advanced into a Zone I vessel, the continuous column of blood between the catheter tip and the left atrium will be compressed and thus interrupted by the alveoli, which are under greater pressure than the surrouding vasculature. In this situation, the catheter tip would register a pressure equal to the alveolar pressure plus the pressure equivalent of the vertical height between the catheter tip and the transducer zero reference point. Because of the lack of flow to this zone, a flow-directed catheter would not be carried out into such vessels.

A catheter that is advanced into a Zone II vessel also would not measure left atrial pressure because as the balloon tip occludes flow, alveolar pressure exceeds left atrial pressure, which interrupts the continuity between the catheter tip and left atrium. Thus, only catheters that are advanced into Zone III vessels will accurately reflect left atrial pressure. Two situations convert more of the lung from Zone III to Zones I and II: hypovolemia and mechanical ventilation with PEEP.[4,5] In animal studies, pulmonary artery catheters that are wedged into vessels lower than the left atrium will accurately reflect left atrial pressure despite increasing levels of PEEP (to 30 cm H_2O) or progressive hemorrhage. Catheters that have been advanced into vessels higher than the left atrium will not accurately record left atrial pressure, however. Recent studies in humans demonstrate that flow-directed catheters usually are carried into a Zone III vessel, and that PWP reflects left atrial pressure despite mechanical ventilation with PEEP up to 15 cm H_2O.[6,7] Despite this correlation between PWP and left atrial pressures measured relative to atmospheric pressure, however, these pressures may be spuriously elevated by PEEP when compared with their transmural counterparts.

The final link in the chain that makes PWP an index of LVEDV is the recording of an accurate PWP. Spurious pressures may be recorded if the catheter is positioned in a peripheral branch rather than the large pulmonary artery.[8] In this situation, balloon inflation may be eccentric, which causes the catheter tip to impinge on the vessel wall. If a continuous flush system is being utilized, the recorded pressure will be dampened and will rise steadily to values that are higher than mean pulmonary artery pressure. This error can be avoided if the catheter position is checked radiographically and if balloon inflation is stopped at the minimal balloon volume required to wedge the catheter.

Pressures will also be incorrect if the zero reference point of the transducer is not the same vertical height as the left atrium. During the calibration procedure, a stopcock attached to the transducer is opened to expose the transducer to atmospheric pressure. This stopcock should be at the level of the left atrium in order to establish a correct zero baseline. If this stopcock is lower than the left atrium, all subsequently recorded pressures will be spuriously elevated by a pressure equivalent to the vertical distance in centimeters of water between the stopcock and the left atrium. Conversely, if the stopcock is higher than the left atrium, pressures will be spuriously low.

Another potential source of error is in calibration of the strain-gauge transducer. After a zero baseline has been established, calibration is usually performed electronically rather than by imposing a known quantity of pressure on the transducer. Electronic calibration is relatively accurate if properly performed. If there is doubt about its accuracy, a known quantity of pressure can be applied to the transducer with a slightly modified sphygmomanometer. Since the height of the bed and transducer can be inadvertently changed and room temperature may drift, frequent calibration checks should be performed in order to ensure that pressures are being accurately recorded.

TECHNIQUES OF PULMONARY ARTERIAL CATHETERIZATION

The Swan-Ganz catheter can be inserted either into an antecubital vein which has been exposed by means of surgical cut-down or into other veins by means of percutaneous puncture. Possible access sites are the subclavian, internal jugular, or femoral veins.[9,10] Use of catheter introducer sets, which include a catheter sheath, a dilator, and a spring guide, facilitates percutaneous insertion. The choice of sites is usually made on the basis of individual preference and experience. If the patient is being mechanically ventilated with PEEP, the consequences of inadvertent visceral pleural puncture (pneumothorax with possible bronchopleural fistula formation) must be considered when contemplating percutaneous subclavian insertion.

Once the catheter tip has been passed into the subclavian vein, the balloon is inflated to facilitate passage. The catheter is gently advanced as the pressure tracing is being monitored. Changes in pressure-wave form serve as nonfluoroscopic verification of catheter position. The balloon serves to carry and guide the catheter through the right heart. As the catheter is advanced into the pulmonary artery, the balloon will become wedged; the pressure-wave form will change from a pulmonary arterial to a left atrial configuration (see Fig. 5-1). The catheter is positioned such that inflation of the balloon results in a left atrial configuration and deflation results in a prompt return of a pulmonary arterial configuration. During advancement of the catheter, some slack may accumulate which, with time, will allow migration of the catheter tip into a permanently wedged position. It is prudent to wait several minutes before suturing the catheter in place in order for the catheter tip position to stabilize.

Determination of Cardiac Output with Thermodilution

Although the thermodilution technique was described in 1954, it did not gain widespread acceptance until the development of the Swan-Ganz thermistor-tipped catheter. The thermodilution method is an indicator dilution technique in which temperature change is the indicator. An exact quantity of chilled dextrose in water is rapidly injected through the right atrial port of the catheter. The thermistor, located near the catheter tip, senses temperature change within the pulmonary artery, which is integrated to calculate cardiac output. Cardiac output measurements obtained by this method correlate well with those obtained by both Fick and dye-dilution techniques. The advantages over the dye-dilution technique are that serial determinations can be performed rapidly, without significant recirculation of the indicator, and without the need for blood withdrawal.

As with any technique, deviation from specifications will lead to spurious results. The volume and temperature of the injectate should be precise, and the appropriate constant should be entered into the computer. The syringe of injectate is quickly removed from the ice bath and is rapidly injected into the right atrial port as a bolus. Because of the potential decrease in venous return during the inspiratory phase of positive pressure ventilation, the bolus should be injected during the expiratory phase. Several determinations should be performed, and the mean value should be recorded as the cardiac output.

Complications of Pulmonary Artery Catheterization

Flow-directed pulmonary artery catheterization, like any invasive diagnostic procedure, carries a risk which must be weighed against the benefits of employing the technique. However, these risks are low when both medical and nursing staffs are aware of potential problems and strive to avoid them by strict adherence to proper technique.[11] Transient arrhythmias that may occur during catheter insertion usually resolve with proper positioning to minimize the looping of the catheter in the right ventricle. However, on occasion the catheter must be removed because of persistence of the arrhythmia. Balloon rupture may occur if the balloon volume is exceeded or if inflation is continued beyond the minimal volume required to wedge the catheter tip. Injection of 1 to 2 ml air into the pulmonary circulation is probably harmless; however, air embolism into the systemic circulation may result in serious damage. If a right-to-left shunt is suspected, the balloon should be inflated with carbon dioxide.

As with any indwelling catheter, Swan-Ganz catheters may become colonized with infectious organisms, especially if the patient has a source of infection prior to catheterization. While colonization does not necessarily lead to bacteremia or local infection, the incidence of such colonization can be minimized if the duration of the catheterization is less than 72 hours and if the catheter is not advanced.[12] The only acceptable repositioning maneuver is slight withdrawal from a permanent wedge position; catheter advancement after the initial insertion should be avoided. Local thrombosis of the antecubital or subclavian vein may occur, but the incidence of this is low. A more serious complication is pulmonary infarction, which may occur if the catheter tip remains wedged owing to either unrecognized catheter migration or failure to deflate the balloon.[13] Fatal pulmonary arterial rupture has been reported. Prevention of distal migration of the catheter and rapid inflation of the balloon will probably eliminate this disastrous situation.[14]

BEDSIDE ARTERIAL CATHETERIZATION

Since the safety of arterial puncture has become apparent, knowledge of arterial blood gases is considered essential in the management of the critically ill patient. If frequent serial samples are needed or if continuous monitoring of arterial pressure is necessary, an indwelling catheter may be inserted. The two major risks of this procedure—infection and thrombosis—can be minimized if appropriate precautions are taken.[15,16] After Allen's test is performed to demonstrate ulnar artery patency, an 18- to 20-gauge Teflon catheter is inserted percutaneously into the radial artery. Surgical cutdown may be performed but is associated with a higher incidence of local infection. Patency of the catheter is maintained with continuous infusion of heparinized saline through a Sorenson intraflow device. To-and-fro movement of the catheter is decreased by suturing the catheter hub to the skin.

To minimize infection, the catheter should not be left in place more than four days.[16] If continuous monitoring is needed, the other radial artery is used. Arterial thrombosis occurs more frequently if catheters are left in place six days or more, if hypotension is present, or if vasoactive drugs are given.[15] This complication occurred in 0.6% of the series reported by Gardner et al. All cases were successfully managed with thrombectomy.

MIXED VENOUS BLOOD GAS ANALYSIS

Mixed venous blood drawn through the Swan-Ganz catheter may be analyzed for hemoglobin saturation ($S\bar{v}O_2$) or oxygen tension ($P\bar{v}O_2$) as an index of tissue oxygenation. These mixed venous values may be interpreted alone or in combination with arterial values (Table 5-1). The basic goal in the management of ARDS is to maintain adequate tissue oxygenation (see Chap. 8). Systemic oxygen transport, the product of cardiac output and arterial oxygen content, is the absolute value of oxygen available to the body. This value requires cardiac output determination, which may not be practical if a thermodilution Swan-Ganz catheter has not been employed. Mixed venous blood drawn through a standard Swan-Ganz catheter may be

TABLE 5-1. Parameters of Tissue Oxygenation

Term	*Symbol*	*Normal**	*Comments*
Arterial oxygen tension	PaO_2	97 mm Hg	
Mixed venous oxygen tension	$P\bar{v}O_2$	38 to 42 mm Hg	May approximate tissue oxygen tension
Oxygen hemoglobin saturation			
Arterial	SaO_2	0.95–0.97	
Mixed venous	$S\bar{v}O_2$	0.70–0.75	
Blood oxygen content			
Arterial	CaO_2	19.5 ml/dl	Equals hemoglobin concentration × 1.34 × saturation
Mixed venous	$C\bar{v}O_2$	15.0 ml/dl	
Oxygen consumption (Tissue demand)	$\dot{V}O_2$	250 ml/min	
Cardiac output (Fick Principle)	$\dot{Q}T$	4–7 L/min	Equals $\dot{V}O_2/(CaO_2 - C\bar{v}O_2) \times .1$
Oxygen transport (Tissue supply)	—	1100 ml/min	Equals $\dot{Q}T \times CaO_2 \times 10$
Coefficient of oxygen delivery (Supply/demand ratio)	COD	4–4.5	Equals $CaO_2/(CaO_2 - C\bar{v}O_2)$

* Refers to a healthy resting adult at sea level breathing room air.

analyzed for hemoglobin saturation or oxygen concentration, however. These values may be interpreted alone or in combination with arterial values as an index of tissue oxygenation.

Theoretic models suggest that mixed venous oxygen tension approximates mean tissue tensions.[17] The coefficient of oxygen delivery is a ratio of tissue oxygen supply to tissue oxygen demand.[18] This value is calculated by measuring arterial and mixed venous hemoglobin saturations simultaneously. To adjust therapy on the basis of arterial oxygen tension alone completely disregards the effect that therapy may have on cardiac output. If one suspects that cardiac output is being adversely affected, oxygen transport, mixed venous oxygen content, or coefficient of oxygen delivery should be monitored as an index of tissue oxygenation. Therapy can then be altered to optimize this situation. Venous blood should be sampled from the pulmonary artery in order to ensure that there has been adequate mixing of blood from both superior and inferior vena cava and from the coronary sinus.

In critically ill patients, oxygen tension or hemoglobin saturation of blood obtained from the superior vena cava may not approximate values from the pulmonary artery.[19] If a large volume of blood is rapidly aspirated from the Swan-Ganz catheter, it is possible that the sample may contain pulmonary capillary or pulmonary venous blood, the oxygen content of which may equal that of systemic arterial blood.[20,21] In order to minimize the possibility of spurious results, the pressure tracing is analyzed to ensure that the tip is sensing pulmonary arterial pressure rather than pulmonary wedge pressure. Two to three milliliters of fluid are aspirated from the catheter and discarded as dead space. Two to three milliliters of blood are then aspirated over a 60-second period for analysis as a mixed venous sample.

MECHANICAL VENTILATION AND HEMODYNAMIC MONITORING IN THE ADULT RESPIRATORY DISTRESS SYNDROME

The adult respiratory distress syndrome (see Chap. 8) is used to describe the abrupt onset of respiratory failure in a patient who has recently suffered a catastrophic insult, such as shock, multiple trauma, extensive burns, sepsis, and so forth. The patient rapidly becomes dyspneic; severe hypoxemia and radiographic evidence of pulmonary edema are subsequently detected. Mechanical ventilation is invariably necessary, but high inspired concentrations of oxygen do not correct the hypoxemia. Pulmonary wedge pressure is within a normal range; mild to moderate pulmonary hypertension is usually present. Occasionally, copious quantities of edema fluid may be aspirated from the trachea. The protein concentration of this fluid, expressed as a ratio to total plasma protein concentration, is high relative to the edema-fluid protein concentration in cardiogenic pulmonary edema.[22] This increase in fluid protein concentration is thought to represent increased permeability of the pulmonary capillaries.[23] The pathogenic mechanisms by which this increase in permeability occurs remain obscure, however.

Systemic capillary endothelial injury and thrombosis is a common denominator of many of the catastrophic events that precede ARDS. Microembolization of these capillary thrombi could result in increased permeability of the pulmonary capillaries. Indeed, small glass-bead embolization can alter permeability by permitting overperfusion of the nonobstructed portion of the pulmonary capillary bed.[24] This overperfusion may result in abnormally high stresses at capillary bifurcations with a subsequent increase in fluid and protein flux. An alternative explanation is that a humoral agent released during the thrombotic or ensuing fibrinolytic process may increase pulmonary capillary permeability. Animal studies have suggested that fibrin–fibrinogen degradation products may injure the pulmonary vasculature.[25] We have demonstrated that patients who develop ARDS have much higher levels of D-D dimer fibrin degradation product than patients who have equally severe burns or trauma but who do not develop the syndrome (see Chap. 8).[26] The pathogenic sequence of events must be more precisely elucidated before prophylactic or specific therapy can be developed.

The increase in pulmonary capillary permeability permits accumulation of interstitial solute and fluid. If the rate of interstitial fluid formation exceeds the rate of lymphatic reabsorption, the edema progresses to the stage of alveolar flooding. Edema fluid interferes with the action of surfactant to enhance alveolar collapse. Shunting of mixed venous blood through these collapsed segments of the lung results in severe hypoxemia. Mechanical ventilation with PEEP may lessen the severity of this alveolar collapse in such a way that arterial oxygenation is improved. It is important to realize that such therapy is only supportive: Experimental evidence suggests that PEEP does not decrease the extent of the pulmonary edema.[27] Until more specific therapy is available, mechanical ventilation with PEEP should be used to maintain adequate tissue oxygenation without exposing the patient to prolonged periods of high oxygen concentration. As therapy is directed toward the predisposing illness, the relative rate of fluid formation and reabsorption may be reversed so that the edema is slowly cleared.

Mechanical Ventilation with Positive End-Expiratory Pressure in ARDS

It is important to understand the potentially adverse effects of PEEP in order to utilize this type of mechanical ventilation effectively. Although PEEP may improve arterial oxygen content, PEEP tends to reduce cardiac output, an effect that may offset any improvement in oxygen transport. PEEP within the alveoli results in transmission of pressure to the surrounding capillary network and to the pleuropericardial space. Compression of the capillary network increases pulmonary vascular resistance, which, by increasing right ventricular afterload, may increase right atrial pressure. Likewise, the increase in pleuropericardial pressure is transmitted passively through the heart to increase right atrial pressure. Venous return depends upon existence of a pressure gradient between the systemic venous system and the right atrium; thus, PEEP results in a decreased venous return by causing an increase in the right atrial pressure.[28] The resultant decrease in stroke volume elicits a reflex increase in heart rate and in systemic vasoconstriction.[29] The latter response raises the mean capillary pressure, which minimizes the decrease in venous return. Hypovolemia will accentuate the tendency toward cardiac output reduction with PEEP ventilation. In a hypovolemic state, baseline venous return may be borderline. With the addition of PEEP, the compensatory vasoconstriction may not be effective in raising mean circulatory pressure.

Some studies have concluded that PEEP depresses left ventricular contractility. These conclusions are based upon the observation that for a constant transmural atrial or left ventricular end-diastolic pressure, cardiac output (or stroke work) is decreased by PEEP ventilation.[2,28] These conclusions are based on the premise that diastolic pressure–volume characteristics are not altered by PEEP. However, PEEP does alter this relationship in such a way that a given transmural pressure in the setting of PEEP corresponds with a lower end-diastolic volume. These PEEP-induced alterations in left ventricular pressure–volume relationships may result from ventricular interdependence. As the right ventricle distends in response to a PEEP-induced increase in pulmonary vascular resistance, the interventricular septum is also distended; however, this localized septal distention affects the overall pressure–volume characteristics of the left ventricle. Echocardiographic measurements, which demonstrate an increase in right ventricular dimensions with a simultaneous decrease in left ventricular dimensions, support such a theory.[30] If the left ventricular dimensions are used as an index of preload pressure rather than of transmural pressure, no decrease in left ventricular function is detected: As PEEP is applied, both left ventricular end-diastolic area and stroke area decrease.[1] If sufficient dextran is infused to restore end-diastolic area to control values, stroke area is also normalized. This normalization of stroke area, with volume restoration alone, is inconsistent with the theory that PEEP depresses ventricular function.

Assisted Mechanical Ventilation with PEEP versus Intermittent Mandatory Ventilation with CPAP (CPPB)

The acronyms PEEP and CPAP (same as CPPB, see Chap. 4) are used in respiratory therapy to describe different types of airway pressure patterns. Yet these differences are not apparent from the acronym. With assisted mechanical ventilation (AMV) with PEEP, the patient triggers the ventilator with slight inspiratory effort. As the ventilator delivers the tidal volume, airway pressure becomes more positive, but during passive expiration it returns to the level of PEEP that has beeen selected, as controlled by a threshold resistor (see Chap. 4). With intermittent mandatory ventilation and PEEP, the patient breathes spontaneously except for a preselected number of breaths that are delivered by the ventilator. During the spontaneous breaths, the patient must make an inspiratory effort to generate a pressure gradient between the mouth and the alveolus. With expiration, airway pressure rises back to the level of PEEP that has been selected. With CPAP, the patient breathes from a low-pressure source and performs almost all the work of breathing. Exhalation is done against a threshold resistor, similar to PEEP. Thus, CPAP, like PEEP, tends to prevent expiratory alveolar collapse and to increase lung compliance. However, if the work of breathing remains difficult, the patient may tire rendering spontaneous tidal volumes inadequate.

The potential advantage of CPAP is that the negative pleural pressure generated by spontaneous inspiration may enhance venous return in such a way that cardiac output may be comparatively preserved. Clinical studies in ARDS patients have produced conflicting results.[31-33] For a given level of end-expiratory pressure, some patients clearly have a higher cardiac output with CPAP than with PEEP; however, there is no obvious predictor of which patient will demonstrate such an improvement. The majority of patients demonstrate either an improvement or no change in cardiac output with CPAP as compared with PEEP. If PEEP results in a significant decrease in cardiac output, CPAP may be considered. However, the patient must be able to maintain an adequate spontaneous minute ventilation. If high IMV rates are required, one should not expect much difference between cardiac output with CPAP and mechanical ventilation with PEEP.

Optimal PEEP

Because the increasing arterial oxygen content resulting from PEEP may be offset by a concomitant reduction in cardiac output, it is advantageous to define an optimal level of PEEP. If PEEP reduces the severity of the pulmonary edema, one might define optimal PEEP as that level that results in the lowest shunt fraction. By this definition, little emphasis is placed upon changes in cardiac output, and levels of PEEP up to 30 to 40 cm H_2O may be selected.[34] However, in that animal studies suggest that PEEP does not decrease pulmonary edema, it seems more logical to define optimal PEEP as that level which maximizes systemic oxygen transport.[27] Calculation of this or of similar clinical parameters requires that a Swan-Ganz catheter be inserted. In an effort to define optimal PEEP noninvasively, Suter and associates have demonstrated that the level of PEEP that results in maximal systemic oxygen transport is usually the level that optimizes total compliance.[35] However, others have not been able to demonstrate this close correlation.[36] Thus, although invasive techniques are required for its calculation, systemic oxygen transport is probably the optimal parameter upon which to select levels of PEEP.

A Practical Approach to the ARDS Patient

The diagnosis of ARDS should be established based upon the criteria listed in Chapter 8. If cardiogenic causes of the pulmonary edema cannot be definitely excluded upon the basis of age, clinical presentation, and physical examination of the patient, Swan-Ganz catheterization must be performed in order to measure PWP. The finding of a low to normal PWP is consistent with the diagnosis of ARDS. Specific therapy is directed toward the catastrophic event which frequently precedes the onset of ARDS. If there is a possibility of gram-negative sepsis, appropriate antimicrobial drugs and corticosteroids are administered until culture results are available.

For a given state of pulmonary capillary permeability, the lower the capillary pressure, the less severe the edema.[37] Thus, fluid therapy should be reduced to low maintenance levels (50 to 75) ml/hr) if possible. There is no concensus of opinion regarding the type of fluids—crystalloids versus colloids—that are used. The permeable pulmonary capillary bed can no longer sieve proteins in order to generate an osmotic force: thus, it appears more logical to use crystalloids, but this has not been established by clinical trials. In fact, colloid use appears to offer no advantage over crystalloid fluid replacement.[38]

The patient will almost universally require intubation and assisted mechanical ventilation in order to decrease the work of breathing necessary to ventilate the poorly compliant lungs. Usually, high-inspired oxygen concentrations are required, but administration of 100% oxygen should be avoided after the first few hours if possible. Increasing oxygen concentrations above 70 to 80% usually results in only slight improvement in arterial oxygen tension and may actually worsen the shunt fraction through absorptive atelectasis.[39] Likewise, oxygen toxicity is proportional to both the oxygen concentration and duration of that therapy. Ideally, the inspired oxygen concentration should be reduced to 50% or less by 48 to 72 hours. In general, PEEP is required because of persistently low arterial oxygen tensions. If a Swan-Ganz catheter is not in place, the initial level of PEEP can be selected empirically or upon the basis of lung compliance measurements. The initial value should probably be between 5 and 10 cm H_2O. If arterial oxygenation improves and indirect parameters of cardiac output, such as urine output and blood pressure, are adequate, this level is continued for the next 24 to 48 hours.

During this period, the pulmonary edema may be partially reabsorbed, and PEEP can be reduced. However, if arterial oxygenation is not improved or if urine output or blood pressure deteriorates, a Swan-Ganz catheter should be inserted. A baseline PWP is measured from PEEP as an index of intravascular volume. If the volume is low and the blood pressure has fallen with PEEP, fluids should be given to raise this value to the low-normal range. Then simultaneous cardiac output and arterial oxygen tensions are measured at several levels of PEEP. The level of PEEP that maximizes systemic oxygen transport is chosen. If a thermistor-tipped Swan-Ganz catheter is not available, PEEP can be selected based upon mixed venous oxygen tension or upon the coefficient of oxygen delivery. This level of PEEP is maintained 24 to 48 hours, at which time the cardiopulmonary status is reassessed. If improvement has occurred, the inspired oxygen concentration is reduced to 40%, followed by a gradual reduction in PEEP at 3- to 4-cm H_2O increments.

Mechanical ventilation is discontinued when the patient can support his own respirations.

The prognosis for ARDS depends largely upon its cause. The overall survival is approximately 40%, but if ARDS occurs following gram-negative sepsis, the survival rate is only 10%.[40] Patients who do not demonstrate overall improvement within 24 hours have a much poorer prognosis than those who demonstrate a prompt response.[41] Death usually results from either the underlying illness or hemodynamic collapse.

The pathophysiology of ARDS and principles of management are fully discussed in Chapter 8.

REFERENCES

1. Haynes, J.B., Carson, S.M., Whitney, W.P., Zerby, G.O., Hyers, T.M., and Steele, P.: Positive End-Expiratory Pressure shifts left ventricular diastolic pressure-area curves. J. Appl. Physiol., *48:*670, 1980.
2. Prewitt, R.M., and Wood, L.D.H.: Effects of Positive End-Expiratory Pressure on ventricular function in dogs. Am. J. Physiol., *236:*H534, 1979.
3. West, JB., Pallery, C.T., and Naimark, A.: Distribution of blood flow in isolated lung. Relation of vascular and alveolar pressure. J. Appl. Physiol. *19:*713, 1964.
4. Todd, T.R.J., Baile, E.M., and Hogg, J.C.: Pulmonary arterial wedge pressure in hemorrhagic shock. Am. Rev. Resp. Dis., *118:*613, 1978.
5. Tooker, J., Huseby, J., and Butler, J.: The effects of Swan-Ganz catheter height on the wedge pressure-left atrial pressure relationship in edema during positive-pressure ventilation. Am. Rev. Resp. Dis., *117:*721, 1978.
6. Davison, R., Parker, M., and Harrison, R.A.: The validity of determination of pulmonary wedge pressure during mechanical ventilation. Chest, *73:*352, 1978.
7. Cross, C.J., Cain, H.D., Deaton, W.J., Sumerhill, S., and Stevens, P.M.: Vertical relationships of the pulmonary arterial catheter tip and transducer reference point in estimation of the left atrial pressure. Am. Rev. Resp. Dis., *117*[Suppl.]:105, 1978.
8. Shin, B., Ayella, R.J., and McAslan, T.: Pitfalls of Swan-Ganz catheterization. Crit. Care Med., *6:*36, 1978.
9. Rodman, G.H., and Civetta, J.M.: Bedside pulmonary artery catheterization. Arch. Surg., *109:*840, 1974.
10. Civetta, J.M., and Gabel, J.C.: Flow directed-pulmonary artery catheterization in surgical patients: Indications and modifications of technique. Am. Surg., *176:*753, 1972.
11. Elliot, C.G., Zimmerman, G.A., and Clemmer, T.P.: Complications of pulmonary artery catheterization in the care of critically-ill patients. Chest, *76:*647, 1979.
12. Applefeld, J.J., Caruthers, T.E., and Reno, D.J.: Assessment of the sterility of long term cardiac catheterization using the thermodilution Swan-Ganz catheter. Chest, *74:*377, 1978.
13. Foote, G.A., Schabel, S.I., and Hodges, M.: Pulmonary complications of the flow-directed balloon-tipped catheter. N. Engl. J. Med., *290:*927, 1974.
14. Chun, G.M.H., and Ellestad, M.H.: Perforation of the pulmonary artery by a Swan-Ganz catheter. N. Engl. J. Med. *284:*1041, 1971.
15. Gardner, R.M., Schwartz, R., Wong, H.C., and Burke, J.P.: Percutaneous indwelling radial artery catheters for monitoring cardiovascular function. N. Engl. J. Med., *290:*1227, 1974.
16. Band, J.D., and Maki, D.G.: Infections caused by arterial catheters used for hemodynamic monitoring. Am. J. Med. *67:*735, 1979.
17. Tenney, S.M.: A theoretical analysis of the relationship between venous blood and mean tissue oxygen pressures. Resp. Physiol., *20:*283, 1974.
18. Mithoefer, J.C., Holford, F.D., and Keighley, J.F.H.: The effect of oxygen administration on mixed venous oxygenation in chronic obstructive pulmonary disease. Chest, *66:*122, 1974.

19. Scheinman, M.M., Brown, M.A., and Rapapart, E.: Critical assessment of use of central venous oxygen saturation as a mirror of mixed venous oxygen in severely ill cardiac patients. Circulation, *40:*165, 1969.
20. Suter, P.M., Lindaner, J.M., Fairley, B., and Schlobohm, R.M.: Errors in data derived from pulmonary artery blood gas values. Crit. Care Med., *3:*175, 1975.
21. Shapiro, H.M., Smith, G., Pribble, A.H., Murray, J.A., and Cheney, F.W.: Errors in sampling pulmonary arterial blood with a Swan-Ganz catheter. Anesthesiology, *40:*291, 1974.
22. Fein, A., Grossman, R.F., Jones, J.C., Overland, E., Pitts, L., Murray, J.F., and Staub, N.C.: The value of edema fluid protein measurement in patients with pulmonary edema. Am. J. Med., *67:*32, 1979.
23. Staub, N.C.: Pulmonary edema due to increased microvascular permeability to fluid and protein. Circ. Res., *43:*143, 1978.
24. Ohkuda, K., Nakahara, K., Weidner, W.J., Binder, A., and Staub, N.C.: Lung fluid exchange after uneven pulmonary artery obstruction in sheep. Circ. Res., *43:*152, 1978.
25. Manwaring, D., Thorning, D., and Curreri, P.W.: Mechanisms of acute pulmonary dysfunction induced by fibrinogen degradation product D. Surgery, *84:*45, 1978.
26. Haynes, J.B., Hyers, T.M., Giclas, P.C., Franks, J.J., and Petty, T.L.: Elevated fibrin(ogen) degradation products in the Adult Respiratory Distress Syndrome. Am. Rev. Resp. Dis., *122:*841, 1980.
27. Hopewell, P.C.: Failure of Positive End-Expiratory Pressure to decrease lung water content in alloxan-induced pulmonary edema. Am. Rev. Resp. Dis., *120:*813, 1979.
28. Scharf, S.M., Caldim, P., and Ingram, R.H.: Cardiovascular effects of increasing airway pressure in the dog. Am. J. Physiol. *232:*H35, 1977.
29. Scharf, S.M., and Ingram, R.H.: Influence of abdominal pressure and sympathetic vasoconstriction of the cardiovascular response to Positive End-Expiratory Pressure. Am. Rev. Resp. Dis., *116:*661, 1977.
30. Cassidy, S.S., Eschenbucher, W.L., Robertson, C.H., Nixon, J.V., Blomquist, G., and Johnson, R.L.: Cardiovascular effects of positive pressure ventilation in normal subjects. J. Appl. Physiol., *47:*453, 1979.
31. Hudson, L.D., Tooker, J., Haisch, C., Weaver, J., and Carrico, C.J.: Comparison of assisted ventilation and PEEP with IMV and CPAP in ARDS patients. Am. Rev. Resp. Dis., *117*[Suppl.]:129, 1977.
32. Scoggins, W.G., Zocco, J.W., Greenfield, L.J., and O'Donohue, W.J.: Critical comparison of Positive End-Expiratory Pressure and Continuous Positive Airway Pressure with IMV in ARDS. Am. Rev. Resp. Dis., *115*[Suppl.]:161, 1977.
33. Shah, D.M., Newell, J.C., Dutton, R.E., and Powers, S.R.: Continuous Positive Airway Pressure versus Positive End-Expiratory Pressure in respiratory distress syndrome. J. Thorac. Cardiovasc. Surg., *74:*557, 1977.
34. Kirby, R.R., Downs, J.B., and Civetta, J.M.: High level Positive End-Expiratory Pressure (PEEP) in acute respiratory failure. Chest, *67:*156, 1975.
35. Suter, P.M., Fairley, H.B., and Isenberg, M.D.: Optimal end-expiratory airway pressure in patients with acute pulmonary failure. N. Engl. J. Med., *292:*284, 1975.
36. Hudson, L.D., Tooker, J., Haisch, C.E., and Carrico, C.J.: Does compliance reflect optimal oxygen transport with Positive End-Expiratory Pressure (PEEP)? Chest, *72:*401, 1977.
37. Brigham K., Woolverton, W., Blake, L., and Staub, N.C.: Increased sheep lung vascular permeability caused by Pseudomonas bacteremia. J. Clin. Invest., *54:*792, 1974.
38. Stothert, S.C., and Carrico, C.J.: Fluid therapy in Adult Respiratory Distress Syndrome: A pathophysiologic approach. Sem. Resp. Med., *2:*123, 1981.
39. McAslon, T.C., Matjasko-Chin, J., Turney, S.Z., and Cowley, R.A.: Influence of inhalation of 100% oxygen in intrapulmonary shunt in severely traumatized patients. J. Trauma, *13:*811, 1973.
40. Kaplan, R.L., Sahn, S.A., and Petty, T.L.: Incidence and outcome of respiratory distress syndrome in gram-negative sepsis. Arch. Intern. Med., *139:*867, 1979.
41. Shimada, Y., Yoshiya, I., Tanaka, K., Sone, S., and Sakurai, M.: Evaluation of the progress and prognosis of the Adult Respiratory Distress Syndrome. Chest, *76:*180., 1979.

Chapter 6

ACID-BASE AND ELECTROLYTE DISTURBANCES IN RESPIRATORY FAILURE

By Thomas L. Petty

Disorders of acid regulation and electrolytes are an integral part of almost all episodes of respiratory insufficiency or failure. Such disorders can develop as a result of (1) primary consequences of respiratory failure, i.e., hypercapnia and hypoxemia, acute or chronic, (2) attempts of the organism to compensate for variations in the carbon dioxide tension, (3) special problems during recovery from hypercapnia, (4) the effects of various modes of therapy, or (5) associated problems such as metabolic acidemia due to poor tissue perfusion and renal failure or metabolic alkalemia. Any combination of acid regulation or electrolyte disturbances can occur when the lungs fail.[1]

ASSESSMENT OF THE PATIENT

Appropriate laboratory evaluation of disorders of acid regulation and electrolytes is imperative for patients with respiratory insufficiency or failure, since bedside assessment of the signs and symptoms is notoriously unreliable. To evaluate the laboratory determinations properly, the physician must have complete knowledge of the clinical situation of the patient. A physiologic approach must be applied to these complex disturbances, and the physician must understand the expected response of the normal intact organism to changes in pH, P_{CO_2}, bicarbonate concentration, and other electrolytes. Only with such knowledge can the physician interpret the labortory data properly and direct therapy appropriately.

Serial monitoring of the arterial pH as a measurement of hydrogen ion concentration (H^+) is imperative for all patients with respiratory insufficiency or failure. One must not rely on other so-called "acid-base measurements" to infer the pH. The physician must remember that respiratory acidosis or hypercapnia does not necessarily indicate that the pH will be low. Case examples will illustrate this point. Measurement of the arterial P_{CO_2} is likewise important, since it is the only way to establish how effectively the lungs are eliminating CO_2. As discussed below, other measurements with CO_2 in their title cannot be substituted for the arterial P_{CO_2}. The bicarbonate is then determined by an indirect calculation employing the Henderson-Hasselbalch equation

$$pH = 6.1 + \log \frac{HCO_3-}{H_2CO_3}$$

(interchangeable with H_2CO_3 is the product of the solubility coefficient of CO_2, 0.03 multiplied by the P_{CO_2}). The bicarbonate is usually read from a nomogram.

Physicians have used the measurement of CO_2 content in venous blood for many years.[2] The *CO_2 content* is defined as the concentration of the total CO_2 in the whole blood, which includes bicarbonate (HCO_3), H_2CO_3 plus other small amounts of CO_2 which circulate as carbamino compounds. Ordinarily, essentially all the carbon dioxide content consists of bicarbonate, with the dissolved forms of carbon dioxide usually contributing no more that 2 or 3/mmol/L. Therefore, for practical purposes carbon dioxide content and "actual" bicarbonate concentration are interchangeable. It should be appreciated that the term *CO_2 content* tells essentially nothing about the P_{CO_2}. The CO_2 combining power is another measurement that has frequently been used in venous blood to measure essentially the same components as the CO_2 content. This measurement was introduced as an attempt to eliminate the respiratory effects on acid regulation and thereby allow one to assess the metabolic effects of the particular disturbance. The *CO_2 combining power* is a measure of the total CO_2 of the plasma, which is separated from the cells at the patient's actual P_{CO_2} and then equilibrated with P_{CO_2} of approximately 40 mm Hg.[3] This measurement has nothing to contribute to modern understanding of blood gas abnormalities.

In recent years, several new indices have been introduced for the measurement of metabolic disturbances of acid-base equilibrium. The first of these was the concept of *whole-blood buffer base*, which is defined as the sum of the concentrations of all buffer anions which include the bicarbonate in the plasma and in the red cells, hemoglobin, plasma proteins, and the phosphate in the plasma and red cells.[4] Nearly all this buffering capacity is contributed by hemoglobin and bicarbonate. More recently, two additional measurements have been introduced for the measurement of metabolic disturbances: standard bicarbonate and base excess.[5,6] *Standard bicarbonate* is defined as a concentration of bicarbonate in plasma when fully oxygenated whole blood has been equilibrated with carbon dioxide at a P_{CO_2} of 40 mm Hg at a standard temperature of 38°C. The standard bicarbonate is determined by interpolation from the in vitro carbon dioxide titration curve of the patient's blood. This is plotted on a nomogram, and the value is read directly from this nomogram.[7] *Base excess* (or *base deficit*) is a term which is designed to express directly the amount of strong base (or acid) added per liter of blood, with the normal mean excess arbitrarily set at zero. Therefore, zero base excess corresponds to the normal mean for standard bicarbonate, and when the term *base excess* is used, the positive values will express the excess of base and negative values the deficit in base.

We agree with others who believe that these newer indices add very little to the knowledge of pH, P_{CO_2}, and bicarbonate of the arterial blood.[8] Without knowledge of the patient's clinical problem and a physiologic approach to the disorder, the physician can often be misled by these new terms. Furthermore, since these values are determined by in vitro CO_2 titration curves, they do possess inherent errors. It has been demonstrated that the in vivo and in vitro carbon dioxide titration curves differ.[9] Nevertheless, we do acknowledge that for the new student of acid-base disturbances, the base excess value may be of some assistance in separating metabolic from respiratory disorders and in assessing the relative degree of the metabolic abnormality. It is again stressed that this should only be done with complete knowledge of the patient's clinical situation and the arterial pH, P_{CO_2}, and bicarbonate.

In addition to arterial pH and P_{CO_2} determinations, plasma electrolytes and bicarbonate must also be evaluated. As will be discussed, these are frequently altered, often in a profound manner, as the kidney attempts to compensate for the respiratory disorder or as a result of various therapeutic efforts. Whereas most physicians will frequently observe plasma electrolyte determinations, the concentrations of these electrolytes in the urine are frequently overlooked. Patients who have replacement problems and those receiving various medications which enhance urine electrolyte losses should have determinations of urine electrolytes done. The knowledge of urine losses can greatly enhance the physician's judgment as he directs therapy. A case example later in this chapter (Case 1) will reinforce this point.

TERMINOLOGY

Somewhat confusing terminology continues to be an important problem facing physicians who must use the concepts discussed in this chapter. We use the terminology outlined by the New York Academy of Science Symposium.[10] The term "acidosis" or "alkalosis" is used to describe the abnormal process causing the acid-base disturbance. Acidosis refers to the abnormal process that causes accumulation of acid in the body; alkalosis implies the converse. These abnormalities can then be referred to by type, i.e., either metabolic or respiratory. The terms may also specify the stage of the development of this disorder, acute or chronic, as well as whether secondary or compensatory changes have occurred. The term "acidemia" refers to pH determinations below 7.35 and "alkalemia" for those above 7.45. It will be readily appreciated that acidosis does not necessarily mean acidemia, as Case 2 will show. For practical purposes, *hypercapnia* may be used interchangeably with respiratory acidosis and *hypocapnia* with respiratory alkalosis.

VENOUS VS ARTERIAL BLOOD

Physicians frequently inquire about substituting venous measurements of pH and P_{CO_2} for arterial blood. Methods have been described for making these determinations on capillary blood as well as determining the P_{CO_2} of mixed venous blood by rebreathing techniques.[11–13] A comparison of simultaneous venous and arterial values is shown in Table 6-1. One venous sample was drawn from a vein of an uncongested limb, and the other from an arm after a tourniquet had been applied and the hand was "pumped." Obviously, a venous sample gives no information regarding the oxygen saturation of arterial blood, so that it is important to take an arterial sample from patients with respiratory insufficiency or failure. It is true that a close correlation exists between arterial and venous P_{CO_2} and pH when the venous sample is taken from an uncongested extremity in the normal person. It has been shown that a correlation between arterial and central venous blood in the normal individual and in those with

TABLE 6-1. Venous vs Arterial Blood

	ARTERIAL	*VENOUS Uncongested Extremity*	*VENOUS Tourniquet, after "Pumping" Hand*
P_{O_2} (mm Hg)	76	36.5	23
pH	7.45	7.39	7.25
P_{CO_2} (mm Hg)	36	41	68
HCO_3 (mEq/L)	24.8	24.4	29.0

Normal values for Denver (5200 ft. above sea level): P_{O_2}, 65 to 75 mm Hg; P_{CO_2}, 34 to 38 mm Hg.

metabolic disorders exists, but the relationship is less reliable in patients with respiratory disturbances.[14] As can be readily appreciated, however, once an extremity has had a tourniquet applied and muscular activity has taken place, the values change rapidly. Studies have shown that arterialized capillary blood has close correlation with central arterial blood in the normal.[11] In the sick patient with poor tissue perfusion, however, obtaining capillary blood is not always simple, and manipulations in drawing the sample may cause distortions similar to those demonstrated by the two venous samples recorded in Table 6-1. The technique of measuring mixed venous P_{CO_2} by the rebreathing technique gives quite reliable determinations of this isolated value, but this determination gives no information regarding the pH or oxygen saturation. As previously mentioned, the degree of P_{CO_2} elevation may have little or no relationship to the pH. Therefore, we always insist on measuring arterial blood. Many hospitals have now realized that specially trained nurses or technicians can draw arterial blood with ease (see Chap. 1). Consequently, there is no reason for substituting other less accurate or informative determinations.

THE ACID-BASE STATUS OF THE BLOOD

F. Beerel and J.W. Vance of Buffalo have offered a visual and practical method of showing the relationship among pH, HCO_3^- and P_{CO_2} in uncompensated and compensated states.[15] This method shows the pH as a balance between P_{CO_2} (controlled by the lungs) and bicarbonate (controlled by the kidneys) in a pictorial relationship that is easily grasped by medical students. In their system, the standard bicarbonate value (i.e., the value in fully oxygenated blood and at a P_{CO_2} of 40) is used. One might prefer to use the actual bicarbonate values instead (Figs. 6-1 to 6-7). In addition, values for buffer base and base excess are included.[4] For illustrative purposes, the renal acid-base balance and classic acute compensated respiratory and metabolic states are depicted in Figures 6-2 through 6-7. Each state is described in more detail later.

Respiratory Acidosis

When the respiratory system fails to eliminate CO_2 as rapidly as it is produced by metabolism in the tissues of the body, the blood P_{CO_2} rises and respiratory acidosis develops.[16] The intact organism immediately attempts to defend itself from the invading H_2CO_3. Hemoglobin is a most important buffer and has great affinity for binding hydrogen ion. Hemoglobin allows the normal transport and elimination of 13,000 to 15,000 mEq CO_2 per day. Evidence of the great buffering capacity of hemoglobin is seen in the small difference between venous and arterial pH (0.05 units). As hemoglobin unloads oxygen at the tissue level, it becomes a strong base (Hb −) capable of binding hydrogen ion as the tissues produce CO_2 and form H_2CO_3. Consequently, as CO_2 production exceeds CO_2 elimination, hemoglobin provides the immediate extrarenal defense against the rising hydrogen concentration. Additional extrarenal buffering comes from tissue contributions within the extracellular fluid, which is mediated by bicarbonate transfer, transfer of chloride across the erythrocyte membrane, shifts of sodium and potassium across an extracellular boundary other than the red cell, transfer of inorganic phosphate, and significant alterations in lactate metabolism.[17] Acute rises in P_{CO_2} induce a rise in extracellular bicarbonate before renal factors come into play.[9] This pattern is illustrated in Figure 6-2.

Within a short time after hypercapnia develops, renal responses to this change take place.[18,19] A rise in P_{CO_2} of the body's fluid is the effective stimulus for bicarbonate generation by the kidneys. In patients with chronic hypercapnia, the generation of bicarbonate may go on several days in an attempt to compensate for respiratory acido-

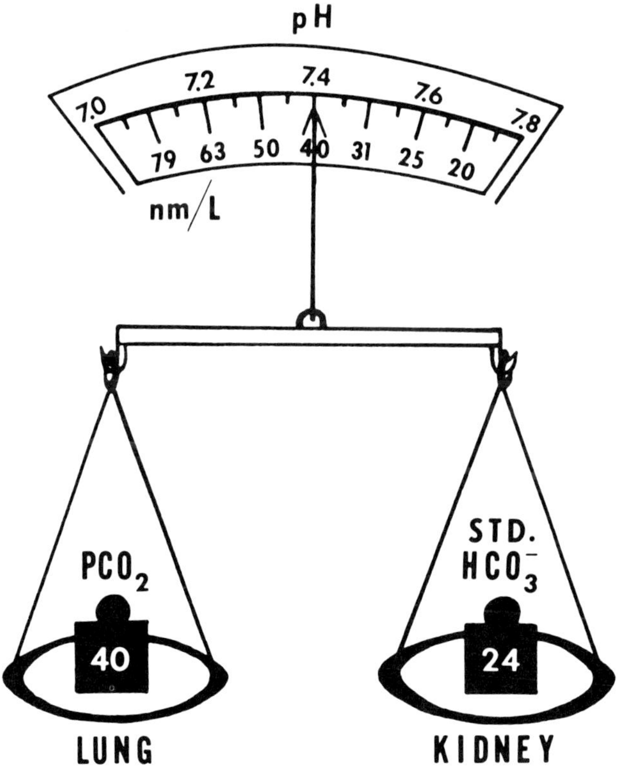

Fig. 6-1. Normal relationship between P_{CO_2} and HCO_3^- resulting in normal pH of 7.4 (hydrogen ion concentration of 40 nanomoles/L). In this illustration, as in others, standard bicarbonate value was used. (From Beerel, F.R., and Vance, J.W.: A simplified method of presenting acid base situations. Chest, *57*:480, 1970.)

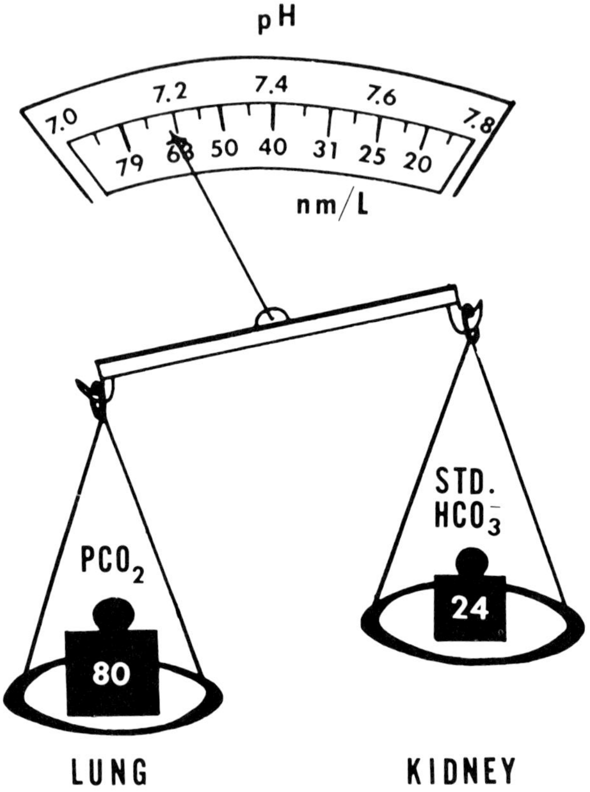

Fig. 6-2. Uncompensated respiratory acidemia. (From Beerel, F.R., and Vance, J.W.: A simplified method of presenting acid base situations. Chest, *57*:480, 1970.)

sis and acidemia. Since the stimulus for bicarbonate production may be high arterial P_{CO_2} and not pH per se, it has been our experience that at lower levels of P_{CO_2} elevation (50 to 75 mm Hg), compensation may be complete or nearly complete (see Fig. 6-3).[20] Compensation is usually incomplete at high levels of arterial P_{CO_2}; i.e., $>$ 75 mm Hg when these elevations occur acutely. Full compensation to higher levels of P_{CO_2} occurs in patients with severe chronic airway obstruction who receive continuous oxygen.[16]

The pattern of primary respiratory alkalemia (acute hyperventilation) is presented in Figure 6-4. There are a number of additional renal responses occurring in respiratory failure that have therapeutic implications. The titratable acidity of the urine is increased along with ammonium excretion. In addition, a marked chloruresis occurs as well as an initial increase in the potassium excretion.[19] In animal studies, it appears that potassium loss continues only during the first one or two days of hypercapnia. However, in patients, especially those receiving drugs which enhance potassium loss such as cortico-

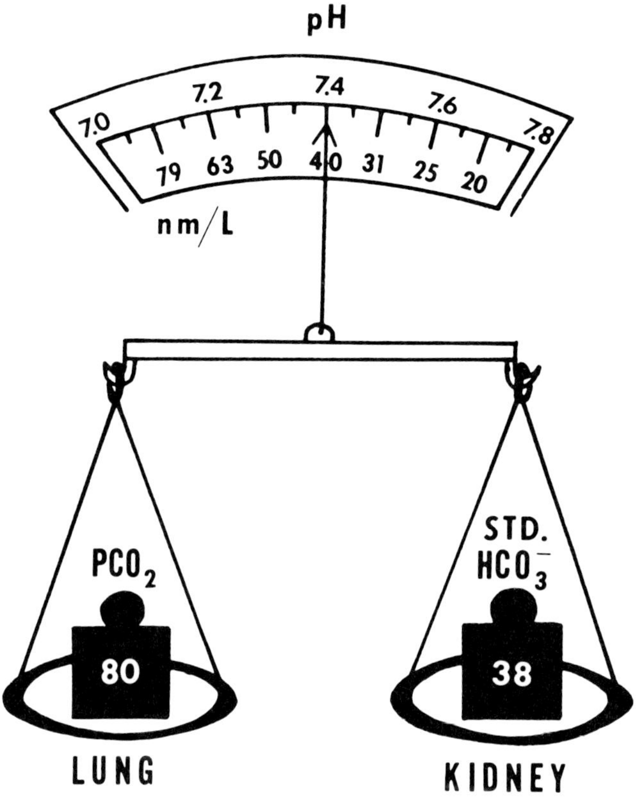

Fig. 6-3. Complete bicarbonate compensation following slow carbon dioxide retention.[16] This occurs in severe chronic airflow limitation (COPD, Chap. 10). Since the originating clinical event is in the lung, the term "respiratory acidosis" is appropriate (see text). (From Beerel, F.R., and Vance, J.W.: A simplified method of presenting acid base situations. Chest, *57:*480, 1970.)

steroids or diuretics, potassium losses are frequently profound and require specific and quantitative replacement. Likewise, the chloruresis is significant and recovery from hypercapnia requires chloride replacement.[20]

During acute metabolic acidosis with acidemia, serum potassium invariably rises (at least transiently) as potassium comes out of the cell in exchange for sodium and hydrogen.[5,20,21] Animal studies during respiratory acidosis show a variable response with regard to potassium shifts during acidemia.[5,9,17,19] Our experience has shown that in humans the potassium response is variable. At times, serum potassium rises abruptly in response to acute respiratory acidosis and acidemia (as it does in metabolic acidosis); at other times the change may be minimal. Problems of electrolyte replacement will be discussed in case examples later in this chapter.

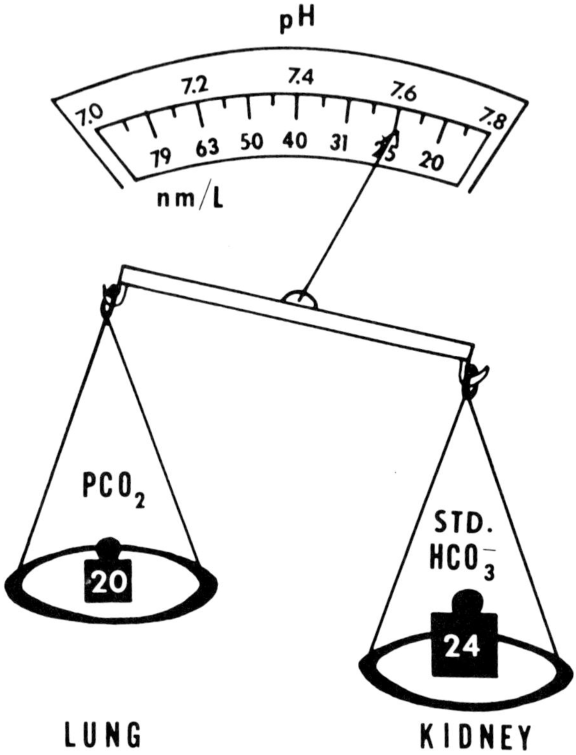

Fig. 6-4. Uncompensated respiratory alkalemia, such as in hyperventilation syndrome. In this example, hypocapnia has occurred through hyperventilation before kidneys have had sufficient time to excrete bicarbonate. The compensated state (compensated respiratory alkalosis, lower bicarbonate level) balances the scales. (From Beerel, F.R., and Vance, J.W.: A simplified method of presenting acid base situations. Chest, *57:*480, 1970.)

Primary metabolic disorders are illustrated in Figures 6-5, 6-6, and 6-7.

Combined Disturbances

Problems with acid-base regulation and electrolytes occasionally occur in pure form. However, in patients with respiratory insufficiency or failure, disturbances are often combined. Combined disorders commonly found in clinical practice are illustrated by the cases that follow.

Acute respiratory acidosis with severe uncompensated acidemia is a common problem; an example is Case 1. Respiratory acidosis with moderate P_{CO_2} elevations and complete or nearly complete compensation has recently been recognized particularly in patients with obstructive pulmonary disease who are receiving long-term continuous oxygen (see Chaps. 3 and 18). An example of this problem is illustrated in Case 2. Profound alkalemia after mechanical ventilation

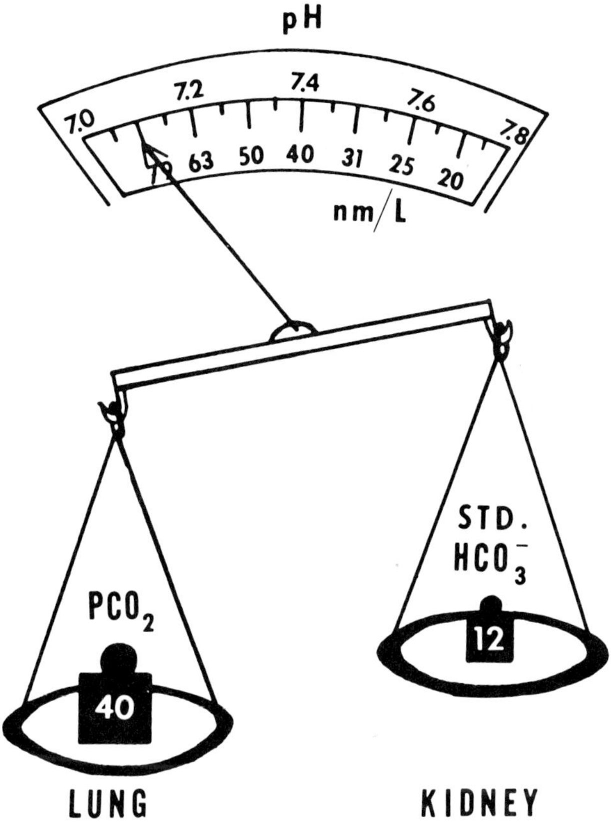

Fig. 6-5. Uncompensated metabolic acidemia, such as in an uncontrolled diabetic patient with ketoacidosis or in an acute uremic state. Generally pH compensation occurs rapidly via hyperpnea (see Fig. 6-6). (From Beerel, F.R., and Vance, J.W.: A simplified method of presenting acid base situations. Chest, *57:*480, 1970.)

of patients with respiratory acidosis and renal compensation can occur; the serious consequences will be discussed further in Chapter 15, on the complications of respiratory failure. However, Case 2 also illustrates the problems of alkalemia during recovery from respiratory acidosis. Combined problems of respiratory acidosis and metabolic acidosis do occur in patients with poor tissue perfusion or renal insufficiency, or both. However, we have not observed metabolic acidosis as a regular concomitant of respiratory acidosis.[9]

Case 3 illustrates the fact that elevated levels of CO_2 retention can be well tolerated and are compatible with long-term survival.

Case 4 illustrates combined respiratory and metabolic acidosis.

Respiratory alkalosis with profound alkalemia can occur in comatose patients who receive excessive minute volumes during mechanical ventilation. This will be considered in more detail in

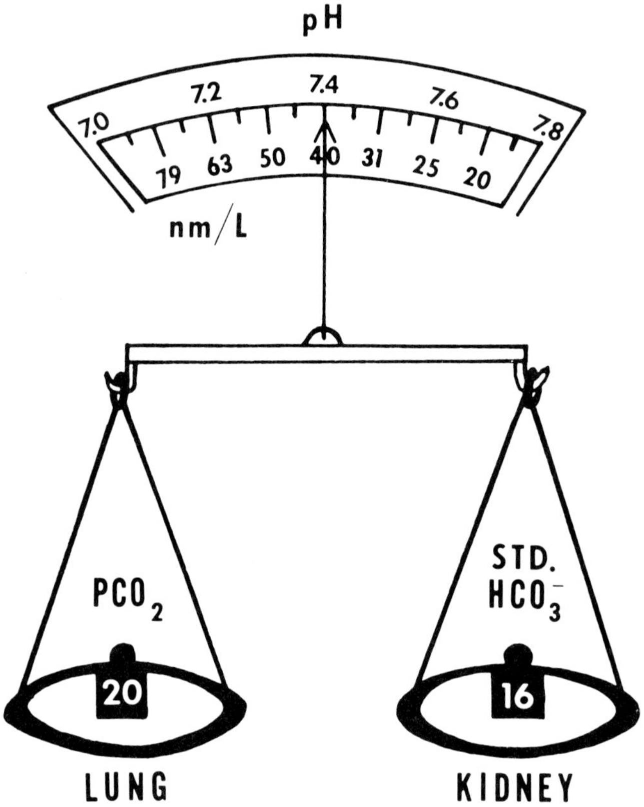

Fig. 6-6. Compensated metabolic acidosis. Full compensation via hyperventilation produces normal pH or hydrogen ion concentration. Since the original clinical problem was metabolic (e.g., diabetes mellitus or uremic acidosis), the term "metabolic acidosis" is still appropriate. (From Beerel, F.R., and Vance, J.W.: A simplified method of presenting acid base situations. Chest, *57:*480, 1970.)

Chapter 15. Other patients with hypoxemia and decreased lung compliance secondary to fibrosis, pneumonia, or congestive heart failure may develop respiratory alkalosis due to excessive ventilatory drives. Patients with a variety of central nervous system disorders can also have excessive ventilation due to abnormal central drives.

Occasionally severe hypercapnia occurs as a result of severe metabolic alkalosis. In this situation the CO_2 retention is a compensation for the alkalemia and occurs in the absence of chronic obstructive lung disease.[22] Elevations of P_{CO_2} of 60 mm Hg or greater may occur, particularly in vomiting, dehydration, and azotemia.[22] This respiratory adjustment is also enhanced by diuretics which increase renal hydrogen ion (ethacrynic acid and furosemide).[23] It must be stressed that this form of CO_2 elevation requires metabolic repair with fluid replacement, chloride, and potassium and is not an indication for mechanical ventilation, which would increase the alkalemia.[22]

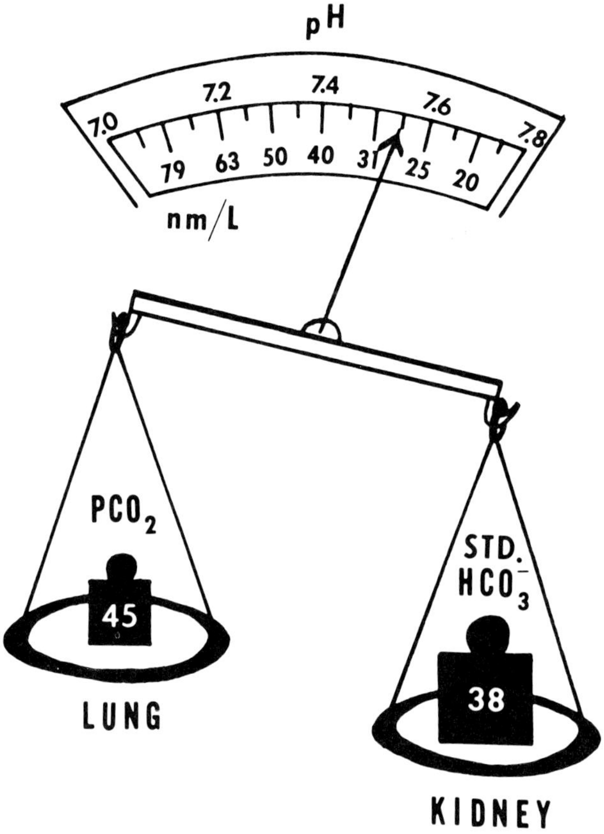

Fig. 6-7. Uncompensated metabolic alkalemia such as occurs in excessive bicarbonate ingestion for relief of ulcer pain or if given intravenously during a cardiac arrest. In full compensation (not illustrated), hypoventilation results in carbon dioxide retention, resulting in a near-normal pH. P_{CO_2} as high as 70 mm Hg or more may occasionally occur. This pattern is properly termed "compensated metabolic alkalosis" rather than "respiratory acidosis" (high but compensating P_{CO_2}). Sometimes the term "respiratory failure" is inappropriately applied to states of full respiratory compensation.

Finally, we are often asked to evaluate patients with disease process involving metabolic acidosis and acidemia who also have marked respiratory compensation (hypocapnia). These patients are then occasionally overtreated with sodium bicarbonate given as an "intravenous push," resulting in metabolic alkalosis and alkalemia. This condition is aggravated by the sustained respiratory drive causing respiratory alkalosis (hypocapnia), which has not had a chance to readjust after the sudden shift from acidemia to alkalemia.

No attempt is made to show examples of all disorders of acid regulation and electrolytes which can occur in patients with respiratory insufficiency or failure, but the following four cases illustrate the most commonly encountered situations.

CASE EXAMPLES

Case 1. A 43-year-old alcoholic white woman was admitted to the hospital with a history and physical examination compatible with acute pancreatitis. This diagnosis was supported by elevated amylase and lipase values. The patient's abdomen was tender and rigid, and the diaphragm was elevated. During the first two hospital days the patient had no apparent abnormality of the respiratory system. No history or physical finding suggestive of chronic airway obstruction was found. At approximately 1:00 A.M. on the third hospital day, the patient was noted to be tachypneic and was seen in consultation. An arterial blood gas sample obtained while the patient was breathing room air showed a mild oxygen unsaturation at 84% with a mild metabolic acidosis and acidemia (Table 6-2). It was suggested that the patient receive low-flow oxygen of 2 or 3 L/min and be observed closely for increasing metabolic acidosis, which can complicate pancreatitis. The patient was then seen by the respiratory care staff at approximately 7:30 A.M. In the intervening time, the patient had deteriorated significantly. After complaining of abdominal pain, she had received a small amount of morphine sulfate. A short while later, she was considered to have possible impending delirium tremens and was given 25 mg chlordiazepoxide (Librium) intramuscularly. By 7:30 A.M. the patient had become stuporous and had a tachycardia of 180 to 200/min and had had a decrease in her urinary output. The oxygen had been increased from low flow to 10 L/min.

On examination at the bedside at 7:30 A.M., no cyanosis was found. The respiratory rate was 22 to 24/min. Chest expansions appeared more than adequate, and on auscultation "good air exchange" was believed to be occurring. No evidence of decreased ventilation or suppressed respirations was observed clinically. Bedside observers did not feel that the deterioration was pulmonary, but most likely was due to complications of acute pancreatitis.

Table 6-2 shows the arterial blood gases obtained at 7:30 A.M.; these determinations are compared with a venous sample taken at exactly the

TABLE 6-2. Case 1

	Hospital Day 3			
	1:00 A.M.	7:30 A.M.	10:00 A.M.	3.30 P.M.
Arterial				
Saturation	84%	62%	96%	97%
pH	7.34	7.06	7.25	7.45
P_{CO_2} (mm Hg)	37	115	65	44
HCO_3^- (mEq/L)	18.9	33.5	28.5	30
Venous				
CO_2 content (mEq/L)		24		
Na^+ (mEq/L)		139		
K^+ (mEq/L)		3.7		
Cl^- (mEq/L)		98		

same time. Marked arterial oxygen unsaturation (62%) was present at this time. Even though the patient appeared to be ventilating well in clinical observations, carbon dioxide elimination was impaired, with P_{CO_2} elevated to 115 mm Hg and pH lowered to 7.06. The patient was immediately intubated and placed on a respirator to improve oxygenation and carbon dioxide elimination.

By 10:00 A.M. that morning, the P_{CO_2} had been lowered to 65 mm Hg; the pH had risen to 7.25. By 3:30 P.M. the P_{CO_2} was nearly normal (44 mm Hg) and the pH, 7.45.

The slightly elevated bicarbonate reflects one ampule of $NaHCO_3$ the patient received as "an intravenous push" given as an immediate measure, while the initial resuscitative measures were being made to improve CO_2 elimination.

Comment. This case of acute uncompensated respiratory acidemia illustrates a number of important points: (1) respiratory failure can occur in a wide variety of clinical situations and in patients other than those with chronic airflow limitation (see Chap. 10); (2) sedatives must be considered potential precipitators of respiratory insufficiency or failure; (3) the signs and symptoms noted at the bedside are unreliable in alerting the physician to the presence of hypoxemia or hypercapnia; and (4) only arterial blood gas analyses clearly revealed that the patient had severe hypoxemia, hypercapnia, and acidemia. The venous electrolytes obtained at the same time as the second set of arterial determinations are completely within normal limits and in no way suggest either an elevation in the P_{CO_2} or acidemia.

Case 2. A 61-year-old white man with a long history of asthma had airway obstruction that was considered to be largely reversible although there was an element of chronic, irreversible obstruction. He had been hospitalized previously, at which time he demonstrated airway obstruction plus the findings compatible with cor pulmonale and "right-sided heart failure." After the patient's discharge, his therapy included 10 mg prednisone and 50 mg hydrochlorthiazide daily. A 3- or 4-day history of progressive dyspnea and wheezing was reported prior to the patient's admission. Blood gas determinations at the time of admission are shown in Table 6-3. The arterial oxygen saturation was normal, with the patient receiving oxygen via nasal prongs. The pH of 7.37 is at the lower limits of normal; the P_{CO_2} was elevated to 65.5 mm Hg; and bicarbonate was elevated to 36.8 mEq/L. This is an example of chronic respiratory acidosis that is compensated with a pH at the lower limits of normal. The venous electrolyte determinations show low chloride and low potassium. The low serum sodium level was considered to be a result of dilution due to water retention.

Following his admission, the patient's dosage of prednisone was increased to 40 mg daily and the hydrochlorthiazide continued at 50 mg. Aminophylline was given by continuous intravenous infusion using approximately 500 mg q 8 h. In addition, 60 mEq intravenous potassium chloride were given per day.

Within 48 hours, the severe airway obstruction noted at the time of admission had improved significantly. Arterial blood gases showed normal arterial oxygen saturation with low-flow nasal oxygen; P_{CO_2} was almost normal at 43 mm Hg; the pH had risen to 7.54; the bicarbonate was almost unchanged. The venous electrolytes demonstrate that the chlorides and potassium were lower than at the time of admission.

The patient was still alkalemic on the eighth hospital day. Chloride, sodium, and potassium remained low. Because of the problems with electrolyte replacement, analysis of urinary electrolytes was advised. Chloride, sodium, and potassium losses were significant during the administration of 60 mEq intravenous potassium chloride daily. Analysis revealed that 55 mEq potassium were lost each 24 hours through the urine.

After increasing the patient's intake of potassium chloride to approximately 120 mEq/day and adding a small dose of ammonium chloride, significant improvement occurred by the tenth hospital day. As the level of plasma chlorides was increased, the kidneys were able to excrete the excess bicarbonate which had been generated earlier. As renal bicarbonate excretion increased, the blood pH returned to normal and plasma electrolyte levels improved concomitantly.

Comment. This case also illustrates several important factors: (1) moderate rise in the P_{CO_2} can be completely compensated, if the patient is receiving supplemental oxygen; (2) hypochloremia and hypokalemia are frequent complications of hypercapnia, especially if the patient is receiving steroids or diuretics, or both; (3) the replacement of chloride during the recovery from hypercapnia is important; (4) potassium loss can continue in the urine and stool despite a deficiency of this ion, a loss expedited by steroids or diuretics; (5) as

TABLE 6-3. Case 2

	Hospital Day 1	*Hospital Day 3*	*Hospital Day 8*	*Hospital Day 10*
Arterial				
Saturation	98%	96%	96%	99%
pH	7.37	7.54	7.51	7.46
P_{CO_2} (mm Hg)	65.5	43	48.5	46
HCO_3^- (mEq/L)	36.8	36.9	38	32
Venous				
Cl^- (mEq/L)	85	76	79	88
Na^+ (mEq/L)	128	126	125	132
K^+ (mEq/L)	3.2	2.6	3.0	3.9
Urine				
Cl^- (mEq/24 hr)			47	
Na^+ (mEq/24 hr)			70	
K^+ (mEq/24 hr)			55	

chloride and potassium are replaced, the excess bicarbonate can be excreted during the recovery phase; and (6) significant alkalemia can occur in patients with compensated respiratory acidosis as P_{CO_2} returns to normal.[20,21,24,25] Alkalemia in itself has potentially severe complications.

Case 3. A 57-year-old white man with chronic airflow limitation was hospitalized, at approximately 10:00 A.M. There had been a several-day history of worsening of his symptoms, and on the morning of admission, he was found to be stuporous. He was given oxygen on the way to the hospital, and at the time that the first arterial blood sample was obtained, he was receiving oxygen (Table 6-4). The patient was in a semicomatose condition. The arterial saturation was only 40%; P_{CO_2} was 150 mm Hg; and pH, 7.08. He was placed on a respirator following a tracheostomy, and was administered intravenous bicarbonate. Approximately 3 hours later, the P_{CO_2} had been reduced to 111 mm Hg. The following day the patient was alert and requested removal of the respirator. While receiving oxygen through a tracheostomy collar, the patient was able to maintain adequate arterial oxygen saturation and an arterial P_{CO_2} between 75 and 80 mm Hg. During this period, therapy was directed at the combating of infection and the removal of secretions. Nine days following admission, the patient was entirely weaned from the mechanical respirator, and infection and secretions were well controlled. An arterial oxygen saturation of 91% was maintained with supplemental oxygen through nasal prongs. However, the patient readjusted his ventilation to a point that P_{CO_2} was elevated to 90 mm Hg. The resultant respiratory acidemia was only partially compensated for, and there was a significant reduction in pH. The patient remained amazingly alert with arterial P_{CO_2} ranging from 90 to 110 mm Hg. The arterial blood gas analysis showed a continued high level of P_{CO_2} 50 days after admission, the day that the patient was transferred to a domiciliary Veterans Administration Hospital in another city. It was believed that the patient could not survive for any length of time with this degree of respiratory insufficiency. However, the patient's condition remained stable for approximately 10 months. He was then returned to our hospital at his request. Arterial blood gas levels on the day he returned are shown in Table 6-4. Apparently, the patient had maintained a significant elevation in arterial P_{CO_2} and acidemia for the entire intervening period. He survived at this level of respiratory insufficiency 3 more months before he expired.

TABLE 6-4. Case 3

	Admission Day					*11 Months*
	10:00 A.M.	*1:00 P.M.*	*Day 1*	*Day 9*	*Day 50*	*After Admission*
Arterial						
Saturation	40%	97%	92%	91%	90%	92%
pH	7.08	7.25	7.33	7.26	7.25	7.29
P_{CO_2} (mm Hg)	150	111	77	90	110	85
HCO_3^- (mEq/L)	42.8	47.9	39.9	39.2	35.2	30.0

Comment. This case illustrates the fact that high levels of arterial P_{CO_2} and acidemia can be tolerated by some patients for prolonged periods of time if they remain well oxygenated. Complete compensation of the acidemia is not possible with high levels of P_{CO_2}, however.

Case 4. A 62-year-old man known to have chronic airflow limitation was admitted to the hospital after several days of worsening of the symptoms at home. The results of blood gas analysis on the day of admission are shown in Table 6-5. The arterial pH of 7.38 also demonstrates complete compensation of hypercapnia. The patient was also receiving oxygen. After 4 days of therapy directed at controlling infection and secretions, the P_{CO_2} dropped to normal limits (38 mm Hg). The patient continued to improve until the seventh hospital day, when rapid deterioration occurred. The pH dropped to 7.20, and P_{CO_2} rose to 55 mm Hg. The bicarbonate was 21 mEq/L, which was lower than it had been previously and lower than one would anticipate from a P_{CO_2} of 55 mm Hg.[9] The base excess value is included to show how some physicians use this value to aid in recognizing the presence of a combined disorder. As stated earlier, the disproportionately low bicarbonate concentration should lead one to the same conclusion.

Comment. This is an example of combined respiratory and metabolic acidosis with acidemia. The cause for this patient's abrupt change was not completely clear, but a pulmonary infarction was suspected. Mild hypotension was present; this most likely created poor tissue perfusion and subsequent anaerobic metabolism with lactic acid production. Metabolic acidosis is not a regular feature of respiratory acidosis.[9]

In spite of vigorous therapeutic efforts, this patient expired. An autopsy revealed panlobular emphysema, chronic bronchitis, and many small pulmonary emboli, both old and new, which had not been clinically or radiographically apparent during life.

TABLE 6-5. Case 4

	Hospital Day 1	*Hospital Day 4*	*Hospital Day 7*
Arterial	*Receiving O_2*	*Breathing Room Air*	*Receiving O_2*
Oxygen saturation	96%	77%	91%
pH	7.38	7.46	7.20
P_{CO_2} (mm Hg)	52	38	55
HCO_3^- (mEq/L)	30	26	21
Base excess (mEq/L)	+4	+4	−7.5

Almost any type of acid-base disturbance can accompany respiratory failure and its blood gas abnormalities.. These may be in part compensatory or complicating factors requiring specific therapy. The physician must be alert to a wide variety of possibilities and guide his therapy by repeated arterial blood gas analyses and serum and urine electrolyte determinations.

Recent reports have shed additional light on acid-base disturbances in the critically ill. The overwhelmingly high incidence of significant ,metabolic alkalemia in hospitalized patients has been noted.[26] Often, a metabolic alkalemia either following the use of excessive or unnecessary doses of bicarbonate or during a cardiac resuscitation—thus iatrogenic problems—are all too commonly superimposed onto already serious clinical situations.[27] Any form of acute metabolic alkalosis will naturally complicate the course of patients with severe chronic airflow obstruction and will aggravate or perpetuate hypercarbia.[28] Excessive bicarbonate can be rapidly eliminated by using acetazolamide to promote a brisk bicarbonate diuresis in states where this is desirable to help restore a more normal pH.[28]

It has also been pointed out that venous CO_2 values obtained during routine electrolyte determinations cannot be used to replace the arterial bicarbonate concentration in calculating pH or P_{CO_2} from the Henderson-Hasselbalch equation.[29]

REFERENCES

1. Simmons, D.H., and Shkolnik, S.: Acid-base alterations in pulmonary disease. Dis. Chest, *45:*175, 1964.
2. Van Slyke, D.D., and Cullen, G.E.: Studies of acidosis I. Bicarbonate concentration of blood plasma; its significance and its determination as a measure of acidosis. J. Biol. Chem., *30:*289, 1917.
3. Peters, J.P., and Van Slyke, D.D.: Quantitative Clinical Chemistry. Volume I, Interpretations. Baltimore, Williams & Wilkins, 1931.
4. Singer, R.B., and Hastings, A.B.: An improved clinical method for the estimation of disturbances of the acid-base balance of human blood. Medicine, *27:*223, 1948.
5. Astrup, P., Siggaard Andersen, O., Jorgensen, K., and Engel, K.: The acid-base metabolism: a new approach. Lancet, *1:*1035, 1960.
6. Astrup, P.: New approach to acid-base metabolism. Clin. Chem., *7:*1, 1961.
7. Siggaard Andersen, O.: The pH-log P_{CO_2} blood acid-base nomogram revised. Scand. J. Clin. Lab. Invest., *14:*598, 1962.
8. Schwartz, W.B., and Relman, A.S.A.: A critique of the parameters used in the evaluation of acid-base disorders. N. Engl. J. Med., *268:*1382, 1963.
9. Cohen, J.J., Brackett, N.C., Jr., and Schwartz, W.B.: The nature of the carbon dioxide titration curve in the normal dog. J. Clin. Invest. *43:*777, 1964.
10. Winters, R.W.: Terminology of acid-base disorders. Ann. N.Y. Acad. Sci, *133:*211, 1966.
11. Brooks, D., and Wynn, V.: Use of venous pH and carbon dioxide studies. Lancet, *1:*227, 1959.
12. MacDonald, J.S., Laughlin, D.E., and Bedell, G.N.: Direct approach to evaluation of patients with acid-base imbalance. JAMA, *188:*9, 1964.
13. Griggs, D.E., Hackney, J.D., and Collier, C.R.: The rapid diagnosis of ventilatory failure with the carbon dioxide analyzer. Am. J. Med., *25:*31, 1958.

14. Phillips, B., and Peretz, D.I.: A comparison of central venous and arterial blood gas values in the critically ill. Ann. Intern. Med., *70:*745, 1969.
15. Beerel, F.R., and Vance, J.W.: A simplified method of presenting acid-base situations. Chest, *57:*480, 1970.
16. Neff, T.A., and Petty, T.L.: Tolerance and survival in severe chronic hypercapnia. Arch. Intern. Med., *129:*591, 1972.
17. Giebisch, G., Berger, L., and Pitts, R.F.: The extrarenal response to acute acid-base disturbances of respiratory origin. J. Clin. Invest., *34:*231, 1955.
18. Dorman, P.J., Sullivan, W.J., and Pitts, R.F.: The renal response to acute respiratory acidosis. J. Clin. Invest., *33:*82, 1954.
19. Polak, A., Haynie, G.D., Hays, R.M., and Schwartz, W.B.: Effects of chronic hypercapnia on electrolyte and acid-base equilibrium. I. Adaptation. J. Clin. Invest., *40:*1223, 1961.
20. Schwartz, W.B., Hays, R.M., Polak, A., and Haynie, G.D.: Effects of chronic hypercapnia on electrolyte and acid-base equilibrium. II. Recovery with special reference to the influence of chloride intake. J. Clin. Invest., *40:*1238, 1961.
21. Kilburn, K.: Movements of potassium during acute respiratory acidosis and recovery. J. Appl. Physiol., *21:*679, 1966.
22. Tuller, M.A., and Mehdi, F.: Compensatory hypoventilation and hypercapnia in primary metabolic alkalosis. Am. J. Med., *50:*281, 1971.
23. Goldring, R.M., Cannon, P.J., Heinemann, H.O., and Fishman, A.P.: Respiratory adjustment to chronic metabolic alkalosis in man. J. Clin. Invest. *47:*188, 1968.
24. Evans, B.M., Hugh-Jones, N.C., Melne, M.D., and Steiner, S.: Electrolyte excretion during experimental potassium depletion in man. Clin. Sci., *13:*305, 1954.
25. Womersely, R.A., and Darragh, J.: Potassium and sodium restriction in the normal human. J. Clin. Invest., *34:*456, 1955.
26. Hodgkin, J.E., Soaprono, F.F., and Chan, D.M.: Incidence of metabolic alkalemia in hospitalized patients. Crit. Care Med., *8:*725, 1980.
27. Bishop, R.L., and Weisfeldt, M.L.: Sodium bicarbonate administration during cardiac arrest (effect on arterial pH, P_{CO_2} and osmolality). JAMA, *235:*506, 1976.
28. Miller, P.D., and Berns, D.S.: Acute metabolic alkalosis perpetuating hypercarbia (a role for acetazolamide in chronic obstructive pulmonary disease). JAMA, *238:*2400, 1977.
29. Brashear, R.E., Oei, T.O., Rhodes, M.L., Fatty, D.E., and Hostetler, M.L.: Relationship between arterial and venous bicarbonate values. Arch. Intern. Med., *139:*440, 1979.

Chapter 7

RESPIRATORY CARE TECHNIQUES

(Intensive Nursing, Respiratory Therapy, and Physical Therapy)

By Louise M. Nett

GENERAL CARE OF THE PATIENT WITH ACUTE RESPIRATORY FAILURE

It is obvious that the care of critically ill patients with advanced COPD requires an integrative skillful approach. Perhaps the most important aspects of care are human and personal considerations, without which recovery would not be possible in many cases. This includes the important human values of patience, acceptance of frustration, and kindness at all times to help carry the patient through an extremely difficult life-threatening emergency. Attention should be paid to "creature comforts" in terms of personal hygiene, mouth care, frequent and appropriate changes of bed linens, and the maintenance of a bright cheery atmosphere even in the intensive care unit setting. Patients must be placed by the window and encouraged to maintain contact with the environment, which not only encourages the will to recovery, but also is effective in preventing or combating "intensive care delirium." The family should be allowed to visit essentially at all times, and in fact, they may play an important role in the care. They can comfort the patient, bring news, read letters and cards, and provide other diversions from an otherwise uncomfortable and almost untenable situation. The patient should have a transistor radio or television set in order to maintain contact with the outside world and interest in life in general. By all means, the patient must be treated in a dignified, friendly, and hopeful fashion. All too often, these crucial aspects of care are forgotten or not followed by those more oriented to technical or pharmacologic considerations. This is most common in the inexperienced and immature personnel, but in fact those who do not have the experience, judgment, and balance to handle these situations must themselves have the guidance of more experienced individuals who are able to add the extra element that results in survival in many patients who otherwise would have died.

Personnel

The enormous expansion of knowledge and technology and the development of new equipment for the care of the acutely ill patient have been accompanied by an increased responsibility for the personnel in today's hospitals. Therefore, it is not surprising to find that the patient with acute respiratory failure is being cared for by individuals with a variety of training backgrounds, including nurses, respiratory therapists and technicians, and physical therapists.

In the interest of better care for patients today, the roles of all involved must be coordinated. In many smaller hospitals, all the care described in this chapter is given by nurses; nurses in this situation must be skilled in all the necessary therapeutic maneuvers employed in the care and treatment of all forms of respiratory failure. The physician who directs treatment must be able to depend on intelligent applications of care and on accurate reporting of adverse physical and psychologic signs and symptoms. In some units, nurses and therapists institute changes in therapy independently; therefore, they must be highly skilled and knowledgeable individuals who have the trust and confidence of the physician in charge. He must become heavily involved in the training necessary to update care in this relatively new specialty.

Location

The provision of a well-equipped intensive care unit in which respiratory failure can be quickly diagnosed and treated is also fundamental to good care. For example, blood gas values should be quickly available. The nurse or therapist who suspects that a sudden change in the patient's condition is indicative of respiratory failure (or worsening of gas transport in the already diagnosed case) should have access to a laboratory for immediate blood gas determinations. Then, if the values of the blood gases are worsening, the physician is quickly provided with the information that enables him to order appropriate changes in therapy. This unit need not be separate from already-established medical or surgical intensive care units.

Attitude

Development of a team spirit among the personnel of the respiratory care unit is also a fundamental step to good care. Several factors should be considered. The leadership of the staff must reside with a highly trained and respected nurse. The head nurse must have the obvious support of the physician-director of the unit. In-service education needs must be met promptly, and new personnel must be oriented adequately. Well-known morale sustainers such as a reasonable salary and time off cannot be ignored. Providing an outlet for staff frustrations, perhaps by psychiatric consultation at a regular staff meeting, should be tried. Seeing formerly desperately ill patients when they return for clinic visits is always gratifying to the team, since they can then appreciate that all those tedious hours of care were worthwhile. Humor is also important and is perhaps one of the most often-forgotten fundamentals of good care.

Nurses seem to be the logical ones to coordinate therapies, because they have the most complete picture of the patient's overall needs. Effective coordinated care begins with respect for the other team members' areas of expertise. Conferences that include all team members, besides promoting good care, are frequently successful in establishing lines of communication that can be called upon if personality or interdisciplinary clashes arise. It is our belief that the care of these patients requires the close cooperation and skills of *all* the respiratory care team.

Conferences

The team conference is usually concerned with a specific patient. All members of the health team bring to the conference information and observations of the patient derived from their own vantage points. Presumably a synthesis of these views will provide a workable and more complete picture of the patient's personality and life style. A personal history from the family often adds considerable information on which to base the patient's care plan. The goal of these conferences should be to develop an approach that will be warm, affectionate, and human in the midst of the cold and sterile atmosphere often found in a respiratory intensive care unit.

PRINCIPLES OF NURSING CARE AND RESPIRATORY THERAPY

Patients in the respiratory care unit will range from those requiring total care to those just beginning independent activity. The patient with acute respiratory failure may or may not require ventilatory support. We have had increasing success in the management of respiratory failure in chronic pulmonary patients without a ventilator, using the methods described in detail in Chapters 9 and 10. However, these patients, like those who need mechanical ventilation, require skilled intensive care.

Airway Care

Maintenance of a patient's airway is of primary importance.[1–3] (See also Chap. 2.) Skills involved in maintaining the natural airway include moisture therapy, assistance with coughing, postural drainage, and, if required, nasotracheal suctioning. If a tracheostomy is performed, special care and suctioning techniques are required. (See discussion of tracheostomy tubes in this chapter.)

Natural Airway. Nasotracheal suctioning should be preceded by having the patient rinse his mouth and gargle, if possible, with mouthwash. He should also blow his nose if he is able. A sterile catheter is gently inserted into one of his nares while the patient protrudes his tongue. The catheter is advanced only when the patient inspires, as the epiglottis will be open at this time. Except in the most obtunded patient, vigorous coughing will result when the catheter passes into the trachea. Suction is applied intermittently. The catheter may be left in the airway, but the patient should be given opportunity to reoxygenate between suctioning episodes. If the patient is receiving oxygen, the nasal prongs may be adjusted so that a single nare is occupied or the cannula may be placed to introduce the oxygen through the mouth. Oxygen flow may be increased several liters during this period. A self-inflating bag and mask with added oxygen should be used for the patient who is unable to take a deep breath. When a patient requires frequent nasotracheal suctioning, a nasopharyngeal airway is sometimes helpful. It guides the catheter into the trachea and prevents trauma to the nasal mucosa.[1]

The frequency of nasotracheal suctioning will depend on the clinical situation, and the development of severe hypoxemia during suctioning must be avoided.[4] The procedure should be ordered by the physician, but experienced personnel can decide how often to suction by assessing the accumulation of retained secretions with the aid of chest auscultation.

Artificial Airway. Keeping an artificial airway patent employs many of the same skills. With adequate moisturization, the occlusion of the tube due to encrustation by dried secretions is uncommon. All team members must be aware of the reasons for moisture therapy and must see to it that the equipment used is properly functioning at all times.

Endotracheal Tubes. Suctioning through endotracheal tubes is sometimes difficult because of their length. After x-ray confirmation of proper placement, any excess tubing should be cut off the proximal end and the connector reinserted. Obviously, the suction catheter must be longer than the endotracheal tube for proper suctioning.

Even apparently unconscious patients should be informed about the procedure to avoid unnecessary anxiety. It should be stressed that suctioning is required to remove secretions that they are unable to cough out and that they may feel temporarily short of breath, but that they will be given the opportunity to take a deep breath with oxygen or will be assisted with a self-inflating bag.

Those patients who have severe problems in oxygen transport should be given several deep breaths of 100% oxygen prior to suctioning. Patients who have obviously accumulated a large amount of mucus in the tube should be quickly suctioned first and then oxygenated.

Tracheostomy Tubes. Suctioning the patient with a tracheostomy tube in place is technically easier than through an endotracheal tube. In all variations of suctioning the tracheobronchial tree, the basic anatomic and physiologic principles remain the same. Since the lung is normally sterile, precautions must be taken to prevent contamination or mucosal trauma that might aid colonization or bacterial invasion of the airways.

A standardized suctioning procedure should be formulated for use with all patients throughout the hospital.[2]

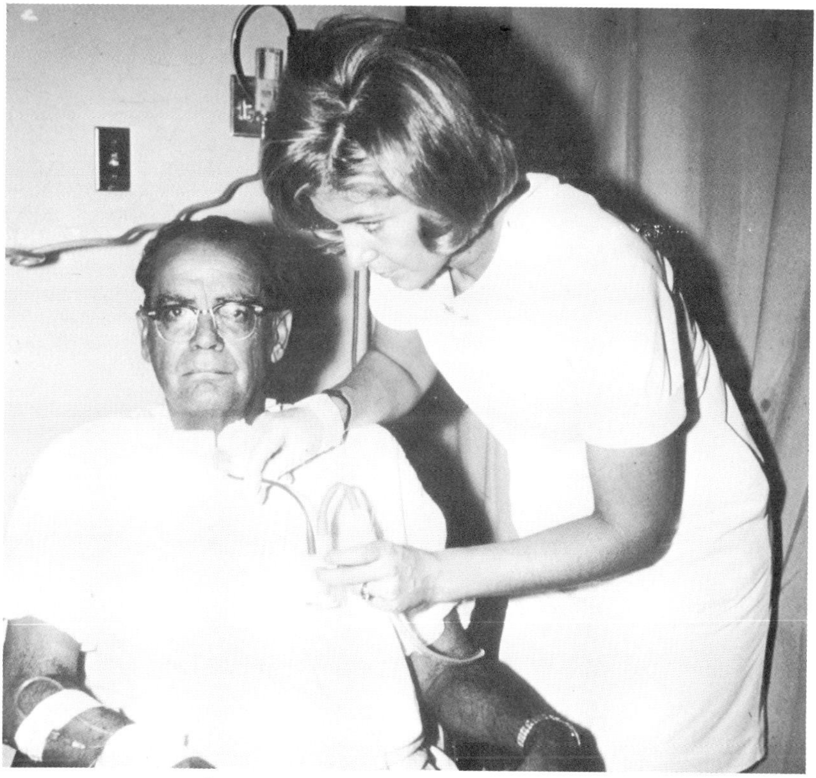

Fig. 7-1. Technique of tracheostomy suctioning and the collection of sputum for culture (note left hand). A sterile catheter and a sterile trap are used for this procedure.

The nurse's hands should be washed. A sterile catheter is selected, and a sterile glove is placed on the manipulating hand. After informing the patient, the catheter is inserted as deeply as it will pass without forcing (Fig. 7-1). If the catheter adheres to the side of the tube, it should be withdrawn and moistened with sterile solution to ease insertion. The catheter is withdrawn in a rotary fashion, with suction applied at this time *only*. Selective control of the suctioning force is best effected by using a T-connector or by using a tube that has a built-in by-pass port that is controlled by closure with the thumb (Fig. 7-2). Suction should not be applied on insertion because the catheter will adhere to the tracheal mucosa in a potentially traumatic "poking fashion." The one exception to this rule is when secretions are obviously present in the tube itself. Suction is then applied when the catheter is inserted, but only until the catheter reaches the end of the tube. This practice will prevent the secretions from adhering to the catheter and being carried back into the lungs. If the secretions are tenacious, tracheal lavage using 3 to 5 ml normal saline solution instilled directly into the tracheostomy tube may be

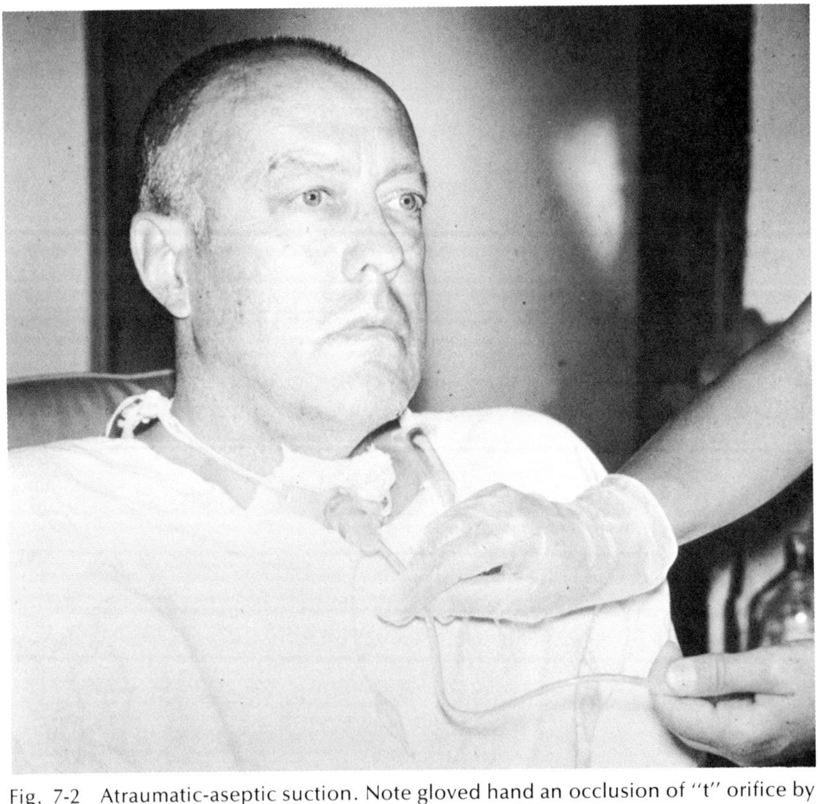

Fig. 7-2 Atraumatic-aseptic suction. Note gloved hand an occlusion of "t" orifice by the left thumb with suctioning only on withdrawal of the catheter.

useful in releasing the material (Fig. 7-3). Care must be taken to insure sterility of the solution introduced into the airway.

On completion of each suctioning maneuver, the patient is given deep breaths with a self-inflating bag with oxygen added. Alternately, the ventilator may be reattached to the patient and deep breaths given with the machine. Most self-inflating bags can provide only a 50% (approximate) oxygen fraction in the inspired air. In our unit we prefer using a bag modified to provide a 95 to 100% inspired oxygen concentration to hyperoxygenate the patient during suctioning (Fig. 7-4). The sequence of suctioning and giving deep breaths can be repeated until the secretions are cleared. If a cardiac monitor is being used, close observation of rhythm will give an additional indication of the patient's tolerance of this procedure.

Many institutions have found that the practice of reusing a catheter placed in a "sterilizing" solution at the bedside is dangerous. These solutions can lose efficacy because of infrequent changes, or the solution itself can become contaminated. When sufficient sterile cathe-

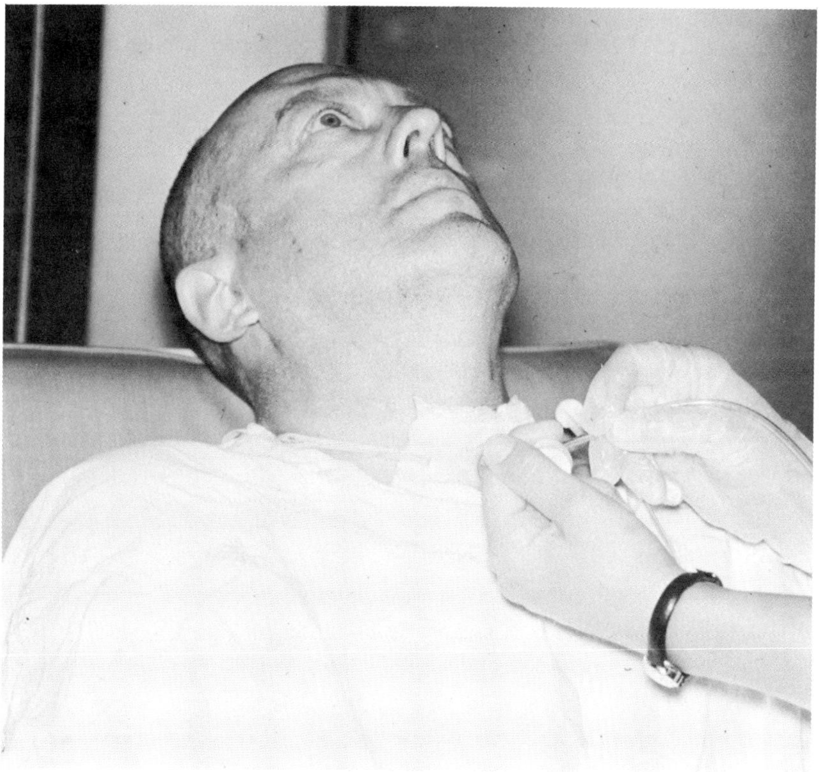

Fig. 7-3. Tracheal lavage using 3 to 5 ml saline solution instilled directly into tracheostomy tube. This is followed immediately by suctioning. This procedure, although widely used, remains controversial.

ters are not immediately available at the bedside, the temptation is to ignore breaks in technique, a factor to be considered honestly and carefully.

On completion of the entire suctioning session, the ventilator (if used) is reattached to the tracheostomy tube using a standard 15-mm adaptor, and the delivery pressure and tidal volume are checked and recorded (Fig. 7-5).

Cuffs. Tracheal stenosis and erosion are serious complications associated with cuffed transtracheal tubes. Prevention of these complications requires careful attention to intraluminal cuff pressures. High pressures can be transmitted to the tracheal wall, and the resultant ischemia may lead to inflammation, ulceration, erosion, and later to stenosis.

In attempting to prevent this type of damage, some authors advocate a controlled leak technique.[5] The cuff is inflated to occlusion; then a small amount of air is withdrawn until an audible inspiratory leak is heard. Losses in tidal volume are made up for by readjusting the bellows or the cycling pressure, depending on the type of ventilator being used. ("Terminal flow" may also be needed to cycle a pressure-cycled ventilator properly.)

The use of high residual volume "low-pressure" cuffs is now considered preferable.[6–8] (See also Chap. 2.) To measure accurately the intracuff pressure (which closely approximates the tracheal wall pressure in this type of cuff), a four-way stopcock is required.[9] Air is injected into an evacuated cuff through one limb of the stopcock. The

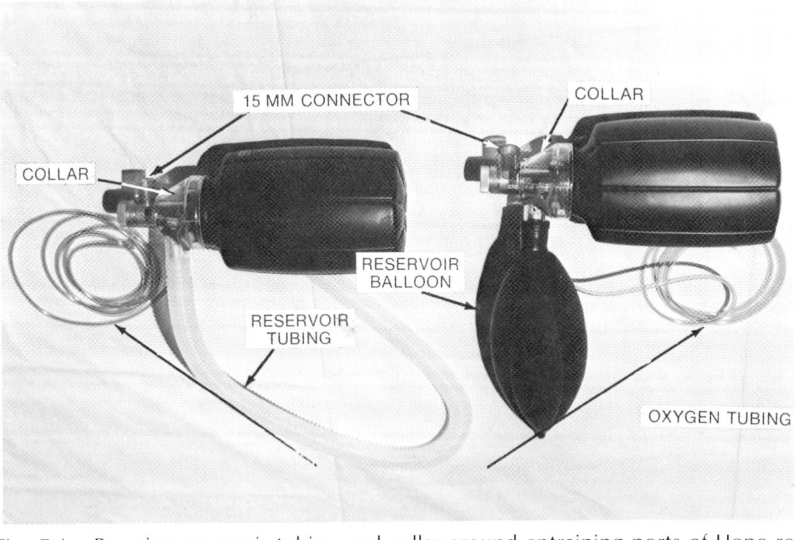

Fig. 7-4. By using reservoir tubing and collar around entraining ports of Hope resuscitator (*left*) or reservoir balloon with collar (*right*), oxygen is supplied to the entraining mechanism and a high F_{IO_2} is achieved.

other two limbs are simultaneously open to a mercury manometer and the cuff inflation line (Fig. 7-6). When the cuff reaches occlusion, the height of the mercury in the manometer reflects the intracuff pressure. Cuff pressures should be remeasured and recorded every eight hours or whenever the cuff has been deflated.

Inhaled Moisture

The patient with a respiratory disturbance frequently needs special attention to fluid administration. Do not discount the contribution of inhaled moisture to overall water balance. When the natural upper airway is by-passed, high-density mist or high humidity in the inspired air is needed to prevent mucus impaction. Since the alveolar gas is always completely saturated at body temperature, a moisture deficit in the large airways is possible if steps are not taken to add adequate moisture to inhaled gases. In fact, the tracheal mucosa can become seriously dried out and friable with inadequate moisturization. Even the gentlest suctioning will then cause bleeding wherever the catheter touches the mucosa.

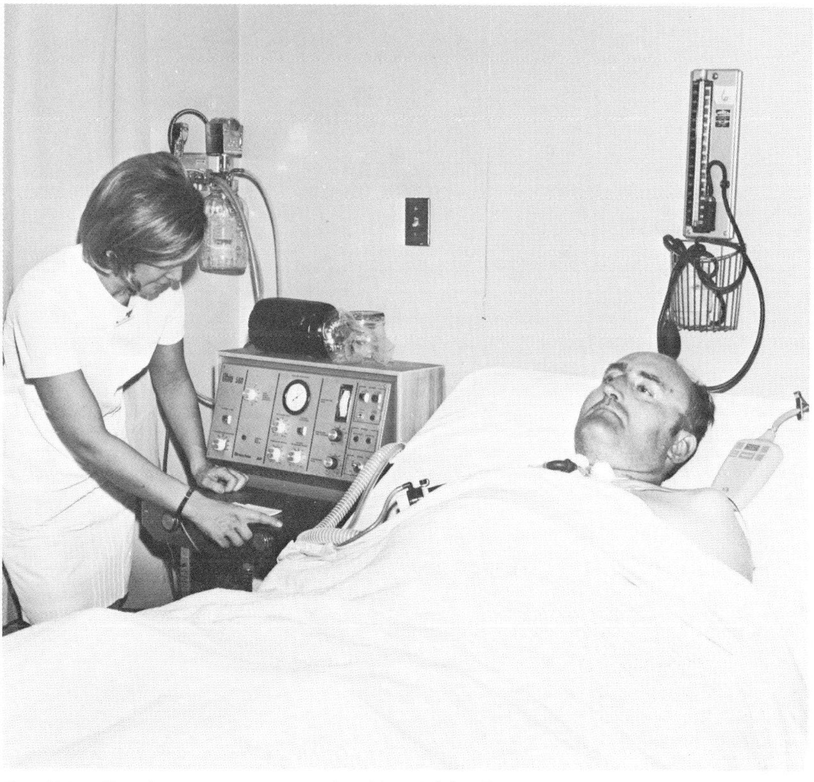

Fig. 7-5. Respiratory care nurse checking tidal volume rate and delivery of pressure from Ohio respirator.

The moisture needed to prevent these complications is supplied as molecular water (high humidity) or as particulate water (aerosol). Many adequate commercial devices are available for providing these forms of moisture. Routines should be established to insure that humidifiers or nebulizers are operating properly. Most of these devices are heated to increase the moisture-carrying capacity of the gas, and it is thus possible to cause rapid drying of the mucosa if the device is allowed to run dry.

Another danger is the possibility of bacterial growth within the nebulizer.[10] Only a sterile nebulizer should be used. When it needs refilling, residual water should be discarded, and the container should be rinsed out and then refilled with sterile water. Condensation that collects in the tubing should be discarded rather than

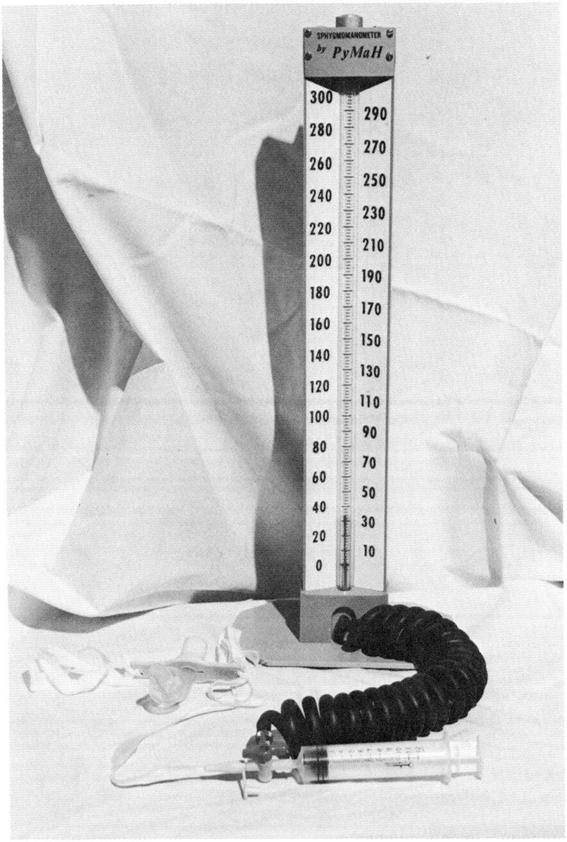

Fig. 7-6. Four-way stopcock arrangement for measurement of occluding balloon pressure. Occluding balloon and manometer deadspace must be filled simultaneously to indicate the true pressure within the cuff. Use of only a three-way stopcock allows for air from the occluding balloon to fill the deadspace of the mercury manometer; thus, inaccurately low pressures are indicated on the manometer. (Also see Chap. 2.)

drained back into the reservoir because it may contain contaminating bacteria.

It is beyond the scope of this chapter to give all details of intravenous or oral therapy, but in the absence of overt heart failure, a high urinary output (up to 100 ml/hr) resulting from liberal intake of fluids is desired.

Respirators

It is imperative that the nurses caring for the respiratory patient have a thorough understanding of the theory and principles of artificial respiration. Although numerous mechanical ventilators are available, the basic principles of operation are similar. Until nurses are technically competent with the respirators, they should not be made responsible for a patient requiring ventilatory support. The administrative policies of the hospital should include obligatory educational programs for the staff prior to assignment in the intensive respiratory care unit.

The respiratory therapy department can present formal and informal programs for others on the respiratory care staff to acquaint them with the complex equipment used in the unit. Their technical support should be valued and not be considered a threat by others.

Many useful texts on the subject of mechanical ventilation are now available, and machine manufacturers also publish complete manuals about their respirators. There are, however, a few points about ventilator use that we have found particularly helpful.

When working with a volume ventilator, frequent observation of the pressure gauge alerts personnel to changes in total pulmonary resistance. In normal lungs, for every centimeter of H_2O pressure applied to the airway, the tidal volume increases 100 ml. One can easily make a rough calculation of effective compliance by adjusting the respirator so that inflation is held static for a brief period, i.e., inflation held for 1 to 2 sec. Inflation can also be momentarily held by occluding the tube to the mushroom catheter of the exhalation manifold following delivery of the tidal volume. The tidal volume divided by the end inflation pressure is the effective compliance. For example, if the tidal volume is 700 ml and the pressure reading is 35 cm H_2O, compliance in this situation is 20 ml/cm H_2O.

These observations should be included in assessing the patient's status. A sudden increase in total pulmonary resistance may indicate a mucus plug, pneumothorax, pulmonary embolus, or kinked tubing. A gradual increase might be associated with pulmonary edema, bronchospasm, or development of the adult respiratory distress syndrome (see Chap. 8).

The patient pressure gauge on pressure-cycled respirators should also be observed at frequent intervals. These machines differ in principle from volume respirators because the pressure is preset to give a desired tidal volume; thus, they always register the same cycling pressure (see Chap. 4). However, the time required for each inspiration will vary as pulmonary resistance changes. This can be judged by the speed with which the patient indicator needle reaches the preset cycling pressure. A shortened inspiratory time with this type of ventilator may therefore indicate the same problems of increasing pulmonary resistance.

The goal of all artificial ventilation is to provide adequate alveolar ventilation, as judged by arterial blood gas evaluations. Once a tidal volume and rate that provide acceptable blood gas and pH values have been found, care should be taken that these parameters are maintained (unless, of course, the clinical state suddenly changes). With volume-cycled ventilators this is an easy task because the tidal volume is preset; volume will be delivered up to the pressure capability of the machine, barring electrical or other mechanical failures, such as tubing disconnections, leaks, or changes in respirator set-

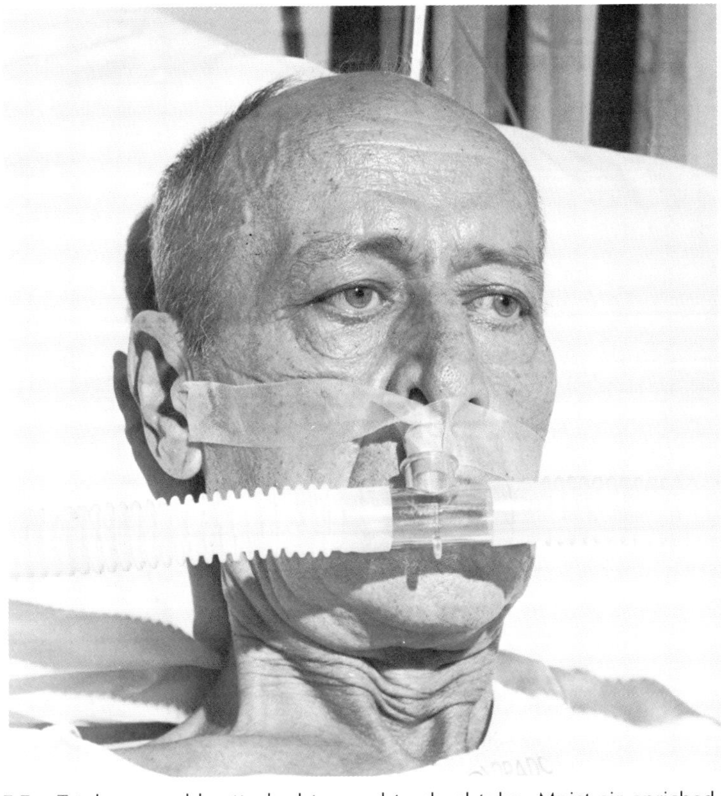

Fig. 7-7. T-tube assembly attached to nasal tracheal tube. Moist air enriched with oxygen comes from patient's right side from wall source and nebulizer. Exhalation occurs through the extention tubing to the left of patient. This is an open system, and CO_2 retention does not occur owing to flushing of the system by the continuous flow. This avoids CO_2 retention because there is no rebreathing.

tings. "Knob twiddling" is best prevented by adequate education of personnel. Electrical failure is usually obvious, and the availability of a "back-up system" with a self-inflating bag with each respirator is always helpful. Tube disconnections or leaks can be detected by an alarm system, which can be obtained as auxiliary equipment if it is not built into the particular ventilators being used (Figs. 4-3, 4-4, and 4-7).[11]

When using a pressure-cycled ventilator, maintaining adequate alveolar ventilation is more complex and requires even closer attention. As discussed previously, changes in pulmonary resistance cause changes in the speed with which the cycling pressure is reached. As volume is gas flow × unit time, the duration of each inspiration has a direct effect on the volume. If the respiratory rate does not change, increased resistance can lower minute ventilation. It is therefore important to monitor the expired tidal volume frequently with a hand-held respirometer (Wright). When presssure respirators are used, the physician should leave orders indicating a desired tidal volume range, with instructions to change the pressure setting as needed to achieve this goal. Adjustments are then made

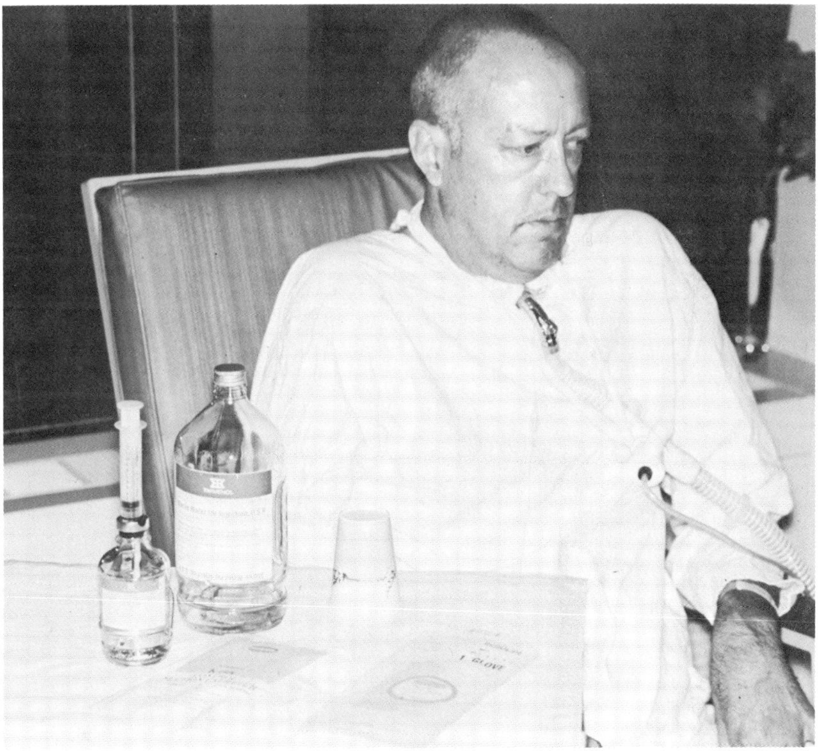

Fig. 7-8. Patient with COPD being ventilated and rested in a chair in the intensive care unit. Same patient as in Figures 7-2, 7-3, 10-1, and 10-6.

without frequent consultation with the physician unless there appears to be a change in total pulmonary resistance that requires immediate intervention by the physician.

Fluctuations in rate can also cause significant changes in minute ventilation. Therefore, it is important to note the respiratory frequency even when the patient is receiving mechanical support. We customarily allow a breathing patient to set his own respiratory rate. A "safety rate," usually less than the patient's spontaneous rate, is always preset. This rate will provide an adequate minute ventilation if the patient fails to trigger the machine. Those patients who hyperventilate are easily managed by adding dead space tubing between the patient's airway and the exhalation manifold.

Leaks anywhere in the system can cause significant loss of minute volume. These frequently occur at the humidifier connections, or they can be caused by incomplete seating of the balloon on the exhalation manifold. Particularly in patients with high pulmonary resistance, complete disconnection at the tracheostomy or endotracheal tube connection may occur. This problem can usually be prevented

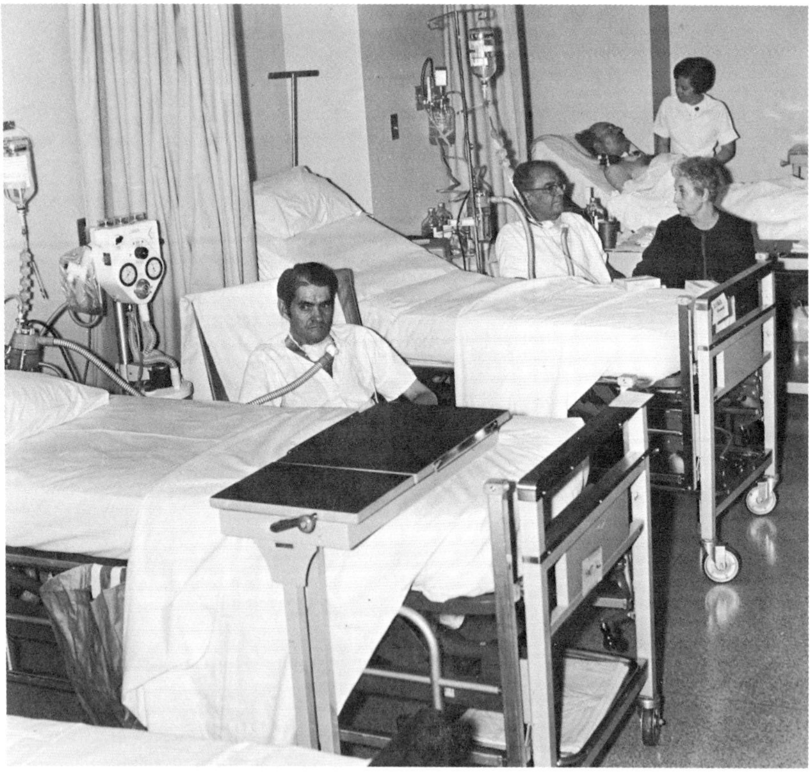

Fig. 7-9. Patient requiring ventilatory support or weaning, or both, in intensive care unit seated at the bedside. Notice wife visiting second patient with COPD.

by the use of tubes with well-fitting standard 15-mm connectors. Leaks may also occur within the patient's trachea when the balloon on the tracheostomy or endotracheal tube is inadequate. Occasionally, a small leak is tolerated in this area so that undue pressure is not exerted in the tracheal mucosa, but there must be close monitoring of the exhaled tidal volume to be sure that the patient is receiving sufficient ventilation.

The effectiveness of humidification is judged by noting the nature of the patient's secretions. If the tracheal aspirate is thick, additional humidification is necessary. With humidifiers, an increase in temperature provides more moisture delivery and may result in thinner secretions. If this is still not adequate, greater volume of moisture can be provided by nebulizers, which can be added to any respirator.

In any properly functioning moisturizing system, condensation will be apparent throughout the entire length of the tubing, and "rain out" will occur. One should not be misled by the moisture that

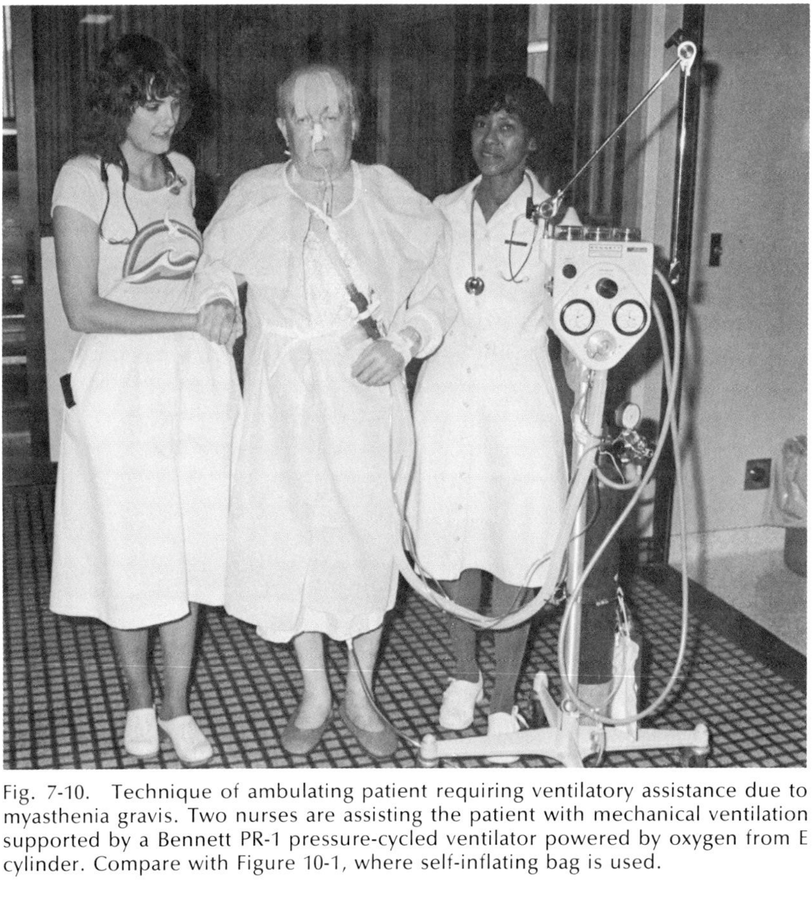

Fig. 7-10. Technique of ambulating patient requiring ventilatory assistance due to myasthenia gravis. Two nurses are assisting the patient with mechanical ventilation supported by a Bennett PR-1 pressure-cycled ventilator powered by oxygen from E cylinder. Compare with Figure 10-1, where self-inflating bag is used.

appears only in the dead space or exhalation tubing and which comes from the patient's exhaled moisture. Excessive "rain out" in the main tubing should be frequently discarded, and it should not be drained back into the humidifier since this will result in contamination.

We feel strongly that all patients requiring respiratory support should be cared for in an intensive care unit. The requirements of providing proper care and maintaining a life-support system cannot be met in the open ward or in private rooms. It is far too demanding for nurses and therapists and, more importantly, unsafe for the patient to compromise this principle. In spite of alarms and monitors, nothing can replace the watchful, intelligent eye of the nurse or therapist.

Practical sessions in the unit are useful to supplement formal seminars in inhalation therapy. Respirators equipped with test lungs are very effective teaching tools, since the nursing staff can observe

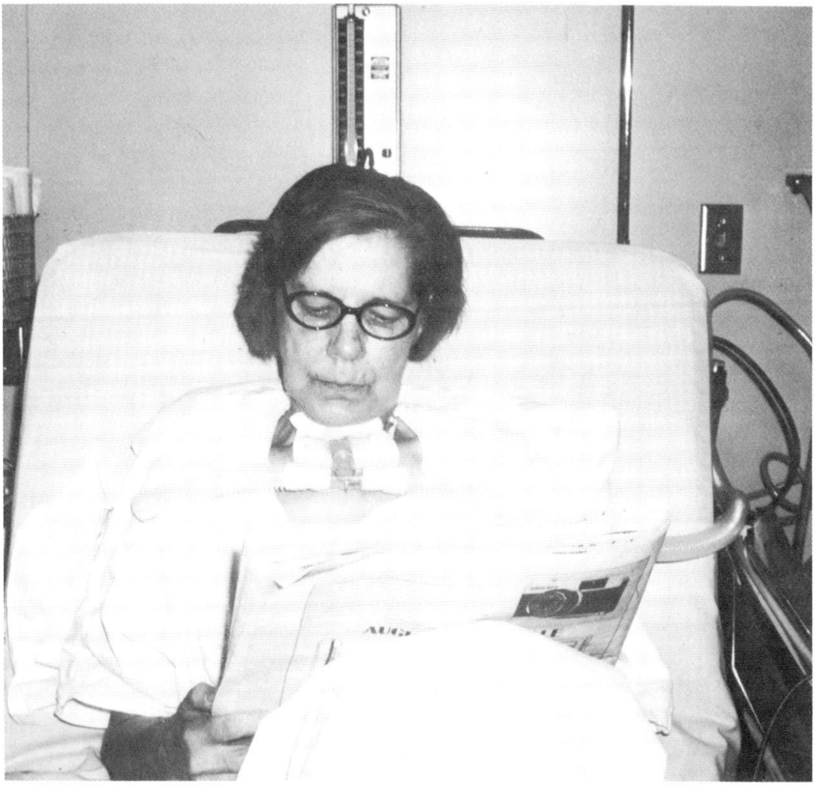

Fig. 7-11. Weaning system with T-tube assembly attached to tracheostomy. In this case, oxygen and moisture come from patient's left-hand side from wall nebulizer source, and exhalation occurs via patient's right-hand side. The extention tubing provides a reservoir that is useful if the patient's minute ventilation exceeds the flow of oxygen from the source.

the functions of the various knobs and dials. Practice in animal ventilation can also demonstrate pulmonary dynamics under laboratory conditions.

Weaning from the Respirator

Weaning from the respirator requires patience, skill, and an alertness to subtle changes in the patient's condition. Analyses of blood gases should always be obtained to serve as a baseline before weaning is attempted. Obviously, the values should be acceptable and appropriate for the clinical situation prior to weaning. The patient's own tidal volume should be near that produced by the respirator, and his "forced breath" (which can be measured at the bedside) should ideally be two to three times his necessary tidal volume. Weaning should not be attempted if the patient requires PEEP (see Chap. 5) or more than 40% inspired oxygen on the ventilator.

Other parameters helpful in making the decision to wean are resting minute ventilation and maximum voluntary ventilation. Both can be measured at the bedside with a respirometer (see Chap. 4).[12]

The initial period off the respirator should be carefully selected. Because physical activity should be at a minimum, the period should not include either the bath or mealtime. A calm atmosphere should be maintained with a team member at the bedside offering encouragement and support. During the weaning period, deterioration of the vital signs and volume measurements may indicate the need for a return to the respirator. Blood gas values must be obtained at appropriate intervals (often every 30 to 60 minutes). If they remain stable, time off the respirator can be extended. Patients with normal lungs who have required temporary ventilatory assistance, e.g., postoperative surgical patients or those recovering from drug overdose, may be weaned much faster than the patient with underlying lung disease.

All patients should have supplemental oxygen and mist supplied during weaning. All necessary equipment, including a tracheostomy collar or T-piece, large-bore tubing, and a nebulizer, should be gathered in preparation (Fig. 7-7). Oxygen should never be provided by a catheter inserted into the endotracheal or tracheostomy tube. Not only does this practice desiccate the mucosa—since bubble-through humidifiers can only produce approximately 30% relative humidity—but also, of greater importance, exhalation is made difficult by the constant flow of oxygen into the tube. This resistance will greatly increase the work of breathing and may rapidly tire the patient. If oxygen support is still necessary after the tracheostomy or endotracheal tube has been removed, it can be supplied via nasal cannulae at flows that produce an acceptable arterial oxygen tension ($>$60 mm Hg).

If secretions continue to be a problem, a Kistner tracheostomy button may be substituted for the tracheostomy tube to maintain a portal for suctioning (Figs. 2-11, 10-3, and 10-4). These buttons may be occluded to allow speech except when suctioning is needed. We will not suggest a schedule for weaning periods, since it is best to individualize the process rather than have the nurse and the patient become frustrated and discouraged if they cannot meet *preconceived* time tables. The popular technique of IMV has not offered any advantage in weaning and only delays the process or fatigues the patient. It is extremely important not to exhaust the patient during weaning. Rest periods back on the respirator for one hour must be strategically placed in the weaning plan (Fig. 7-8).

Cardiovascular and Renal Problems

The severely ill patient should receive close observation of his cardiovascular status and renal functions. The incidence of cardiac arrhythmias in patients with chronic lung disease is the same as that in patients in the coronary care unit. Therefore, cardiac monitoring is necessary, and prompt action in the case of arrhythmias may be life saving. It should be stressed, however, that correction of the arrhythmia must include the reversal of blood gas or pH abnormalities. When this is accomplished, pharmacologic therapy of the type used in acute myocardial infarction is not usually necessary.

Renal tract infections are common in patients whose respiratory failure is due to paralysis, since the necessary catheter drainage provides an opportunity for bacterial invasion. The use of catheters should be discontinued as soon as possible. Use of a closed drainage system with frequent changes of sterile equipment will reduce the infection hazard. Urinary problems are minimized when the patient can be nursed in the upright position in a chair.

Central Nervous System

Confusion and irrational behavior may be exhibited by the patient with a high P_{CO_2} or a decreased P_{O_2}, or both. The patient may seem obstinate and cantankerous or even psychotic. It is important that the nurse realize that this can be a manifestation of an underlying *blood gas* disturbance, the correction of which most often results in a return to normal behavior. A history from the family will usually reveal whether or not mental changes are recent. In severe cases it is not unusual for the patient to have become combative at home, and, in fact, hospital admission may be sought because of this behavior rather than because of any suspicion of respiratory failure. Often, personnel are threatened with physical abuse and legal action if they do not comply with the patient's wishes immediately. Some patients are aware that they are behaving bizarrely but are not able to control themselves.

The long-term patient in the intensive care unit may project his anxieties, fears, and hopelessness so strongly that members of the nursing staff may need counsel from a psychiatric physician or nurse to combat their own feelings of hopelessness or hostility toward the patient.

The subject of "intensive care delirium" has been recently studied.[13] The incidence of this complication can be minimized by simply placing the patient near a window to aid his day-night orientation and contact with his environment.[13]

Oxygen

Oxygen is most frequently administered through nasal prongs (see Chap. 3), since this system allows the patient to eat, converse freely, and take other treatments without interrupting his oxygen therapy. As with any medication, there should be a definitive oxygen order. Occasionally, when high flows are uncomfortable through the nasal prongs, a face mask can be substituted. It should be remembered that the patient using a mask should also be provided with nasal cannulae for use while eating or having oral hygiene.

On the rare occasions when a nasal catheter is required, one must be careful to ascertain the position of the catheter tip at frequent intervals. If the catheter becomes placed lower into the oropharynx, there is a possibility of gastric dilatation. Cleaning or replacement of the catheter at eight-hour intervals, or more often if the patient has a large amount of nasal secretions, is imperative.

Oxygen tents for the adult are obsolete except as air conditioners. In pediatric practice, tents are still used, more often for moisture therapy than for oxygen administration.

Activity

Maintaining the function of the musculoskeletal system is a prime concern with any acutely ill patient. Even though patients with respiratory failure are often surrounded by complex equipment, the nurse should not forget the time-honored principles of exercise (passive or active) and ambulation if this is at all possible.

The paralyzed patient will need a detailed program including maintenance of motion and function and prevention of decubitus ulcers. Today this aspect of care is the responsibility of the physical therapist in most larger hospitals, but this in no way relieves nurses of their continuing responsibilities in total patient care.

For patients who are able, sitting upright in a chair should begin as soon as possible. With a little assistance, the patient can be helped out of bed without disconnecting the respirator. Some patients are more comfortable sitting in a chair that provides good support than they are in bed (Figs. 7-1 to 7-3, and 7-8). Intensive care units need comfortable chairs. The patient's morale may also be raised by getting out of bed (Fig. 7-9). The period out of bed needs to be carefully gauged so that the patient does not become overtired and discouraged.

The next step is to assist the patient in ambulation. Even patients with severe respiratory insufficiency can be successfully ambulated when ventilation is augmented with a self-inflating bag with added oxygen. A size "E" oxygen tank with a mobile stand or the portable liquid oxygen system is valuable in aiding ambulation (Fig. 7-10; also see Chap. 10). Ambulation is particularly important in maintaining the muscular strength of patients with a chronic respiratory problem. Muscular activity requires more oxygen than does sedentary activity. A patient with severely limited pulmonary function may become bed- or chairbound if steps are not taken to maintain muscular strength.

Nutrition

The malnutrition of patients receiving mechanical ventilatory support is finally receiving appropriate emphasis.[14,15] Average daily vitamin, protein, and caloric intake is inadequate in almost all patients. Any degree of starvation weakens the respiratory muscles and reduces natural defenses against bacterial invasion, making these deficits of crucial importance in the patient requiring even modest periods of mechanical ventilation, e.g., five or more days. Although intravenous hyperalimentation has been proposed to counterbalance the effects of starvation, enteral hyperalimentation using a small-bore pediatric feeding tube is preferred.[16,17] Enteral hyperalimentation is more physiologic because it employs the wisdom of the body. It is safer and more economical then intravenous hyperalimentation.

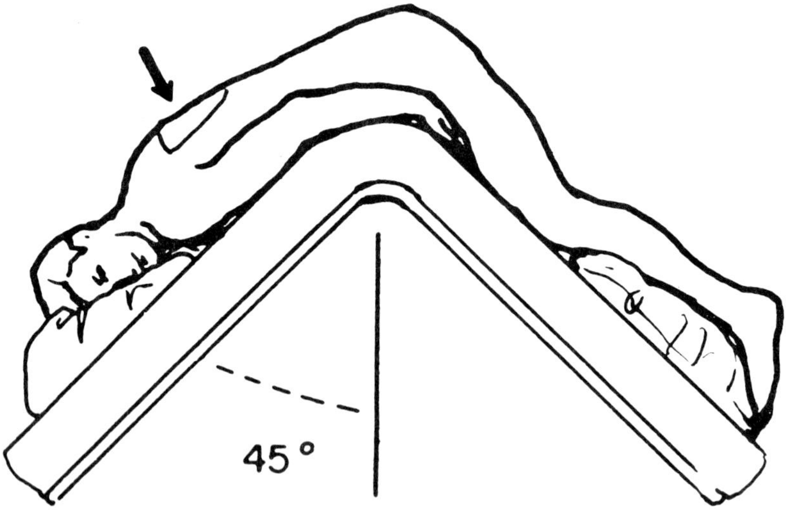

Fig. 7-12. Position for draining lower lobe and posterior basal segments. This can be accomplished by adjusting standard hospital beds or by using pillows.

It avoids atrophy of the gastrointestinal tract, which results in diarrhea and poor food tolerance. Thus, for may reasons it is preferred. Many patients who are awake and alert and who require long-term mechanical ventilation via a tracheostomy can eat regular food, which is the best possible way to receive oral nutrition. It also provides some pleasure for the critically ill patient.

Visitors and Comfort

The value of placing the patient near a window has been mentioned earlier in this chapter, as has the provision of a transistor radio or television, which is also helpful for many patients. Allowing unrestricted visiting, encouraging visits by the clergy, and employing friends and relatives in certain aspects of care such as feeding seems of obvious benefit, but this practice is unfortunately overlooked in many intensive care units. Something as simple as reading the newspaper is beneficial. The alert and well-groomed patient in Figure 7-11 was also able to eat a full diet. She was discharged from the unit after three more days of care with the tracheostomy tube removed.

PRINCIPLES OF PHYSICAL THERAPY

The purpose of chest physical therapy is prevention of respiratory complications and improvement of pulmonary function in patients with acute pulmonary problems. The physical therapist will find that the following techniques are helpful in reaching these goals: postural

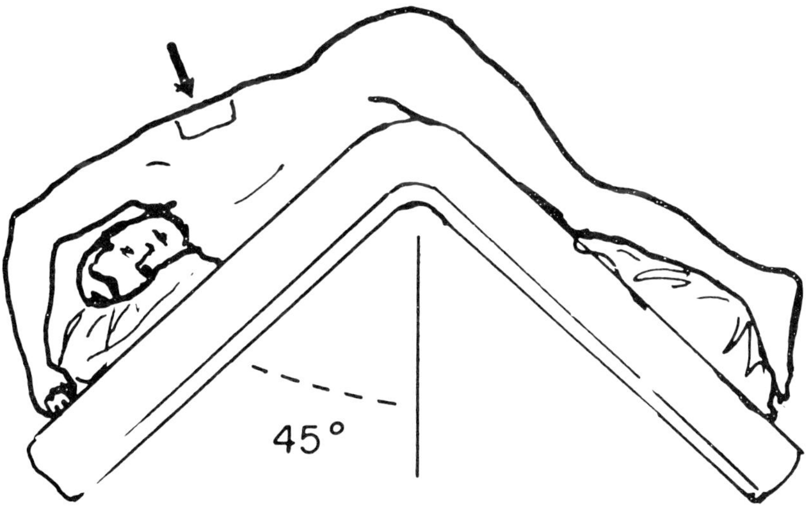

Fig. 7-13. Position for draining lateral basal segment of left lower lobe. The patient is rolled to the left for drainage of right lower lobe and to the right for drainage of left lower lobe.

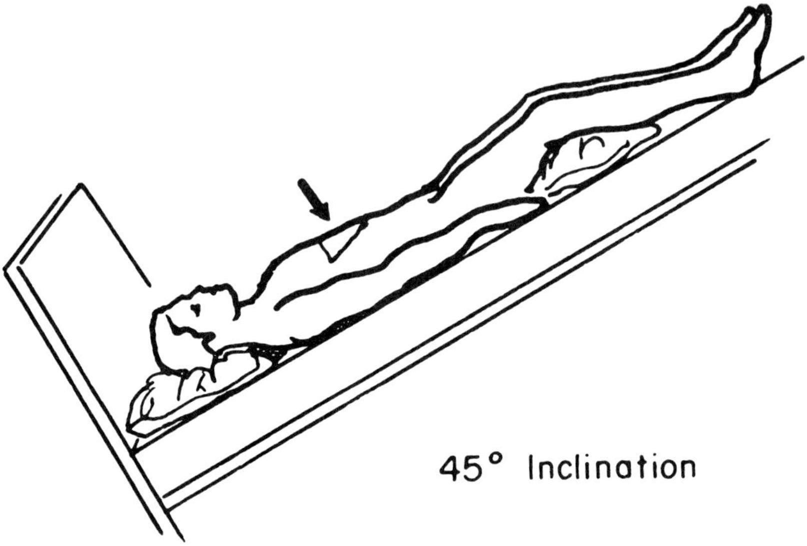

Fig. 7-14. Trendelenburg position for draining anterior basal segments of right and left lower lobes. This can be done by elevating the foot of the bed.

drainage with or without percussion and vibration, breathing retraining, and a program of progressively more strenuous exercise activity.[18]

Postural Drainage

Postural drainage is a physical means of forcing secretions from the lung toward the trachea so that they can be removed by expulsive coughing or aseptic suctioning. The aim of postural drainage is to promote more efficient clearing of the bronchial tree in less time and

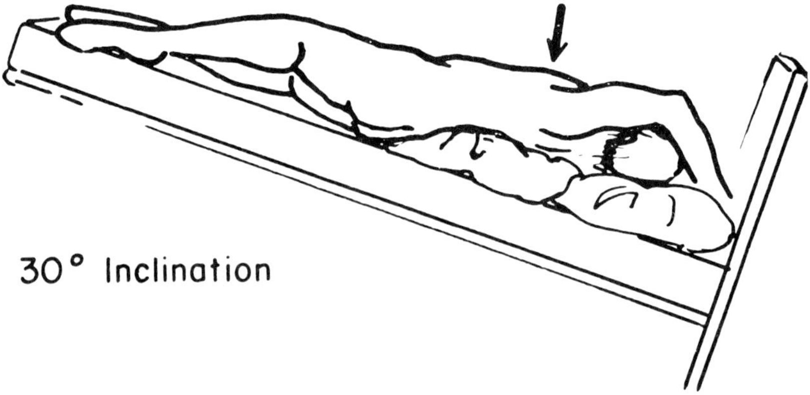

Fig. 7-15. Position for draining lingula. Right middle lobe can be drained similarly by rolling the patient onto the left side.

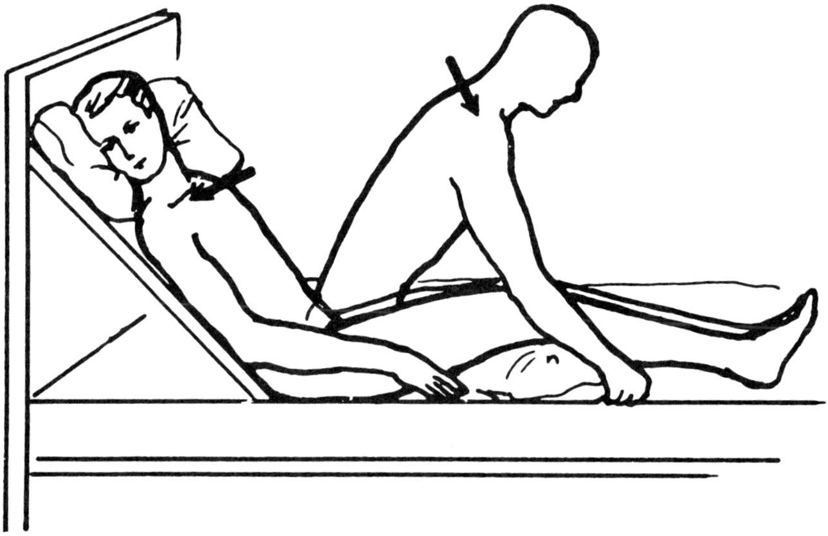

Fig. 7-16. Draining upper lobe segments. Leaning forward helps drain apical and posterior segments of the right and the apical and posterior segments of the left upper lobe.

with less energy expenditure and stress for the patient than is otherwise possible.

Posturing enlists the aid of gravity in draining local areas of the lungs. The various positions required to produce effective drainage are based on the anatomy of the bronchial tree. They involve positioning the patient so that the segmental bronchi are in a vertical position, and gravity can then assist drainage of that specific segment. Generally, five basic positions are used in postural drainage. These are shown in Figures 7-12 to 7-15. These positions allow drainage of each segment of the lung individually with the exception of

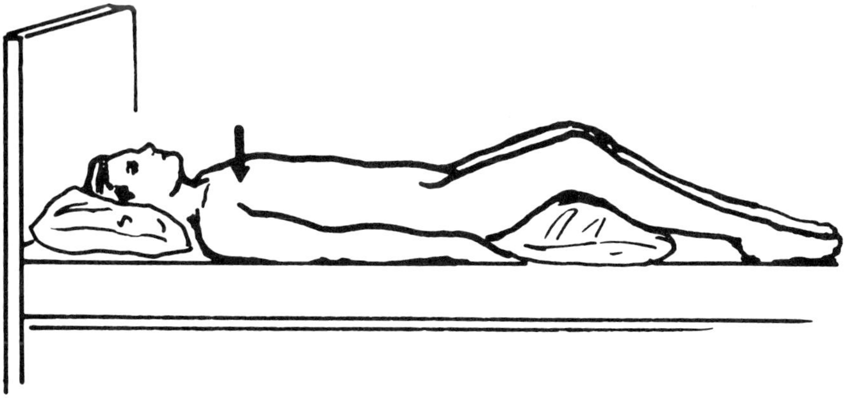

Fig. 7-17. Draining anterior segments of the upper lobes.

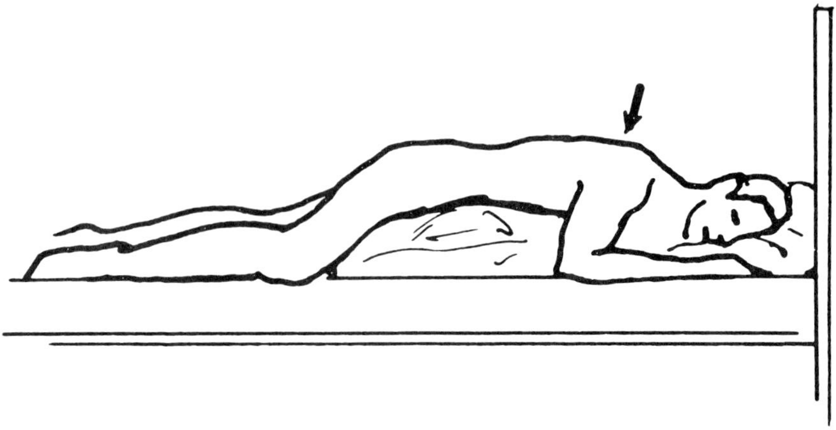

Fig.. 7-18. Draining posterior segment of right upper lobe as an adjunct to the procedure used in Figure 7-16.

the apical segments of the lower lobes. To drain each segment of the upper lobe selectively, four additional positions are employed (Figs. 7-16 to 7-20). To accomplish drainage in all these positions at one session would be time-consuming and fatiguing; specific positions should be chosen to suit each individual's needs. The complete sequence should be used cautiously and only in those patients with diffuse disease. One chooses each individual position by auditory and tactile clues and chest roentgenograms that indicate the location of retained secretions.

The total treatment time should generally not exceed 30 to 45 minutes. In special cases the patient's limited tolerance will make fre-

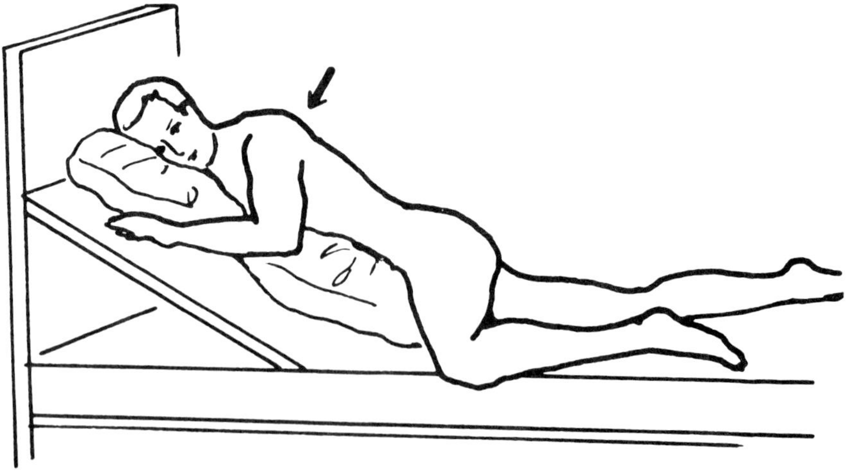

Fig. 7-19. Draining apical-posterior segment of left upper lobe as an adjunct to position in Figure 7-16.

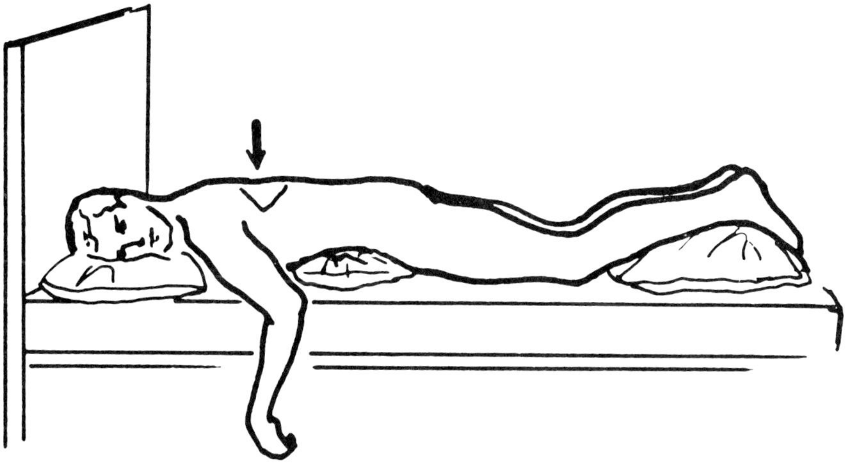

Fig. 7-20. Position for draining apical segments of lower apical (superior) segments of lower lobes.

quent but shortened treatment periods more desirable. On the other hand, occasionally a patient's pulmonary status will require that he remain in a drainage position 24 hours a day, with treatment periods used to relieve problem areas. Percussion is then given by the nurse or therapist for short periods and only over the most obstructed area to minimize fatigue. A good routine for drainage when a patient has moderate amounts of secretions is three times a day—before breakfast, before lunch (or late in the afternoon), and before bedtime.

Excessive handling of the patient should be avoided, and posturing for drainage can be incorporated into the routine for general turning and repositioning. Just before turning, deep breathing and controlled expulsive coughing should be encouraged.

Depending on the patient's condition, strength, and pulmonary function, he may require a modified program of bronchial drainage. If the patient is extremely dyspneic the angle of tilt may be reduced, or postural drainage may be accomplished with the patient in a horizontal position. Dyspnea may also be relieved by the use of an IPPB device or self-inflating bag while the patient is in the postural drainage positions. The patient with a tracheostomy tube or some other artificial airway in place may be unable to tolerate the prone position. For these individuals, extreme side-to-side positioning is substituted for the prone Trendelenburg position to drain the posterior basal segments of the lower lobes. For weak patients, the program may be alternated with rest periods to avoid unnecessary fatigue.

The results of postural drainage can be dramatic in the patient with impending respiratory failure from insufficient alveolar ventilation caused by the accumulation of secretions. Intubation and tracheostomy may sometimes be avoided by frequent and vigorous physical therapy.

Postural drainage is indicated in many clinical situations, including the following:

1. In the preoperative patient with excessive secretions from any cause.
2. In the postoperative patient when excessive secretions have accumulated because of a decrease in cough due to pain.
3. In patients with pneumonia.
4. In all disease states in which abnormal sputum production makes the patient subject to recurrent infection (e.g., cystic fibrosis).
5. When bronchospasm or extreme thickness of sputum makes it exhausting for the patient to raise his own secretions.
6. When a musculoskeletal abnormality makes the patient's cough mechanism mechanically inadequate (quadriplegia, scoliosis, myopathies).

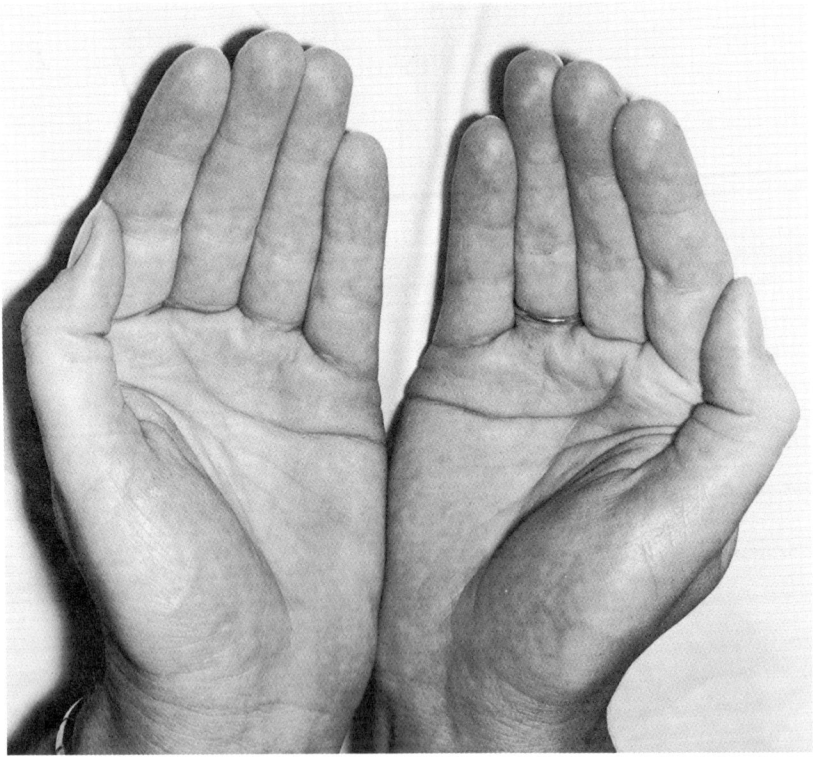

Fig. 7-21. Position of cupped hands for clapping maneuver. Hands should not slap the chest.

7. When the patient is unable to initiate a voluntary cough (comatose state, infancy).
8. In the obese or otherwise inactive individual.

Postural drainage is also used prophylactically to prevent retention of secretions when a patient is supported by mechanical ventilation or is unconscious. When intubation and mechanical ventilation are required, the obstruction to airflow by secretions or bronchospasm may require undesirably high inflation pressures to obtain adequate ventilation. Also, retained secretions increase the possibility of bacterial invasion. The suction catheter can only remove secretions from major airways; suctioning does not reach the distal airways. By adding postural drainage to the other techniques of airway maintenance, secretions can usually be delivered from specific segments of

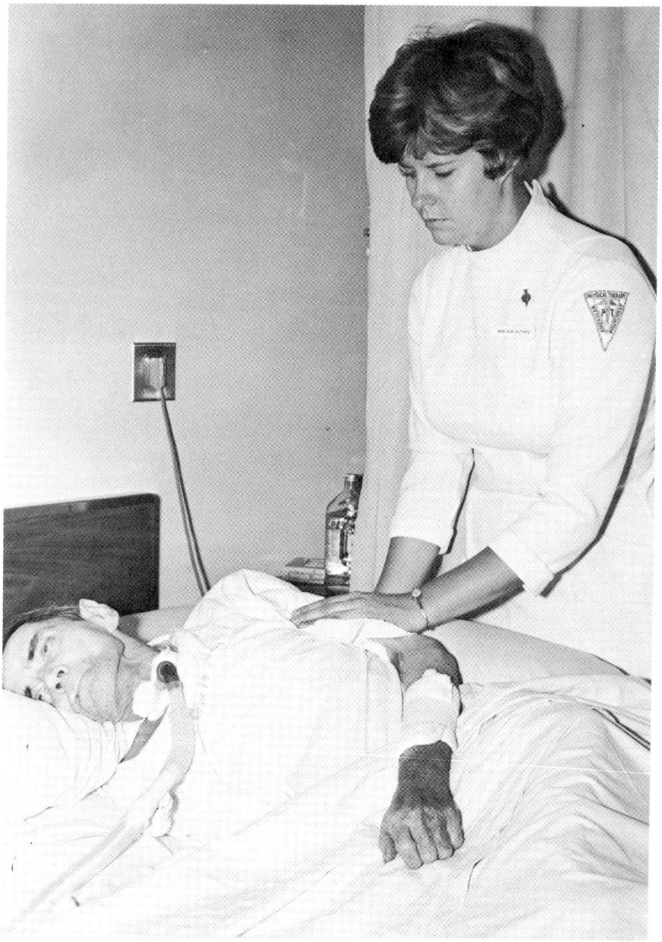

Fig. 7-22. Technique for shaking and vibrating a ventilator patient.

the lung to the bronchi, where they can be effectively removed by suctioning.

Postural drainage may be contraindicated in patients with unstable vital signs (extremes of blood pressure), directly after meals, and whenever suction equipment is unavailable.

Certain positions present a particular problem when a pressure-cycled respirator is being used to support ventilation. The efficiency of the respirator is greatly reduced when the patient's head is 30° below his hips because of an increase in total pulmonary resistance caused by the pressure of the abdominal contents (see Figs. 7-12 to 7-15).

By using the self-inflating bag for manual ventilation during this period, one nurse or therapist can control the pressures required for

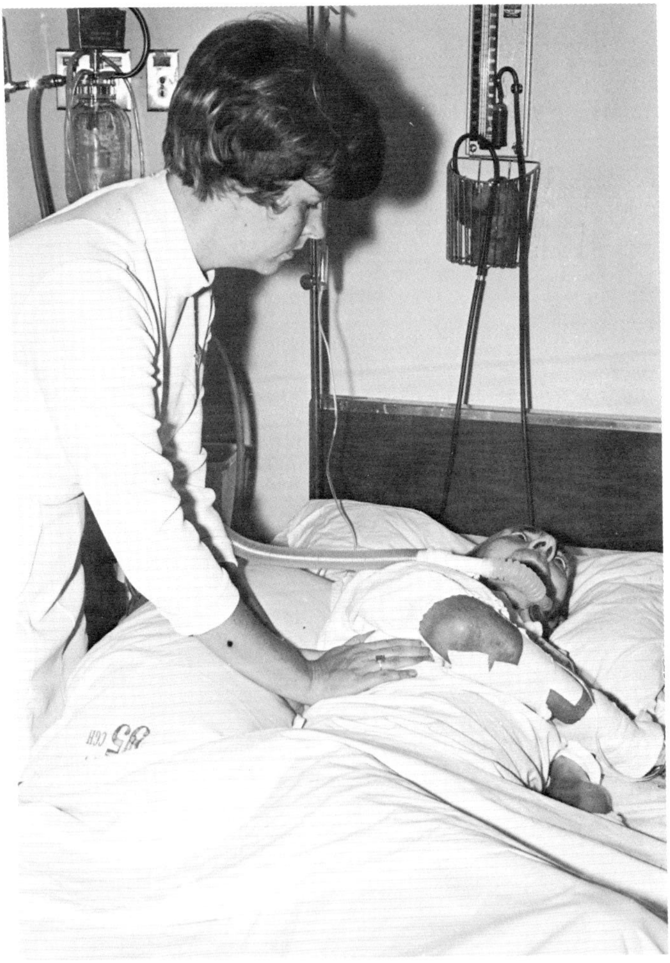

Fig. 7-23. Technique for shaking and vibrating a ventilator patient.

ventilation as the patient is changed from position to position; this staff member can thus maintain an adequate tidal volume while another aids the patient with drainage. When using the self-inflating bag to support ventilation, care must be taken to assure proper oxygenation. There are a variety of bags available which deliver varying percentages of oxygen. Choose the self-inflating bag that delivers the appropriate amount of oxygen.

The self-inflating bag can also help the patient to "sigh." When patients are able to breathe by themselves, an important adjunct to drainage is voluntary deep breathing by the patient. The small airways dilate slightly in inspiration; since mucus is more cohesive than adhesive, it will tend to peel off the walls of the airways allowing the force of the airflow on expiration to move plugs toward the trachea. The squeezing and vibrating by the physical therapist also aid this movement. The respirator or the self-inflating bag can be used to increase inflation volumes for the patient who is unconscious or paralyzed.

Percussion; Shaking; Vibration

Percussion, shaking, and vibration of the chest augment the effect of gravity in the removal of secretions. Percussion is the act of striking the chest wall rhythmically with cupped hands over the segment

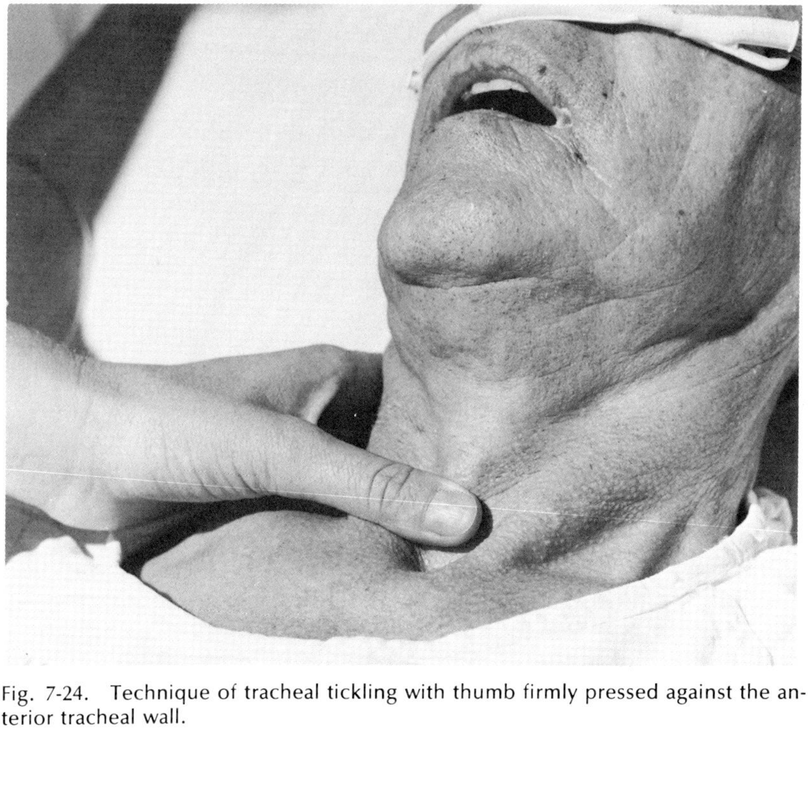

Fig. 7-24. Technique of tracheal tickling with thumb firmly pressed against the anterior tracheal wall.

to be drained. Cupping of the hands creates an air cushion on impact so that tenacious mucus is dislodged without discomfort to the patient.

To achieve the proper position with the hands, one should flex the metacarpal phalangeal joints approximately 30° and extend the interphalangeal joints fully with the thumb held tightly alongside the index finger (Fig. 7-21).

With the hands in this position, the wrists are alternately flexed and extended allowing the cupped hands to strike the chest wall rhythmically. Most of the motion should come from the wrists; the upper arms and shoulders should remain relaxed throughout the procedure. Proper clapping makes a hollow sound and is not painful; clapping is continued for about one and one-half minutes.

It is believed that this series of blows to the chest wall alters pressure within the airways. This percussive action will dislodge plugs of mucus and allow air to penetrate behind the secretions and help move these toward the trachea. The effect can be observed by bronchography. More secretions can be raised in a shorter period of time when percussion is added to posturing.

Clapping should be performed only over the thoracic cage; it should never be performed over the spine or below the thoracic cage, since the percussion can cause injury to the spinal column and internal organs.

Percussion may be contraindicated:

1. When bronchospasm is increased by its use.
2. If the patient is likely to hemorrhage.
3. If the patient is having seizures.
4. If pain is increased by its use.
5. In an obese patient.
6. If the patient has suffered a spontaneous pneumothorax and the risk of developing a tension pneumothorax still exists.

Immediately following percussion, a series of shakes or vibrations should be performed. Shaking and vibration are techniques of applying manual compression and tremor to the chest wall which loosens secretions further and moves them toward the trachea by encouraging the patient to exhale more forcefully. Techniques of shaking and vibrating are being illustrated by the physical therapist in Figures 7-22 and 7-23.

One should tense all muscles of the hands and arms and cause them to vibrate as if experiencing a cold chill. Pressure should be applied in the direction in which the ribs move on exhalation. Vibrations should be confined to the area that has been percussed; they are applied as the patient exhales slowly and steadily through pursed lips. Following full exhalation, the therapist relieves the pressure on the thorax but leaves the hands on the chest, as the patient inhales. Vibration is usually continued for three to five expirations. This technique may be used alone in the immediate postoperative period when pain makes percussion impossible. Vibration is more effective when coordinated with a large breath for the patient who is being mechanically ventilated or "bagged" during the treatment.

Controlled coughing or aseptic suctioning should follow postural drainage in order to clear the loosened secretions. An effective cough begins with a slow, deep inspiration through the nose. The patient is then instructed to open his mouth, to stick his tongue forward, and to cough three times before taking another breath in. This enables the maximum build-up of intrathoracic pressure during inspiration followed by a deep forceful trio of coughs on expiration. In the postoperative patient, the abdominal or thoracic incision must be

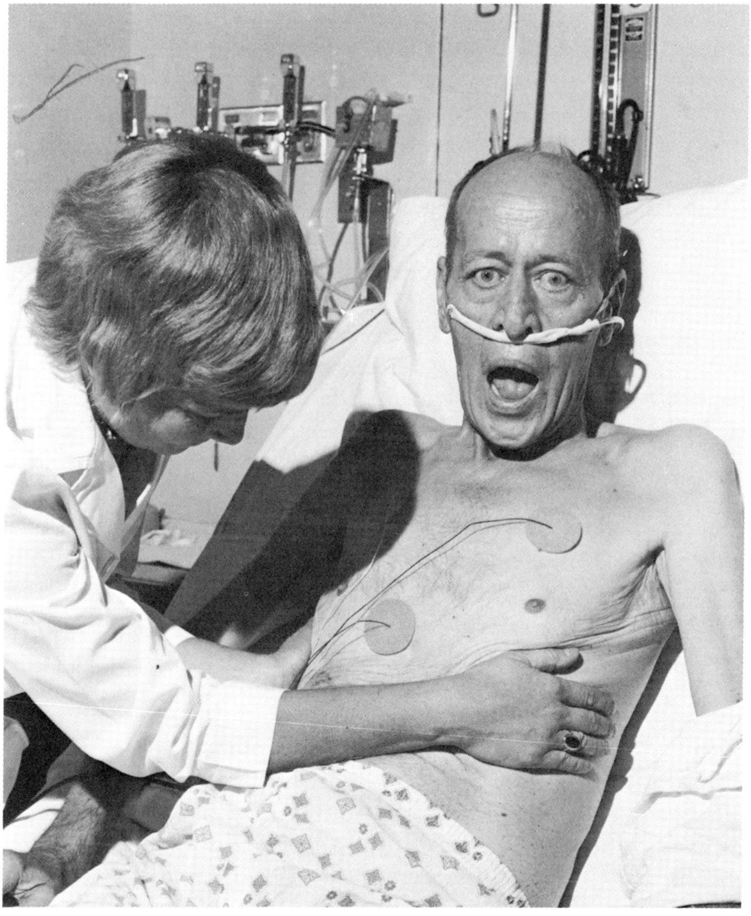

Fig. 7-25. Technique of expulsive coughing by lowered chest compression.

splinted with either pillows or the therapist's hands prior to expulsive coughing to reduce pain.

Tracheal tickling may be required to elicit an effective cough for the infant or the patient who is unwilling to cough because of fear and pain. By applying manual pressure to the trachea above the manubrial notch, an artificial obstruction is created. This obstruction serves to trigger an involuntary cough reflex that overrides the patient's inhibition (Fig. 7-24).[19]

Special supportive maneuvers may be used for the patient suffering from neuromuscular deficits which render his cough mechanism ineffective (i.e., scoliosis, quadriplegia, paraplegia, Guillain-Barré syndrome, myasthenia gravis). The therapist can substitute for weak intercostal and abdominal muscles and a paralyzed diaphragm by applying manual compression to the abdomen and lateral thorax at the exact instant that the patient reaches his peak inspiratory effort, when the patient attempts expulsive coughing (Fig. 7-25).

The percussion, shaking, vibration, and coughing cycle should be continued as long as the patient's condition permits or until coughing is no longer productive of mucus in that position. Allow the patient a moment's rest before proceeding to the next position.

Objective benefit from the techniques of postural drainage with or without the shaking, vibrating, or expulsive coughing maneuvers just described remains somewhat controversial. In one study, pneumonia did not clear more rapidly with either postural drainage or IPPB compared with a control group.[20] This study can be criticized on the basis of patient selection, and most likely the negative outcome can be related to the inclusion of patients with few or no retained bronchopulmonary secretions. Maximum expiratory flow-volume curves have been shown to be improved in both chronic bronchitis and cystic fibrosis using a combination of postural drainage, percussion, and vibrating.[21] The benefit from cough alone, probably the most effective method of clearing secretions, was not evaluated in this study.[21] Benefits must be tempered by possible deficits, and a least one study has shown decreased arterial oxygenation following postural drainage.[22] Another study found no significant change in arterial oxygenation following chest physiotherapy in ventilated patients requiring positive end-expiratory pressure.[23] The chest roentgenogram improved in the majority of patients in this study following use of physiotherapy techniques designed to mobilize and remove retained tracheobronchial secretions.[23]

A striking anecdotal example of improvement in re-expanding an atelectatic segment is illustrated in Figure 7-26. The posterior-anterior view shows an elevated right diaphragm and a small infiltrate at the right cardiophrenic angle (*arrow*, left panel) in an asthmatic patient with thick secretions. Following shaking, vibration, and expulsive coughing, a large mucus plug was expectorated, and a repeat chest roentgenogram obtained 30 minutes later shows the right diaphragm in its normal position and resolution of the shadow, which represented segmental or subsegmental atelectasis (*right panel*).

DISCHARGE FROM THE INTENSIVE CARE UNIT

Discharge from the intensive care unit should occur only when the patient is physiologically and psychologically ready. In general, this means that the patient no longer requires suctioning, chest physiotherapy, or other similar therapy more often than every 4 hours. Independence in breathing, eating, and personal hygiene should be established before the patient leaves the unit. Those few patients who cannot be independent should be placed under custodial care. Over a 16-year period, this practice has resulted in only 4 patients' being discharged from our intensive care unit while still requiring ventilatory assistance. Two were long-term muscular dystrophy patients requiring mechanical ventilation indefinitely (see Chaps. 13 and 19). One patient with severe COPD lived comfortably in a nursing home for 8 months, and another young man with congenital hypogammaglobulinemia was cared for by his mother at home for 6 months before he died.

Team conferences are necessary when the patient is transferred from the intensive care unit to the general unit. The nursing staff, as

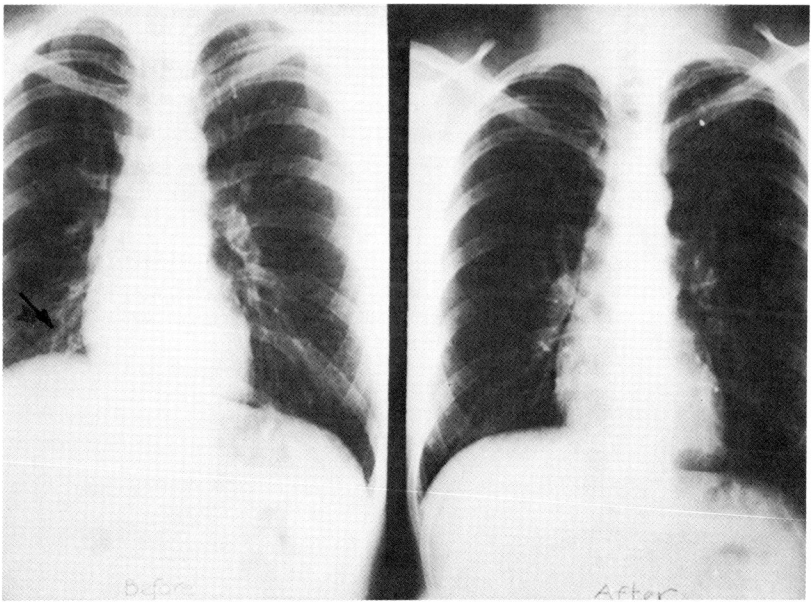

Fig. 7-26. X-ray evidence of segmental or subsegmental atelectasis (*left*) in asthmatic patient with retained secretions. Note elevated right diaphragm and infiltrate in the right costophrenic angle (*arrow*, on left panel). Clearing of infiltrate and return of right diaphragm to normal position 30 minutes following shaking, vibrating, and expulsive coughing that removed a large mucus plug.

well as other specialty staffs, should be included in this conference. The goals are to establish an immediate care plan, to outline the patient's program, and to arrange for home equipment if necessary. The patient with underlying pulmonary disease will require continuing attention (see Chap. 18), as will the respirator-supported patient with progressive neuromuscular disease (see Chap. 19). The patient who is interested in and knowledgeable about his disease is more likely to perform the daily treatments necessary to maintain pulmonary function at its optimum level. Key members of the family should be included in the instruction program, but whenever possible the patient should administer his own treatments. It is not advisable for other family members to mix medicines or to fill nebulizers, and so forth, since this fosters an unnecessary dependence. However, the family's support and understanding of the disease often help patients to adhere to their programs. Some specialized treatments, such as postural drainage, may require a family member's assistance.

The patient who has been so ill as to require assistance in ventilation should be seen by a visiting nurse on his return home. Instructions that were apparently well learned in the hospital often need to be repeated at home. Follow-up visits to the clinic or office may also reinforce home instruction. There should be close communication between the visiting nurse and the primary physician.

SUMMARY

Working together, the nurse, respiratory therapist, and, when available, the physician have vital roles in the successful care of any patient from the onset of acute illness throughout the convalescent and rehabilitative phases leading to recovery. Care is best when all staff members have a knowledge and appreciation of the interrelated disciplines working within the intensive care unit.

REFERENCES

1. Wanner, A., Zighelboim, A., and Sackner, M.A.: Nasopharyngeal airway: a facilitated access to the trachea. Ann. Intern. Med., *75:*593, 1971.
2. Nett, L.M., and Petty, T.L.: Acute respiratory failure (principles of care). Am. J. Nurs., *67:*1847, 1967.
3. Helming, M.G.: Nursing in respiratory diseases. Nurs. Clin. N. Am. *3:*383, 1968.
4. Boutros, A.R.: Arterial blood oxygenation during and after endotracheal suctioning of the apneic patient. Anesthesiology, *32:*114, 1970.
5. Bryant, L.R., Trinkle, J.K., and Dubilier, L.: Reappraisal of tracheal injury from cuffed tracheostomy tubes. Experiments in dogs. JAMA, *215:*625, 1971.
6. Geffin, B., and Pontoppidan, H.: Reduction of tracheal damage by the prestretching of inflatable cuffs. Anesthesiology, *31:*462, 1969.
7. Ching, N.P., Ayres, S.M., Paegle, R.P., Londen, J.M., and Nealon, T.F.: The contribution of cuff volume and pressure in tracheostomy tube damage. J. Thorac. Cardiovasc. Surg., *62:*402, 1971.
8. Cooper, J.D., and Grillo, H.C.: Analysis of problems related to cuffs on intratracheal tubes. Chest, *62:*215, 1972.

9. Cox, P.M., and Schatz, M.E.: Pressure measurements in endotracheal cuffs: a common error. Chest, *65:*84, 1974.
10. Reinarz, J.A., Pierce, A.K., Mays, B.B., and Sanford, J.P.: The potential role of inhalation therapy equipment in nosocomial pulmonary infection. J. Clin. Invest., *44:*831, 1965.
11. Petty, T.L., Nett, L.M., and Schmader, R.D.: A simple ventilator warning device. Ther., *14:*67, 1969.
12. Sahn, S.A., and Lakshminarayan, S.: Bedside criteria for discontinuation of mechanical ventilation. Chest, *63:*1006, 1973.
13. Wilson, L.M.: Intensive care delirium. Arch. Intern. Med., *130:*225, 1972.
14. Driver, A.G., and LeBrun, M.L.: Iatrogenic malnutrition in patients receiving ventilatory support. JAMA, *244:*2195, 1980.
15. Bennetti, P., and Blackburn, G.L.: Protein and caloric or macronutrient metabolic management in the critically ill patient. Crit. Care Med., *7:*520, 1979.
16. Heymsfield, S.B., Bethel, R.A., Ansley, J.D., Nixon, D.W., and Rudman, D.: Enteral hyperalimentation: An alternative to central venous hyperalimentation. Ann. Intern. Med., *90:*63, 1979.
17. Robinson, E.P., Jr., and Cox, P.M.: Feeding tube introduction—an easier way. Crit. Care Med., *7:*349, 1979.
18. Anonymous: Physiotherapy for medical and surgical thoracic conditions. London, Brompton Hospital Physiotherapy Dept., 1967.
19. Unguarski, P.: Mechanical stimulation of coughing. Am. J. Nurs. *71:*2359, 1971.
20. Graham, W.G.B., and Bradley, D.A.: Efficacy of chest physiotherapy and intermittent positive pressure breathing in the resolution of pneumonia. N. Engl. J. Med., *299:*624, 1978.
21. Feldman, J., Traver, G.A., and Taussig, L.M.: Maximal expiratory flows after postural drainage. Am. Rev. Resp. Dis., *119:*239, 1979.
22. Connors, A.F., Jr., Hammon, W.E., Martain, R.J., and Rogers, R.M.: Chest physical therapy: The immediate effect of oxygenation in acutely ill patients. Chest, *78:*559, 1980.
23. MacKenzie, C.F., Shin, B., and McAslan, T.C.: Chest physiotherapy: The effect on arterial oxygenation. Anesth. Analg., *57:*28, 1978.

Section B

Clinical Applications

Chapter 8

ADULT RESPIRATORY DISTRESS SYNDROME

By Thomas L. Petty

The adult respiratory distress syndrome (ARDS) is the final combination of a variety of unrelated but massive insults to the lung that injure its gas-exchanging interface. This often fatal syndrome is characterized by severe dyspnea, hypoxemia, and diffuse bilateral pulmonary infiltrations following lung injury occurring in persons who were previously healthy. The clinical presentation, the pathophysiology, a current understanding of the pathogenesis of the disorder, and an approach to systematic, physiologically oriented management are briefly reviewed in this chapter. Hemodynamic monitoring during mechanical ventilation using a flow-directed Swan-Ganz catheter is considered in Chapter 5.

HISTORIC PERSPECTIVE

The adult respiratory distress syndrome is not new to medicine; it is only now that it is recognized as an important clinical state and is better understood and better managed. Previous clinical reports and reviews of the underlying pathologic state resulted in numerous descriptive terms: congestive atelectasis, traumatic wet lung, postperfusion lung, "white lung," and "Da Nang lung." Table 8-1 lists many of the previous designations, all of which refer to the adult syndrome of acute diffuse lung injury. None are especially accurate or descriptive of all the pathways to the development of ARDS.

TABLE 8-1. Clinical Terms Often Synonymous with ARDS

Acute alveolar failure
Acute respiratory failure*
Adult hyaline membrane disease
Blast lung
Capillary leak syndrome
Congestive atelectasis
Da Nang lung
Postcardiopulmonary bypass perfusion lung (pump lung)
Respirator lung
Shock lung
Stiff lung syndrome
Traumatic wet lung
Whiteout lung or white lung syndrome

* Versus acute ventilatory failure.

My colleagues and I first described ARDS as a clinical syndrome in 1967.[1] Twelve patients were reported to exhibit a syndrome that was believed to be "remarkably similar to the infantile respiratory distress syndrome." The mechanical ventilatory support technique of trapping air within the lung with a threshold resistor (later called positive end-expiratory pressure [PEEP]) was used to improve oxygen transfer across the lung. Five patients survived. Autopsy findings of the seven who died revealed striking alveolar atelectasis, engorgement of capillaries, and hyaline membrane formation.

Shortly after, in 1968, a conference on the effects of nonthoracic trauma on the pulmonary system was conducted by the Committee on Trauma of the Division of Medical Sciences, National Academy of Sciences—National Research Council.[2] It became apparent that in patients in shock, with multiple long-bone trauma, and in those resuscitated with large volumes of fluid, there often developed a pulmonary picture that bore a monotonous regularity and a striking similarity to the original description of the adult respiratory distress syndrome. Many of the presentors were clinicians who had cared for combat casualties in Vietnam. It was believed that many cases came to the attention of physicians because huge numbers of combat casualties were cared for by "alert, informed physicians whose minds have been sensitized to detect the unusual and the unexplained." The excellent battlefield resuscitation and prompt evacuation to surgical care facilities allowed people who previously would have died to receive medical attention.

The mechanisms of the acute lung injury, which was clearly the common denominator in all cases presented at this conference, was unknown, and remains so today. Possibilities included toxic factors or vasoactive substances, the pulmonary effects of fat embolization, lung ischemia, surfactant abnormalities, hemodynamic factors, and exogenous factors such as overtransfusion of fluids.

Over the years, controversy over the appropriateness of the ARDS designation arose, and as our understanding of the process began to unfold, it became likely that the conceptual parallel between the adult respiratory syndrome and that suffered by the newborn infant may have been inappropriate. Specifically, the central role of a surfactant abnormality in the adult is not established, and experimental evidence suggests that a surfactant abnormality is not a primary event but rather a late complication of acute diffuse lung injury. In the infantile respiratory distress syndrome, surfactant abnormality is the primary cause. Whether the lumping together of all forms of injury under the syndrome is feasible continues to be debated. The term "ARDS" does create a conceptual framework on which to base therapy and further serves as a stimulus to understand better the basic mechanisms of injury caused by a variety of acute diverse pulmonary insults.

The remainder of the chapter presents the current understanding of ARDS, beginning with a clearer clinical definition, the current understanding of its pathogenesis, and then its pathophysiology. The contemporary approach to management is briefly reviewed.

DEFINITION

It is important to adhere to the original definition of the adult respiratory distress syndrome, summarized briefly in Table 8-2. ARDS is best recognized in patients with no previous underlying lung disease who have suffered a sudden catastrophic, often multiorgan system insult, which has led to dyspnea, labored

TABLE 8-2. Criteria for Diagnosis of the Adult Respiratory Distress Syndrome (ARDS)

Clinical history of catastrophic event,
Pulmonary or nonpulmonary (e.g., shock, multisystem trauma)
But exclude
Chronic pulmonary disease
Left ventricular failure
Must have clinical respiratory distress
Tachypnea > 20/min
Labored breathing
Central cyanosis when breathing air
With chest showing
Diffuse pulmonary infiltrates
And physiologic measurements of
Pa_{O_2} < 50 mm Hg (6.6 kPa) when F_{IO_2} > .6
Total respiratory compliance < 50 ml/cm, usually 20–30 ml/mm
Increased shunt fraction and deadspace ventilation

breathing, and noncardiogenic pulmonary edema with associated abnormalities of lung mechanics and gas exchange. In defining this syndrome, it is important to exclude primary left ventricular failure, subacute and chronic infiltrative lung disease, and other forms of respiratory insufficiency such as those associated with chronic airflow obstruction.

PATHOPHYSIOLOGY AND PATHOGENESIS

The respiratory distress syndrome is caused by diffuse damage to the gas-exchanging surface—the alveolar-capillary membrane. Damage to either the alveolar or the capillary side of this membrane can cause ARDS.

Diffuse alveolar injury, that is, injury to the alveolar-lining cell (type 1 alveolar cell), results from contact of these cells with a toxic substance. Inhalation of toxic gases, hydrocarbons, or gastric acid can cause such damage.

Diffuse capillary endothelial injury is probably the most common mechanism causing ARDS, but the precise pathogenesis remains unknown. It has been postulated that humoral agents, toxins, components of the coagulation system, activation of the complement system, or excessive sympathetic activity may individually or collectively play a role. Lung injury from infusion of oleic acid; endotoxin, salicylate, or narcotic administration; and central nervous system insults are among the most common methods used to produce ARDS in experimental animal studies designed to explain acute diffuse lung injury in people. However, so far no model of acute lung injury accurately reflects all facets of the human syndrome.

Whether the primary lesion is alveolar or vascular, an increase in vascular permeability occurs. The mechanisms keeping fluid in these capillaries may thus fail, and fluid may leak into the interstitial space and may flood into the alveoli, causing pulmonary edema.

A pathologic examination in the acute stage shows fluid and red blood cells in the interstitial space and in the alveoli. Later, hyaline membranes are seen, which are made up of proteins, mainly fibrinogen, that have leaked into the alveoli.

The response of the lung to injury is limited. The type I alveolar cells do not replicate. The type II cells, which are the producers of surfactant, can replicate and differentiate into type I cells. Thus, hyperplasia of type II cells may be prominent. In addition, the repair reaction in the interstitial space may result in fibrosis.

Lungs become noncompliant (stiff) in ARDS. This is caused by fluid accumulation in the interstitial space and alveoli. Another mechanism that may be responsible is the inactivation of surfactant by edema fluid, leading to an increase in surface tension that can cause alveolar instability and collapse. The noncompliant lungs have greater recoil, a greater "tendency to collapse." Since functional residual capacity is determined by the balance of forces caused by the chest wall recoiling outward and the lungs recoiling inward, the increased recoil of the lungs in ARDS causes a low functional residual capacity (Table 8-3).

Recent research into the pathogenesis of ARDS has focused again on surfactant abnormalities (Table 8-3). This reflects the continued comparison with the respiratory distress syndrome of the newborn, in which deficient surfactant plays a central role. There are certainly many similarities between the infantile respiratory distress syndrome (IRDS) and ARDS:

—Similar abnormalities in lung mechanics and gas transport.
—Indistinguishable pathologic features of congestive atelectasis, alveolar debris, and hyaline membrane formation.
—A comparable approach to supportive therapy.

This analogy remains one of the major reasons why the term "ARDS" was coined to designate this syndrome.

TABLE 8-3. Pathogenesis of ARDS

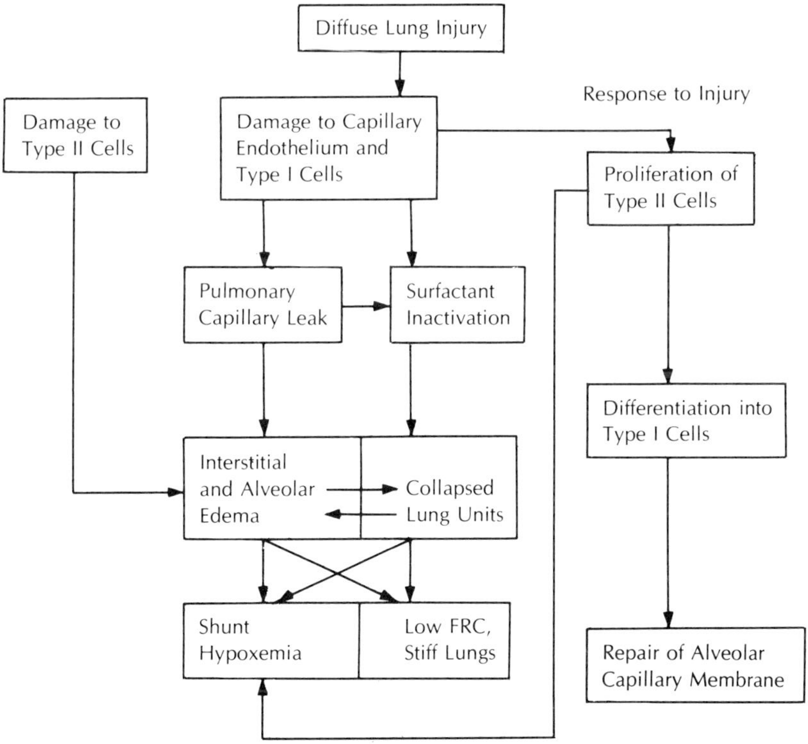

Unlike premature infants with IRDS, previously healthy patients with ARDS must have had normal surfactant function before the acute lung injury occurred. Since surfactant loss may promote alveolar collapse, which in turn may encourage the sequestration of alveolar edema, this could lead to further inactivation of surfactant function, so that a vicious circle might be set up. Thus, surfactant abnormalities found in ARDS may influence the secondary pathogenesis of the syndrome. If a convenient means of monitoring surfactant function or chemistry, or both, could be established, this might serve as a marker of injury or recovery. It is also conceivable that surfactant function could be restored pharmacologically or artificially by means of infusion or nebulization.

Hypoxemia is a cardinal feature of ARDS. The hypoxemia can be difficult to treat but is not often the cause of death. The major cause of hypoxemia in ARDS is shunting—continued perfusion of alveoli that are filled with fluid or collapsed and thus not ventilating. Hypoxemia caused by shunting is relatively resistant to oxygen therapy.

Because hypoxemia stimulates ventilation, and because the lung disease stimulates receptors that cause rapid shallow breathing, hyperventilation is common in ARDS. Hypercapnia is not usually the major problem.

CLINICAL SETTING

Many etiologic factors lead to ARDS, including major insults such as:

—Shock from any cause.
—Multisystem trauma.
—Overwhelming infection.
—Overdoses of drugs or other substances likely to damage the pulmonary circulation.
—Inhaled toxic substances.
—Infectious alveolar insults, including bacterial and nonbacterial pneumonia.

Table 8-4 lists the clinical states most commonly resulting in ARDS, but most often these clinical events occur without this complication.

DEVELOPING CLINICAL FEATURES

ARDS usually occurs in previously healthy people. Characteristically, there is a latent period between the occurrence of the insult and the development of the full-blown clinical picture, which is usually 18 to 24 hours (with extremes of 12 to 48 hours). After this interval, tachypnea, labored breathing, air hunger, and cyanosis are observed, and arterial blood gas analysis confirms the presence of hypoxemia. The abnormalities in lung mechanics and oxygen transfer are readily estimated once the patient is intubated

TABLE 8-4. Clinical States Associated with ARDS

Shock
Septic
Hemorrhagic
Cardiogenic
Anaphylactic
Trauma
Direct pulmonary contusion
Nonpulmonary, multisystem
Infection
Viral pneumonia
Bacterial pneumonia—staphylococcal or streptococcal
Miliary tuberculosis
Legionnaire's pneumonia
Disseminated intravascular coagulation
Fat emboli
Amniotic fluid emboli
Aspiration: especially of highly acid gastric contents ($pH < 2.5$)
Near-drowning
Inhaled toxic agents
Smoke
Phosgene
Oxides of nitrogen
Pancreatitis
Oxygen toxicity
Narcotic drug abuse
Heroin
Methadone
Propoxyphene
Radiation pneumonitis
Drugs
Ethchlorvynol
Salicylates

and receiving mechanical ventilatory support. It is likely that monitoring the respiratory rate and simple bedside measurements of respiratory mechanics during ventilatory support or of indices of gas transfer will yield important clues to the impending development of the fully established syndrome.

Three important clinical indices that could be continuously monitored in those patients thought to be at risk are:

—A fall in total respiratory compliance, as shown by an increase in the pressure necessary to inflate the stiff lungs ($\Delta V/\Delta P$ in ml/cm H_2O) at their maximal tidal volume.

—Tachypnea—often causing the patient to fight the respirator.

—An increase in the concentration of inspired oxygen (F_{IO_2}) or tension (P_{IO_2}) necessary to maintain an adequate arterial P_{O_2}.

The chest roentgenogram shows diffuse bilateral, usually symmetric, interstitial and alveolar infiltrations, characteristically sparing the costophrenic angles (Figs. 8-1 and 8-2).

MANAGEMENT

Today, the management of ARDS is empirical and supportive. Mechanical ventilatory support is essential, which requires:

—A definitive airway—an endotracheal tube placed through either the nose or the mouth, or a tracheostomy.

—A volume-cycled ventilator that allows exquisite control of the inspired oxygen concentration and modification of pressure-wave forms, as well as sufficient power to provide high levels of mechanical work.

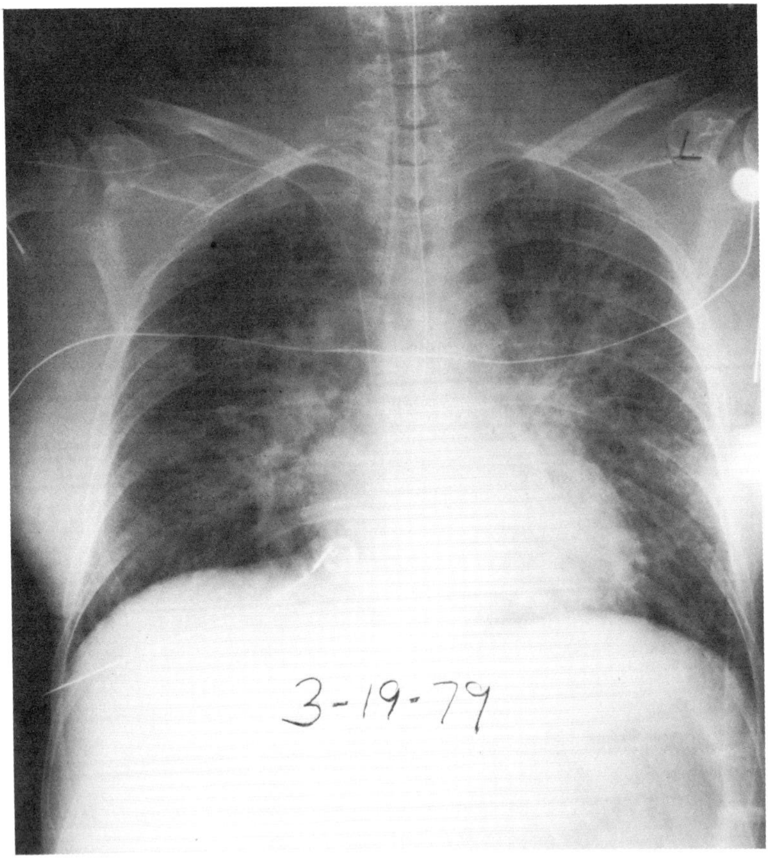

Fig. 8-1. Admission film from 42-year-old patient transferred from another hospital because of ARDS resulting from septic shock as well as hemorrhagic shock due to second massive gastrointestinal bleeding caused by esophageal varices. ARDS, hepatic failure, and diffuse intravascular coagulation were all background factors, along with aspiration of gastrointestinal contents. Endotracheal tube is in place.

The tidal volume is usually set at 10 to 12 ml/kg body weight at first, with a patient-initiated respiratory rate. Chosen by the patient's respiratory center, this may be relatively rapid owing to reflexes received from stretch receptors of the stiff (noncompliant) lungs.

PEEP

The use of positive end-expiratory pressure (PEEP) has continued to receive considerable attention. This technique maintains an end-expiratory pressure of 8 to 15 cm H_2O by imposing a threshold resistor during exhalation. PEEP keeps open lung units that are otherwise likely to collapse and be unavailable for gas transfer. These lung units may be "unstable" or collapsed owing to surfactant abnormalities. PEEP raises functional residual capacity and improves arterial

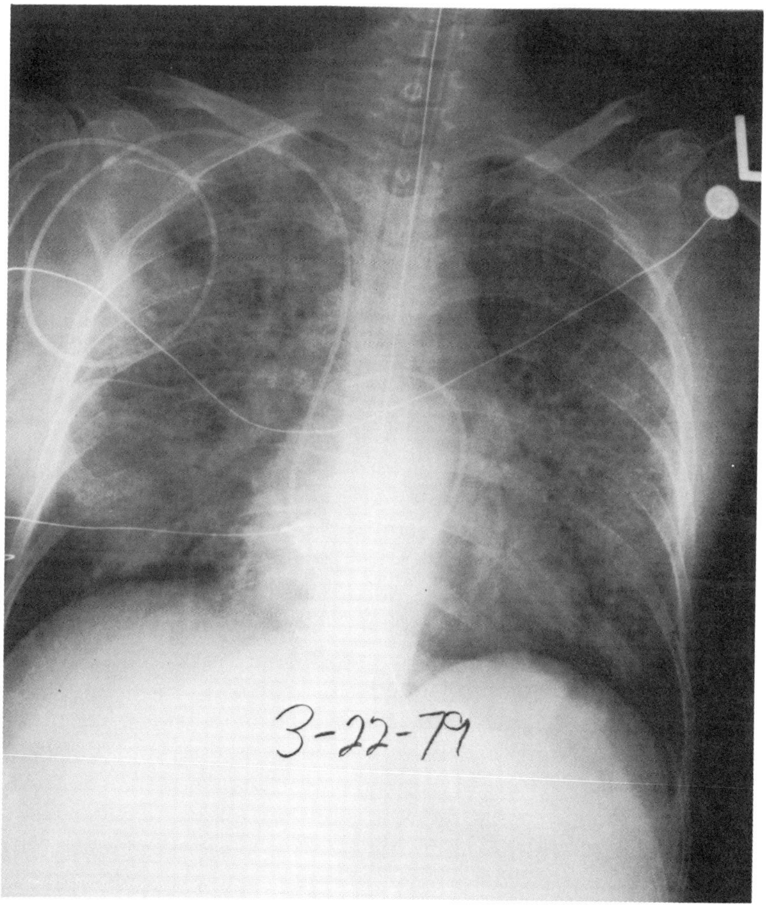

Fig. 8-2. Worsening alveolar infiltrates during third hospital day. Note characteristic sparing of costophrenic and cardiophrenic angles, which is a classic roentgenographic feature of ARDS.

oxygenation by opening up nonventilating units, effectively reducing shunting and thus allowing mechanical ventilation with a lower inspired oxygen concentration (FIO_2). Reducing the FIO_2 may prevent or delay oxygen-induced pulmonary damage that may take place after 24 to 48 hours of ventilation with an FIO_2 of more that 60%, or after only 12 to 24 hours with an FIO_2 of 100%. The benefit of PEEP is counterbalanced by the potential disadvantages of reducing cardiac output and the risk of further damage to the lungs caused by excessive intra-alveolar pressure (barotrauma). These two considerations are seldom problems in the case of markedly impaired pulmonary compliance, when conventional levels of PEEP (8 to 15 cm H_2O) are used. Although some advocate use of higher levels of PEEP, these are reasons for caution:

—There is no good experimental evidence to support this risky maneuver.

—Recent evidence suggests that there is an increased accumulation of lung water at higher levels of PEEP in isolated perfused lungs.

—Higher levels of PEEP may impair left ventricular function, adding a circulatory burden that would be undesirable in the face of the increase in pulmonary capillary permeability, which is the hallmark of ARDS.

Whether or not PEEP actually improves survival rates has also been recently questioned in a retrospective analysis, but unfortunately this study included patients with all forms of acute respiratory failure and not only patients with well-defined ARDS. (See also Chaps. 4 and 5.)

Pharmacologic Therapy

Pharmacologic therapy is discussed here only briefly and in principle. Almost all investigators agree that antibiotics should be used only for specific identified infections. The author has not found that so-called prophylactic antibiotics reduce bacterial colonization or invasion. In addition, the uncontrolled use of antibiotics has not been shown to reduce the burden of sepsis, which often results from infection with resistant gram-negative bacilli.[5]

Inotropic agents, such as dopamine, which increase cardiac output, would seem appropriate in the face of a failing circulation. Theoretically, a combination of inotropic agents and drugs that would promote peripheral vasodilatation, such as nitroprusside, would allow adequate tissue perfusion and oxygen delivery, even with a low left ventricular filling pressure. This approach might lower pulmonary microvascular pressure and, despite increased capillary permeability, could reduce capillary leak. These considerations at present remain theoretical but are the subject of intense investigation in some centers.

The use of corticosteroid drugs remains controversial. Corticosteroids given early in acute lung injury can reduce transcapillary fluid flux, may combat the damage to the capillary endothelium caused by complement fragments such as C5A, and promote membrane "stability."[6] Corticosteroid therapy has a potentially harmful effect on the function of the lung macrophages, which play a major role in the lung's defense against bacterial infection. Whether or not corticosteroids can improve surfactant elaboration in ARDS, as they appear to do in immature lungs, is debatable, but we must suppose that steroids may accomplish this in certain patients. Our group currently uses methylprednisolone sodium succinate in pharmacologic doses, 30 mg/kg body weight for 24 to 48 hours, in an attempt to capitalize on the potential beneficial effects just discussed, yet aiming to minimize side-effects such as bacterial colonization that theoretically should occur after the first 24 to 48 hours. So far, no controlled study has been conducted to either support or challenge the use of corticosteroids in ARDS, but their use is currently widespread.

TABLE 8-5. Etiologic Factors Associated with the Adult Respiratory Distress Syndrome

Factors	*Single Cause**	*Multiple Cause†*	*Total‡ (%)*
Common			
Sepsis	9	16	25
Shock	2	22	24
Trauma	2	21	23
Fluid overload	2	19	21
Aspiration	2	13	15
Major virus pneumonia	6	4	10
Disseminated intravascular coagulation syndrome	0	8	8
Fat embolism	0	7	7
Uncommon	7 patients	4 patients	
Drug overdose	2		
Drowning	2		
Pulmonary embolism and transplant		2	
Hemorrhage and transplant		2	
Air embolism	1		
Pancreatitis	1		
Inhaled irritant	1		

* 23 patients.
† Resulting from 57 different combinations of 66 patients.
‡ 100 consecutive cases.

OUTCOME

It is of interest to review the outcome of ARDS in 100 recent consecutive cases selected from one of our five hospitals, over a period of just more than 5 years. Patients were selected retrospectively by my colleagues and me, according to the definition in Table 8-2. The etiologic factors underlying these cases were analyzed and classified as major (common) and minor (uncommon) causes (Table 8-5). Although in some patients only a single etiologic factor was present, in the majority there was a combination of causes: A total of 57 different combinations of etiologic factors was found in this group of patients. This is why it is impossible to categorize patients with ARDS in terms of a single lung insult; in most patients not one, but many factors operate.

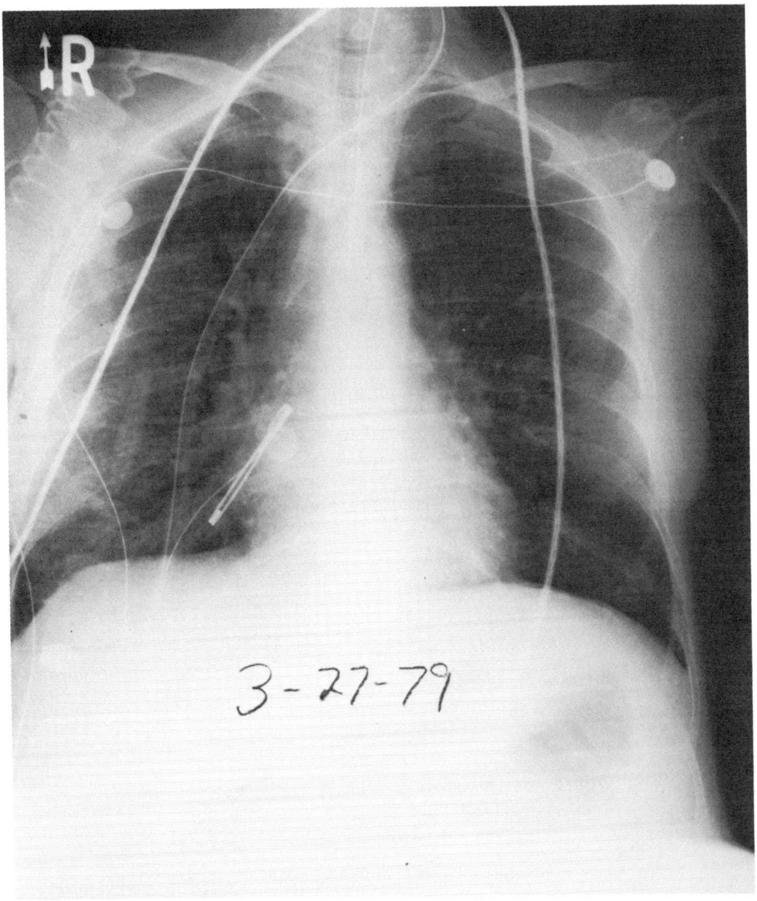

Fig. 8-3. Nearly complete clearing of infiltrates. Patient still required mechanical ventilation, but this could be discontinued on the next day. The patient was discharged on the eleventh hospital day. This is a remarkable outcome considering the adverse background factors resulting in ARDS.

Only 44 of these 100 patients survived, which is similar to other large series, although no other well-defined prospective study of this type has been reported. The outcome for these 100 consecutive patients, analyzed in terms of the 8 major etiologic factors, suggests that sepsis and shock are most clearly associated with a poor prognosis. Overall, the outcome must depend not only on the type of the original injury but also on the effectiveness of the initial respiratory support and the avoidance of such subsequent complications as oxygen toxicity, sepsis, and barotrauma. Initial respiratory support is usually successful, so that in avoiding complications an additional margin of success might be achieved:

—Using the lowest possible oxygen fraction (preferably $FIO_2 < 0.4$).

—Using meticulously clean techniques to avoid infecting the patient's unprotected airway.

—Keeping a careful watch for infection by means of daily clinical assessment, paying particular attention to fever, leukocytosis, new pulmonary infiltrates, and culture of tracheobronchial secretions.

—Avoiding excessive levels of PEEP or ventilation with an unnecessarily high level of tidal volume to prevent barotrauma, which can result in pneumothorax or pneumomediastinum, or both, with subsequent septic complications.

SEQUELAE

A rapid resolution of the x-ray manifestations of ARDS is evident in patients who make a rapid recovery, but this resolution is not immediate and often requires a week or more. Figure 8-3 shows nearly complete resolution of the alveolar and interstitial infiltrates,

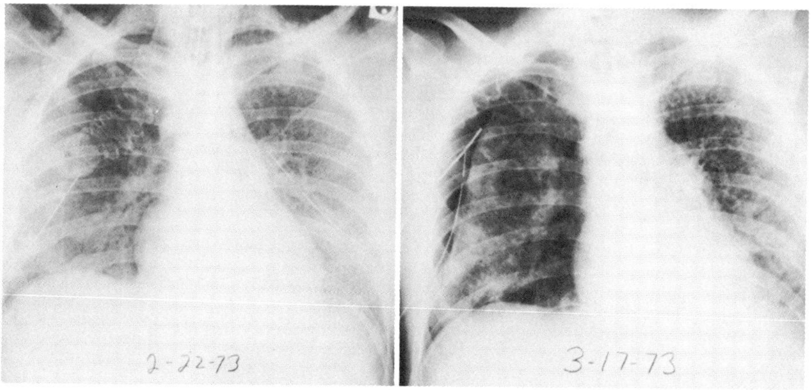

Fig. 8-4. *Left,* x-ray picture of pulmonary infiltration from ARDS after a month of mechanical ventilatory support in 25-year-old man suffering from amphetamine and other intravenous drug abuse and vasculitis. Note bilateral chest tubes for bilateral pneumothoraces (*left*). *Right,* slight clearing 4 weeks later and persistence of right-sided pneumothorax.

following the x-ray appearance of Figures 8-1 and 8-2. (See legends to all three figures).

Patients can be weaned from mechanical ventilation when they no longer require either PEEP or an F_{IO_2} of > 0.4, and when they can provide the necessary effort for breathing without fatigue.

Patients in a group followed more than seven years have shown progressive functional improvement, except for one patient who had a substantial degree of underlying chronic airflow limitation before ARDS was diagnosed. It is surprising that radiographically apparent interstitial fibrosis does not progress; in fact, the reverse is true. Figures 8-4 to 8-6 show slow x-ray resolution over a period of time in one of the cases in this follow-up series.

This series of patients demonstrated a progressive improvement in forced vital capacity (FVC), total lung capacity (TLC), and single-breath carbon monoxide transfer a period of months or years. Thus,

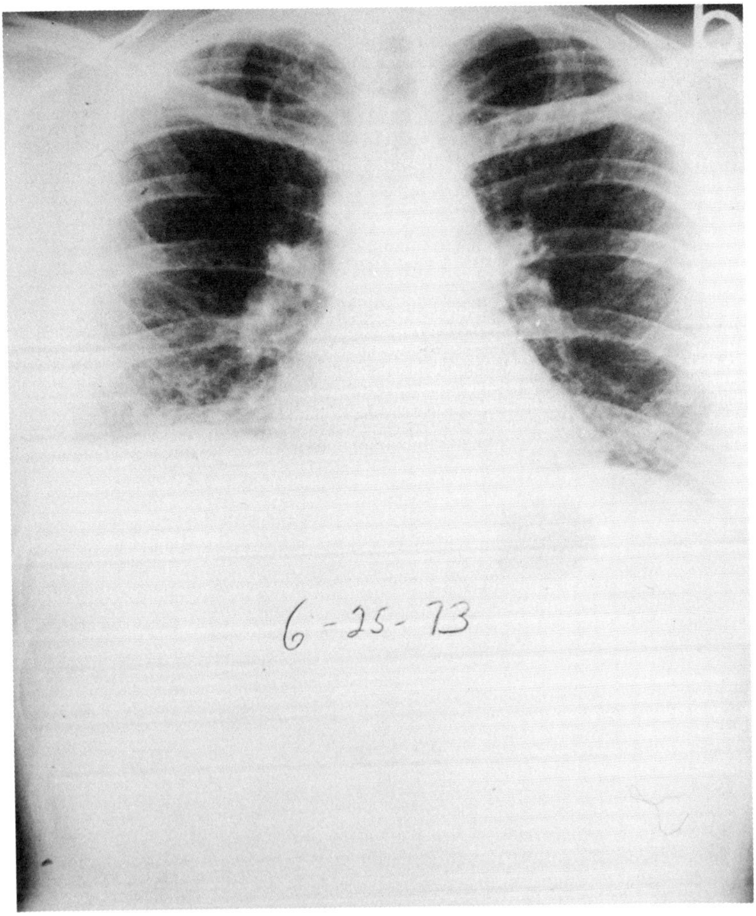

Fig. 8-5. Further roentgenographic clearing at time of discharge.

although in the early stages of recovery a patient may have moderate to severe respiratory insufficiency, further improvement in overall lung mechanics and gas transfer can be expected.[7,8]

The probable explanation for the progressive improvement in gas transfer is that although type I cells die after injury, this is followed by a proliferation of type II cells, which then line the alveolar spaces. These metabolically active cells may, of course, create an impediment to gas transfer. Later, however, the type II cells differentiate into type

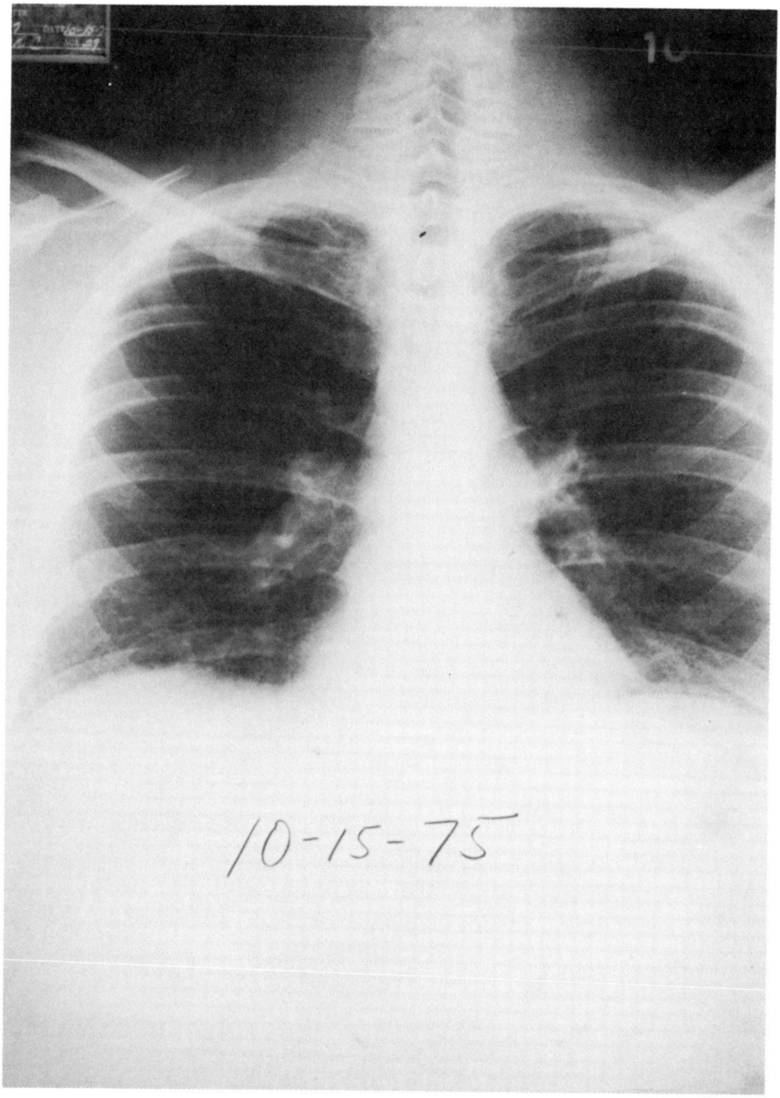

Fig. 8-6. Excellent resolution of roentgenographic evidence of fibrosis with only minimal basilar infiltration remaining approximately 2½ years following initial insult resulting in ARDS. Patient remains well 8 years following discharge.

I cells, thus perhaps "reconstituting" the alveolar epithelium.[9] This is most likely to occur if the basement membrane is intact. A great deal of fibrosis is also present relatively early in the course of ARDS. The pathologic picture, found at open lung biopsy, bears a good relationship with recovery.[10] Since such excellent resolution of residual x-ray and physiologic features occurs over months or years following recovery, considerable remodeling of the lung must take place.

THE FUTURE OF ARDS

Many unanswered questions and challenges remain. We urgently need to find a circulating marker for ARDS in order to identify those patients who are likely to develop the syndrome. If markers can be found that relate to pathogenesis, perhaps pharmacologic blockers can be developed. Recently, members of our investigational team have found the level of a fibrin or fibrinogen degradation product, the D-dimer, to be markedly increased in patients developing ARDS following a variety of difficult lung insults.[11] The level of this same

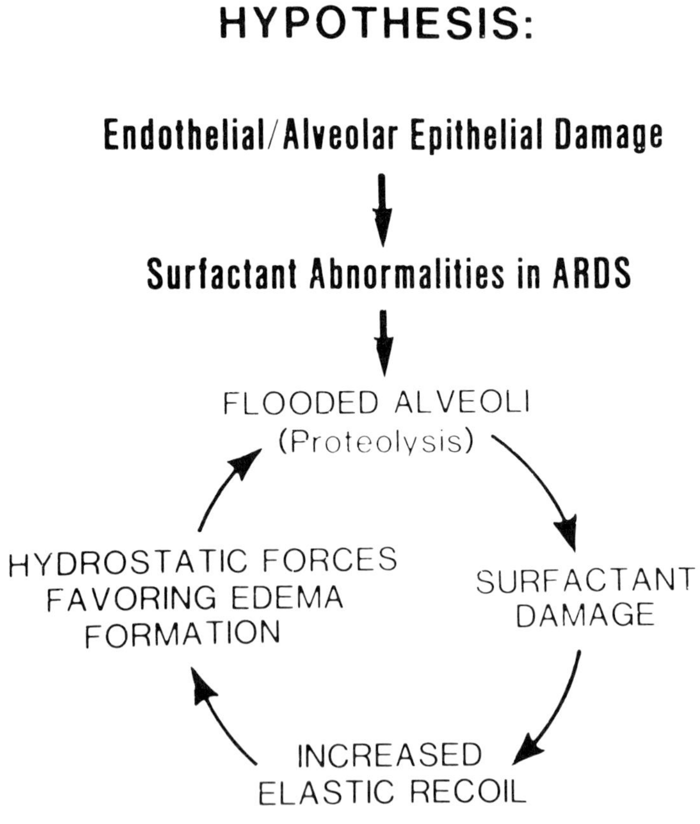

Fig. 8-7. Hypothesis linking endothelial-epithelial injury to surfactant damage in ARDS.

D-dimer was not increased or was only mildly increased in patients with similar injuries. These patients had almost identical risk factors for the development of ARDS but did not develop the full-blown syndrome.[11] Another group of investigators found evidence of complement activation, and this may be the mechanism of leukocytic aggregation and sequestration that occludes the pulmonary capillary bed and releases protolytic enzymes to cause lung damage.[12,13] This offers a rationale for the prompt and aggressive use of corticosteroids, which have been shown to block complement-mediated leukocytic aggregation.[14]

In addition to mechanical compromise of the pulmonary circulation, release of prostaglandins and other mediators is most likely operative in the development of pulmonary hypertension. A search for new agents to combat this mechanism is ongoing. Preliminary information suggests that a prostaglandin inhibitor, ibuprofen, may be useful, and it is currently under study.[15]

Complement activation, leukocytic aggregation, and release of elastase and vasoactive amines, along with activation of the clotting cascade, may occur simultaneously. Together these factors insult the alveolar capillary membrane, resulting in pulmonary edema. It is likely that the final common pathway is an attack on surfactant. With surfactant deficiency, the lungs are flooded further and become stiff. Antibacterial defenses are impaired, and sepsis almost invariably ensues. The possible vicious cycle of lung injury, surfactant damage or destruction, increased elastic recoil, and edema formation is presented as a hypothesis in Figure 8-7. Thus, the steps in pathogenesis are compatible with the usual concepts of pathogenesis and of transvascular fluid and protein movement in pulmonary edema in ARDS.[16–18]

Experimental models are also needed for controlled studies designed to offer better pharmacologic approaches to the problem. For example, can the lung be encouraged to tolerate a high inspired oxygen concentration for longer periods of time? Can early pulmonary fibrosis be avoided? Can lung surfactant production be stimulated? Can surfactant be replaced by natural or synthetic material? Most important, can septic complications be avoided or better treated? All these challenging questions remain for the clinical investigator of the future. In the meantime, supportive therapy and empirical approaches that have been established during the past 14 years should continue to be applied in a systematic and physiologically oriented way, for experience has shown that they can save approximately 40% of patients suffering from ARDS.

REFERENCES

1. Ashbaugh, D.G., Bigelow, D.B., Petty, T.L., and Levine, B.E.: Acute respiratory distress in adults. Lancet, *2*:319, 1967.

2. Eiseman, B., and Ashbaugh, D.G.: Pulmonary effects of nonthoracic trauma. J. Trauma, *8:*624, 1968.
3. Petty, T.L., Reiss, O.K., and Paul, G.W.: Characteristics of pulmonary surfactant in adult respiratory distress syndrome associated with trauma and shock. Am. Rev. Resp. Dis., *15:*531, 1977.
4. Petty, T.L., Silvers, G.W., Paul, G.W., and Stanford, R.E.: Abnormalities in lung elastic properties and surfactant function in adult respiratory distress syndrome. Chest, *75:*571, 1979.
5. Ashbaugh, D.G., and Petty, T.L.: Sepsis complicating the acute respiratory distress syndrome. Surg. Gynecol. Obstet., *136:*865, 1972.
6. Luce, J.M., and Pierson, D.J.: Corticosteroids and antibiotics in adult respiratory distress syndrome. A review. Sem. Resp. Med., *2:*151, 1981.
7. Lakshminarayan, S., Stanford, R.E., and Petty, T.L.: Prognosis after recovery from adult respiratory distress syndrome. Am. Rev. Resp. Dis., *113:7*, 1976.
8. Simpson, D.L., Goodman, M., Spector, S.L., and Petty, T.L.: Long-term follow-up and bronchial reactivity testing in survivors of the adult respiratory distress syndrome. Am. Rev. Resp. Dis., *117:*449, 1978.
9. Bachoven, M., and Weibel, E.R.: Basic patterns of tissue repair in human lungs following nonspecific lung injury. Chest, *65:*145, 1974.
10. Lamy, M., Fallat, R.J., Koeniger, E., Harm-Peter, D., Ratliff, J.L., Eberhart, R.C., Tucker, H.J., and Hill, J.D.: Pathological features and mechanisms of hypoxemia in adult respiratory distress syndrome. Am. Rev. Resp. Dis., *114:*267, 1976.
11. Haynes, J.B., Hyers, T.M., Giclas, P.C., Franks, J.S., and Petty, T.L.: Elevated fibrin (ogen) degradation products in the adult respiratory distress syndrome. Am. Rev. Resp. Dis., *122:*841, 1980.
12. Jacob, H.S., Craddock, P.R., Hammerschmidt, D.E., and Moldow, C.F.: Complement-induced granulocytic aggregation. N. Engl. J. Med. *302:*789, 1980.
13. Hammerschmidt, D.E., Weaver, L.J., Hudson, L.D., Craddock, P.R., and Jacob, N.S.: Association of complement activation and elevated plasma C5a with adult respiratory distress syndrome. Lancet, *1:*947, 1980.
14. Hammerschmidt, D.E., White, J.G., Craddock, P.R., and Jacob, H.S.: Corticosteroids inhibit complement-induced granulocytic aggregation. J. Clin. Invest., *63:*789, 1979.
15. Hempel, F.G., and Lenfant, C.J.M.: Current and future research on adult respiratory distress syndrome. Sem. Resp. Med., *2:*165, 1981.
16. Hyers, T.M.: Pathogenesis of adult respiratory distress syndrome: Current concepts. Sem. Resp. Med., *2:*104, 1981.
17. Albert, R.K., Lakshminarayan, S., Huang, T.W., and Batlin, J.: Fluid leaks from extra alveolar vessels in living dog lungs. J. Appl. Physiol. Resp. Envir. Exer. Physiol., *44:*759, 1978.
18. Albert, R.K.: Factors affecting transvascular fluid and protein movement in pulmonary edema and ARDS. Sem. Resp. Med., *2:*109, 1981.

Chapter 9

STATUS ASTHMATICUS IN ADULTS

By Thomas L. Petty

Status asthmaticus represents an immediate, life-threatening medical emergency in adults and children. Appreciation of this fact, and prompt, systematic, and aggressive management can be life saving in many patients. This chapter deals with the pathogenesis, pathophysiology, recognition, and treatment of status asthmaticus in adults. The problem of emergent asthma in children is reviewed in Chapter 16.

DEFINITION

Classically, status asthmaticus is defined as severe asthma not responsive to inhaled or injected sympathomimetic amines or to oral, rectal, or intravenous administration of theophylline (such as aminophylline).

PATHOPHYSIOLOGY

Figure 9-1 summarizes the pathophysiologic features of severe acute asthmatic attacks leading to status asthmaticus. The central problem is increased airway resistance due to bronchospasm, mucous secretion, and inflammation. The increased airway resistance increases the work of breathing, which in turn increases oxygen consumption and carbon dioxide production (not shown in the figure). Ventilation-perfusion mismatch is present in the areas of bronchial obstruction, resulting in hypoxemia. Hypoxemia also occurs when alveolar ventilation fails. Both hypoxemia and respiratory acidosis (acidemia) can cause reactive pulmonary hypertension.[1] Finally, when ventilation fails further, profound carbon dioxide retention, respiratory acidemia, and refractory hypoxemia may terminate in a fatal arrhythmia. It is recognized that the proposed scheme represents an oversimplification of the effects of blood gases and pH abnormalities on airways and pulmonary vasculature.

Additionally, asthma experts recognize that severe asthma attacks are *self-perpetuating* and tend to worsen steadily and become more refractory to treatment. Most patients who develop status

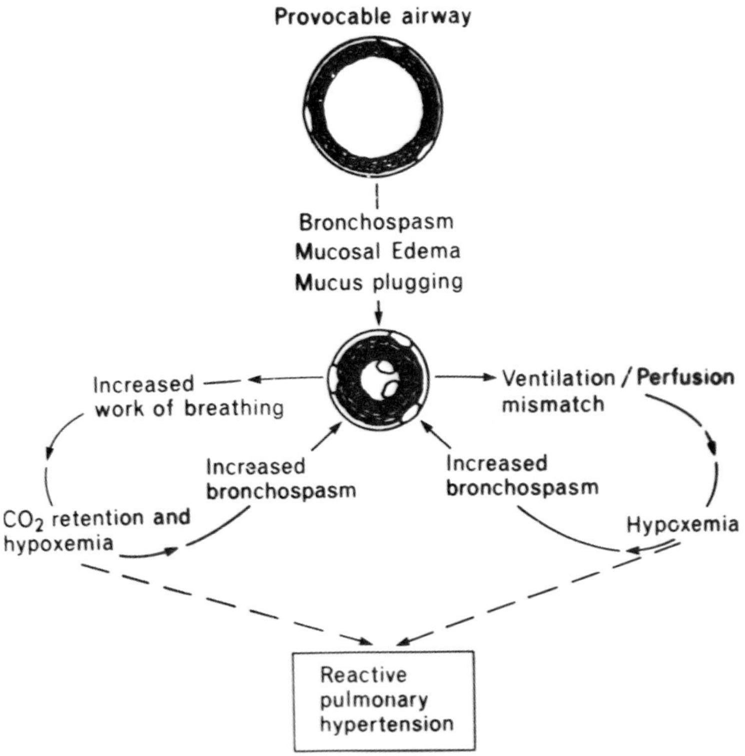

Fig. 9-1. Scheme hypothesizing pathophysiology of severe bronchial asthma. Increased airways resistance leads to ventilation-perfusion mismatch and hypoxemia, which in turn increases airways resistance (*right*). Increased work of breathing, ultimate carbon dioxide retention due to alveolar hypoventilation with accompanying hypoxemia, and increased airways resistance by this mechanism are indicated on left. (*From* Recent Advances in Asthma Therapy. Kenilworth, NJ, Schering Corp. Copyright 1976 by Schering Corporation. All rights reserved.)

asthmaticus have suffered from increased coughing, wheezing, and dyspnea for several days before they seek medical attention. Understanding the pathologic changes in the air passages helps the physician to plan treatment. The obstruction is not merely the result of severe bronchospasm but is due to mucous plugging and bronchial wall inflammation as well.

Status asthmaticus in advanced stages actually approaches irreversibility; that is, it is reversible only with great difficulty. Irreversible asthma is dramatically illustrated in Figure 9-2*A*, which shows the postmortem bronchograms of a patient who died of status asthmaticus. In this postmortem bronchogram (Fig. 9-2*A*), taken during simulated breathing in an artificial thorax, marked narrowing of major segmental airways (*arrows*) is seen, compared with the normal airway diameter of a patient without lung disease who died of a myocardial infarction (Fig. 9-2*B*).

A similar degree of bronchospasm is revealed in the bronchogram of an asthmatic patient referred from another hospital, who suffered an exacerbation of asthma during this procedure (Fig. 9-3). Bronchography is rarely performed in asthmatics and should *never* be done during an asthma attack. In this case, bronchospasm was probably worsened during the bronchographic procedure. The

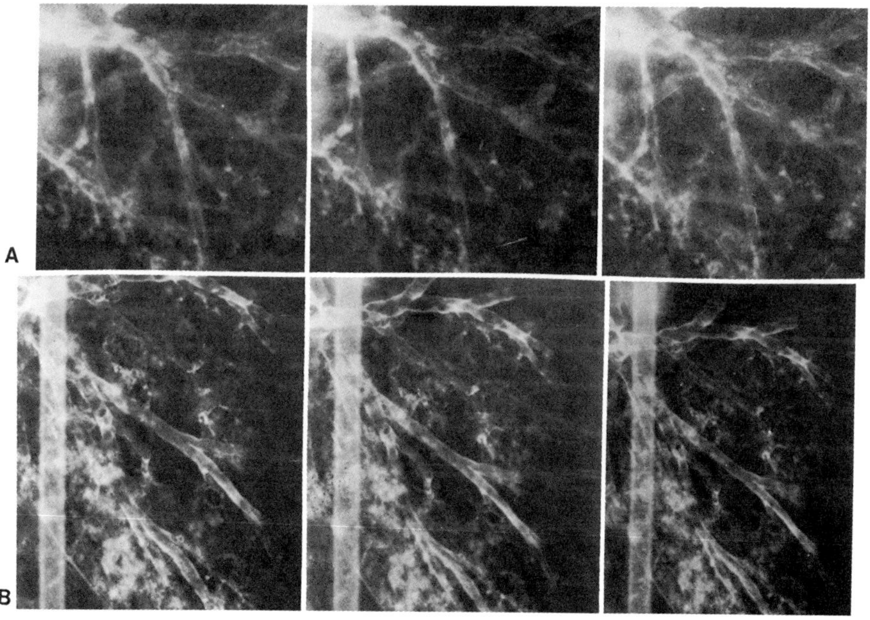

Fig. 9-2. *A*, Postmortem bronchogram from 19-year-old patient dying of status asthmaticus obtained during simulated breathing in artificial thorax. *B*, Postmortem bronchogram of patient who died with myocardial infarction but had normal lungs postmortem. Shown at same magnification. (*From* Cohen, E.P., Petty, T.L., Szentivanyi, A., and Priest, R.E.: Ann. Intern. Med., *62:*103, 1965.)

patient recovered with administration of intravenous aminophylline and steroid therapy.

Thus, in status asthmaticus, airway obstruction may be progressive and profound, and management is directed at the basic mechanisms of airway narrowing that lead to increased airway resistance.

MANIFESTATIONS

Generally, the patient with status asthmaticus presents a dramatic picture and should receive continuous EKG monitoring until improved. Wheeze is audible with the unaided ear, labored respirations are obvious, and tachycardia and diaphoresis are frequently present. In far-advanced status asthmaticus, the chest will be overexpanded and quiet. Signs and symptoms which are present in varying combinations and degrees are as follows:

1. Tachypnea
2. Wheezing or quiet chest (severe)
3. Dyspnea
4. Air hunger
5. Retractions

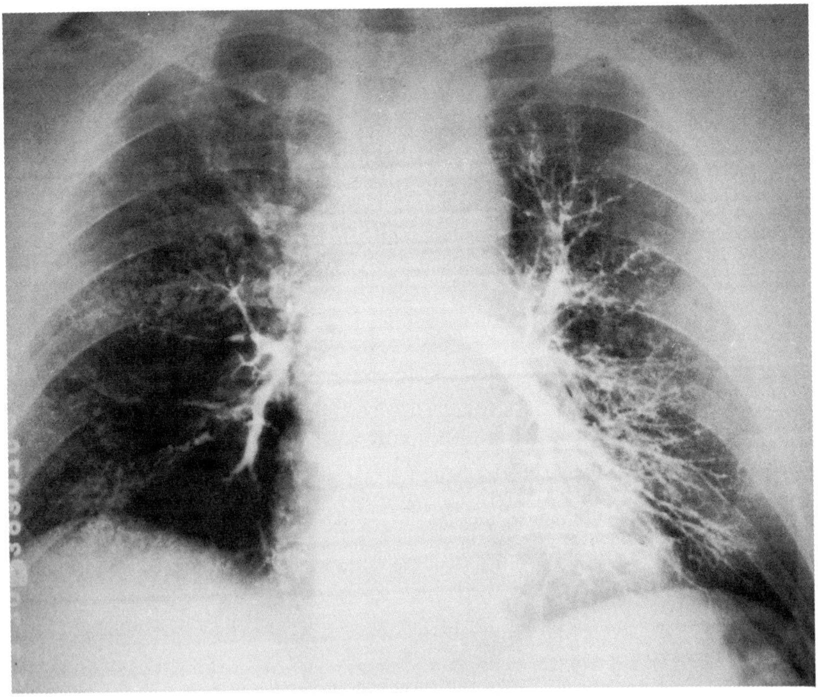

Fig. 9-3. Bronchogram of asthmatic patient referred from another hospital who suffered asthma attack during bronchographic procedure for hemoptysis. Marked narrowing of large central conducting airways is noted.

6. Overexpanded chest
7. Restlessness
8. Fatigue, stupor (coma)
9. Ineffective cough
10. Irritability
11. Hypotension
12. Tachycardia
13. Pulsus paradoxus
14. Diaphoresis
15. Dehydration
16. Cyanosis

Simple bedside spirometry such as measurement of FEV_1, peak flow, and vital capacity will document the severity of derangement of lung mechanics if the patient is able to perform the test. The degree of pulsus paradoxus correlates well with the severity of airway obstruction and blood gases.[3,4]

Arterial blood gas determinations are absolutely fundamental in assessing the severity and progression of the clinical situation. In the early stages of status asthmaticus, the usual blood gas manifestations are hypocapnia due to hyperventilation, and hypoxemia due to ventilation-perfusion abnormalities (mismatch).[5] The hypoxemic stimulus as well as neurogenic reflex stimulation produces an increased respiratory drive. Humoral mediators may also play a role in the increased respiratory drives of asthma. The hypocapnia is accompanied by an elevated pH (respiratory alkalemia). With progression, the work of breathing exceeds the capacity of the respiratory "pump" and alveolar hypoventilation develops, resulting in carbon dioxide retention and ultimately acidemia. A rise in $Paco_2$ from the range of 35 to 45 mm Hg to the range of 45 to 55 mm Hg is cause for alarm. This means that the effort to breathe is failing to keep pace with the metabolic production of carbon dioxide. When the carbon dioxide tension becomes greater than the oxygen tension (room air), the so-called crossover point, mechanical ventilation may be necessary or else progressively rapid and severe deterioration may take place.[6] (See discusssion on mechanical ventilation, following.)

Table 9-1 displays the normal relationship between pH, $Paco_2$, bicarbonate, and Pao_2. This is contrasted with examples of common blood gas abnormalities observed during status asthmaticus when the patient is seen early in the attack, when hypoxemia is corrected with administration of supplemental oxygen, and when there is severe alveolar hypoventilation with carbon dioxide retention and respiratory acidemia. The bicarbonate can be further reduced owing to accompanying lactic acidosis resulting from the excessive muscular activity or from anaerobic metabolism (in the case of severe hypotension). When this occurs, however, arrhythmia and

TABLE 9-1. Examples of Blood Gas Values during Severe Progressive Status Asthmaticus

	Normal	*Early Status Asthmaticus*	*Nasal Oxygen*	*Respiratory Failure*
Pa_{O_2}	90	55	75	50
Pa_{CO_2}	40	27	35	77
pH	7.40	7.48	7.42	7.04
HCO_3^-	24	22	22	20

circulatory collapse with or without respiratory arrest are imminent. Few asthmatics tolerate pH values of less than 7.10 for long.

MANAGEMENT

General

After a brief review of the historical events leading to the attack, including a review of current medications either prescribed or self-administered, and a quick but systematic physical examination (often done during the brief history-taking and assessment of the situation), an arterial puncture should be immediately performed for blood gas and pH analysis (see Chap. 1). Even before results are available, oxygen administration should be started via nasal cannula at 4 L/min. In contrast to chronic obstructive pulmonary disease and hypercapnia, there is no danger of depressing the hypoxemic ventilatory drive with the administration of oxygen. Because of the severe degree of ventilation-perfusion mismatch, higher flow rates of oxygen may be needed as compared with those needed for emphysema and chronic bronchitis (see Chap. 3). The oxygen flows can be adjusted later as necessary based on the blood gas determinations repeated after approximately 20 min, a time interval that allows the patient to achieve a new steady state. The physician should be especially alert to the rate of increase in Pa_{CO_2} rather than the actual amount of change.

A large intravenous catheter or needle (e.g., # 18 or 19) should also be placed and fluid administration begun, usually 5% dextrose in one-fourth or one-half normal saline solution. Most patients with status asthmaticus are dehydrated, and a liter of fluid over the first 1 or 2 hr is generally appropriate. Care should be taken not to overhydrate. The intravenous set-up will also be required for the use of intravenous medications described in the following sections.

Beta-Adrenergic Agonists

The definition of status asthmaticus includes a refractory reaction to all sympathomimetic agents including oral, inhaled, and injected drugs. Thus, in status asthmaticus the further administration of sympathomimetic agents as initial therapy is not likely to be useful and carries the possibility of serious adverse effects (arrhythmia). If the patient arrives in the emergency room, clinic, or physician's office and has not had excessive amounts of sympathomimetics and, furthermore, if tachycardia greater than 120 beats/min and arrhythmias are not present, a single subcutaneous injection of epinephrine (Adrenalin) 1/1000, 0.3 ml, or terbutaline, 0.5 ml, should be given. These agents are preferred for younger individuals and generally should not be given to patients with severe hypertension, a history of cardiac arrhythmia, or recent symptomatic coronary artery disease. Certainly, their repeated use should be condemned if there is no clear benefit immediately.

Intravenous Theophylline

After epinephrine, the first and frequently most effective form of immediate emergency room management is the intravenous use of theophylline in the form of aminophylline (theophylline ethylenediamine). The availability of determination of theophylline levels in plasma and saliva has added to the understanding of the proper use of aminophylline.[8–10] It is reported and generally accepted that the usual therapeutic level of 10 to 20 μg/ml can be achieved with a loading dose of 5 to 6 mg/kg infused over a 20 min period. Use of this loading dose must take into consideration the patient's prior use of theophylline compounds. If the patient had already been receiving oral theophylline and if the theophylline plasma level is in the therapeutic range, further infusions should be used with great caution. Weinberger et al. recently evaluated a new method for estimating the initial loading dose and a maintenance dose to arrive at acceptable therapeutic levels.[11]

The problem of aminophylline toxicity must be kept in mind at all times. Excessive levels may be accompanied by gastrointestinal side effects, abdominal discomfort, nausea, and vomiting, which in themselves are not dangerous. As plasma levels increase further, seizures occur.[12] Furthermore, as a result of congestive heart failure, or other causes, liver impairment may lengthen the half-life of theophylline, rendering the possibility of serious side effects more likely.[12]

A common practice is to give a loading intravenous dose as previously described, followed by a maintenance dose of 0.9 mg/kg/hr for patients who have not previously received methylxanthines. Clinical examination together with theophylline blood levels should determine proper dosage, however.[11]

Corticosteroids

Intravenous corticosteroid therapy should be instituted immediately on admission unless prompt control of the acute attack is achieved. These agents reduce inflammation over a period of hours to days. Short-term administration of steroids in high dosage is rarely accompanied by adverse effects. The exact dose that should be given cannot be specified at this time, since there are no satisfactory studies of dose–response relationships in the use of steroids in status asthmaticus. Clearly, the dose should be that which aborts the asthma attack as quickly as possible. A commonly employed dose that is effective in the majority of patients is 200 mg hydrocortisone given intravenously every 4 to 6 hours or 40 mg methylprednisolone given intravenously every 4 to 6 hours. These doses should be continued until the patient has improved and lung function approaches normal or the patient's best function. At this time, administration of an oral steroid (e.g., prednisone) should be started in equivalent doses. Measurement of pulmonary function (e.g., FEV_1, MMEF) should be followed by daily bedside spirometric examination.

An alternate and effective choice based on my unpublished studies is the use of intravenous methylprednisolone sodium succinate, giving at least 250 mg intravenously at once. Experience gained over the past 15 years indicates that high doses are well tolerated and apparently more effective from a clinical point of view. An additional dose of 500 mg can be given after 6 to 8 hours. Recent evidence suggests that intravenous prednisolone may be effective within an hour, with a peak effectiveness in 8 hours.[13] Even higher doses of corticosteroids can be used for patients whose asthma is severe enough to require intubation and mechanical ventilation. The rationale for use of this large dose is demonstrated steroid resistance in certain asthmatics, the high degree of effectiveness, and the lack of side effects with short-term use.[14] Specifically, severe steroid-induced hypokalemia or hyperglycemia has not been observed. It is wise, however, to monitor levels of electrolytes and blood sugar daily during the use of massive doses of corticosteroids.

Intravenous Albuterol (*Salbutamol*)

The use of intravenous albuterol (salbutamol) in the form of a continuous drip has achieved some popularity in the United Kingdom.[15] This selective $beta_2$-agonist has little of the undesirable cardiovascular side effects of older sympathomimetics such as isoproterenol. It has only about one-tenth the chronotropic effect of isoproterenol and little effect on the force of left ventricular ejection.[15,16] Only limited experience with this drug is available in the United States. Preliminary experience indicates that this form of therapy is not apt to be useful in advanced cases and probably should not be considered if proper doses of theophylline and corticosteroids are used early in treatment. Future studies should establish whether intravenous albuterol will be useful early in the management of status asthmaticus.

Sodium Bicarbonate

The use of intravenous sodium bicarbonate to combat occasionally severe respiratory acidemia and any accompanying metabolic acidosis in status asthmaticus has been suggested.[17-19] The correction of acidemia is believed to restore responsiveness to epinephrine and also to aid in the relief of bronchospasm.[17] Of course, the Pa_{CO_2} will rise after bicarbonate administration because the bicarbonate combines with hydrogen ions to produce carbonic acid, which in turn dissociates to water and carbon dioxide (i.e., $H_2CO_3 = H_2O + CO_2$). Nonetheless, the buffering capacity of bicarbonate produces a significant rise in pH. The elevation of pH is small in a closed system, but in status asthmaticus there is still significant elimination of carbon dioxide by the lungs, even though carbon dioxide homeostasis is not normal.[20] If the infused bicarbonate causes a significant rise in pH, fatal arrhythmias may be prevented and airway resistance lessened, which of course represents a therapeutic dividend even if the Pa_{CO_2} rises further. In clinical practice it is customary to infuse 88 mEq in 5 min and repeat in 30 min as dictated by the clinical situation. It must be stressed, however, that the definitive method of treating respiratory acidemia is to establish adequate ventilation, and that bicarbonate infusion is only an adjunct to therapy and is often a temporizing measure used during the brief period before mechanical ventilation is instituted.[21]

Mechanical Ventilation

When patients enter the hospital in advanced stages of disease, or if the modes of therapy discussed thus far in this chapter are not effective, then fatigue, alveolar hypoventilation, respiratory acidemia, and unconsciousness may develop. Under these conditions, immediate intervention with an airway and mechanical ventilation is mandatory. Ventilatory support provides the work of breathing and thus "buys" the necessary time for the specific pharmacologic agents to reverse the basic pathologic changes of status asthmaticus.[21]

When to Ventilate. With the exception of coma and apnea, no simple criteria can be set forth as absolute indications for the institution of mechanical ventilation in status asthmaticus. In these extreme situations, it is obvious that death will occur if skillful mechanical support of ventilation is not achieved immediately. Blood gas criteria are useful but are not absolute guidelines. The so-called crossover point, that is, when the Pa_{CO_2} exceeds the Pa_{O_2} is a useful point of reference, but it must be stressed that any pattern of blood gas values must be interpreted within the context of the dynamic clinical situation judged at the bedside.[6] For example, a patient may have normal or near-normal arterial blood gas levels but may be exhausted and on the verge of collapse. This patient should be intubated and ventilated immediately before severe blood gas abnormalities occur. Conversely, a patient's general clinical condition, including hemodynamic measurements and estimates of respiratory work, may appear satisfactory in the face of moderate blood gas abnormalities. The blood gas values indicate what the patient's condition is but tell nothing about the physical cost, such as the respiratory work and cardiovascular responses that have occurred.

Choice of Airway. The most appropriate definitive airway for mechanical ventilation is an endotracheal tube placed through either the nose or the mouth. Nasotracheal intubation is preferred by some and is possibly more comfortable for the patient. Whether this is so is a widely debated point. Certainly, oral intubation is the most rapid and direct approach and should be used in all patients who are rapidly deteriorating; otherwise, a nasal endotracheal tube can be placed by an experienced physician on a semielective basis (see Chap. 2).

Choice of Mechanical Ventilator. A wide selection of mechanical ventilators with high capability is currently available to provide the necessary ventilatory work. Volume-cycled respirators with high pressure and flow capability are preferred, primarily because their volume and cycling delivers the necessary tidal volume against changing resistance, which may be variable in status asthmaticus. Table 4-1 lists the most popular volume-cycled respirators in common use and their individual capabilities.

These modern ventilators offer the important features of accurate control of inspired oxygen fraction, flow-rate control, variable inspiratory/expiratory ratios, and an alarm system in case of ventilator failure. Thus, all these machines are versatile and generally can be adjusted to meet the needs of the patient in spite of the necessity of rapidly delivering fairly large tidal volumes against high resistance.

In general, the necessary tidal volume proves to be 10 to 12 ml/kg. A slow respiratory rate of 10 to 12/min is desirable. It is best to allow the patient to cycle the ventilator; thus, his respiratory system maintains partial control of the mechanical support of ventilation by "closing the loop," i.e., allowing the patient to initiate each tidal breath. Therefore, the assist mode is preferred by most experts in respiratory care. Additionally, a relatively fast inspiratory time, allowing a longer expiratory time for lung emptying, meets the needs of most patients. High inspiratory flows, however, may cause a significant element of dynamic airway resistance, causing airway pressures to be high.

The priorities in mechanical ventilation must be: (1) adequate alveolar ventilation and oxygen transport, (2) avoidance of complications such as pneumothorax, and (3) patient comfort.

Most patients with status asthmaticus who are exhausted from the enormous work of breathing are comfortable once the endotracheal tube has been placed and the ventilator skillfully programmed to take over the work of breathing. As a matter of fact, the majority of such patients often relax and even fall asleep when this important aspect of care is accomplished. If pain or restlessness is troublesome, it is acceptable to give analgesic drugs such as morphine or meperidine; sedatives or tranquilizing drugs can also be given during mechanical ventilation. It must be stressed that these drugs are absolutely contraindicated in status asthmaticus patients who are not supported by mechanical ventilation, since these drugs are respiratory depressants, and their use may make the patient fail to meet the work requirements necessary for alveolar ventilation. There is absolutely no evidence that tranquilizers or sedatives are useful in aborting an attack of status asthmaticus. They may be useful adjuncts, however, once patients are receiving assisted or controlled mechanical ventilation.

In a patient who "fights the respirator," analgesics and sedatives may also be useful. Paralyzing agents such as curare derivatives or succinylcholine are also necessary and are a poor substitute for the skillful adjustment of the ventilator to meet the needs of the patient. This is one situation in which the technique of intermittent mandatory ventilation (IMV) may be found useful (see Chap. 4).

Prognosis in Patients Requiring Mechanical Ventilation. That status asthmaticus is potentially fatal is well established. Mortality has been attributed to the excessive use of isoproterenol-containing aerosols in high concentration, and the use of sedatives and analgesics.[22-24] The question of increasing mortality in England as compared with Canada and the United States resulted in a comprehensive editorial review and a caution regarding the serious consequences of inadequately or inappropriately treated asthma.[25]

The major systematic measures detailed earlier in this chapter are effective in controlling most severe asthmatic attacks. In a small number, the attack is so rapidly progressive or already advanced at the time of hospitalization that acute respiratory failure, arrhythmia, or complications will result in death unless mechanical ventilation can be utilized to provide adequate ventilation and gas transfer. The prognosis in such severe cases is much worse than in the majority of patients in whom mechanical support is not required.[26-29]

The experience with status asthmaticus patients managed by our University Hospital intensive respiratory care unit is illustrative of the severe nature of the disease when it requires mechanical ventilation. From July 1967 to July 1975, 811 patients entered the Colorado University Hospital with a diagnosis of status asthmaticus, indicative of the large number of asthmatic patients managed by this center.[27] Many had acute respiratory failure as defined by an arterial oxygen tension of less than 50 mm Hg while breathing air or a concomitant carbon dioxide tension of greater than 50 mm Hg, or both (not an absolute definition). The mildest cases were managed on the medical wards, while those requiring intensive care were managed in the intensive respiratory care unit.[30] Of the serious cases, 20 patients required mechanical ventilation as a result of exhaustion, unconsciousness, severe and progressive blood gas abnormalities, or respiratory or cardiac arrest. Table 9-2 presents background data from this retrospective analysis. Of 20 patients, 8 died, including one death following anoxic brain damage after discharge from the hospital to a nursing home. Deaths resulted from terminal arrhythmias, tension pneumothorax, and sepsis. Although the experience of our center in managing large numbers of asthma cases, including those referred to our intensive care unit from other nearby hospitals specializing in asthma treatment, has resulted in an average of only one death per year from status asthmaticus, a fatal outcome in 8 of 20 patients who required mechanical ventilation is higher than that reported from other centers.[29,30] This reflects the pernicious nature of advanced and uncontrolled asthma. Most deaths occurred in older patients with long-standing asthma.

Before focusing on these 8 deaths, however, one should study the entire series, as illustrated in Table 9-3. Of the 20 patients who required mechanical ventilation, as judged by clinical criteria, 8 died in spite of intubation and use of a ventilator. However, none of the 791 patients *not* judged to require ventilation died. We could hardly have improved on the fact that *all* these 791 patients were discharged from the hospital following a severe bout of acute respiratory failure due to status asthmaticus.[27]

In another recent series, 80 of 770 asthmatic patients had sudden and largely unexpected life-threatening (status) asthmas.[29] These 80 patients required 111 admissions for severe asthma during a 10-year period. The unpredictable features of life-threatening asthma were noted and included long-standing disease and the tendency toward recurrence following a severe episode of asthma.[29] These patients require especially careful supervision and management.

Weaning. The time to discontinue mechanical ventilation is when the patient can do his own work of breathing. This might be after a rather short interval, or it may not be possible for a prolonged period in advanced cases with a greater degree of underlying chronic obstructive lung disease and in older patients with greater degrees of impairment.

In general, discontinuance of mechanical ventilation can be considered when the patient can maintain his own necessary tidal volume, double it on command, and provide evidence of a good inspiratory force measured at the airway of −30 cm H_2O. A prospective study of ventilation weaning criteria was recently done at the University of Colorado, as discussed in Chapter 4. Briefly, the

TABLE 9-2. Analysis of 20 Patients Requiring Mechanical Ventilation

	Survivors (12)	*Nonsurvivors (8)**
Sex		
Male	3	2
Female	9	6
Age		
Less than 35 years	4	2
More than 35 years	8	6
Age of onset		
Less than 20 years	5	5
More than 20 years	7	3
Duration		
Less than 10 years	1	0
More than 10 years	11	8

* Includes one posthospital death after anoxic brain damage.

study indicated that if a patient's requirement for resting minute ventilation is low (less than 10 L) and if the patient can demonstrate a reserve, such as more than doubling the resting value on command, then discontinuation of the mechanical ventilator is possible. The term *"weaning"* is largely a misnomer because this implies the gradual discontinuance of mechanical ventilation. In asthma particularly, when airway resistance lessens, patients can rapidly take over the work of breathing. They can be extubated promptly with the high expectation that they will be able to breathe on their own. IMV has not been found useful in weaning in this situation and may only delay the decision to extubate.

Continuing Care

A discussion of status asthmaticus would be incomplete without a consideration of after-crisis care. Clearly, the precipitating events and mechanism may still be active, and thus further pharmacologic therapy will be required. In general, the xanthines should be continued in the form of oral theophylline. Oral theophylline sufficient to maintain therapeutic blood levels should be continued and may form the cornerstone of long-term maintenance pharmacologic therapy. Theophylline, 200 mg (or equivalent) or more, 4 times daily will usually be required.

TABLE 9-3. Outcome of Patients with Status Asthmaticus

	Ventilator Required	*Ventilator Not Required*
Survived	12	791
Died	8	None

Today a variety of sustained-release preparations are available, allowing for twice daily dosing and, perhaps, better patient acceptance. Blood levels of theophylline are more sustained with fewer "peaks and valleys." Whether or not strict control of blood levels of theophylline is preferable from an overall standpoint of symptomatic and objective control of asthma, however, compared with some variation in blood levels with use of immediate-release tablets or capsules, has not been established by controlled clinical trials.

The large doses of corticosteroids required for management of status asthmaticus are not necessary and should not be continued. The appropriate maintenance dose must be determined and continued. In a patient who has previously required steroids as part of the maintenance management program, it is unlikely that lesser levels of steroids could be used after recovery from a severe episode. Massive doses, described earlier in this chapter, can immediately be decreased to 60 to 100 mg prednisone (or equivalent) daily. From this time on, tapering should be slow and should be dictated by the clinical course of the patient and any side effects encountered. Most patients recovering from status asthmaticus will require oral theophylline, steroids, and, at times, beta-agonists for maintenance management for weeks, months, or even years after the attack. It is usually possible, however, to arrive at a program that is well tolerated by the patient and effective in controlling or preventing asthma exacerbations. Before discharging the patient from the hospital, the physician should be sure that the patient understands how to recognize that the severity of the disease is increasing and how to obtain additional advice and treatment promptly, before the attack develops into status asthmaticus. Various additional strategies that can prevent a recurrence of life-threatening status asthmaticus have been outlined in a recent monograph.[28] The goal of maintaining the patient in a "wheeze-free" or otherwise asymptomatic state without undue side effects due to necessary pharmacologic agents is stressed.[28]

In summary, status asthmaticus is a life-threatening problem that could be better recognized and treated. Pharmacologic therapy, supplemented as needed with mechanical ventilation, can be expected to be lifesaving in the majority of patients. The outcome is most hopeful when patients are identified and treated early. When patients deteriorate to the point of requiring mechanical ventilation, the prognosis remains guarded.

REFERENCES

1. Harvey, R.M.: The influence of hydrogen ion in the control of pulmonary artery pressures in patients with obstructive disease of the lungs. Med. Thorac., *22*:108, 1965.
2. Dworetzky, M., and Philson, A.D.: Review of asthmatic patients hospitalized in the pavillion service of the New York Hospital from 1948 to 1963, with emphasis on mortality rate. J. Allergy, *41*:181, 1968.

3. Knowles, G.K., and Clark, T.J.H.: Pulsus paradoxus as a valuable sign indicating severity of asthma. Lancet, *2:*1356, 1973.
4. Rebuck, A.S., and Pengelly, S.D.: Development of pulsus paradoxus as in the presence of airway obstruction. N. Engl. J. Med., *288:*66, 1973.
5. McFadden, E.R., Jr., and Lyons, H.A.: Arterial blood gas tension in asthma. N. Engl. J. Med., *278:*1027, 1968.
6. Weiss, E.B., and Faling, L.J.: Clinical significance of $Paco_2$ during status asthma: the cross-over point. Ann. Allergy, *26:*545, 1968.
7. Petty, T.L., Bigelow, D.B., and Levine, B.E.: The simplicity and safety of arterial puncture. JAMA, *195:*693, 1966.
8. Jenne, J.W., Wyze, M.S., Rood, R.S., and McDonald, F.M.: Pharmacokinetics of theophylline: Application to adjustment of the clinical dose of aminophylline. Clin. Pharmacol. Ther., *13:*349, 1972.
9. Koysooko, R., Ellis, E.F., and Levy, G.: Relationship between theophylline concentrations in plasma and saliva of man. Clin. Pharmacol. Ther., *15:*454, 1974.
10. Mitenko, P.A., and Ogilvie, R.I.: Rational intravenous doses of theophylline. N. Engl. J. Med., *289:*600, 1973.
11. Weinberger, M.M., Matthay, R.A., Ginchansky, E.J., Chidsey, C.A., and Petty, T.L.: Serum theophylline measurement as a determinant of intravenous aminophylline dosage. JAMA, *235:*2110, 1976.
12. Zwillich, C.W., Sutton F.D., Neff, T.A., Cohn, W.M., Matthay, R.A., and Weinberger, M.M.: Theophylline induced seizures in adults (correlation with serum concentrations). Am. J. Med., *82:*784, 1975.
13. Ellul-Micallef, R., and Finech, F.F.: Intravenous prednisolone in chronic bronchial asthma. Thorax, *30:*312, 1975.
14. Schwartz, H.J., Lowell, F.C., and Melby, J.C.: Steroid resistance in bronchial asthma. Ann. Intern. Med., *69:*493, 1968.
15. Paterson, J.W.: Human pharmacology: Comparison of intravenous isoprenaline and salbutamol in asthmatic patients. Postgrad. Med. J., *47*[Suppl]:38, 1971.
16. Gibson, D.G., and Coltart, D.J.: Hemodynamic effects of intravenous salbutamol in patients with mitral valve disease: Comparison with isoprenaline and atropine. Postgrad. Med. J., *47*[Suppl.]:40, 1971.
17. Addis, G.J.: Bicarbonate buffering in acute exacerbation of chronic respiratory failure. Thorax, *20:*337, 1965.
18. Mithoefer, J.C., Porter, W.F., and Karetzky, M.S.: Indications for the use of sodium bicarbonate in the treatment of intractable asthma. Respiration, *25:*201, 1968.
19. Lakshminarayan, S., Sahn, S.A., and Petty, T.L.: Bicarbonate therapy in severe acute respiratory acidosis. Scand. J. Resp. Dis., *54:*128, 1973.
20. Ostrea, E.M., and Odell, G.B.: The influence of bicarbonate administration on blood pH in a "closed system": Clinical implication. J. Pediatr., *80:*671, 1972.
21. Misuraca, L.: Mechanical ventilation in status asthmaticus. N. Engl. J. Med., *275:*318, 1966.
22. Fraser, P.M., Speizer, F.E., Waters, S.D.M., Doll, R. and Mann, N.M.: The circumstances preceding death from asthma in young people in 1968 to 1969. Br. J. Dis. Chest, *65:*71, 1971.
23. Stolley, P.D.: Asthma mortality: A possible explanation of international variations. Chest, *63:*185, 1973.
24. Dworetzky, M., and Philson, A.D.: Review of asthmatic patients hospitalized in the pavillion service of the New York Hospital from 1948 to 1963 with emphasis on mortality rate. J. Allergy, *41:*181, 1968.
25. Editorial: Morbidity from bronchial asthma. Can. Med. Assoc. J., *100:*405, 1969.
26. Hetzel, M.R., Clark, T.J.H., and Branwaith, M.W.: Asthma analysis of sudden death and ventilatory arrests in hospital. Br. Med. J., *1:*808, 1977.
27. Scoggin, C.H., Sahn, S.A., and Petty, T.L.: Status asthmaticus (a nine year experience). JAMA, *238:*1158, 1977.
28. Scoggin, C.H., and Petty, T.L.: Clinical Strategies in Adult Asthma. Philadelphia, Lea & Febiger, 1982.
29. Williams, M.H.: Life-threatening asthma. Arch. Intern. Med., *140:*1604, 1980.
30. Shechy, A.F., DiDenedetto, R., Lefroc, S., and Lyons, H.A.: Treatment of status asthmaticus (a report of 70 episodes). Arch. Intern. Med., *130:*37, 1972.

Chapter 10

CHRONIC AIRFLOW LIMITATION

(Emphysema, Chronic Bronchitis, and Cystic Fibrosis)

By Thomas L. Petty

Acute respiratory failure is a common complication of advanced chronic obstructive pulmonary disease (referring to emphysema and chronic bronchitis, fulfilling the American Thoracic Society's 1962 definitions).[1] Although acute respiratory insufficiency progressing to overt acute respiratory failure is most apt to occur in advanced stages of disease, i.e., with FEV_1 of 1.0 or less, life-threatening acute respiratory failure may occur in less severe stages of disease when a major precipitating event such as viral or bacterial pneumonia, thromboembolism, heart failure, or chest trauma adds an additional overwhelming burden to the pulmonary apparatus. The pathophysiology of acute respiratory failure has been the subject of numerous specific articles and reviews.[2-4] In brief, acute respiratory failure is a result of a marked impairment in ventilation-perfusion matching, impaired ventilatory drives, weakness or fatigue of the respiratory muscles, or both, and associated hemodynamic abnormalities including reactive pulmonary hypertension, right ventricular failure, and impaired tissue oxygen transport. These related abnormalities are present in various combinations and degrees.

The manifestations of acute respiratory failure in COPD are those of the precipitating event such as pneumonia, the contributions of the underlying pulmonary obstructive disease as measured by airflow, and the manifestations of blood gas abnormalities themselves. These signs of hypoxemia and hypercarbia are listed in Table 1-2. They are often present in varying degrees in most patients with acute respiratory failure in COPD. Similar manifestations are present when acute respiratory failure occurs in cystic fibrosis, another disease state characterized by chronic progressive obstruction or limitation to expiratory airflow.

This chapter focuses upon approaches to management in the advanced COPD patient with acute respiratory failure. Some similarities in management strategy as well as some distinct differences are included relative to the growing problem of cystic fibrosis in this chapter, as well as in Chapter 16. This chapter deals with specific modalities of care including controlled low-flow oxygen, humidity, methods to improve alveolar ventilation without mechanical ventilation such as by use of pharmacologic agents, IPPB treatments and physical therapy measures, and intubation with ventilatory management for patients requiring and likely to benefit from this form of supportive care. Techniques of weaning from mechanical ventilation and approaches to early steps in pulmonary rehabilitation are included.

CONTROLLED OXYGEN

It is now well established that hypoxemia can be effectively corrected with the use of controlled oxygen enrichment of the inspired air. This can be accomplished by use of either double nasal cannula or masks that fix the inspired fraction of oxygen, so-called "Venturi masks" (see Chap. 1).[3,4,6,7] Both accomplish the same thing, i.e., the correction of hypoxemia without the development of hyperoxia, and both may be successfully used usually without significant CO_2 retention. Controlled oxygen can be safely administered even if substantial hypercarbia is present.[6,7] I prefer the use of a nasal cannula for the advantages of: (1) comfort, (2) ability to eat and talk, and (3) a greater likelihood of keeping the oxygen device in place than with the Venturi mask. No question remains about the efficacy of double nasal prongs, and the oxygen flow is guided by frequent arterial blood gas analyses performed at appropriate intervals. If masks are used, arterial blood gas monitoring is equally important at approximately the same intervals. It makes little or no difference whether patients are mouth breathers, since the nasopharynx effectively entrains the oxygen flow from the nasal prongs. Additionally, the nasal prongs have a hidden advantage in the face of emerging hypoventilation since, in fact, a reduced minute ventilation will result in an elevation of the inspired oxygen fraction, thus acting as a hedge against insidiously developing hypoxemia. Of course, when this occurs the likelihood of the necessity of mechanical ventilatory assistance is obvious.

By contrast, with the use of Venturi masks the inspired oxygen fraction remains fixed, and hypoxemia may ensue during subtle periods of hypoventilation. In any case, either technique of controlled oxygen administration may be effective in controlling hypoxemia if properly used. At times readjustments in flow are required, as illustrated in Table 10-1. Even in this extreme example, however, hypoxemia could be effectively controlled and CO_2 retention avoided with controlled low-flow oxygen. Careful adjustments of flow with frequent arterial blood gas monitoring were required to achieve correction of hypoxemia without progressive worsening CO_2 retention, however. In the case cited, severe hypoxemia was present associated with an exacerbation of chronic bronchitis. Bicarbonate compensation of chronic CO_2 retention was present resulting in partial correction of the respiratory acidosis associated with the admission P_{CO_2} of 66. The initial liter flow chosen by the admitting house officer was 3 L/min. This resulted in hyperoxia (P_{O_2} 110) and an uncompensated rise in the P_{CO_2} (86 mm Hg). Nonetheless, the patient's state of consciousness improved owing to the correction of severe hypoxemia. Reduction in the liter flow resulted in improvement in CO_2 hemostasis, and the final flow of 1 L/min produced satisfactory correction of hypoxemia and a P_{CO_2} roughly equal to that present on admission. Of course, these results most likely reflect the effects of the total care of the patient including measures to open the conducting airways, as discussed later.

Similar care must be exercised with the use of Venturi masks. Selecting a mask that brings the P_{O_2} to just the desired level of 55 to 65 mm Hg will offer an oxygen saturation of 88 to 92%. A series of masks providing various concentrations, offering F_{IO_2} of 0.24, 0.28, 0.35, and 0.40, is available. Even higher oxygen concentrations may be needed in a few patients. Correction of hypoxemia is fundamental

TABLE 10-1. Response to Controlled Oxygen Via Double Nasal Prongs in Acute Respiratory Failure in COPD

	Admission	*1 hr*	*2 hr*	*3hr*
	State of Consciousness			
	Confused Disoriented	Oriented Semi-alert	Alert and cooperative	Alert and cooperative
O_2 L/minute	0	3	2	1
P_{O_2}	31	110	80	65
P_{CO_2}	66	86	69	64
pH	7.35	7.21	7.32	7.31
HCO_3^-	36	34	35	36

to care and results in improved oxygen availability to tissues and treatment of the consequences of hypoxemia on the circulation, i.e., reactive pulmonary hypertension and impaired cardiac output.

METHODS OF OPENING CONDUCTING AIRWAYS

Compromise of the conducting air passages is a fundamental problem in COPD, resulting in respiratory insufficiency or failure. Mechanisms of airflow limitation include both impairment of elastic recoil and compromise of both large and small conducting air passages. Little can be done to combat the effects of reduced elastic recoil in emphysema, but correction of disturbances of airflow due to retained secretions, bronchospasm, and mucosal edema may improve overall ventilation and ventilation-perfusion matching. Techniques to improve airflow include a variety of measures comprising both pharmacologic and nonpharmacologic therapy.

Moisture

The use of moisture is a time-tested method that is aimed at thinning and mobilizing secretions. Whether or not already-formed mucus can be in fact thinned by water or saline solution is questioned, but most physicians, nurses, and therapists believe that this can be accomplished with the use of inhaled moisture. Moisture may be inhaled from either molecular water provided by humidifiers or particulate water provided by nebulizers. More water is delivered by particles, but whether or not this is desirable has never been proven by any well-controlled study. Most intensive care units use heated nebulizers, which have the effect of delivering small-sized particles at approximately body temperature with the temperature being controlled by a heating system at the source. Extensive clinical experience indicates that this form of moisture delivery is well tolerated and appears to be helpful in the clearing of secretions, at least in some patients. A high-density water mist is provided by ultrasonic nebulizers and is also used in some centers. Certain studies have indicated, however, that this high-density mist may in fact increase airway resistance in patients with chronic bronchitis or asthma.[8] This fact, in addition to extensive experience indicating that moisture supplied by this route is not well tolerated by many patients, has essentially eliminated the use of ultrasonic nebulizers for moisture administration at most hospitals. Some patients do not tolerate mist therapy at all, and it must not be used in these patients.

Physiotherapy Techniques (see Chap. 7)

Hand in hand with moisture administration must be the use of methods to improve mobilization of secretions. Although controversy remains over the effectiveness of various posturing, vibrating, shaking, and pummeling techniques, particularly in pneumonia, recent studies do show improved mucus clearance and improved airflow by use of physiotherapy techniques in both chronic bronchitis and cystic fibrosis.[9–11] Certainly, there is a definite art in the effective application of these techniques, and the various effects of these time-tested approaches are debated by experts. Many experienced physicians, nurses, and therapists conclude, however, that most or all of these methods are effective in the context of the other care necessary in the management of advanced COPD with acute respiratory failure. Similar techniques are considered useful in cystic fibrosis (see discussion later in this chapter). It also appears that cough is the most efficient method of mobilizing and removing secretions.[12]

Mucolytic and Expectorant Drugs

Mucolytic agents are often used in some centers in conjunction with physiotherapy techniques and IPPB to aid in the removal of retained secretions. Acetylcysteine is the only truly mucolytic drug available today in the United States, but it may be too irritating and can evoke bronchospasm.[13] This can be avoided by the concomitant administration of a bronchodilating aerosol.[14] Nonetheless, nonpharmacologic methods employing water as a bland aerosol with careful hydration of the patient in conjunction with physiotherapy techniques is preferred by most, including myself.

IPPB

IPPB is probably the most controversial technique for clearing secretions.[9,15,16] No study has shown that IPPB alone helps mobilize secretions better than other methods, although it is likely that IPPB followed by expulsive coughing is far more effective than no therapy. But it is cough and mobilization of the patient through positioning and exercise, if possible, that have the greatest effect upon mucus clearance.[12] IPPB devices are still widely used to deliver bronchodilating aerosols, but again, there is no convincing evidence that they are more effective in bronchodilator administration than simpler nebulization devices.[17] IPPB is also used in conjunction with mucolytic agents and physiotherapy techniques as well as bronchodilating aerosols.[18,19] Thus, assigning benefit to one component of therapy, namely the IPPB, is difficult at best. The final word on IPPB therapy will have to come from controlled clinical trials, some of which are currently underway and others of which are in the planning stages.[17] Suffice it to say that although this is one method of bronchodilator administration and, properly applied, probably helps in mucus clearance, there is nothing particularly magic about IPPB used as a measure of delivering pharmacologic agents or as a vehicle to aid in the mobilization of secretions.

Bronchodilators

Pharmacologic agents, including methylxanthines and beta agonists, are effective in improving airflow by combating muscular bronchospasm and probably also by improving mucociliary clearance.[20] This phenomenon has been found in all bronchodilators and has been particularly well studied in terbutaline.[20] Intravenous aminophylline, widely used in asthma, is also used in patients with COPD because of the belief that significant muscular bronchospasm may also be present. The standard loading dose of 5 to 6 mg/kg is probably appropriate for patients with COPD, but this should be reduced if patients are already receiving oral theophylline. One should be certain that effectiveness is being achieved and that excessive blood levels are not occurring, particularly if gastrointestinal upset, cardiac arrhythmias, or any convulsive disorders are identified.

Oral beta agonists are probably less important than methylxanthines given by the systemic route. Thus, although metaproterenol or terbutaline may be given and, in fact, may be effective when given by mouth, the likelihood of oral bronchodilators playing a major role in acute respiratory failure in COPD is relatively small.

Inhaled beta agonists are another matter. These drugs are effective in rapidly improving airflow in responsive patients. Isoetharine (Bronkosol), metaproterenol (Alupent or Metaprel), and inhaled terbutaline from ampules (Brethine or Bricanyl) are widely used today. Albuterol (salbutamol; Ventolin, Proventil) has just been released and is available in a metered-dose cartridge. Simple nebulization devices such as those powered by compressed gas sources used in conjunction with a Y-tube assembly or IPPB are the common method of administration of inhaled beta agonist solutions. Occasionally, atropine is also used in an inhaled bronchodilator by similar nebulization techniques.

Corticosteroids

A recent study of acute respiratory failure due to COPD has clearly indicated that systemic corticosteroids improve airflow, compared with placebo administration.[21] This is the first incontrovertible evidence that steroids, also time tested by experienced physicians, really produce objective benefit in acute respiratory failure.[21] Methylprednisolone sodium succinate, 0.5 mg/kg given every 6 hours, was used in this important study.[21] In clinical terms, a "burst of steroids" in doses of 100 to 200 mg daily would seem appropriate in most patients.

It is often a combination of steroids, inhaled beta agonists, and systemic bronchodilators, usually methylxanthines, that offers a tripartite approach to improving airflow. These pharmacologic agents are used in conjunction with both inhaled moisture and physical therapy techniques. Thus, it is sometimes difficult to assign benefit to one therapy vs another, and in fact it may be all therapies in concert that ultimately result in improvement of the patient.

The overall effectiveness of the therapeutic measures just listed, i.e., the so-called "conservative approach" to acute respiratory failure and COPD, is high. This approach to therapy is so common and well established that most units no longer keep outcome records unless particular research questions are being asked. The paper by Albert and associates, who used corticosteroids in controlled fashion, again revealed the high proportion of patients who can recover from acute respiratory failure in COPD.[21] According to these researchers, 43 of 44 patients survived with or without corticosteroids.[21] An in-hospital mortality rate of only 6% has also been reported in another study dealing with the nonventilator management of acute respiratory failure in advanced COPD.[22]

MANAGEMENT OF SPECIFIC PRECIPITATING EVENTS

Acute Purulent Bronchitis

Acute exacerbations of bronchitis with purulence are probably the commonest and most readily identified feature of disease. Common organisms are usually involved, including *Haemophilus influenzae* and *Streptococcus pneumoniae.* It is likely, however, that an acute virus infection is the initiating event, with the bacterial invasion occurring secondarily. Nonetheless, numerous studies have established the presence of these common bacteria in the clinical setting of acute purulent bronchitis in patients with advanced COPD. Antibiotics should be given promptly and empirically. It is best to examine a stained sputum smear, but it is unlikely that sputum cultures will be crucially informative. Ampicillin is generally the drug of choice in patients able to take penicillin derivatives. Tetracycline or chloramphenicol given parenterally would be alternate choices in patients allergic to penicillin. Chloramphenicol is the drug of choice for severe infections with *H. influenzae.* Antibiotics are administered five to seven days until purulence is reduced, as judged by the examination of expectorated sputum, along with lessening of fever and leukocytosis.

Pneumonia

Acute bacterial pneumonia is also common in patients with advanced COPD. Again, common aerobic organisms are the most likely etiologic agents. *S. pneumoniae, H. influenzae,* an occasional mycoplasma pneumonia, Legionnaire's bacillus, and other less common organisms are frequently encountered. Depending upon the origin of the infection, penicillin G, ampicillin, or erythromycin would be agents of choice, directed at *S. pneumoniae* and *H. influen-*

zae or *S. pneumoniae,* mycoplasma, and *Legionella pneumophila,* respectively. There appears to be little doubt that erythromycin is the drug of choice for *Legionella pneumophila.* Rifampin is an alternative. Chloramphenicol might be employed as an alternative to ampicillin and is the drug of choice in *H. influenzae* pneumonias.

Pulmonary Thromboembolism

The problem of thromboembolism in the setting of COPD is well established. Diagnosing this complication, however, is difficult owing to ventilation and ventilation-perfusion abnormalities associated with underlying advanced COPD. Isolated perfusion or ventilation/perfusion scans are not helpful in diagnosis of pulmonary embolus in COPD without a baseline for comparison. Even angiography, the so-called "gold standard" for the diagnosis of pulmonary embolus, may not be helpful in the presence of small peripheral pulmonary emboli caused by vascular cut-offs present in advanced COPD. I often diagnose pulmonary embolism based upon knowledge of its frequency in the setting of acute increasing dyspnea, worsening blood gases, and lack of clinical evidence of infection, such as increased sputum purulence, fever, and leukocytosis. Heparin therapy in full dose is required, however, and it is best to establish a definitive or highly presumptive diagnosis using angiography in cases in which diagnosis is questionable or in which the risk of heparin anticoagulation is high, such as in elderly patients or patients with previous bleeding disorders.

Heart Failure

Congestive left heart failure may complicate the mechanical derangements of advanced COPD by adding pulmonary congestion to the problem. In fact, right heart failure may be associated with significant salt and water retention and edema formation, which itself complicates pulmonary mechanics. When the heart failure is diagnosed on clinical grounds, salt restriction, potent diuretics, and oxygen are required. Prescribing digitalis would be useful primarily for the control of tachycardiac atrial arrhythmias and for clear-cut left ventricular failure.

Pneumothorax

Spontaneous or traumatic pneumothorax is common in advanced COPD. Depending upon the degree of involvement, pulmonary mechanics may be substantially worsened except in the case of a minimal pneumothorax, i.e., if 10 or 15% small anterior or axillary chest tube placement with underwater seal or suction is required. At times, the duration of continued air leak is long, requiring continuous chest tube drainage. During these periods, patients tend to be immobilized and fail to clear secretions owing to pain. Judicious use of analgesic drugs may help the patient cough and mobilize secretions. Patients should be as active as possible, even walking in halls and corridors either with the chest tube bottle on a portable stand or with use of a one-way Heimlich valve, which allows the egress of air without a bottle connection.

VENTILATORY MANAGEMENT

When fatigue, exhaustion, or cardiac or respiratory arrest occurs, the decision to institute mechanical ventilatory assistance must be made. The objectives of mechanical ventilation are to gain time and to rest the patient in order to allow for either treatment of precipitating events in acute respiratory failure or recovery of respiratory muscle function and general strength and vigor. By no means, however, should all patients with advanced or so-called "end-stage" COPD receive intubation and mechanical ventilation. The majority of these patients die of the respiratory disease or attendant cardiovascular complications, and the use of supportive means after all forms of systematic therapy, including rehabilitation techniques, have failed, is unfair to most patients. In these patients, ventilatory care actually extends death rather than prolonging life. (See Chap. 20.) By contrast, in patients who have not had optimum care, in those who are relatively young, and particularly in those in whom there is an identifiable precipitating event that is at least potentially reversible, mechanical ventilatory assistance is not only proper but beneficial and lifesaving.

The approach to mechanical ventilatory assistance described here is well established. Immediate intubation by the nasal or oral route offers an immediate definitive airway.[23] Mechanical ventilation with a high-performance volume ventilator is most commonly used. A short inspiratory and long expiratory ratio is desired, and tidal volumes of 10 to 12 ml/kg are generally employed at the onset. This may, however, represent a higher tidal volume than the patient can sustain later during early stages of weaning. It must be pointed out that careful surveillance of the known complications of mechanical ventilation must be done, and all patients mechanically ventilated must receive care in an intensive care unit.[24,25]

The mechanical ventilator, of course, is simply used to buy time. During this period, however, it is imperative that patients maintain muscle strength and nutrition. These aspects of care are most often overlooked. Thus, emphasis is placed upon these vital measures of management during mechanical ventilation.

Most patients can be ventilated upright in a chair during waking hours. In fact, it is commonplace for patients to ambulate with assistance during mechanical ventilation, with ventilation provided by a portable self-inflating bag with supplemental oxygen (Fig. 10-1). Although it is possible to keep an endotracheal tube in place many days, as based upon a recent prospective study from this center,

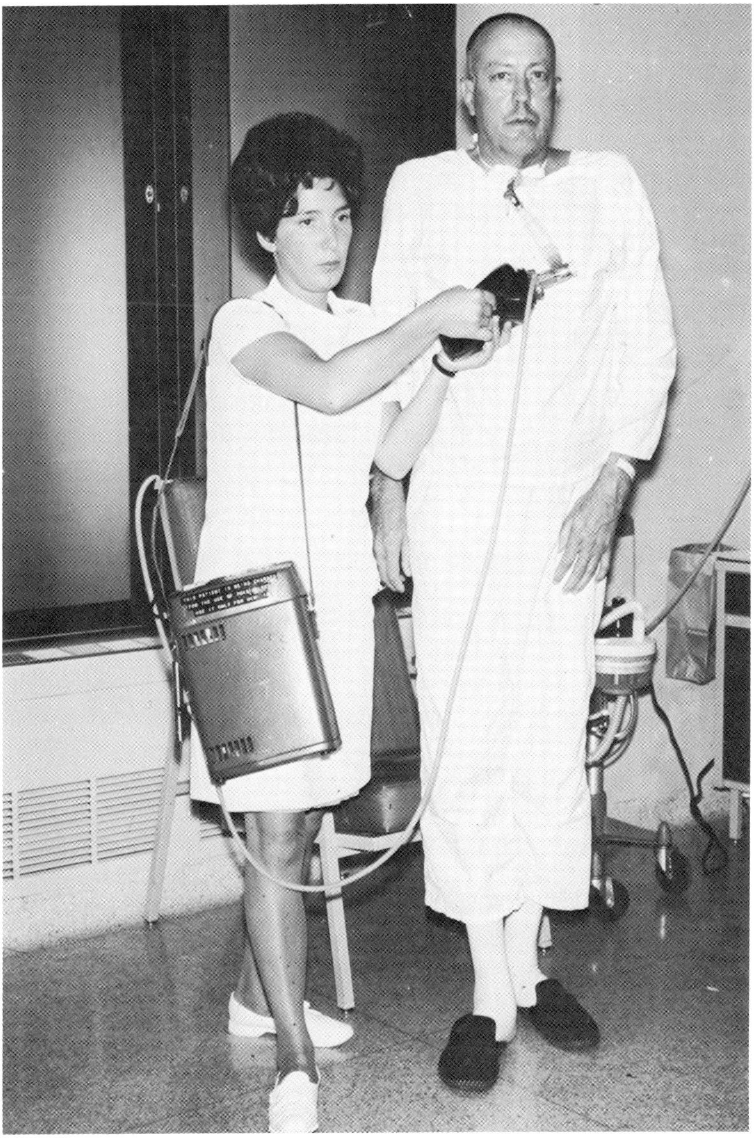

Fig. 10-1. Technique of progressive ambulation with ventilation still supported by self-inflating bag and supplemental oxygen. This technique maintains muscle tone, strengthens respiratory muscles, helps breathing coordination, and maintains interest in survival. Compare with Figure 7-10. This patient's care was also illustrated in Figures 7-2, 7-3, and 7-8. (From Hosp. Med., 9:36, 1970.)

when it is anticipated that needs for mechanical ventilation will be prolonged, i.e., greater than 3 to 4 days, it is far better to switch to a tracheostomy for comfort and for ease of feeding.[23] During the interim, i.e., during the first few days that an endotracheal tube is used, feeding can take place through a small nasogastric feeding tube. At least 3000 calories should be given in small aliquots, being careful to avoid gastric distention or vomiting. The product, Ensure, contains a balanced calorie mixture equivalent to 1 cal/ml. Thus, 3000 ml nutrient-containing fluid should be administered. Enteral nutrition is far better than intravenous from the standpoint of being more physiologic and of avoiding the complications of parenteral nutrition.

It is even better if patients can eat food (see Chap. 7). This offers enjoyment, gratification, and control of the rate of food intake by the patient, and employs the wisdom of the body in handling nutrients. It is easy for patients to eat once a tracheostomy is in place. Patients are assisted at first, but it is better if they can feed themselves. Often, a regular tray can be ordered and the patient simply allowed to eat by whatever methods seem appropriate.

WEANING FROM MECHANICAL VENTILATION

Few aspects of ventilatory care engender more controversy than the technique of weaning the respiratory cripple. Certainly, no simple formula exists. The key to success is a systematic approach that involves patient participation, the maintenance of muscle strength, and nutrition. This must be coordinated by the nurse or therapist in a regular fashion each day. Certain parameters measured at the bedside can assess the likelihood of the patient's ability to discontinue mechanical ventilation. These are: a minute ventilation of less than 10 L/min, the ability to double this on command, a low spontaneous respiratory rate (i.e., less than 20), and the ability to generate an instantaneous inspiratory force of greater than -20 cm H_2O.[26,27]

The effectiveness of these observations in predicting patients who can be rapidly disconnected from the ventilator has been determined in a prospective study.[26] When these criteria are met, the patient is awake and alert, and, most important, when the patient wants to be off the ventilator, it is time to extubate him. This is accomplished following a 30-min T-tube trial using 40% oxygen with moisture. The T-tube trial is to make certain that the patient will not become rapidly fatigued. It is recognized that during this period, the patient has to breathe against the additional burden of the resistance of the endotracheal tube. Although this resistance is not great, particularly with large-bore tubes, this is added to the patient's own airway resistance, which itself is usually high. Thus, this is an important consideration for obvious reasons in patients with marginal respiratory capability. Once it is evident that the patient can support his own ventilation, it is far better to have the tube out than to go through any ritual of progressive "near weaning" such as the use of intermittent mandatory ventilation (IMV), which may only delay the final decision to extubate.[28]

The pros and cons of IMV are discussed further in Chapter 4. Extubation is advantageous because it reduces the resistance to breathing, allows the patient to cough and clear secretions, allows for pursed-lip breathing, and allows for eating food and drinking liquids. The ability to communicate should not be underestimated. There are many patients with advanced COPD, of course, that cannot meet these criteria. These are the individuals with most marked respiratory insufficiency. It is nonetheless important to monitor tidal volume and respiratory rate as well as inspiratory force to obtain a baseline and to be able to observe trends. If the patient can never meet the tidal volume of the machine, the latter should be gradually reduced to match what the patient can accomplish. This aims to get the patient comfortable while breathing on a fixed low tidal volume, which will be compatible with the patient's own pulmonary mechanics once weaning takes place. Usually, tidal volume is reduced at 50 to 100 ml/day down to a range of 300 to 400 ml, depending upon the size of the patient. Minute ventilation is usually maintained by an increased respiratory rate chosen by the patient and assisted by the machine.

Another maneuver that will help insure success in weaning is allowing for chronic compensated CO_2 retention. The simple act of reducing the tidal volume on the respirator may accomplish this; adding mechanical dead space may do so as well. It is desirable for slow CO_2 retention to occur at a level compatible with the patient's own pulmonary mechanics. Often, P_{CO_2} of 60 to 70 mm Hg with appropriate bicarbonate reclamation and generation, allowing for a normal pH, will allow the patient to "adjust" minute ventilation to a low level commensurate with his ability to perform respiratory work. The adaptive nature of chronic compensated CO_2 retention has been known by experts in the field for many years.[29,30]

The timing of extubation is crucial. This is considered the "golden moment" in our unit. One needs to focus upon timing and the coincidence of all necessary factors that insure successful extubation—the patient's ventilatory mechanics, state of nutrition, lack of fatigue, interest in life, and desire for the "final push" to acheive early extubation. The most encouraging situation is a rested, alert patient with a twinkle in the eye seen on early morning rounds. When these observations indicate that the "golden moment" is at hand, the patient is given a 30-min trial of spontaneous breathing via the endotracheal tube attached to a T-tube assembly or trach cover supplying moist oxygen-enriched air (Fig. 10-2; see also Figs. 7-7 and 7-11). The patient is told that he will not be allowed to become fatigued, and will be obliged to breathe on his own only 30 min. At the end of 30 min, the patient's general appearance, pulse, respiratory rate, and blood gas determinations are considered all together. The absence of diaphoresis, of tachycardia, and of tachypnea with a respiratory rate

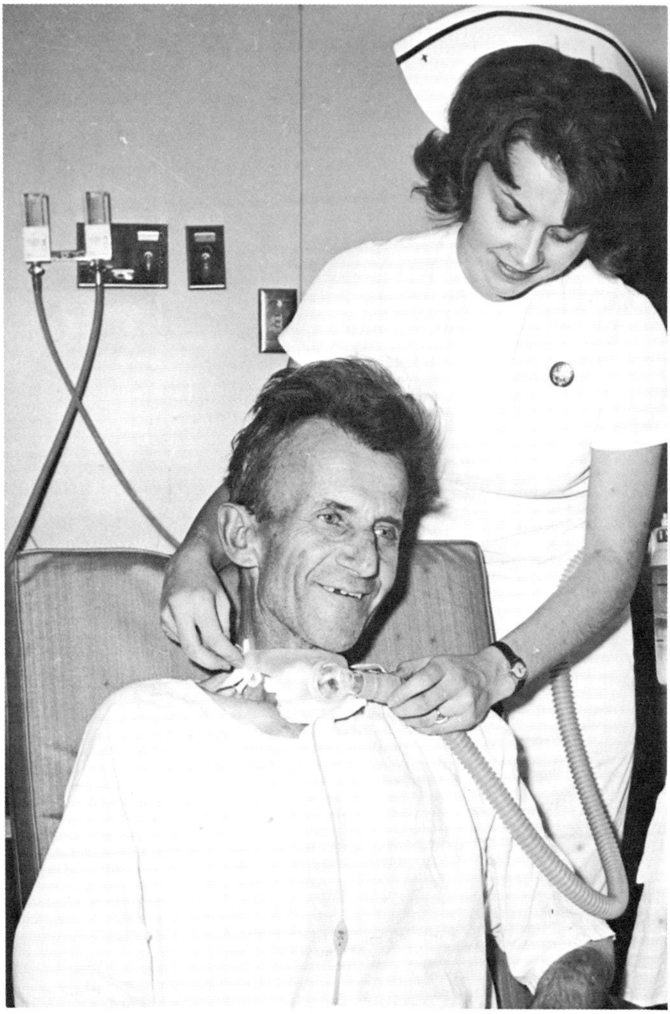

Fig. 10-2. Technique of weaning using moist, enriched oxygen from a tracheostomy collar, which avoids traction on the tracheostomy. Compare with Figures 7-7 and 7-11. (From Am. J. Nurs., *62*:1847, 1967.)

of more that 20, and the maintenance of acceptable blood gases, i.e., P_{O_2} of 55 to 70 and P_{CO_2} in the desired range, including chronic compensated CO_2 retention and no essential change during the 30-min trial, are desirable before extubation. At this point, however, the patient is placed back on the respirator in order to insure rest. Following one hour of rest, if all looks well, extubation is immediately accomplished.

Careful suctioning of the airway and nasopharynx is performed just before extubation. Following this, the nasal prongs are placed, and coughing and coordinated abdominal diaphragmatic breathing are encouraged by the nurse or therapist. Careful observations with reference to the presence of respiratory distress, diaphoresis, tachycardia, tachypnea, and blood gases are once again made. The patient is managed sitting upright in a chair during these procedures in order to capitalize upon the slight improvement in pulmonary mechanics in the upright sitting position. This approach to extubation is almost always successful if the observations just detailed are carefully made and the sequence of planning for and accomplishing extubation faithfully followed. This systematic approach capitalizes upon the patient's own resources and is encouraging to the patient from the standpoint of his being able to continue to live and to return to his previous activities. This is a period in which psychologic support from the nurse, therapist, or physician is most crucial. Patients are assured that should reintubation be necessary, this will be accomplished promptly. This is almost never the case, however.

For more prolonged weaning, one needs to consider that from this point onward, the technique of weaning will be almost entirely an art and not a science. The principles of using progressively prolonged periods of T-tube spontaneous breathing, always avoiding fatigue, must be scrupulously followed. In these situations, a tracheostomy should be used to minimize resistance caused by a wider bore, shorter tube, to facilitate management of secretions, and to encourage eating (see Chap. 7). The same T-tube trials just described are performed in a systematic manner. Lengthening the period off the respirator is the goal. The patient always rests one hour after each period of weaning. At first, the patient sleeps the entire night with assisted ventilation provided by the respirator. When the patient is able to perform all his breathing during daytime hours, the evening hours are included, working up to midnight, but still allowing the hours of sleep to insure rest. At times, a simple afternoon respite for one hour with assisted ventilation during a nap is also useful. Again, the same principles of removing the tracheostomy are employed. Often, removal of the tracheostomy takes place after weeks of this form of weaning. An interim step is believed to be valuable—placement of a Kistner button for the purpose of maintaining the tract or allowing suctioning should things suddenly and unexpectedly deteriorate (Figs. 10-3 and 10-4). It is also reassuring to the patient to know that the tracheostomy tube could be replaced through the stoma maintained by the Kistner button if necessary. This again is almost never the case. Most patients weaned by this method have left the hospital, and a few have lived many years.

Perhaps other weaning techniques could be equally successful, but the authors have never been impressed by any other method that

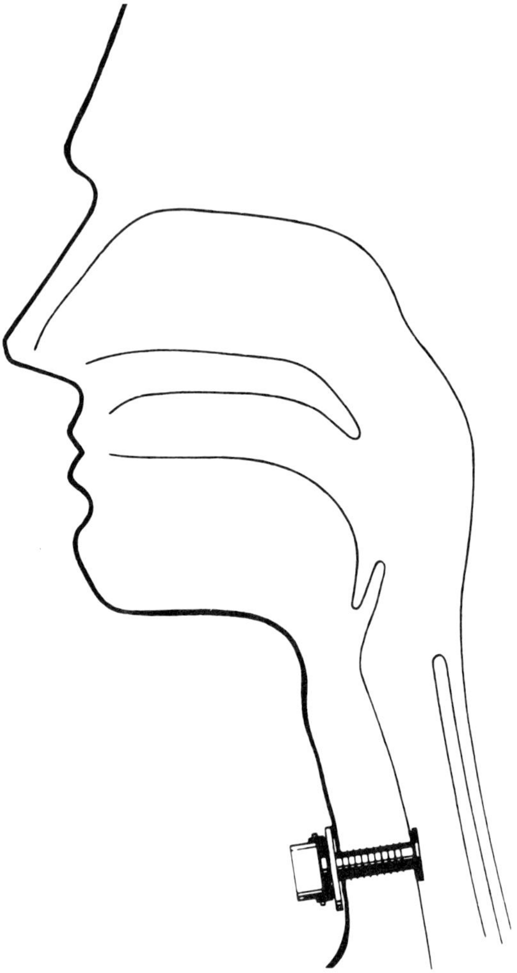

Fig. 10-3. Diagram of Kistner button in place. This resides in the anterior tracheal wall and does not compromise air space. It is capped, and breathing occurs through nose and mouth. This allows for coughing, talking, and so forth. The Kistner button should be maintained in place with an umbilical tie.

works as well as the one described. The recent enthusiasm for weaning by intermittent mandatory ventilation (IMV) has been criticized by the author, but ventilating with IMV is better than with controlled ventilation.[28] This is because the patient is able to breathe at all times, either spontaneously or assisted by the ventilator. If IMV is the only systematic weaning technique that can be practically used, it may be successful. Fatigue must be avoided at all times, however.

With our weaning approach of progressive T-tube breathing, careful recording in a systematic way is also important. The morning

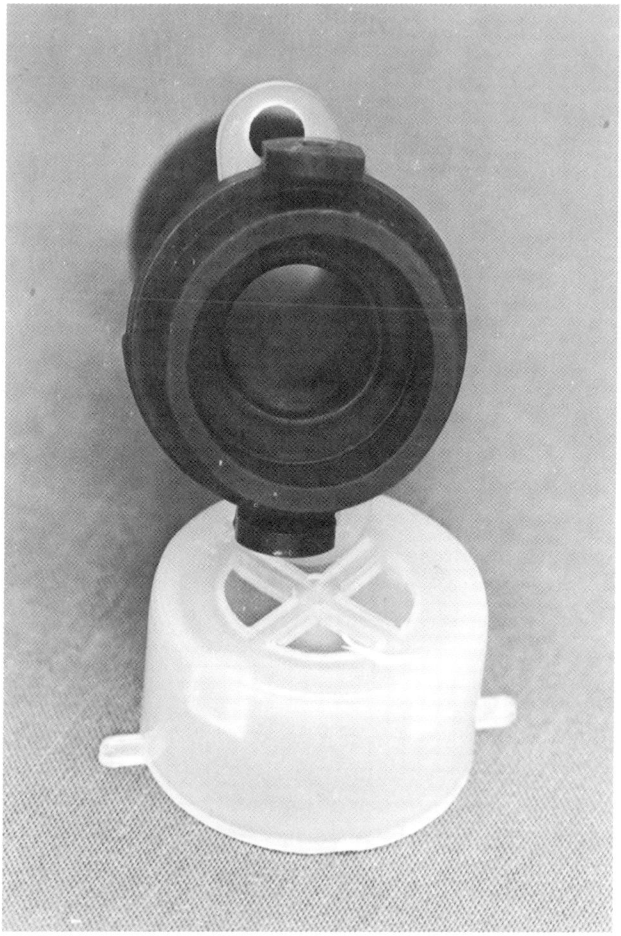

Fig. 10-4. Close-up view of Kistner button with strait shaft viewed on cross section while it is resting on the cap of the button.

checklist is always used. The duration of weaning with notation of progress is documented. Of paramount importance is avoidance of fatigue in general and respiratory muscle fatigue in particular. Fatigue always represents a setback and actually results in respiratory muscle dysfunction. The important thing is sustained nonfatiguing respiratory muscle activity. This activity, in addition to the use of food to improve strength and stimulate respiratory center activity, has been successful in assisting the weaning of all except 3 patients with COPD managed at the University of Colorado Hospital in the past 18 years. These 3 patients were finally discharged, 2 to continued care at home and the other to a nursing home. Thus, the success of the weaning program described is self-evident.

Table 10-2 lists the numbers of patients with COPD managed by mechanical ventilation since the opening of our intensive respiratory care unit.[31] The details of our most recent experience from the University of Colorado Hospital are listed. This is only one of 4 hospitals of a Health Sciences Center capable of providing both intensive and rehabilitative respiratory care. An overall survival rate of 82% is noted. These data include only patients with acute respiratory failure due to disease exacerbation such as acute purulent bronchitis, pneumonia, heart failure, and thromboembolism. Patients requiring surgery are not included.

OUTCOME OF THE MANAGEMENT OF ACUTE RESPIRATORY FAILURE IN COPD

It is important, however, to focus on the survival rate of those who recover from acute respiratory failure. Further background information on this, representing consecutive series of 48 patients, is cited in Tables 10-3, 10-4, and 10-5. The long term outcome of this group of patients is presented in Figure 10-5. This late outcome is consistent with previous reports documenting the poor prognosis of patients with advanced COPD following an episode of acute respiratory failure requiring mechanical ventilation.[32–35]

EARLY PULMONARY REHABILITATION

The management of acute respiratory failure by either ventilator or nonventilator techniques is only one facet of the care of patients with advanced COPD. The presence of acute respiratory failure, however, generally indicates extremely severe underlying lung disease. Most patients recovering from acute respiratory failure are candidates for rehabilitative techniques. The modalities found valuable over the

TABLE 10-2. Outcome of All Patients with COPD Managed by Mechanical Ventilation for Acute Respiratory Failure

Year(s)	*Total*	*Died*	*Survived*	*Percentage Survived*
1964–1974	134	27	107	79.8 (early experience)
1975	13	2	11	
1976	17	3	14	
1977	13	4	9	
1978	14	0	14	87 (recent)
1979	8	0	8	
1980	4	0	4	
Total	203	36	167	82 (overall)

TABLE 10-3. Mechanical Ventilation in COPD (48 Patients—First Episode)

Data	*Range*	*Mean*
Age	34–83	64
Male	—	40
Female	—	8
Duration of disease (years)	1–46	13
Prev. hosp. for RD	0–15	2.6
Prev. pulm. funct. (N = 35)		
FVC % of normal	26–111	64
FEV_1 % of normal	23–65	39
MVV % of normal	7–85	31
Prev. art. blood gas (N = 46)		
P_{O_2}	29–96	58.5
P_{CO_2}	31–96	49.5
pH	7.30–7.51	7.41

past 18 years include patient and family education, breathing retraining, bronchial hygiene techniques aimed at bronchial dilatation and secretion clearance, systemic exercise, and administration of oxygen[36] (see Chap. 18). The importance of each of these techniques is briefly described.

TABLE 10-4. Mechanical Ventilation in COPD (Prior Clinical Features)

Data	*Number (N = 48)*
Chest roentgenogram	
Hyperinflation	43
Bullae	9
Cardiomegaly	17
Electrocardiogram	
RVH	34
P-Pulmon	27
Clinical peripheral edema	40
Medications	
Methylxanthines	36
Oxygen	33
Diuretics	33
Inhaled beta agonists	33
Cardiac glycosides	27
Oral beta agonists	22
Glucocorticoids	16

TABLE 10-5. Arterial Blood Gas Determinations Immediately Before Mechanical Ventilation

Data	*Range*	*Mean*
Pa_{O_2}	24–250	67
P_{CO_2}	52–158	78
pH	6.95–7.42	7.27

Education of the patient is fundamental to the successful management of all patients with chronic disease. This is particularly true in COPD because the patient, requiring detailed therapy, must understand and become a participant in his own health care scheme. Breathing retraining increases the efficacy of ventilation and relieves dyspnea. Systemic exercise expands horizons and increases the ability to participate in activities of daily living. Bronchial hygiene techniques using simple nebulization devices morning, midday, and night, if needed, help relieve bronchospasm and mobilize secretions. Often, a simple metered-dose device or hand-bulb nebulizer is used.

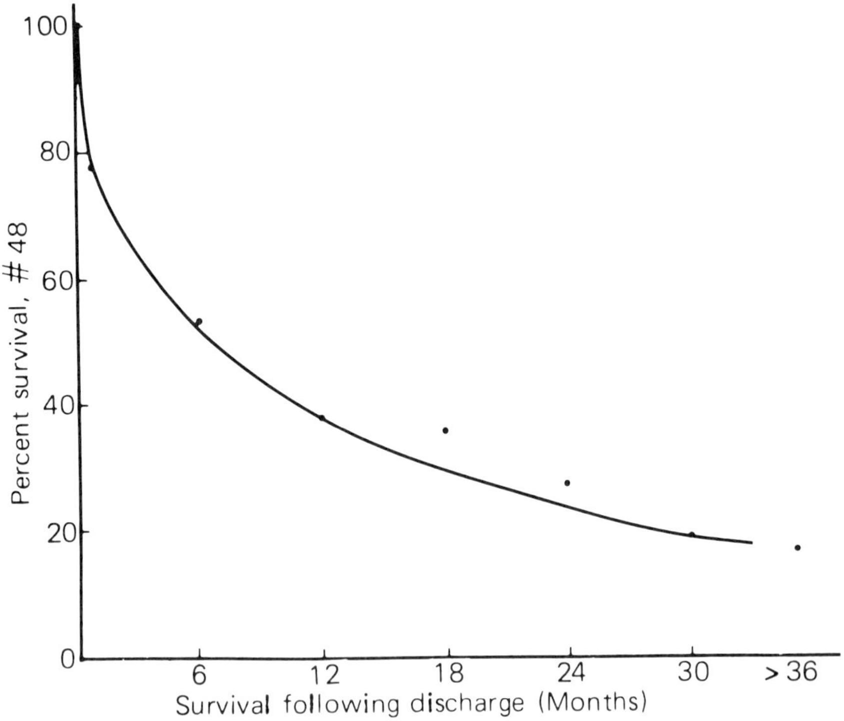

Fig. 10-5. Survival curve for 48 consecutive patients after first episodes of mechanical ventilation. Patients were followed for 3 years.

Other maintenance pharmacologic agents will continue to be used, including oral bronchodilators, antibiotics, and corticosteroids (effective in maintaining improved airflow). Home oxygen is valuable in selected patients with sustained significant hypoxemia, i.e., $Po_2 <$ 55 mm Hg, with cor pulmonale and other evidence of disability. Together, these facets of a comprehensive care program for advanced COPD can be effective in rehabilitation and can forestall or eliminate further hospitalization. Most important, the disease can be palliated, survival can be improved, and the quality of life can be substantially enhanced!

An evaluation of the effectiveness of pulmonary rehabilitation programs has clearly shown that this approach to therapy reduces the symptom impact of disease, improves exercise tolerance, enhances the quality of life, and reduces the need for hospitalization.[37, 38] A suggestion of improved survival in comparison groups has also been reported.[39] How to develop the most effective method of offering rehabilitative care on an outpatient basis remains a challenge for the future.[40]

Cystic fibrosis is another disease characterized by chronic airflow limitation or obstruction. Since the pathophysiologic features and approaches to management are in many ways similar to those in COPD, some comments regarding cystic fibrosis are included in this chapter.

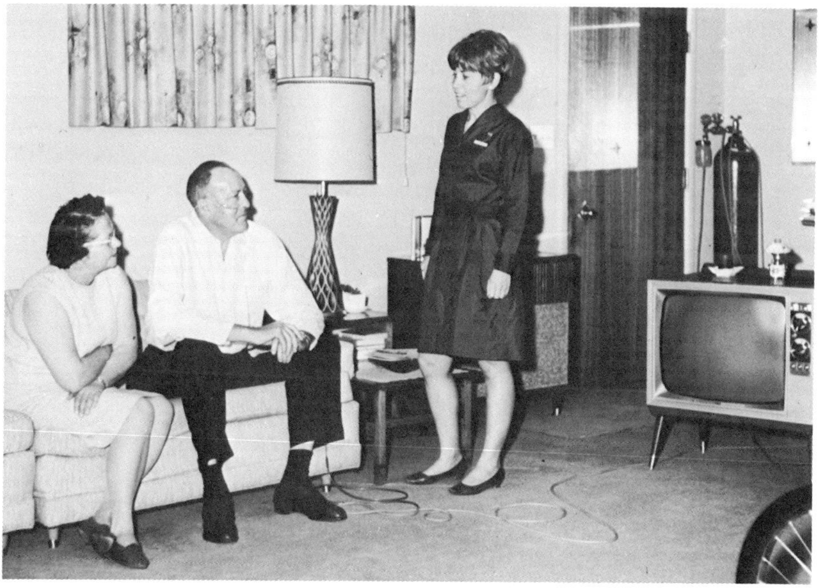

Fig. 10-6. Home care nurse visiting patient, whose details of care were illustrated in Figures 7-2, 7-3, 7-8, and 10-1. Home oxygen is continued because of severe emphysema and hypoxemia with cor pulmonale.

The therapeutic approach to cystic fibrosis in pediatric practice is discussed further in Chapter 16. Today the median age for survival in cystic fibrosis is more than 20 years. Thus, adult physicians, be they internists, pulmonologists, or allergists, are more and more often called upon to care for these patients. Immediate parallels between cystic fibrosis and COPD exist. Like COPD, the cystic fibrosis patient has airflow obstruction, hyperinflation, ventilation-perfusion mismatch, hypoxemia, and reactive pulmonary hypertension. Exacerbations and partial remissions are common. The cystic fibrosis patient, however, is far more burdened by identifiable bacterial pathogens than the patient with COPD. Here, *Pseudomonas aeruginosa*, *Staphylococcus aureus*, and *Haemophilus influenzae* predominate. It is almost, if not absolutely, impossible to eradicate organisms even with the liberal use of potent antibiotic agents. Antibiotics are frequently used almost continuously or on a rotational basis. Ampicillin, erythromycin, chloramphenicol, tetracycline, and trimethoprim-sulfa (Bactrim; Septra) are widely used and are effective against *H. influenzae* and other organisms.

All too often, however, *Pseudomonas* overgrowth predominates. When this occurs and is clinically significant, admission to hospital and the use of aminoglycosides directed against *Pseudomonas* species or, if appropriate, antistaphylococcal semisynthetic penicillins or combination approaches are useful. Again, it is almost impossible to totally eradicate the organism. In severe exacerbations, however, in which *Pseudomonas* or *Staphylococcus* species, or both, appears to predominate on the basis of sputum smears and cultures, admission to hospital and a seven- to ten-day course of intravenous antibiotics is believed to be clinically useful. In addition, controlled low-flow oxygen, expulsive coughing, and chest physiotherapy techniques with or without the use of inhaled moisture are believed to be beneficial by most. Ambulation and good diet are of fundamental importance in maintaining muscle strength and coordination.

The real difference in terms of approach occurs when patients suffer acute respiratory failure and are moribund, apneic, or exhausted. Certainly, the ability to intubate and ventilate these patients is similar to that in the COPD patient. The problem is that these patients usually develop acute respiratory failure late in the natural course of disease, and the likelihood of successful extubation and rehabilitation is small, on the basis of a nationwide clinical survey.[41] This certainly has been our experience in the limited number of cystic fibrosis patients ventilated in our unit. The reason for these differences between cystic fibrosis outcome and COPD are not entirely clear. Usually, the patients are cachectic and psychologically depleted before acute respiratory failure occurs, and they simply give up their tenacious grasp on life. Intubation and mechanical ventilation rarely stem this progress. If, by contrast, a major external precipitating event such as acute respiratory failure in the postoperative period, a major pneumothorax, or a massive pneumonia occurs, some of the same principles of supportive care would be appropriately applied to gain time. It is the opinion of the author that only when a specific treatable event can be identified and when the patient has the will and stamina to struggle for survival should intubation and mechanical ventilation be instituted in the hope of recovery.

In summary, acute respiratory failure in advanced COPD is a common event. A conservative approach employing nonventilator techniques, including controlled low-flow oxygen, measures to open the conducting airways and clear secretions, breathing training and conditioning, and maintenance of nutrition, along with the judicious use of pharmacologic drugs, will salvage the vast majority of patients. Pharmacologic agents alone are not adequate. In immediate life-threatening emergencies, establishment of a definitive airway and mechanical ventilatory support with a ventilator of high capability are required. The patient's nutrition, muscle strength, and will to live must be maintained throughout the management period. Weaning is more of an art than a science and is based upon a systematic approach to maximize the patient's utilization of limited respiratory resources. Even then, almost all patients requiring mechanical ventilation who survive the initial episode can be weaned from the ventilator and return home. These patients are candidates for rehabilitative techniques which have proved to be effective. Similar approaches are useful in patients with cystic fibrosis, but it is doubtful if intubation and mechanical ventilation should be used if acute respiratory failure has occurred insidiously and without a major precipitating factor, which may be amenable to definitive therapy. Certainly, cystic fibrosis remains a tremendous challenge for all pediatricians, internists, and respiratory care personnel.[42]

REFERENCES

1. American Thoracic Society Committee, Definitions and Classification of Chronic Bronchitis, Asthma and Pulmonary Emphysema. Am. Rev. Resp. Dis., *85:*62, 1962.
2. Williams, M.H.: Ventilatory failure. Medicine, *45:*317, 1966.
3. Campbell, E.J.M.: The management of acute respiratory failure in chronic bronchitis and emphysema. Am. Rev. Resp. Dis., *95:*626, 1967.
4. Smith, J.P., Stone, R.W., and Muschenheim, C.: Acute respiratory failure in chronic lung disease. Am. Rev. Resp. Dis., *97:*791, 1968.
5. Petty, T.L.: Acute Respiratory Failure. *In* Intensive and Rehabilitative Respiratory Care. 2nd Ed. Edited by T.L. Petty. Philadelphia, Lea & Febiger, 1974.
6. Cherniack, R.M., and Hakimpour K.: The rational use of oxygen in respiratory insufficiency. JAMA, *199:*178, 1967.
7. Bigelow, D.B., Petty, T.L., Levine, B.E., Filley, G.F., and Finigan, M.M.: The effort of oxygen breathing on arterial blood gases in patients with chronic airway obstruction living at 5,200 feet. Am. Rev. Resp. Dis., *96:*28, 1967.
8. Cheney, F.W., and Butler, J.: The effects of ultrasonically-produced aerosols on airway resistance in man. Anesthesiology, *29:*1099, 1968.
9. Graham, W.G.B., and Bradley, D.A.: Efficacy of chest physiotherapy and intermittent positive-pressure breathing in the resolution of pneumonia. N. Engl. J. Med., *299:*624, 1978.
10. Feldman, J., Traver, G.A., and Taussi, L.M.: Maximal expiratory flows after postural drainage. Am. Rev. Resp. Dis., *119:*239, 1979.

11. May, D.B., and Munt, P.W.: Physiologic effects of chest percussion and postural drainage in patients with stable chronic bronchitis. Chest, *75:*29, 1979.
12. Oldenburg, F.A., Dolovich, M.B., Montgomery, J.M., and Newhouse, M.T.: Effects of postural drainage, exercise and cough on mucus clearance in chronic bronchitis. Am. Rev. Resp. Dis., *120:*739, 1979.
13. Bernstein, L.I., and Ausdenmode, R.W.: Iatrogenic bronchospasms occurring during clinical trials of a new mucolytic agent, acetylcysteine. Dis. Chest, *46:*469, 1964.
14. Kory, R.C., Kirsch, S.R., and Giraldo, J.: Nebulization of N-acetylcysteine combined with a bronchodilator in patients with chronic bronchitis. Dis. Chest, *54:*504, 1968.
15. Fouts, J.B., and Brashear, R.E.: Intermittent positive-pressure breathing: A critical appraisal. Postgrad. Med., *59:*103, 1976.
16. Respiratory Care Committee of the American Thoracic Society, Intermittent Positive Pressure Breathing (IPPB). Clin. Notes Resp. Dis., *18:*3, 1979.
17. Conference on the Scientific Basis of Respiratory Therapy, Intermittent Positive Pressure Breathing Therapy. Am. Rev. Resp. Dis., *110*[part 2]:13, 1974.
18. Gormezano, J., and Branthwaile, M.A.: Pulmonary physiotherapy with assisted ventilation. Anaesthesia, *27:*242, 1972.
19. Gormezano, J., and Branthwaile, M.A.: Effects of physiotherapy during intermittent positive pressure ventilation. Anaesthesia, *27:*258, 1972.
20. Mossberg, B., Strandberg, K., Philipson, K., and Camner, P.: Tracheobronchial clearance and beta-adrenoceptor stimulation in patients with chronic bronchitis. Scand. J. Resp. Dis., *57:*281, 1976.
21. Albert, R.K., Martin, T.R., and Lewis, R.W.: Controlled clinical trial of methylprednisolone in patients with chronic bronchitis and acute respiratory insufficiency. Ann. Intern. Med., *92:*753, 1980.
22. Campbell, E.J.M.: The J. Burns Amberson Lecture: The management of acute respiratory failure in chronic bronchitis and emphysema. Am. Rev. Resp. Dis., *96:*626, 1967.
23. Stauffer, J.L., Olson, D.E., and Petty, T.L.: Complications and consequences of endotracheal intubation and tracheostomy: A prospective study of 150 critically ill patients. Am. J. Med., *70:*65, 1981.
24. Zwillich, C.W., Pierson, D.J., Creagh, C.F., Sutton, F.D., Schatz, E., and Petty, T.L.: Complications of assisted ventilation (a prospective study of 354 episodes). Am. J. Med., *57:*161, 1974.
25. Petty, T.L.: Complications occurring during mechanical ventilation. Heart Lung, *5:*112, 1976.
26. Sahn, S.A., and Lakshminarayan, S.: Bedside criteria for discontinuation of mechanical ventilation. Chest, *63:*1002, 1973.
27. Sahn, S.A., Lakshminarayan, S., and Petty, T.L.: Weaning from mechanical ventilation. JAMA, *235:*2208, 1976.
28. Petty, T.L.: IMV vs IMC. Chest, *67:*630, 1975.
29. Riley, R.L.: The work of breathing and its relation to respiratory acidosis. Ann. Intern. Med., *41:*172, 1954.
30. Barach, A.L.: The Adaptive Function of Hypercapnia. *In* Chronic Obstructive Pulmonary Disease. Edited by T.L. Petty. New York, Marcel Dekker, 1978.
31. Petty, T.L., Lakshminarayan, S., Sahn, S.A., Zwillich, C.W., and Nett, L.M.: Intensive respiratory care unit (review of ten years' experience). JAMA, *233:*34, 1975.
32. Gottlieb, L.S., and Balchum, O.J.: Course of chronic obstructive pulmonary disease following first onset of respiratory failure. Chest, *63:*5, 1973.
33. Burk, R.H., and George, R.B.: Acute respiratory failure in chronic obstructive pulmonary disease (immediate and long-term prognosis). Arch. Intern. Med., *132:*865, 1973.
34. Sluiter, J.H., Blokzijh, E.J., vanDijh, W., van Haeringen, J.R., Hilvering, C., and Steenhuis, E.J.: Conservative and respiratory treatment of acute respiratory insufficiency in patients with chronic obstructive lung disease. Am. Rev. Resp. Dis., *105:*932, 1972.

35. Asmundsson, T., and Kilburn, K.H.: Survival after acute respiratory failure (145 patients observed 5 to 8½ years). Ann. Intern. Med., *80:*54, 1974.
36. Petty, T.L.: Pulmonary rehabilitation. Resp. Care, *22:*68, 1977.
37. Fishman, D.B., and Petty, T.L.: Physical, symptomatic and psychological improvement in patients receiving comprehensive care for chronic airway obstruction. J. Chronic Dis., *24:*775, 1971.
38. Hudson, L.D., Tyler, M.L., and Petty, T.L.: Hospitalization needs during an outpatient rehabilitation program for severe chronic airway obstruction. Chest, *70:*606, 1976.
39. Sahn, S.A., and Petty, T.L.: Results of a Comprehensive Rehabilitation Program for Severe COPD. *In* Chronic Obstructive Pulmonary Disease. Edited by T.L. Petty. New York, Marcel Dekker, 1978.
40. Petty, T.L.: Pulmonary rehabilitation. Am. Rev. Resp. Dis., *122*[Suppl.]:159, 1980.
41. Davis, P.B., and di Sant'Agnese, D.A.: Assisted ventilation for patients with cystic fibrosis. JAMA, *239:*1851, 1978.
42. Warwick, W.J., and Pogue, R.E.: Cystic fibrosis (an expanding challenge for internal medicine). JAMA, *238:*2159, 1977.

Chapter 11

INTERSTITIAL PNEUMONITIS AND FIBROSIS AND OTHER RESTRICTIVE VENTILATORY DEFECTS

By Thomas L. Petty

Restrictive ventilatory defects are common causes of acute and chronic respiratory failure. The lung parenchyma or chest bellows system, including the diaphragm, may be involved. The basic physiologic problem may be not only impaired ventilation, but also impaired oxygen transport in the case of diffuse interstitial pneumonitis or interstitial fibrosis. Some common and less frequent clinical situations in which restrictive respiratory failure occurs are listed in Table 11-1.

Various common clinical entities result in acute respiratory failure due to restrictive defects and ventilation–perfusion abnormalities. The cases cited in this chapter illustrate some of the diverse types commonly encountered in the practice of respiratory care. The systematic approach to management of the individual special cases cited exemplifies the principles of management that apply to all forms of respiratory failure. The goals of management will be largely determined by the potential for reversibility and the natural history of the underlying disorder.

INTERSTITIAL PNEUMONITIS AND FIBROSIS

This is a heterogeneous group of acute and chronic lung insults with different courses and outcomes. Table 11-2 offers a simplified classification of this group of disorders. The so-called idiopathic

TABLE 11-1. Causes of Restrictive Ventilatory Defects

A. Impaired lung expansion
   1. Interstitial lung diseases (case examples 1–3)
   2. Pulmonary edema
      a. Cardiogenic (Case 4)
      b. Noncardiogenic
      c. ARDS (Chap. 8)
   3. Space pre-empting problems
      a. Pleural effusion
      b. Hemothorax
      c. Pneumothorax

B. Limited thoracic expansion
   1. Kyphoscoliosis (Case 5)
   2. Neuromuscular defects (Chap. 13)
   3. Crushed chest (Chap. 14)

C. Impaired diaphragmatic movement
   1. Massive ascites
   2. Severe obesity (Case 6)
   3. Abdominal surgery

group is most perplexing because so little is known about pathogenesis, treatment (usually with corticosteroids) is less than satisfactory, and progression to disability and death is common. The most common, usual interstitial pneumonitis (UPI) and desquamative interstitial pneumonitis (DIP), probably represent a spectrum of a single major disease process which affects the regulation of inflammation, and collagen biochemistry and deposition within the lung.[1] This group of disorders may run a florid and rapidly fatal course, as originally described by Hamman and Rich.[2] More recent authors have described a more indolent course which at times responds favorably to corticosteroids or immunosuppressive drugs.[3,4] For this reason, it is believed that abnormalities of the lung's regulation of immune-mediated inflammation are fundamental to the pathogenesis. Clinicopathologic correlations in patients treated with prednisone and azathioprine have shown variable responses to therapy, with favorable prognosis most likely in patients with an illness of short duration.[5] In a large series, the 2:1 male-to-female predominance was cited, with an overall mean survival of only 3.2 years in spite of treatment.[6] Still another series has offered additional information about its course and prognosis.[7] In general, although the course varies and is generally unfavorable, histologic classification helps forecast prognosis and response to therapies and is thus considered fundamental to evaluation of the patient. It also has significance in long-range planning, where supportive respiratory care might be considered to be either appropriate or inappropriate (see Chap. 20).

TABLE 11-2. Interstitial Pneumonitis—Fibrosis

A. "Idiopathic"	
1. Usual interstitial pneumonitis (UIP)	Together frequently called "fibrosing alveolitis"—Case 1
2. Desquamative interstitial pneumonitis (DIP)	
3. Lymphocytic interstitial pneumonitis (LIP)—rare	
4. Giant-cell interstitial pneumonitis (GIP)—rarer	
5. Bronchiolitis obliterans (Case 2)	
B. Associated with collagen disease	
1. Rheumatoid arthritis (Case 2)	
2. Lupus erythematosus (Case 3)	
3. Scleroderma	
4. Polymyositis	
C. Hypersensitivity Pneumonitis	
1. Farmer's lung (Case 4)	
2. Many others	
D. Drug related (many)	
1. Nitrofurantoins	
2. Bleomycin and other antineoplastic drugs	
E. Industrial hazards	
1. Asbestosis	
2. Silicosis	
3. Other	
F. Granulomas	
1. Sarcoidosis	
2. Histiocytosis X (eosinophilic granuloma)	

Often, one's first encounter with a challenging clinical entity leaves a most lasting impression. This illustrative Case 1, cited in the first and second editions of this book, remains as classic as it did during the formative years of the Colorado program. It is therefore included once again.

Case 1. B.G., a 58-year-old Spanish coal miner, was admitted to the hospital because of acute progressive dyspnea of one month's duration. Following the acute onset of symptoms, he had been admitted to a hospital where the diagnosis of pneumonia was made, but no lasting improvement occurred after treatment with a variety of antibiotics.

On admission to Colorado General Hospital, the patient was dyspneic, and cyanosis was noted. His temperature was 37° C; pulse rate, 110; respiration rate, 25. His systolic blood pressure was 110; the diastolic, 60. Jugular venous pressure increase was noted when the patient was elevated to a 45-degree angle. Signs of consolidation were present at both lung bases posteriorly; coarse, diffuse crackling rales were heard at all lung fields. The pulmonic closure was increased; a gallop rhythm was not present. Hepatomegaly and mild edema were present. Laboratory tests revealed a hematocrit value of 52% and white cell count of 10,300; sputum culture showed "normal flora." Chest roentgenogram (Fig. 11-1, *left*) revealed dense infiltration in both lower

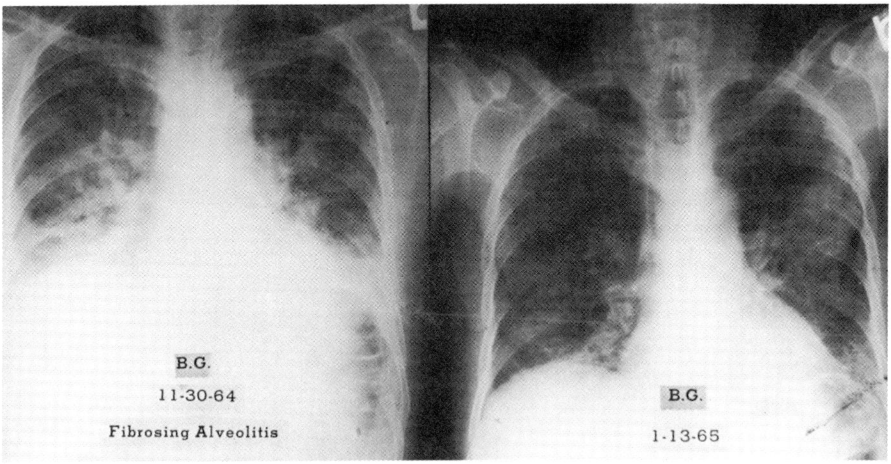

Fig. 11-1. Admission chest roentgenogram (Case 1, *left*). Note lower-lobe diffuse infiltrates bilaterally. Marked clearing response to corticosteroid drugs (*right*). See text and Table 11-3. (From Arizona Med., *23:*655, 1966.)

lung fields and fine, diffuse reticular markings consistent with pulmonary fibrosis. The EKG revealed no abnormality.

The diagnoses were pulmonary fibrosis, chronic pneumonitis, and cor pulmonale with congestive right heart failure.

Ventilation tests and blood gas determinations performed 2 weeks after admission (Table 11-3) revealed both a restrictive and an obstructive ventilatory impairment as well as mild hypoxemia at rest.

Initial management included salt restriction and antibiotic therapy, but little or no improvement followed. Marked clinical improvement occurred after treatment with 15 to 30 mg prednisone daily. Subsequent ventilation tests showed considerable improvement (Table 11-3). The patient was discharged 6 weeks after entry; he was to continue taking 10 mg prednisone daily. A chest roentgenogram taken at the time of discharge (Fig. 11-1, *right*) showed considerable clearing of the basilar infiltrates.

TABLE 11-3. Case 1—Fibrosing Alveolitis

Ventilation Tests and Blood Gas Determinations			
	Initial Tests	*After Cortico-steroids*	*Predicted*
VC	1.52	2.09	3.33 L
FEV_1	0.91	1.61	>75% of VC
MMF	0.50	2.06	3.71 ± 1.00 L/sec
MBC	54	94	114 L/min
SAO_2	88.5		>92%
P_{CO_2}	42		36–38
pH	7.505		7.40

Two months later, congestive right heart failure with jugular venous hypertension and peripheral edema were again noted. Diuresis and improvement in the signs of congestive heart failure occurred after administration of digitalis. One month later, migratory polyarthralgias occurred, and increasing dyspnea required re-hospitalization. On this occasion an open lung biopsy revealed both cellular and fibrotic features of "fibrosing alveolitis," i.e., both features of UIP and DIP.

Following recovery from the operation, the patient was again discharged with instructions to follow a cardiac regimen and to continue taking 10 mg prednisone daily.

Approximately one year after the initial diagnosis was made, increasing dyspnea again occurred with pulmonary edema. Signs of congestive heart failure including mild clubbing of the fingers were again present. No skin abnormalities were observed. A chest roentgenogram (Fig. 11-2) showed "honeycombing" with fibrosis of both lower lung fields. The ECG now revealed a rightward axis and right ventricular and atrial enlargement. Arterial blood P_{O_2} was 38.5; oxygen saturation, 74%; and P_{CO_2}, 42. An esophagogram showed dilation and absence of esophageal peristalsis.

With maintenance digitalis, diuretics, oxygen administered via nasal cannula, and large doses of prednisone, clinical improvement and diuresis of 4 kg occurred. After an increase in the dose of prednisone to 30 mg daily, the patient's clinical course stabilized. Arterial studies one

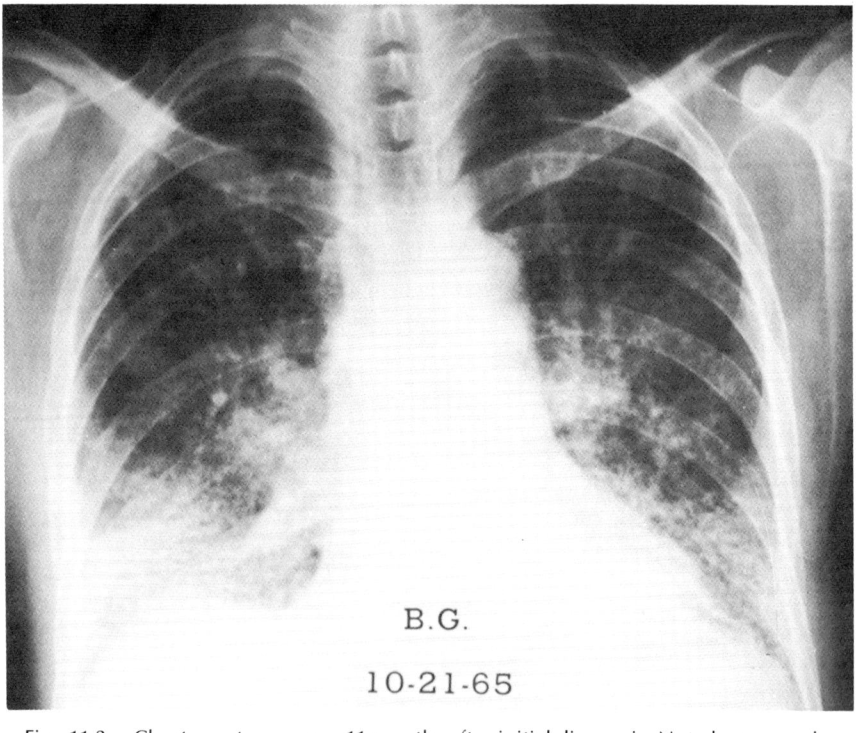

Fig. 11-2. Chest roentgenogram 11 months after initial diagnosis. Note honeycombing and dense infiltration in right lower lung field as well as bilaterally. (From Arizona Med., *23:*655, 1966.)

week following an increased steroid dosage revealed Po_2, 72; oxygen saturation, 95%; Pco_2, 45; pH, 7.42.

Comment. Combined pulmonary and cardiac failure occurred in this patient with pulmonary fibrosis. The patient had many of the signs of fibrosing alveolitis, a condition also frequently called "diffuse interstitial pulmonary fibrosis." The migratory polyarthritis with decreased esophageal motility also implicates progressive systemic sclerosis as a possible underlying disease exemplifying the overlap with a similar clinicopathologic picture found often in patients with collagen diseases.

In this case, impaired oxygen transfer due to both diffusion and ventilation abnormalities as well as possible fibrotic pulmonary vascular obliteration led to pulmonary hypertension and right heart failure. No evidence of vasculitis was found on histologic section.

Improvement occurred with a heart-failure regimen including digitalis and diuretics; supplemental oxygen was administered because of moderately severe hypoxemia. Corticosteroid drugs probably provided improved oxygen transfer, presumably by combating alveolitis.

Both acute and chronic interstitial pneumonitis and fibrosis occur in collagen diseases, particularly in rheumatoid arthritis and lupus erythematosus. The course may be florid and inexorable, ending in acute respiratory failure and death, or it may be reversible with an excellent prognosis, as the next two illustrative cases testify.

Case 2. L.P., a 19-year-old high school student, was admitted to the hospital because of painful arthritis and marked dyspnea. She was first seen six months earlier, when the diagnosis of rheumatoid arthritis and interstitial pneumonitis was made following an open lung biopsy, which also revealed a mild vasculitis. Features of bronchiolitis obliterans were present. The antecedent history of illness covered only 8 months, during which migratory painful swelling of the knees, hips, and other joints occurred, particularly in the morning and with no relation to exercise.

Three months before the present hospital admission, the patient noted the onset of periodic chest pain bilaterally, anteriorly, and posteriorly. She was treated with bed rest at home for one week without relief. Later, she was hospitalized because of pain in the upper chest and beneath the sternum. A biopsy of a subcutaneous nodule over the right elbow showed the lesion to be a typical rheumatoid nodule.

Two months before the present admission to the hospital, dyspnea worsened. The patient was able to walk only one block and climb only one flight of stairs; this limited activity was in contrast to her previous active participation in school athletics. At this time, the patient also noted increased dry coughing without sputum production. Pulmonary function tests gave the following values (normal in parenthesis): FEV_1, 0.49 liter (3.00); maximum mid-expiratory flow (MMF), 0.20 L/sec (3.60 ± 0.88); and maximum voluntary ventilation (MVV), 34 L/min (120).

On physical examination it was noted that the patient was a well-developed young female in obvious respiratory distress. Moderate mental confusion was manifest. Her pulse rate was 140; blood pressure, 110/79; respiration rate, 60. Marked retractions in the suprasternal, supraclavicular, and intercostal regions were noted. Auscultation revealed harsh breath sounds throughout with crackling inspiratory rales. The precordium was hyperactive, and a right ventricular lift was palpated. The pulmonic closure was accentuated. Extremity examination revealed inflammation over both wrists, and a small nodule was found over the right olecranon process.

Initial oxygen tension (Po_2) was 39; carbon dioxide tension (Pco_2), 49; pH, 7.41; and oxygen saturation (SAO_2), 69%. With nasal oxygen the SAO_2 rose to 94% and Po_2 to 65; Pco_2 was 42 and pH, 7.46. The patient's state of orientation improved coincident with oxygen therapy. The respiratory rate dropped to 28; Pco_2 remained at 42. Corticosteroid therapy resulted in transient improvement.

The patient remained improved while being maintained on corticosteroids and continuous nasal oxygen. Oxygen therapy was continued because of her profound hypoxemia (Po_2, 30 to 45 mm Hg) and the intense dyspnea demonstrated when she was not being given oxygen. She later developed progressive dyspnea in spite of continuous oxygen therapy, and her condition became progressively worse owing to chronic ventilatory failure ($Pco_2 > 75$ while on O_2). The patient died 18 months after the original diagnosis of chronic pneumonitis was made.

Comment. This is an example of subacute pulmonary fibrosis presumably related to rheumatoid disease.[8–10] The primary problem in such patients is hypoxemia with relatively normal ventilation. These patients can be initially treated with controlled oxygen therapy sufficient to bring the Po_2 to 50 mm Hg by means of nasal flows without resorting to ventilatory assistance. Progressive fibrosis and development of a progressively noncompliant lung may evolve in spite of corticosteroid therapy and may lead to irreversible ventilatory failure. Use of additional immunosuppressive drugs such as azathioprine and cyclophosphamide should be considered in cases of florid progression of lung involvement resulting in respiratory failure.

Occasionally in acute lupus erythematosus, a sudden picture of pneumonitis occurs, leading to acute respiratory failure. In this case the lung appears to be the "target organ," and kidney involvement is mild or minimal. A dramatic case example is illustrated in Case 3.

Case 3. D.S., an 18-year-old Mexican-American girl, was admitted in September, 1970, with severe shortness of breath and marked cyanosis. Three months prior to admission, the patient had noted an evanescent red rash on her face and transient arthralgias and stiffness with swelling of her distal interphalangeal joints and ankles. One week before admission, while being treated with Azo Gantrisin for a urinary tract infection, she developed a fever (104°F), and oral penicillin was substituted for Azo Gantrisin. Three days prior to admission, the red facial rash reappeared. Progressive severe shortness of breath followed, and she was admitted to the intensive respiratory care unit.

Physical examination revealed a markedly cyanotic, tachypneic woman with a blood pressure of 100/70, pulse 144, respirations 42, and temperature 102°F. An erythematous malar eruption was present. Decreased breath sounds were noted bilaterally with rales at both lung bases. Cardiac examination revealed a right ventricular lift and an accentuated pulmonic closure; no pericardial friction rub was observed. No hepatosplenomegaly or joint involvement was noted.

Laboratory examination showed normal values for hemoglobin, WBC count, and differential. The blood urea nitrogen, serum creatinine, and urinalysis were within normal range. The erythrocyte sedimentation rate (Wintrobe method) was 46 mm/hr, LE prep was positive, antinuclear antibody was positive, revealing a homogeneous pattern, high titers of anti-DNA antibodies were present, and a biopsy of uninvolved skin was positive for immunofluorescence. Admission arterial blood gas values were P_{CO_2}, 21; P_{O_2}, 20; O_2 saturation, 31%, and pH, 7.52, while breathing room air; on high-flow oxygen (12 liters per minute by face mask), the P_{O_2} only increased to 42 mm Hg with a P_{CO_2} of 34 mm Hg (Table 11-4). Anteroposterior chest roentgenogram revealed a diffuse infiltrate, greatest at the lung bases, and bilateral pleural effusions (Fig. 11-3).

Electrocardiogram showed occasional ventricular premature beats. Blood and urine cultures revealed no growth; sputum and throat cultures produced normal flora. Viral cultures of blood, nasopharynx, and stool were negative. The tuberculin skin test (PPD intermediate) gave negative results; the intradermal mumps skin test was positive.

A diagnosis of acute, fulminating lupus pneumonitis was made, and treatment was initiated with nasal oxygen, tetracycline (2 g/day for 7 days), and intravenous hydrocortisone (400 mg/day). The temperature returned to normal by the fourth hospital day, and respirations were less labored. The patient still required high-flow nasal oxygen to maintain an adequate P_{O_2}, and the chest x-ray picture was not improved.

TABLE 11-4. Case 3—Acute Lupus Pneumonitis

		P_{O_2} (mm Hg)*		
Day	O_2	*Rest*	*Exercise*	*FVC (Liters)*†
1	Room air	20		
	12 L (mask)	42		
9				.450
14	10 L (nasal)	62		.580
		Azathioprine		
39	Room air	61		1.00
2 mo	Room air	61	49	1.70
10 mo	Room air	71	68	2.56

* (Range of normal for Denver: 65–75)
† (Range of normal: 3.2 ± .84)

In spite of high doses of corticosteroids for 14 days, the patient's vital capacity was only 580 ml (16% of normal), and high-flow nasal oxygen was still required to maintain adequate oxygenation (Table 11-4). The chest roentgenogram revealed the continued presence of bilateral pulmonary infiltrates and pleural effusions. At this time azathioprine (150 mg/day orally, 2½ mg/kg) was added to the steroid therapy. Marked improvement with less dyspnea and reduced oxygen flow requirements followed. The patient was discharged on the thirty-ninth hospital day on azathioprine (75 mg/day) and prednisone (30 mg/day) with a vital capacity of 1 L (27% of normal) and a P_{O_2} of 61 mm Hg without nasal oxygen (Table 11-4). The chest roentgenogram (Fig. 11-4) showed resolution of the effusions and substantial clearing of the bilateral infiltrates.

Azathioprine and corticosteroids were gradually tapered over the next year, and 3 years after the onset, the patient is entirely asymptomatic and is receiving only 5 mg prednisone each day. Her ventilatory function values, diffusion test, and rest and exercise blood gases are now normal. Evidence of further recovery on follow-up is presented in Table 11-5.

Comment. Acute lupus pneumonitis is a rare manifestation of lupus erythematosus. A second case which also responded well to a combination of azathioprine and corticosteroid medication has been encountered.[12] A review of 12 cases in total, including cases with a more indolent course and variable responses to therapy, has also been reported.[13]

OTHER FORMS OF INTERSTITIAL LUNG DISEASE WITH A MORE FAVORABLE PROGNOSIS

It must be emphasized that the x-ray presentation in interstitial fibrosis does not reliably identify the cause of the abnormality. Except in cases of so-called "end stage" fibrosis with honeycombing of the lung and massive loss of lung volume, the roentgenogram is not a good prognostic indicator. It is beyond the scope of this chapter to present examples of all forms of interstitial lung disease, but four additional case vignettes help make specific points of clinical importance.

Figure 11-5 demonstrates the rapid clearing of the massive alveolar and interstitial infiltrates present in an example of hypersensitivity pneumonitis when exposure to moldy farm silage was avoided and corticosteroids were given in a brief course to relieve severe constitutional symptoms. Note time course and evidence of both x-ray and physiologic improvement. Figure 11-6 shows similar improvement during the use of corticosteroids in a case of sarcoidosis. Figure 11-7 shows that spontaneous clearing can occur, particularly when there is an acute course of the interstitial pneumonitis as in this example of influenza A pneumonia. The nonspecific and nondiagnostic nature of an interstitial process is exemplified by Figure 11-8 from a woman

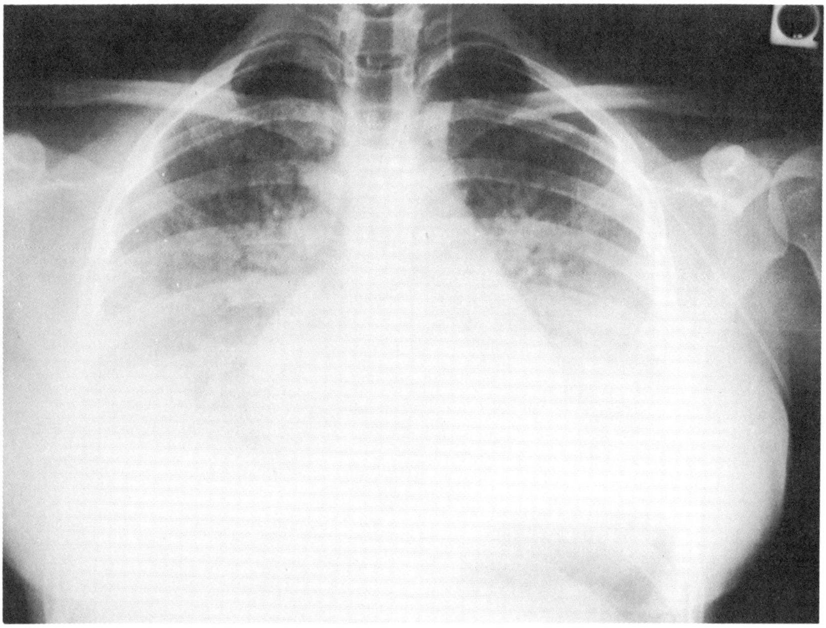

Fig. 11-3. Admission film Case 3, showing massive pulmonary infiltration and poor expansion. (Reproduced with permission from Chest, *63:*117, 1973.)

with a pulmonary drug reaction from nitrofurantoins, taken over a protracted course owing to recurrent urinary tract infections.

PROGRESSIVE FLORID INTERSTITIAL PNEUMONITIS

As discussed briefly in the beginning of this chapter, acute interstitial pneumonitis/fibrosis may follow a florid course, as originally described by Hamman and Rich.[2] In this situation, even ventilatory support will not be lifesaving. The ventilator only buys time to allow therapy to begin to reduce the underlying lung inflammation. If the course is protracted—not responsive to corticosteroids or even immunosuppressive drugs—ventilatory support should not be instituted.

INDIRECT CAUSES OF RESTRICTIVE VENTILATION DEFECTS

Pulmonary Edema

Pulmonary edema due to acute left ventricular decompensation has been associated with marked ventilatory impairment and carbon dioxide retention in patients with otherwise normal lungs. A case example follows.

Case 4. M.W., a 76-year-old woman with no history of pulmonary disease, had had numerous hospital admissions because of angina pectoris and, on 2 occasions, ECG evidence of acute myocardial infarction.

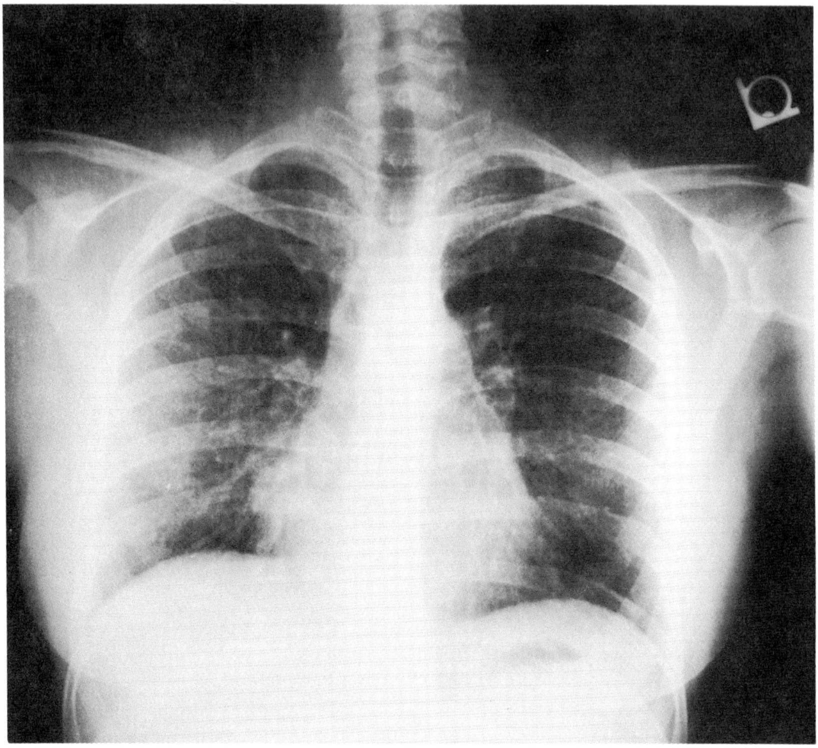

Fig. 11-4. Discharge film after 39 days of treatment with corticosteroids and azathioprine. (Reproduced with permission from Chest, *63*:117, 1973.)

She had recovered from these episodes without evidence of residual cardiac failure. She also had diabetes mellitus, which had been well controlled with small doses of insulin for 25 years. Recent electrocardiograms revealed left bundle branch block, first degree heart block, and left ventricular enlargement. On the evening of admission she had had severe substernal chest pain for which she had taken nitroglycerin tablets without relief. The pain was accompanied by nausea, vomiting, and marked diaphoresis. The patient was found to be lapsing into unconsciousness

TABLE 11-5. Case 3—Acute Lupus Pneumonitis; Pulmonary Function on Recovery

	Day 14	*2 Mo*	*10 Mo*	*37 Mo*
FVC (L)	0.58	1.70	2.56	3.04
FEV_1 (L/sec)	—	1.70	2.42	2.65
P_{CO_2}		8.8	14.6	22
P_{O_2} rest (RA)*		61	71	78
P_{O_2} Ex (RA)		49	68	—

* Normal—Denver 65–75.

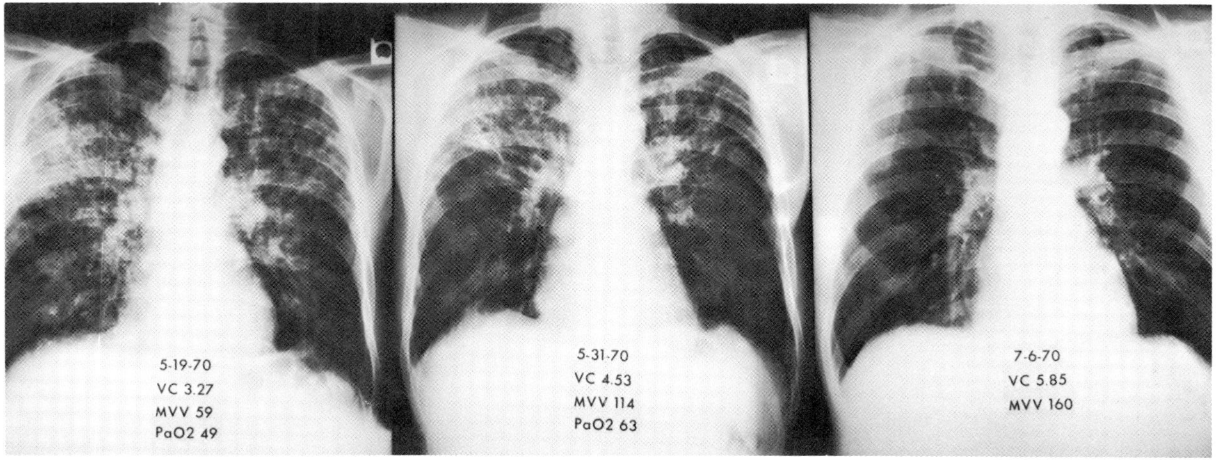

Fig. 11-5. Patient with hypersensitivity pneumonitis. Chest roentgenogram on admission (*left*) shows diffuse bilateral pulmonary infiltrate. Date, VC, MVV, and room air PO_2 shown on each x-ray film. Middle panel shows partial clearing and physiologic improvement after six days of corticosteroids and avoidance of precipitating exposure. Right panel shows complete roentgenographic clearing two weeks after completion of therapy.

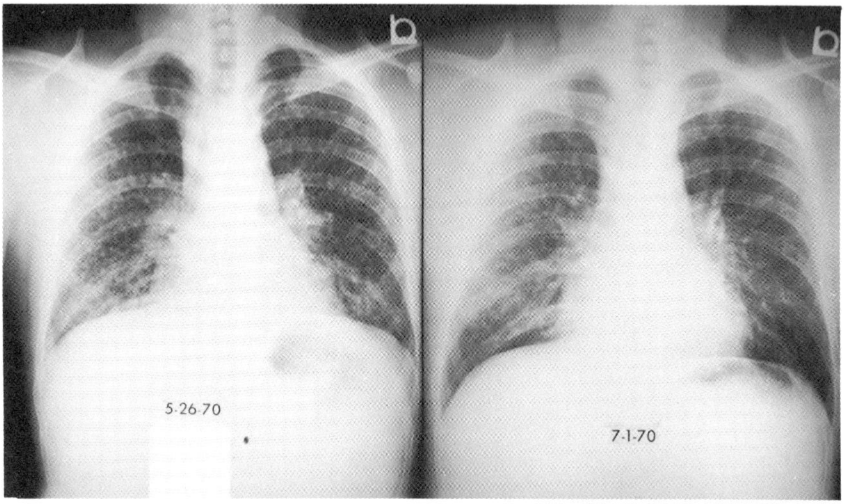

Fig. 11-6. Diffuse interstitial and alveolar infiltrates in biopsy-proved sarcoidosis (*left*). *Right*, roentgenographic clearing following six weeks of low-dose corticosteroid therapy associated with marked symptomatic improvement.

and was brought to the hospital emergency room. On admission she was short of breath, tachypneic, cyanotic, and diaphoretic, with a tachycardia of 150. Central venous pressure measured 22 cm H_2O (upper normal limit = 12–13). Auscultation revealed a loud second heart sound and moist inspiratory rales at the lung bases. Mild pitting ankle edema was present.

Oxygen via nasal cannula was started immediately at 4 L/min. Arterial blood gas values were obtained with the patient breathing oxygen (Table 11-6). Severe hypoxemia and hypercapnia were found with acidemia, due predominantly to CO_2 retention but possibly due in part to a mild degree of lactic acid accumulation.

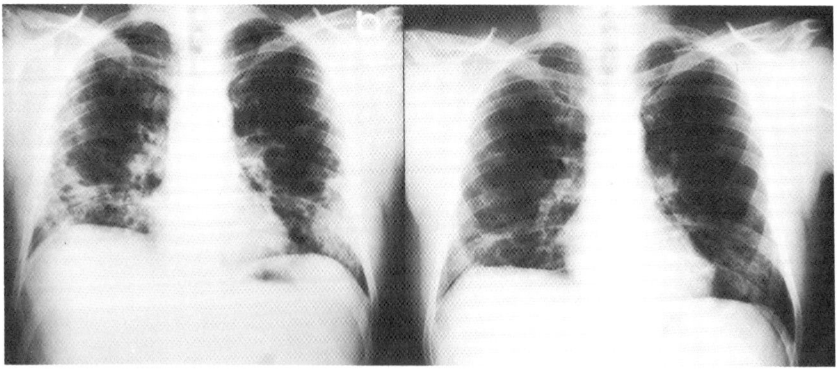

Fig. 11-7. Diffuse patchy alveolar and interstitial infiltrates during peak of critical illness established A type influenza, a virus pneumonia. *Right*, resolution six weeks later without any specific therapy.

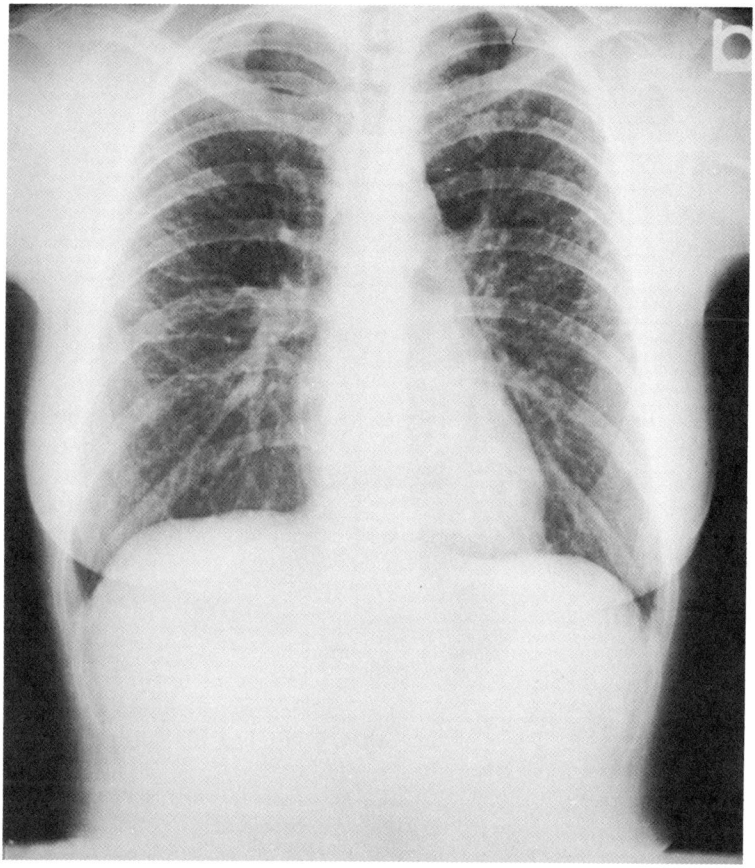

Fig. 11-8. Diffuse fine interstitial infiltrate following nearly six months of nitrofurantoin therapy for recurrent urinary tract infections.

TABLE 11-6. Case 4—Pulmonary Edema

	Admission	*2 Hours*	*12 Hours*	*14 Hours*	*24 Hours*
P_{O_2}	45	75	50	110	120
P_{CO_2}	65	45	43	44	41
pH	7.15	7.35	7.38	7.37	7.40
Bicarbonate	21.5	24	24.5	24.5	24.5
Respiratory support	Nasal oxygen at 4, 1 P.M.	Vol. Vent. 900 ml V_T 60 cm H_2O press 0.6 F_{IO_2}	Vol. Vent. 900ml V_T 65 cm H_2O press 0.6 F_{IO_2}	Vol. Vent. 900 ml V_T 60 cm H_2O press 0.6 F_{IO_2} 10 cm H_2O PEEP	Vol. Vent. 900 ml V_T 40 cm H_2O press 0.4 F_{IO_2} 10 cm H_2O PEEP

Subsequently, the patient developed a slow sinus rhythm followed by a slow idioventricular rhythm and respiratory arrest. Electrocardiogram activity was never lost. She was immediately resuscitated by means of a self-inflating bag with mask. Cardiac rhythm promptly improved. Blood pressure of 60/0 which accompanied the bradycardia rapidly increased to 140/70. It was thought that the patient was suffering from an acute myocardial infarction.

Following resuscitation, the patient was in a state of obvious acute pulmonary edema. She was managed on a volume-cycled ventilator. Initial inflation pressure requirement was high (60 cm H_2O), indicating an effective compliance of only 15 ml/cm H_2O (60 ml delivery pressure per 900 ml tidal volume); normal effective compliance is 50 to 100 ml/cm H_2O. With ventilatory assistance, blood gases were improved by using an inspired oxygen fraction (F_{IO_2}) of 0.6 (Table 11-6).* Thereafter, her heart rhythm stabilized to a supraventricular tachycardia of 140, and digitalis was begun. Twelve hours later, with the same F_{IO_2} of 0.6, the arterial P_{O_2} was reduced to 50 mm Hg despite acceptable alveolar ventilation as indicated by a P_{CO_2} of 43. In spite of frequent suctioning of the endotracheal tube, white frothy foam was continually produced, and severe hypoxemia remained. Because of the severely impaired oxygen transport, 10 cm H_2O of positive end-expiratory pressure (PEEP-see Chap. 5 for explanation) was provided by the ventilator, and blood gases obtained two hours later revealed marked improvement—an arterial P_{O_2} of 110 mm Hg achieved with the same F_{IO_2} of 0.6 and the same ventilator adjustments (Table 11-6). During this period, the patient's pulse rate decreased and blood pressure stabilized at 150/80. The next day, arterial P_{O_2} was 200 mm Hg. The inspired oxygen fraction was reduced to minimize the risk of pulmonary oxygen toxicity.† This still provided an arterial P_{O_2} of 120, indicating improved oxygen transport (narrowed I-a difference).

The patient's course was complicated by a pneumothorax. Pulmonary edema was in evidence on the roentgenogram at this time. (Fig. 11-9.) A chest tube was placed, because of this pneumothorax, which bubbled transiently and then ceased. The patient required 4 days of ventilatory assistance. Thereafter, following a brisk diuresis averaging 3500 to 4000 ml/day, the patient's condition improved, ventilatory assistance was no longer necessary, and the tracheostomy tube that had been placed the second day was removed. The patient made an uneventful recovery and was discharged on the forty-first hospital day. Four months later, she was at home and able to do light gardening.

---

* The arterial oxygen tension of 75 mm Hg from an F_{IO_2} of 0.6 (inspired oxygen tension of 350 mm Hg) indicated an inspired-to-arterial tension difference (I-a difference) of 275 mm Hg (normal I-a difference is 50 to 80). This inspired-arterial oxygen tension difference is a rough index of the alveolar-arterial (A-a) oxygen tension difference and an indication of the degree of impairment of pulmonary O_2 transport.

† In normal circulatory states, inspired oxygen fraction (or tensions) should be reduced to a level where the arterial oxygen tension does not exceed 100 mm Hg. In shock states, however, high oxygen F_{IO_2} up to 1.0 is *needed* to aid oxygen transport. One hundred percent oxygen is well tolerated for at least 24 hours. (Singer, M.: N. Engl. J. Med., *283:*1473, 1970.)

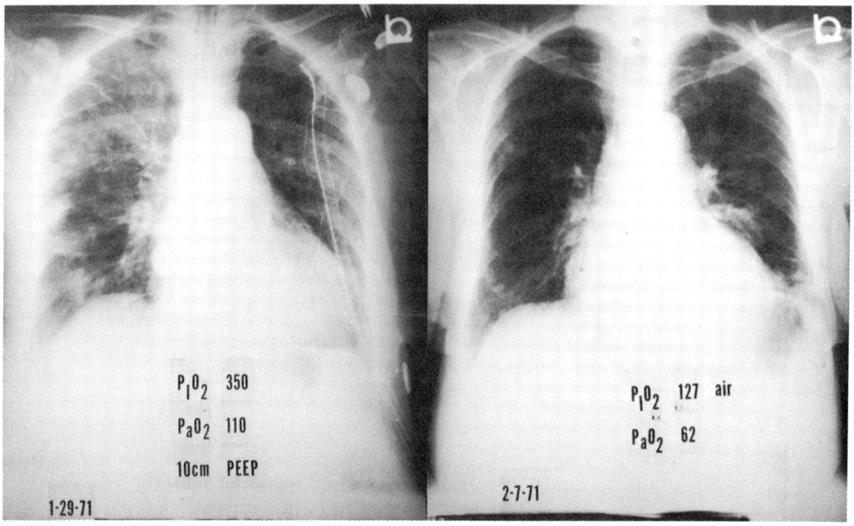

Fig. 11-9. Left bilateral parenchymal infiltrates due to pulmonary edema and cardiomegaly (Case 4), 14 hours following resuscitation. Left lung pneumothorax has been re-expanded by chest tube. *Right*, clearing of lung parenchyma. Chest tube was removed on recovery. Patient recovered.

Comment. This patient had profound respiratory failure associated with pulmonary edema. The impaired oxygen transport required ventilatory assistance, which was lifesaving in her case. The use of positive end-expiratory pressure may be valuable in improving oxygen transport in states of pulmonary edema by improving arterial oxygenation without interfering with cardiac output (see Chap. 5).

As with the case cited, entirely normal pulmonary function can be restored on recovery of cardiac output.[14]

Noncardiogenic causes of pulmonary edema include uremia and poisoning, such as that due to heroin or smoke inhalation. The underlying physiologic abnormality in these cases is primarily impaired oxygen transport and not underventilation. Ventilatory assistance is required not only when ventilatory failure occurs (i.e., uncompensated P_{CO_2} higher than 65), but also to improve oxygen transport by modifications of pressure wave forms (Chap. 5). In milder cases, controlled oxygen may suffice.

It is unusual for pleural effusion or even a complete pneumothorax to be the sole cause of acute respiratory failure, but in states of underlying lung disease, these complications may contribute to acute respiratory failure.

Limited Thoracic Excursion

Although limited thoracic expansion frequently accompanies any form of respiratory failure, it is rare for primary thoracic disease alone to lead to acute respiratory failure. In patients with ankylosing spondylitis (Case 5), however, severe impairment of the thoracic bellows may be a major contributor to ventilatory insufficiency.

Case 5. L.A., a 51-year-old business executive, was admitted to the hospital because of marked dyspnea and focal seizures. The diagnosis of rheumatoid spondylitis had been made 20 years earlier on the basis of progressive pain and stiffness in the back and calcification of the sacroiliac joints. One year before entry, the patient suffered an episode of influenza followed by staphylococcal pneumonia. At that time, he required ventilatory assistance for 14 days. Subsequently, he required continuous oxygen therapy for dyspnea accompanying profound hypoxemia (P_{O_2}, 40 to 45 at rest), but he was able to live at home and lead an active life, even going on occasional fishing outings.

He developed progressive problems in raising secretions in spite of inhaled bronchodilator drugs, moisture, and attempts at expulsive coughing. On the morning of hospital admission, his wife noted that he had a focal seizure involving the right side of his face and his right hand.

On physical examination, the patient was seen to be a somewhat wasted, elderly-appearing man in marked respiratory distress. His blood pressure was 160/80; pulse rate 112; and respiration rate, 26. He was employing accessory muscles as well as abdominal muscles in order to breathe. Funduscopic examination revealed some blurring of the lateral margins of the optic disks as well as marked pulsations of the retinal veins. The chest was fixed, and decreased breath sounds were heard throughout; rhonchi were heard at the right base. Cardiac examination revealed an increased pulmonic component of the second sound as well as a palpable pulmonic closure. A decrescendo diastolic murmur was also heard at the base of the heart, primarily over the aortic valve. The abdomen was distended and tympanitic. The extremities were normal.

Initial laboratory tests made with the patient breathing oxygen revealed a pH of 7.21; P_{CO_2}, 117; P_{O_2}, 67; hematocrit, 52%; and white count, 21,000. A Gram stain of a tracheal aspirate revealed gram-positive cocci. The patient was transferred to the intensive care unit, and penicillin was administered. With frequent nasal tracheal suction, the P_{CO_2} dropped to 87; the P_{O_2} rose to 84; oxygen saturation to 95%; and pH to 7.42 in 2 hours. Thereafter, the patient was more alert and cooperative. A period of moisture inhalation was followed by expulsive coughing and postural drainage aided by nurses and physical therapists in the respiratory care unit. On the second hospital day he was alert; P_{CO_2} was 71 and P_{O_2}, 65. He was discharged from the intensive care unit on the third day and from the hospital on the fifth day.

Comment. This is an example of impaired thoracic excursions due to rheumatoid spondylitis with respiratory failure precipitated by pneumonia and retained secretions. The patient entered with an elevated P_{CO_2}, which can only be present with continuous oxygen therapy.[14a] In spite of the high P_{CO_2}, the patient was conscious on entry because he was adequately oxygenated. The patient had previous pulmonary function tests revealing a VC of 0.94 L (3.54); FEV_1 of 0.40 L/sec (2.65); MMF of 0.32 L/sec (3.82); and MVV of 18 L/min (118). This patient also had obstructive lung disease. Tracheostomy and ventilatory care were not needed because he could cooperate, and immediate therapy produced marked improvement.

Massive chest trauma from the increasing number of automobile accidents can also lead to ventilatory insufficiency. This form of respiratory failure is discussed in Chapter 14.

Impaired Diaphragmatic Excursion

It is unusual for impaired diaphragmatic excursions alone to cause acute respiratory failure in the absence of underlying pulmonary disease. When obesity with hypoventilation, the so-called Pickwickian syndrome, impairs both diaphragm and thoracic function, acute respiratory failure can occur in patients with otherwise normal lung function.[15,16]

Case 6. F.B., a 38-year-old housewife, was admitted to the hospital because of marked dyspnea. She had been obese for at least 15 years and also had suffered from systemic lupus erythematosus, manifested by migrating polyarthritis and transient attacks of pleurisy. "Lupus cells" had been found frequently in the peripheral blood. Her weight averaged 290 lb.

During the year before hospital admission, the patient had suffered repeated bouts of congestive heart failure; treatment consisted of salt restriction and administration of digitalis and diuretics. During the 6 months prior to admission, she had gained 50 pounds in weight; during this period she also experienced periods of somnolence at inappropriate times, such as while talking on the telephone, eating, visiting with friends, or reading a novel. Progression of the dyspnea, somnolence, and ankle edema led to hospital admission.

On examination, the patient was found to be obese, pleasant, and in moderate respiratory distress with a respiratory rate of 42 and mild cyanosis. Her pulse was 110; blood pressure 150/90. Immense obesity hampered the chest examination; her weight was 340 lbs and height, 5 ft, 4 in. Breath sounds were decreased throughout. The heart rhythm was regular, and heart tones were distant. No murmurs, gallops, or rubs could be heard. Peripheral pulses were normal; 2 + pitting edema was present.

Treatment included bed rest and the nasal administration of oxygen; the use of digitalis and diuretic drugs was continued. A 32-lb weight loss occurred. The hospital course was marked by intermittent right upper quadrant pain and fever. When cholecystitis was suspected, the patient was taken to the x-ray room for a cholecystogram. She was obliged to lie flat on the x-ray table, and a firm binder was attached to keep her from falling off. She lapsed into sleep, and the x-ray technician realized there was a sudden cessation of cardiac activity. Closed chest massage and mouth-to-mouth resuscitation revived her, and the patient was returned to the intensive care unit following endotracheal intubation. A constant volume respirator was used with a cuffed endotracheal tube for the first 48 hours, after which a tracheostomy was performed. Peak delivery pressures were 50 to 60 cm H_2O to deliver a tidal volume of 650 ml. The patient was alert, but she had breathlessness during periods of attempted weaning from the respirator. Respiratory assistance was necessary for 14 days, after which time the vital capacity measured by a Wright Respirometer* was 1.4 L, and satisfactory blood gas levels could be maintained with moist oxygen delivered to the tracheostomy opening. The tracheostomy tube was removed, but the use of nasal oxygen was continued. Uneventful recovery followed. Following an 80-lb weight loss, vital capacity increased to 2.4 L; MVV to 45 liters. Blood gas analysis (of samples taken with the patient breathing room air) revealed arterial Po_2 of 61; Pco_2 of 44; and oxygen saturation, 88%.

Comment. This case fulfills the criteria of the so-called Pickwickian syndrome. The essential problems of this abnormality are increased work of breathing, hypoventilation, hypoxemia, reactive pulmonary hypertension, and cor pulmonale.[15,16] The clinical features are obesity with associated congestive right heart failure. Whereas respiratory failure in this patient was present on hospital admission, the x-ray procedure led to further respiratory failure because the patient was required to lie quietly in a position which impairs ventilation in obese people, and the binder restricted ventilation further. Cardiopulmonary arrest was probably due to a combination of hypoxemia and acidemia.

Nonetheless, resuscitation was effected promptly, and life was maintained with an artificial ventilator for 14 days until the patient could adequately maintain ventilation and gas exchange. Thereafter, objective functional improvement accompanied by weight loss occurred.

In addition to a restrictive defect, it is now well recognized that many patients with so-called obesity-hypoventilation syndrome have obstructive apnea as a major physiologic abnormality during sleep.[15]

PRINCIPLES OF MANAGEMENT FOR RESTRICTIVE VENTILATORY DEFECTS

The various clinical problems just cited are representative of many of today's medical and surgical problems in which the underlying considerations are ventilatory restriction and impaired oxygen transport. A central theme concerning management emerges from these otherwise unrelated cases and can be crystallized into important principles to be applied to all cases of acute respiratory failure, with necessary modifications for the individual clinical situation.

---

* Harris Calorific, Cleveland, Ohio.

In all cases of acute respiratory failure cited in this chapter and others, management is directed at both supportive and definitive care. Supportive care means (1) to secure the airway, (2) to provide adequate tissue oxygenation, (3) to maintain carbon dioxide removal commensurate with metabolic production, (4) to control hydrogen ion concentration, and (5) to maintain cardiac output. The purpose of supportive care is to gain time and maintain survival until definitive efforts may correct the underlying situation. The details of supportive care vary immensely with each clinical situation, but a few generalities can be made.

A secure airway can be provided with either an endotracheal tube or a tracheostomy tube (see Chap. 2). If the need for ventilatory assistance is likely to be short, the endotracheal tube will suffice. In other cases, if tracheal secretions are a problem or if the need for ventilatory support is anticipated to be prolonged or if feeding is a consideration, a tracheostomy should be performed immediately. A tracheostomy tube is a superior means of removing secretions, and it is actually more comfortable than an endotracheal tube. Although endotracheal tubes have been left in place for many days with success, their complications seem to outweigh the advantages of avoiding a tracheostomy in some patients. This is discussed at length in Chapter 2.

In restrictive pulmonary defects, adequate oxygenation may often be provided by supplemental oxygen alone. In these states, net alveolar ventilation for CO_2 removal is usually adequate, but oxygen

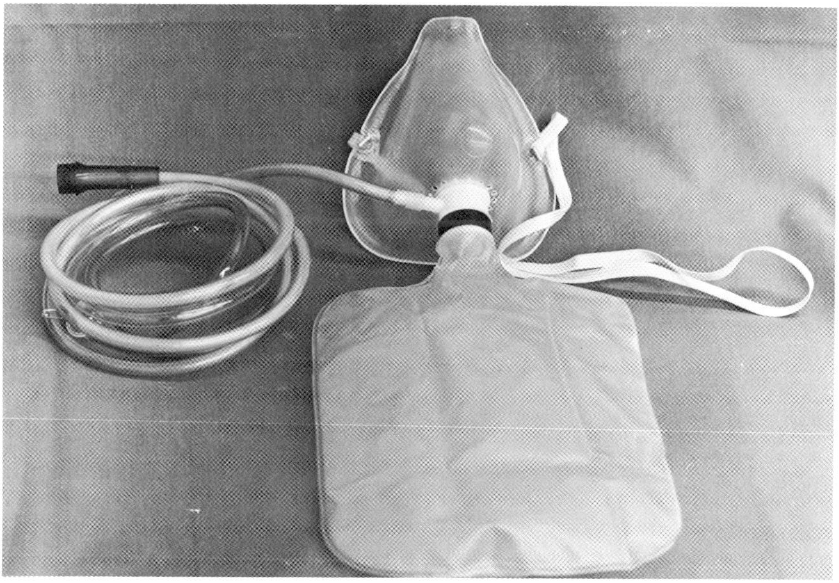

Fig. 11-10. Reservoir mask for high oxygen concentrations. F_{IO_2} of up to 0.7 is possible with well-fitting masks and high-flow oxygen delivery. Useful in states of severe oxygen transport abnormality not requiring ventilatory assistance.

transport is impaired. Reservoir masks (Fig. 11-10) providing high oxygen concentrations may be required. In traumatic states and problems of pulmonary edema, oxygen administration is usually mandatory, often provided by a mechanical ventilator in advanced states.

A variety of mechanical ventilators (see Chap. 4) are available for the respiratory support of patients with all forms of respiratory failure presented in this chapter. Application in cases of chronic airway obstruction is discussed in detail in Chapter 10.

One should not be preoccupied with controlling the carbon dioxide tension. It must be finally established that carbon dioxide elevation is harmful only after hours or days, but hypoxemia may be disastrous in minutes. Nonetheless, carbon dioxide must be adequately eliminated to prevent respiratory acidemia; this can usually be accomplished by clearing the airway and supporting ventilation, either by promoting a higher level of spontaneous ventilation or by applying mechanical assistance.

The hydrogen ion concentration must be maintained within narrow limits. Acidemia from respiratory causes with a pH of less than 7.25 is often harmful from the standpoint of arrhythmia production. Conversely, hyperventilation alkalosis is equally harmful, and pH elevations above 7.5 may cause neurologic cardiovascular complications.[16]

In acute respiratory failure with profound acidemia, intravenous use of bicarbonate will be effective in buffering the hydrogen ion concentration until definitive therapy corrects the underlying situation.[17] Bicarbonate infusion must be guided by frequent pH measurements. Tissue transport of oxygen and carbon dioxide elimination are dependent on adequate circulation. The circulatory burdens of respiratory failure themselves are profound, requiring support of circulation. A listing of details of all the therapeutic efforts in individual cases is beyond the aims of this chapter, but, in brief, effective blood volume must be restored by fluids or blood replacement, or both. Inotropic agents are used in maintaining adequate circulation.

The principles of definitive therapy directed at the underlying precipitating causes of respiratory failure are also exceedingly broad. Infection is common, requiring specific antimicrobial management, particularly for pneumonias, urinary tract infections, and sepsis. The choice of drugs must be guided by an in vitro culture and antibiotic susceptibility tests. The details of infectious disease management for pneumonia and other specific infectious diseases are handled in other chapters. The approach to care for chronic airway obstruction is discussed in Chapter 10.

Bronchial hygiene, which is so important in chronic airway obstruction, is also discussed in Chapter 10, but the techniques of care described are applicable to all situations in which secretions, mucosal edema, bronchospasm, or a combination of these factors are common.

In summary, there is a broad range of insults to the respiratory apparatus that can lead to acute respiratory failure. The major attempt in this chapter has been to develop a set of principles of management. These principles involve maintenance of the airways, support of ventilation, provision of adequate oxygen transport, control of hydrogen ion concentration, provision of adequate carbon dioxide elimination, and maintenance of circulation.

REFERENCES

1. Seyer, J.M., Hutcheson, E.T., and Kang, A.H.: Collagen polymorphism in idiopathic chronic pulmonary fibrosis. J. Clin. Invest., *57:*1498, 1976.
2. Hamman, L., and Rich, A.R.: Acute diffuse interstitial fibrosis of the lungs. Bull. Johns Hopkins Hosp., *74:*177, 1944.
3. Liebow, A.A., Steer, A., and Billingsley, J.G.: Desquamative interstitial pneumonia. Am. J. Med., *39:*369, 1965.
4. Scadding, J.G., and Hinson, K.F.W.: Diffuse fibrosing alveolitis (diffuse interstitial fibrosis of the lung): Correlation of histology at biopsy with prognosis. Thorax *22:*291, 1967.
5. Winterbauer, R.H., Hammar, S.P., Hallman, K.V., Hays, J.E., Pardee, N.E., Morgan, E.H., Allen, J.D., Moores, K.D., Bush, W., and Walker, J.H.: Diffuse interstitial pneumonitis (clinicopathologic correlations in 20 patients treated with prednisone/azathioprine). Am. J. Med., *65:*661, 1978.
6. Turner-Warwick, M., Burrows, B., and Johnson, A.: Cryptogenic fibrosing alveolitis: Clinical features and their influence on survival. Thorax, *35:*171, 1980.
7. Carrington, C.B., Gaensler, E.A., Louta, R.E., Fitzgerald, M.X., and Gupta, R.C.: Natural history and treated course of usual and desquamative interstitial pneumonia. N. Engl. J. Med., *298:*801, 1978.
8. Ellman, P., and Ball, R.E.: Rheumatoid disease with joint and pulmonary manifestations. Br. Med. J., *2:*816, 1948.
9. Ellman, P., and Cudkowitz, L.: Pulmonary manifestations of diffuse collagen diseases. Thorax, *9:*46, 1954.
10. Petty, T.L., and Wilkins, R.M.: The five manifestations of rheumatoid lung. Dis. Chest, *49:*75, 1966.
11. Matthay, R.A., Hudson, L.D., and Petty, T.L.: Acute lupus pneumonitis: Response to azathioprine therapy. Chest, *63:*117, 1973.
12. Matthay, R.A., and Petty, T.L.: Treatment of acute lupus pneumonitis with azathiaprine. Chest, *66:*219, 1974.
13. Matthay, R.A., Schwarz, M.I., Petty, T.L., Stanford, R.E., Gupta, R.C., Sahn, S.A., and Steigerwald, J.C.: Pulmonary manifestations of systemic lupus erythematosus: Review of 12 cases of acute lupus pneumonitis. Medicine, *54:*397, 1974.
14. Antoniensen, N.R., and Smith, N.J.: Respiratory acidosis as a consequence of pulmonary edema. Ann. Intern. Med., *62:*991, 1965.

14a. McNichol, M.N., and Campbell, E.S.M.: Severity of respiratory failure: arterial blood gases in untreated patients. Lancet, *1:*336, 1965.

15. Guilleminault, C., Eldridge, F.L., Tilkiana, A., Simmons, F.B., and Dement, W.C.: Sleep apnea syndrome due to upper airway obstruction. Arch. Intern. Med., *137:*296, 1977.
16. Asmundsson, T., and Kilburn, K.H.: Complications of acute respiratory failure. Ann. Intern. Med., *70:*487, 1969.
17. Lakshminarayan, S., Sahn, S.A., and Petty, T.L.: Bicarbonate therapy in severe acute respiratory acidosis. Scand. J. Resp. Dis., *54:*128, 1973.

Chapter 12

OVERWHELMING PNEUMONIAS

By Thomas L. Petty

Pneumonia, irrespective of its cause, if severe, may lead to acute respiratory failure. In mild to moderate cases, ventilation is usually adequate, but mild to moderate degrees of hypoxemia often occur. With extensive involvement or in patients with pneumonia superimposed upon underlying chronic lung disease, ventilatory failure may also ensue.

In spite of the availability of effective antimicrobial agents, bacterial pneumonia is still a common occurrence. The common pathogens, such as *Streptococcus pneumoniae, Staphylococcus aureus, Haemophilus influenzae,* and beta-hemolytic streptococci, are still encountered, as well as a growing number of gram-negative microorganisms in patients receiving broad-spectrum antimicrobial agents for a variety of problems. In addition, previously uncommon forms of pneumonia are being encountered more often as a result of medical progress in combating common diseases and the improved ability to salvage desperately ill patients. These include the so-called "transplantation" pneumonias.[1] The past five years have ushered in a "new" group of life-threatening pneumonias causing so-called "Legionnaire's disease."[2-5] Thus, the pneumonias, as a group, remain a major challenge in respiratory care.

This chapter discusses general and specific management of patients with certain forms of overwhelming pneumonia in which respiratory failure may occur.

BACTERIAL PNEUMONIAS

Pneumonia continues to rank as the seventh commonest cause of death in spite of all the medical advances of the present era. The majority of deaths continue to be from bacterial causes of pneumonia. The reasons focus on a more vulnerable host, an older patient, and perhaps changing organisms. Nonetheless, this continuing problem remains a challenge for all who care for the critically ill.

Pneumococcal Pneumonia

Lobar or more extensive forms of pneumonia caused by *Streptococcus pneumoniae* continue to be the commonest cause of bacterial pneumonia developing both outside and inside hospitals. The classic presentation of antecedent upper respiratory illness followed a few days later by chills, fever, cough, chest pain, dyspnea, and "hemoptysis" (rusty sputum) may or may not be present, depending on the host. Older patients, those addicted to alcohol, or those receiving corticosteroids for a variety of reasons may not present this usually dramatic response. Bacteremic pneumococcal pneumonia results in a 20 to 30% mortality rate in spite of modern management. Sputum cultures are confirmatory of *Streptococcus pneumoniae* in fewer than 50% of cases with positive blood cultures. The following three brief clinical examples paint the contemporary picture of pneumococcal pneumonia as we see it in the intensive care unit in the 1980s.

Case 1. J.T., a 44-year-old construction worker, was admitted directly from the emergency room to the intensive respiratory care unit because of high fever and a semistuporous state. Seven days before entry, he had developed nasal stuffiness followed by severe myalgias and dry hacking cough. He stayed at home and took salicylates without medical supervision, but 48 hours before admission suffered chills, fever, cough, and pleuritic chest pain. He still failed to avail himself of medical care, but because of headache and severe obtundation his 15-year-old daughter insisted that he "do something" and called the city emergency ambulance. He was taken directly to the emergency room, receiving oxygen en route. The patient had previously joined Alcoholics Anonymous to curb a serious drinking problem 3 months before entry.

Cursory examination revealed a flushed, febrile, disoriented patient with nuchal rigidity. Initial chest roentgenograms revealed infiltration in both lungs with a fluid density and pleural-based density on the right. White count was 2400 with 75% band forms, hemoglobin was 18 g/100 ml, BUN 32, and creatinine 1.1. A lumbar puncture revealed slightly cloudy fluid with 480 polymorphonuclear leukocytes. Sugar was 18 mg/100 ml, protein 64 mg/100 ml.

Admission Po_2 receiving oxygen at 4 L nasal flow was 62 mm, Pco_2 was 41, and pH 7.37.

Nasal oxygen was continued, and a right thoracentesis revealed turbid fluid containing large numbers of white cells and gram-positive diplococci identified on smear. Blood cultures were obtained, and the patient was immediately treated with 12 million U/day aqueous penicillin for the clinically diagnosed pneumococcal pneumonia with pneumococcal empyema and meningitis. Twenty-four hours later, all 6 blood cultures revealed pure growth of strep pneumonia. By this time the patient had become exhausted and further obtunded, and an endotracheal tube was placed. Figure 12-1 shows the extensive pneumonia, the chest tube, the endotracheal tube, and the monitoring leads. The patient then received mechanical ventilation with a MA-1 ventilator for 72 hours, and he improved slightly. Twenty-four hours later, a tracheostomy was performed because the patient was now awake and thrashing around in bed intermittently. At other times, he was cooperative. Moreover, it was considered that it would most likely be possible to feed the patient in the near future. He soon began to take a regular diet and could eat as many as

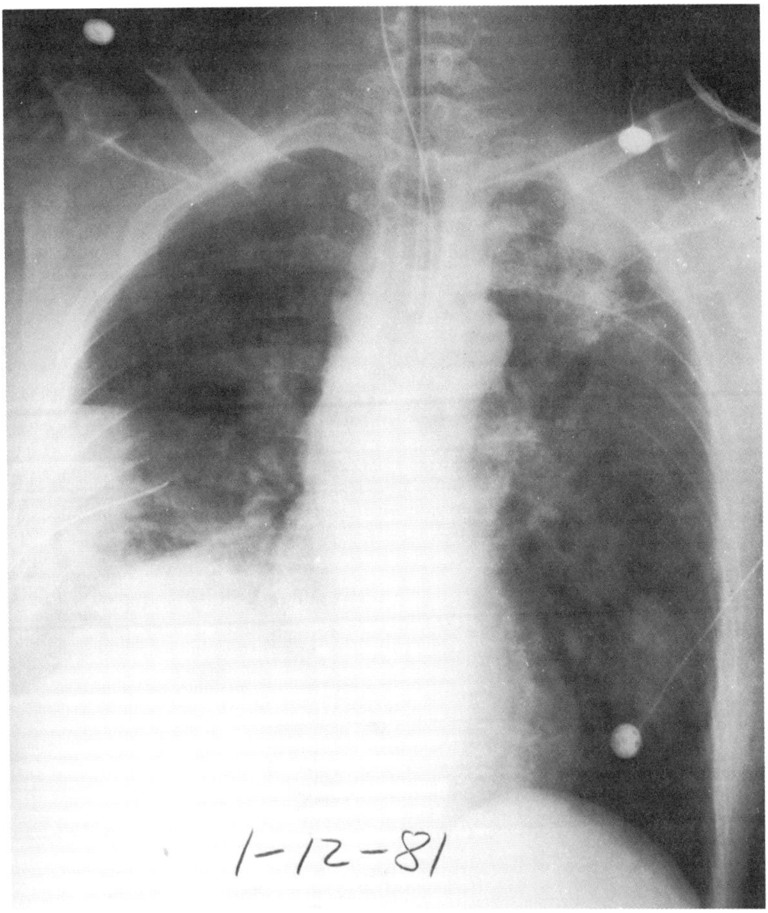

Fig. 12-1. Case 1. Film taken following admission showing extensive pneumonia, chest tube, endotracheal tube, and monitoring leads. Notice pleural-based density and evidence of large pleural effusion as well as left-sided pulmonary infiltration.

3000 calories per day for a total of 14 days as he received mechanical ventilatory assistance. He was then able to support ventilation and oxygenation without assistance. The tracheostomy was closed, and the patient left the hospital 21 days following admission. The follow-up chest roentgenogram taken 5 weeks after admission is shown in Figure 12-2.

Comment. This is a well-established example of bacteremic pneumococcal pneumonia with the complications of empyema and early meningitis. Delay in seeking medical attention most likely resulted in these life-threatening complications, since earlier institution of penicillin G therapy would probably have been immediately curative. The antecedent history of influenza during an influenza epidemic period was classic. The background of previous alcoholism

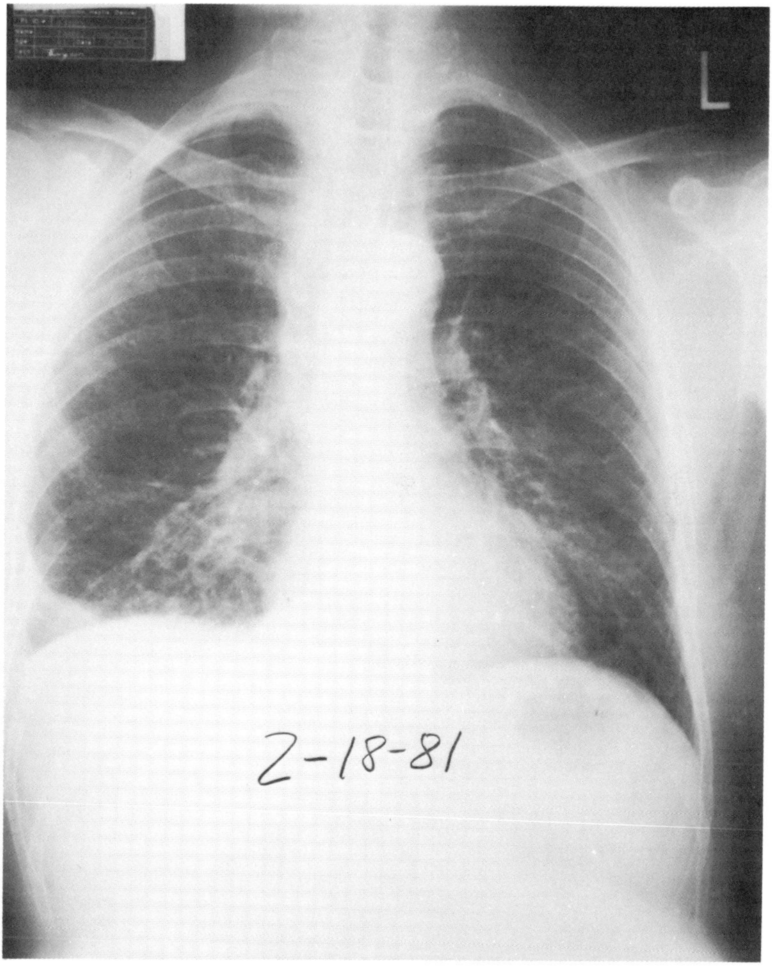

Fig. 12-2. Case 1 on recovery showing excellent resolution of effusion (empyema) and infiltrations. Only a small infiltrate at the right costophrenic angle remains.

probably still played a role in spite of the patient's abstinence from drink for the previous three months. Although the patient had many adverse prognostic factors including bacteremia and meningitis, survival was possible because of effective supportive therapy, good nutrition, and penicillin.

Case 2. W.M., a 62-year-old taxi driver, was found slumped over the wheel of his car while waiting in line at the airport. He was immediately brought to the Colorado University Hospital via ambulance, with oxygen being delivered en route. He had a past history of alcoholism and recurrent urinary tract infections. On admission he was moderately obtunded. White count was 14,000 with 82% lymphocytes, BUN 68, creatinine 2.8, and bilirubin 4 mg/100 ml. Lumbar puncture revealed no cells, normal dynamics, and normal chemistry. Thoracentesis performed because of a

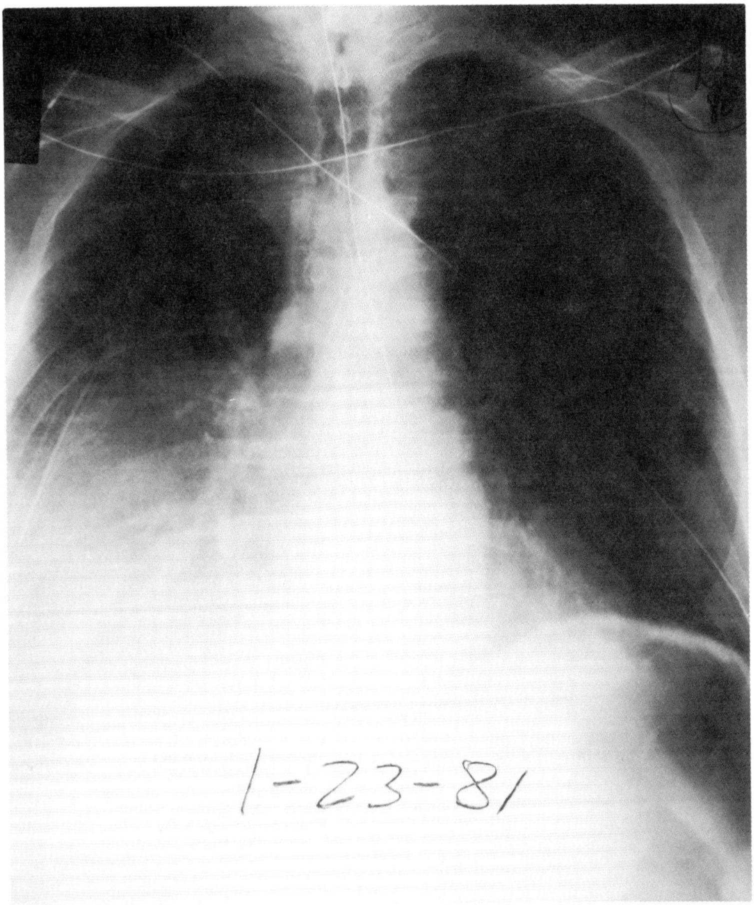

Fig. 12-3. Case 2. Admission chest roentgenogram showing massive empyema and infiltration in right lower lobe as well as chest tube placement, which was accomplished immediately on admission.

right pleural effusion revealed protein to be 3.1 g and pH 7.32, and polymorphonuclear leukocytes were sparse. Chest roentgenogram taken on the day of admission, following chest tube placement, is presented in Figure 12-3. Because of fatigue and a deteriorating blood gas pattern, endotracheal intubation and mechanical ventilation using a volume-cycled ventilator were instituted.

Two of 4 blood cultures revealed *Str. pneumoniae*. In all, the patient required 27 days of mechanical ventilation, hemodialysis on 4 occasions for progressive renal insufficiency, and treatment of delirium tremens. He gradually improved and was discharged. The chest roentgenogram taken at time of discharge is presented in Figure 12-4.

Comment. At his age and with concomitant renal failure and hepatic insufficiency, this patient's outcome was unexpected. Effec-

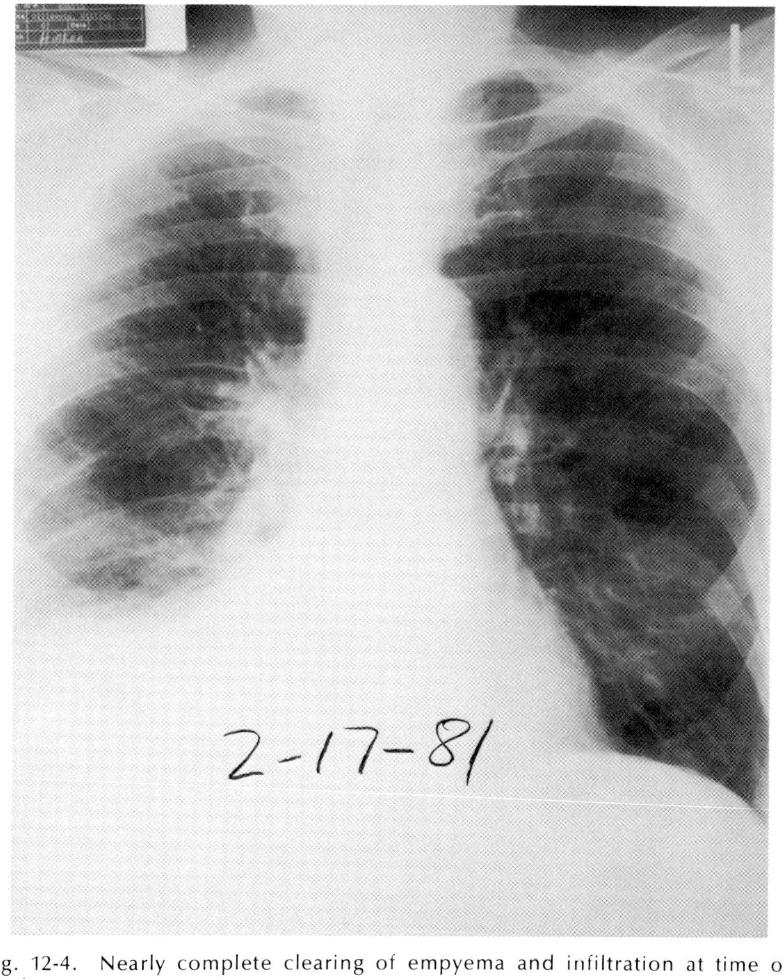

Fig. 12-4. Nearly complete clearing of empyema and infiltration at time of discharge.

tive supportive management and antibiotic management of his infection proved to be effective, however.

Case 3. W.G., a 62-year-old custodian, was brought to the hospital because of fever and anorexia. Chills were not reported. Initially, the patient was admitted to the ward service and was believed to be in good condition. Only a small patchy infiltrate was present in the right costophrenic angle on admission. He became rapidly obtunded over the next 48 hours, however, and developed a cardiorespiratory arrest. He was immediately intubated by the housestaff team and brought to the intensive care unit for mechanical ventilatory assistance. Initially, an F_{IO_2} of 1.0

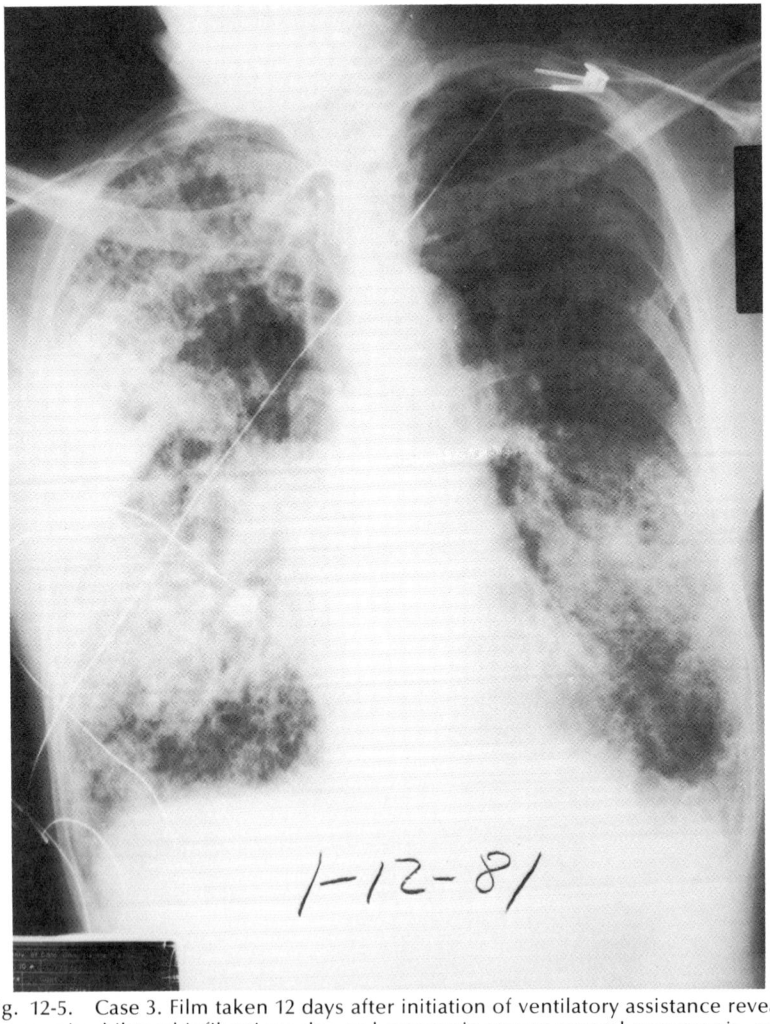

Fig. 12-5. Case 3. Film taken 12 days after initiation of ventilatory assistance revealing massive bilateral infiltrations due to bacteremic pneumococcal pneumonia, and evidence of hyperinflation due to underlying emphysema.

was required for adequate oxygenation. Blood cultures revealed *Str. pneumoniae*. After 12 days of ventilatory assistance, it was realized that long-term mechanical ventilatory assistance would be required, and a tracheostomy was done (Fig. 12-5). He required high oxygen fractions, positive end-expiratory pressure, support of the circulation with dobutamine, and transfusions with whole blood. The patient's course was complicated by a continued need for high oxygen. After 6 weeks of ventilatory assistance, a right-sided pneumothorax, a left-sided one, and finally bilateral pneumothoraces occurred, requiring bilateral chest tube placement. The patient received excellent nutritional support, first by gastric feeding with a pediatric feeding tube averaging 3000 calories and appropriate vitamin and mineral replacement daily. He was also ambulated daily with mechanical assistance and the aid of a nurse and respiratory therapist. In spite of this, the patient failed to thrive, but he also did

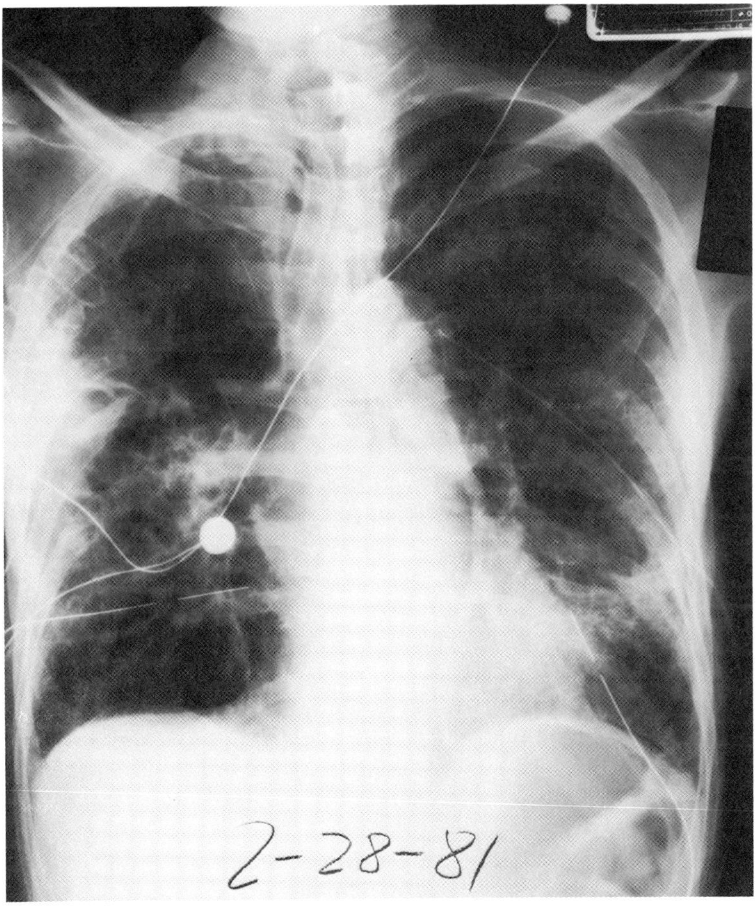

Fig. 12-6. Roentgenographic clearing after nearly two months of mechanical ventilatory support. Bilateral chest tubes in place owing to pneumothoraces. Hyperinflation still present.

not deteriorate. At no time did he lose consciousness. He remained on the ventilator, requiring an oxygen fraction of 40%, but had almost no ability to sustain his own ventilation during brief trials on the T-tube. The chest roentgenogram after nearly 2 months of mechanical ventilation showed some clearing (Fig. 12-6). He then became slightly stronger. Frequent visits from his family and "girl friend" offered encouragement. An all-out attempt to feed, ambulate, and stimulate was maintained. After 3 months, his vital capacity measured with a Wright spirometer increased to 850 ml. Weaning became progressively successful, and he was finally extubated after 3½ months of mechanical ventilation. He was discharged home 4 months following admission.

Comment. It is apparent from the dates that these 3 clinical examples are consecutive cases. (Case 3 was in fact the first of these 3 cases chronologically.) Their severity and apparent hopeless features did not, of course, predict the successful and gratifying outcome documented in this chapter. They illustrate what can be accomplished through meticulous, dedicated, supportive care and antimicrobial and nutritional therapy. The personal and emotional support provided these patients was an important factor in the final outcome. During the same winter, 11 of 12 patients with pneumococcal pneumonia requiring mechanical ventilation survived. The one who died had a total small bowel infarction.

Other Life-Threatening Bacterial Pneumonias due to Aerobic Organisms

It is well known that *Haemophilus influenzae, staphylococcus aureus,* gram-negative organisms, and rarely hemolytic streptococcal pneumonia can also cause life-threatening illnesses similar or identical to the cases just described due to pneumococci. The frequency of *Haemophilus* pneumonia in adults has recently received attention.[6] The diagnosis is most accurately and frequently made by performing a Gram stain of a transtracheal aspirate (Fig. 12-7); this should only be done for good reason and by experienced physicians. Both typable and nontypable strains are involved in acute pneumonia, which otherwise offers no distinguishing features from common pneumococcal pneumonia.

Classically, staphylococcal pneumonia follows a "flu-like illness." It is clearly more common and severe during epidemics of influenza, as are all bacterial pneumonias, particularly pneumococcal. The tendency of the lesions to cavitate is characteristic but not pathognomonic.

Pneumonias caused by gram-negative organisms, often *Klebsiella,* are of increasing importance, particularly in immunologically compromised hosts. The classic bulging fissure is rarely found and is not limited to *Klebsiellae* species.

Hemolytic streptococcal pneumonias are commonly bilateral and associated with pleural effusions and a state of profound prostration. *Pseudomonas* is a most grave etiologic agent of pneumonia and is found primarily in conditions of impaired host defenses, especially in patients with hematologic or reticuloendothelial malignant neoplasm, and is almost always fatal.[7] Other gram-negative pneumonias such as caused by bacteroides (see aspiration pneumonia), *E. coli, serratia,* and *Acinetobacter* have an unfavorable, but variable prognosis.

Legionnaire's Disease

Clearly one of the most challenging problems of infectious pneumonia focuses on a group of bacterial agents that cause an unexpected, pernicious, and often fatal pneumonia, termed Legionnaire's disease following the classic epidemic following the Ameri-

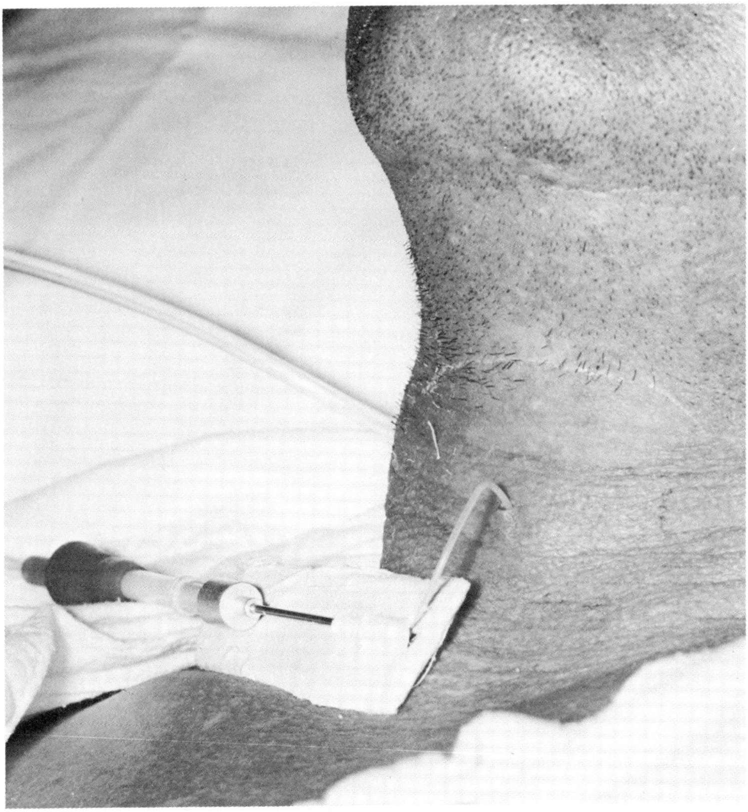

Fig. 12-7. Technique of intracath placement for transtracheal aspiration. Intracath is threaded caudally. Syringe is then used to aspirate tracheal bronchial secretions or to lavage. Immediate sputum stains and cultures should be performed. Occasional hemorrhage and subcutaneous emphysema are serious complications.

can Legion Convention in Philadelphia in 1976.[2-5] The identification of *Legionella pneumophila* as the cause of often florid pneumonia was followed by the identification of similar organisms—acronymically designated WIGA, HEBA, and OLDA—named after their discoverers or in relation to the city of occurrence of a significant outbreak, e.g., Pittsburgh.[8] These related organisms are all gram-negative bacteria that are relatively primitive, live in water or soil, and cannot be cultured using conventional media.[8] Probably the most practical diagnostic method is rapid direct staining with immunofluorescence for sputum smears.[9] Serologic titers by indirect fluorescent antibody testing is a slower and less specific diagnostic method.[3] Culture of transtracheal aspirates is possible on charcoal-yeast infusion agar.

Legionnaire's disease has a predilection for patients who are immunosuppressed owing to underlying disease or use of chemotherapeutic agents. It is common in alcoholics. Although no pathognomonic clinical features exist, Legionnaire's disease commonly occurs in the summer and often in clusters of cases, suggesting a common source of organisms. Generally, high fever is present with a disproportionately low pulse rate and with abdominal symptoms. Legionnaire's pneumonia may follow a devastating course resulting in florid respiratory failure, as the following case exemplifies.

Case 4. M.P., an 18-year-old man, was admitted to Colorado University Hospital for a cadaveric renal transplant. His chronic renal failure was related to congenital nephritis associated with hearing loss. On admission, the chest roentgenogram was normal (Fig. 12-8.). The patient had received chronic hemodialysis since age 14. Immediately following transplantation, the course was uncomplicated, and diuresis occurred over 5 days. The elevated creatinine fell to 2.8. On the sixth postoperative day, urinary output fell, and a renal scan suggested mild rejection. Prednisone was increased to 200 mg daily, and azathioprine was increased from 75 to 100 mg daily.

On the tenth postoperative day, the creatinine had reached 8.2. Hemodialysis was resumed. Prednisone was reduced to 150 mg daily, and azathioprine to 75 mg daily. Renal scan revealed severe rejection. A 1-g bolus of methylprednisolone sodium succinate was given for 3 days with no improvement in renal function.

On the thirteenth postoperative day, the patient complained of weakness and passed a 500-ml melanotic stool. Hematocrit was 10%. An endoscopy suggested an ulcer in the duodenal bulb. After 6 units of blood replacement, the patient began to bleed and underwent a successful vagotomy and pyloroplasty.

On the sixteenth postoperative day, the patient was ambulating but developed an elevated temperature of 38.2°C. The surgical wound looked clean. Prednisone was tapered rapidly to 15 mg daily. Azathioprine was discontinued. White count was 1500 with 80% polymorphonuclear leukocytes.

On the next day, hectic fever developed, and azathioprine was discontinued. Hemoptysis occurred later in the day. Arterial blood gas determinations were Po_2, 39; Pco_2, 29; and pH, 7.5 on air.

A chest roentgenogram was obtained and is shown in Figure 12-9. Ampicillin and tobramycin administration was begun. The patient began to produce frothy brick-red secretions and rapidly deteriorated. Intubation and mechanical ventilation, F_{IO_2} of 1.0 and various levels of PEEP could maintain the Po_2 no higher than 41. Chest roentgenograms showed rapid worsening (Fig. 12-10). Erythromycin was added because of the possibility of existence of *Legionella*. The patient expired 15 hours after institution of mechanical ventilation with deteriorating blood gases and intractable hypoxemia.

Cultures of sputum were positive for *Legionella pneumophila*, and fluorescent antibody staining of tissue was confirmatory of *Legionella*.

Comment. This was an amazingly florid progression of *Legionella* pneumonia. The cause was suspected and erythromycin given in full

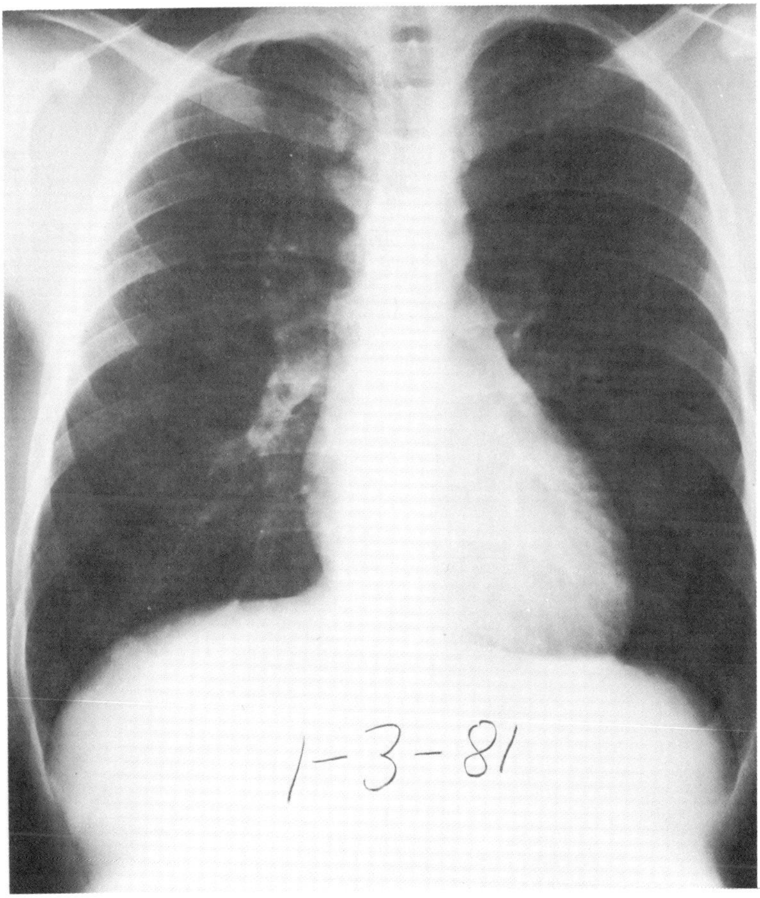

Fig. 12-8. Admission film from Case 4 showing normal lung fields and moderate cardiomegaly due to long-standing hypertension.

dose, but overwhelming pneumonia continued. Very likely, the necessary use of immunosuppressive agents had a bearing on this devastating process.

MYCOPLASMA PNEUMONIA

Mycoplasma pneumoniae is the most common etiologic agent in young adults with pneumonia. It occasionally causes a massive pulmonary involvement and may be life-threatening in isolated instances.[11–13] In fact, mycoplasma may cause overwhelming pneumonia in elderly persons, as illustrated in Case 1, Chapter 17, in which evidence of mycoplasma causing life-threatening pneumonia was found in an 84-year-old woman. There are no absolutely

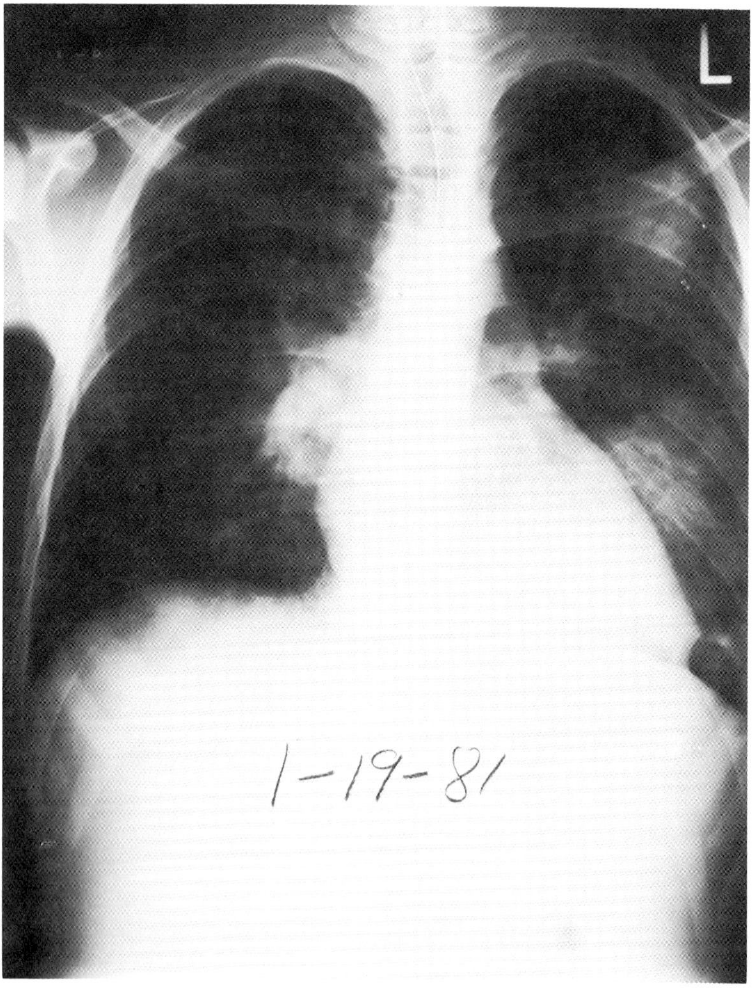

Fig. 12-9. Patchy infiltrates at onset of pneumonia with hectic fever and hemoptysis.

distinctive features of *Mycoplasma* pneumonia except its epidemiology.[13] Pulmonary infiltrates are patchy and often bilateral. Pleural effusion is not common, but may be massive.[11] Cold agglutinin titers elevate upon recovery but are not specific. The organism cannot be readily cultured, and final confirmation rests with the identification of specific elevated serologic titers for *Mycoplasma*. The course is altered with erythromycin and tetracycline. Therapy is otherwise supportive.

SPORADIC INFECTIOUS PNEUMONIAS OF UNCOMMON CAUSES

Life-threatening pneumonia can be caused by a variety of unrelated infectious bacterial or rickettsial agents including

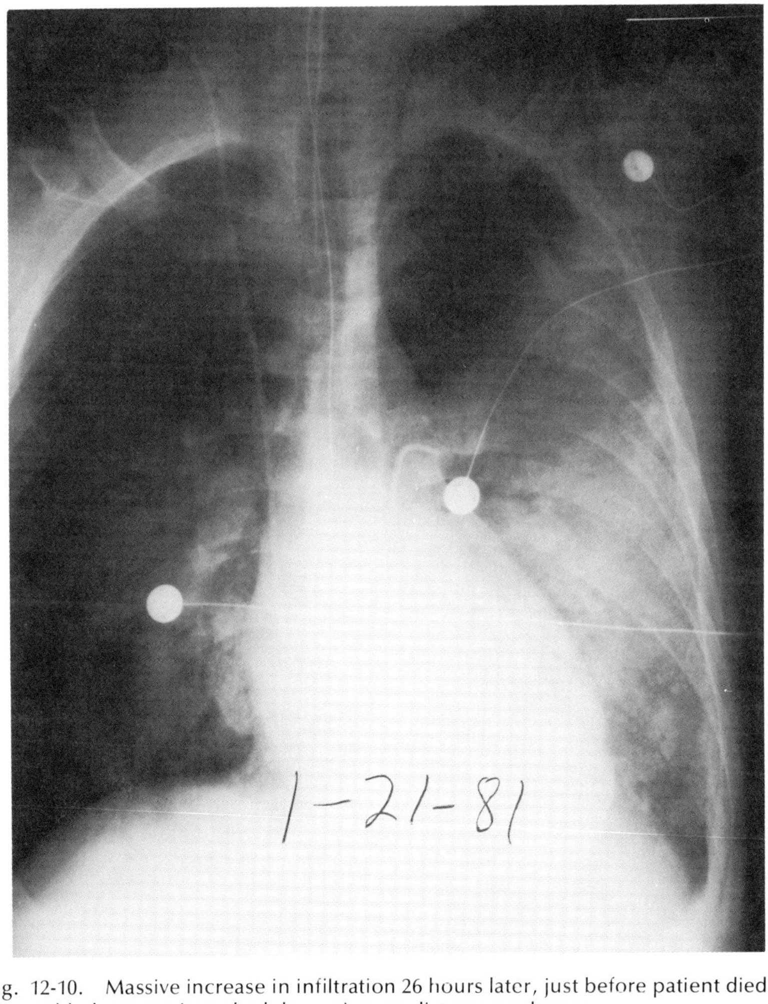

Fig. 12-10. Massive increase in infiltration 26 hours later, just before patient died of intractable hypoxemia and adult respiratory distress syndrome.

tularemia, plague, psitticosis, Q fever, and Rocky Mountain spotted fever. Distinctive features may or may not be present. A pragmatic approach to management is needed before the true cause is known (see "Supportive Management"). Since tetracycline is effective against all these organisms, its prompt use in full doses, e.g., 2.0 g/day, is appropriate. Tetracycline is not the drug of choice in tularemia or in plague, where streptomycin or gentamycin is more effective, but it does modify the cause and may be lifesaving.[14] Since tetracycline is also effective against *Mycoplasma* pneumonias and has shown at least *some* effectiveness against *Legionella,* it is not a bad choice for any undiagnosed pneumonia in which common aerobic organisms such as *Pneumococcus, Staphylococcus, Klebsiellae,* or other aerobic gram-negative rods are not identified in sputum smears (see later). Tetracycline is also a reasonable choice for anaerobic pneumonias often associated with aspiration (see later).

ASPIRATION PNEUMONIAS

Pneumonia following aspiration of gastrointestinal contents is common in hospitals. Pneumonia is caused by both the effects of gastric acid and aspirated organisms. High gastric acidity, however, kills or inhibits most bacteria; thus, most pneumonia caused by pure stomach secretions is sterile and self-limiting. Numerous mouth organisms can cause pneumonia, lung abscess, or empyema. Most of these infectious agents are anaerobic *Streptococcus* and *Bacteroides* species.[15,16]

VIRAL PNEUMONIAS

A variety of viral agents can cause massive pneumonia with acute respiratory failure, most commonly "A" influenzae species, adenovirus type 7, and varicella organisms.[17–19] No specific therapy is available for any of these viral agents, but the early use of amantadine may modify the course of influenza A pneumonia.

Case 5. W.M., a 52-year-old farmer from eastern Colorado, was apparently in excellent health until one day before admission to a local hospital, when he developed a sore throat associated with lethargy and malaise and severe myalgias. He began coughing with production of thick brown sputum. At this time he had severe headache. He was treated with tetracycline and an expectorant with no benefit. The patient was told that he had a "bad case" of influenza, which was common in his community at that time. Three days later he became nauseated and developed dyspnea. Administration of tetracycline was discontinued, and a cephalosporin was begun. Because of production of hemorrhagic sputum, the development of cyanosis, and fever between 102° and 104°F, the patient was transferred to University Hospital. Just before transfer, the patient's sensorium became clouded.

The patient had no past history of illness or disease. Industrial exposure and excessive alcohol intake was denied. He had not smoked a significant number of cigarettes.

On physical examination the temperature was 104°F; the respiration rate was 30; the pulse was regular with a rate of 80; the blood pressure was 100/70. The pharynx was markedly injected. There were diffuse crackling rales throughout both lung fields. Rhonchi and wheezes were not heard. No murmurs were heard, and no signs of congestive heart failure were found. The extremities were normal.

Chest roentgenogram (Fig. 12-11*A*) revealed massive infiltrates occupying both lower lung fields, most marked on the right. The cardiac silhouette was normal. With the patient receiving 5 L nasal oxygen, the P_{O_2} was 44 mm; P_{CO_2}, 41 mm; and pH, 7.41. Hematocrit value was 53%, and white blood count, 33,500; the differential count showed 17% segmented and 4% unsegmented polymorphonuclear leukocytes and 79% lymphocytes. Urea blood nitrogen was 36 mg/100 ml; creatinine, 1.8 mg/100 ml; electrolyte values were within the normal range; urinalysis showed no abnormality except for a trace of protein. With oxygen flows of 10 L, the oxygen tension increased only to 28 mm, attesting to severe problems with oxygen transport. Because of this, a tracheostomy was performed, and the patient was given inspired oxygen fractions of 0.7 with a constant volume respirator. This provided an oxygen tension of only 55 mm (Table 12-1). The chest roentgenogram demonstrated worsening alveolar infiltration (Fig. 12-11*B*). Later in the hospital course, on the second hospital day, 100% oxygen provided an arterial tension of only 37 mm. With positive end-expiratory pressures (PEEP), the arterial oxygen tension rose to 45; on the next day it fell to 34, and the patient developed shock and died.

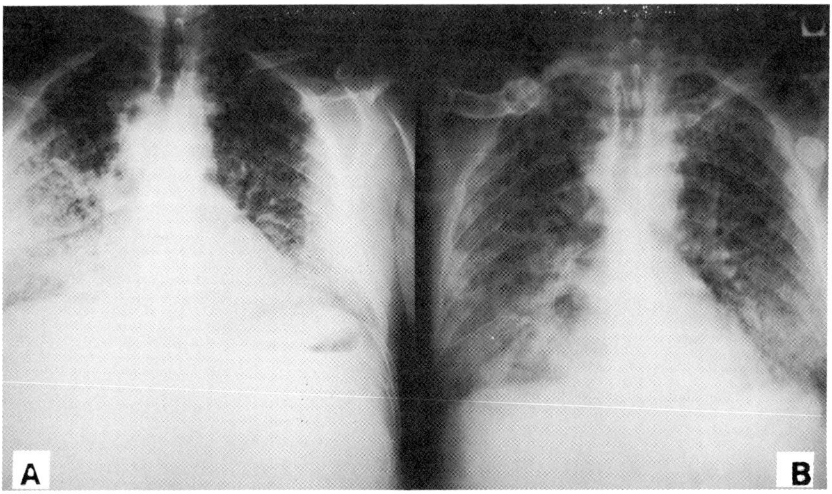

Fig. 12-11. *A*, Case 5 admission film above showing diffuse lower lobe infiltrates. *B*, film one day later after patient is receiving ventilatory assistance. Worsening alveolar infiltrates are noted resulting from A influenza. Patient died.

TABLE 12-1. Effect of Supportive Measures on Blood Gases in Influenza Pneumonia

Hospital Stay	*Admission*	*1 hr*	*2 hr*	*2 day*	*3 day*
Oxygen (liter flow or % by ventilator)	5 L	10 L	70%	100%	100%*
P_{O_2}	24	28	55	37	45
P_{CO_2}	41	43	42	39	38
pH	7.41	7.40	7.42	7.48	7.34

* By PEEP (see Chaps. 4, 5 and 8).

At postmortem examination, the lungs weighed 2570 g; massive amounts of hemorrhagic fluid could be expressed. No pulmonary emboli were found. Cardiac lesions were absent. Cultures and serologic studies done in the virus laboratory were positive for Asian A-2 influenza virus. Examination of the bone marrow and lymph nodes revealed no evidence of leukemia. The massive lymphocytosis was apparently a response to overwhelming viral illness.

Comment. At times, influenzal pneumonia is complicated by bacterial invasion, but overwhelming pneumonia resulting from influenza virus itself can occasionally cause death in previously healthy people, as was demonstrated in this case.[17] Other fatal viral pneumonias are occasionally caused by Adenovirus, Herpesvirus, and cytomegalovirus infections, most commonly in immunosuppressed hosts in the latter two instances.

BACTERIOLOGIC DIAGNOSIS OF PNEUMONIA

A specific bacteriologic diagnosis guides antimicrobial therapy. Material is available for smear and culture tests from expectorated sputum, transtracheal aspiration, or direct aspiration of the pneumonic lung. All are useful in diagnosis in given instances. Sputum study is most readily available, and a careful study of a stained sputum smear will reveal the most likely cause if a good specimen is obtained containing numerous polymorphonuclear leukocytes, and if a predominant organism is found—e.g., gram-positive diplococci (*Pneumococcus*), gram-positive cultures (*Staphylococcus*), pleomorphic small gram-negative rods (*Haemophilus*), or gram-negative rods (*Klebsiella* spp., *Pseudomonas, Seratia, Acinetobacter, Proteus*). Gram-negative aerobic organisms such as *Klebsiella* and *Pseudomonas* are readily cultured from expectorated sputum, as is *Staphylococcus aureus.* Failure to grow these organisms essentially rules them out as the cause of pneumonia. This is not true with *Pneumococcus, Legionella,* or *Mycoplasma,* as mentioned previously.

If no predominant organism is found on initial smear, therapy should be based on epidemiologic considerations, e.g., *Pneumococ-*

cus (most common), *Staphylococcus* (possible and important not to miss), gram-negative pneumonia (devastating in the poorly defended host) or *Legionella, Mycoplasma,* or sporadic uncommon pneumonias. It therefore becomes rational to use a combination of a semisynthetic penicillin for *Pneumococcus* and *Staphylococcus* and an aminoglycoside for suspected gram-negative aerobic organisms. The problem is that this approach will not be effective against *H. influenzae,* some anaerobes, *Mycoplasma,* Legionnaire's disease, or the sporadic pneumonias. Thus, erythromycin is attractive as a good drug for the suspicion of Legionnaire's disease, *H. influenzae,* or *Mycoplasma.* Tetracycline is also reasonable for these considerations as well as the so-called "sporadic" pneumonias.

It should be considered that direct lung aspiration is the most direct approach to an otherwise undiagnosed pneumonia and is most likely to yield a definitive isolation of the offending organism, compared with studies of expectorated sputum or even material obtained by transtracheal aspiration.[20]

Sudden overwhelming bacterial pneumonia may occasionally occur in patients who were previously healthy. Moreover, at times the etiologic agent is in doubt, and initially aggressive efforts must be made to provide chemotherapy for a wide spectrum of bacteria until specific in vitro culture indicates the etiologic basis of the pneumonia. This approach must be aggressive, often empiric, and at times directed at organisms that are not commonly expected to cause pneumonia. The following case illustrates this point.

Case 6. C.H., a 55-year-old Spanish-American farmer, was admitted to the hospital because of fever and dyspnea of 5 days' duration. In addition he had chills, fever, anorexia, and a cough productive of tenacious sputum, as well as chest pain during the 48 hours prior to admission. The illness began with a sore throat and malaise. A history of heavy smoking was also given.

On physical examination the patient's temperature was 39°C; his blood pressure was 120/80; and respiratory rate was 20. The patient appeared to be acutely ill. Chest examination revealed coarse rhonchi throughout the base posteriorly. A friction rub was heard during inspiration along the anterior axillary line on the left. Precordial activity was normal; and no murmurs, gallops, or extra sounds were heard.

Chest roentgenogram revealed massive infiltration involving all lung fields, with air bronchograms (Fig. 12-12*A*).

The sputum contained gram-positive diplococci and numerous gram-negative rods as well as many polymorphonuclear leukocytes. No acid-fast bacilli were found. The white cell count was only 5500 with 16% polymorphonuclear leukocytes, 74 unsegmented neutrophils, and 10 lymphocytes; the hematocrit value was 39%. A lumbar puncture revealed no abnormalities.

Initial blood gas tests made while the patient was breathing room air showed Po_2 of 41.5 mm; with 3 L oxygen delivered via nasal cannula the oxygen tension only increased to 50. The Pco_2 was 32. Oxygen delivered via nasal cannula at 6 L elevated the oxygen tension to 63 and the P_{CO_2} to 36. Later, however, higher flows of oxygen (9 L) produced an oxygen tension of only 48.

Initial chemotherapy was designed to cover the major susceptible potential bacterial pathogens. This included the administration of 10 million U intravenous penicillin G given by continuous infusion (for pneumococci, streptococci, and some strains of *H. influenzae*), 8 g methicillin per day in 2 doses, given by rapid intravenous infusion (for penicillinase-producing staphylococci), and 80 mg gentamycin every 8 hours given intramuscularly. Isonicotinic acid and hydrazide (300 mg) and ethambutol (1200 mg) were also given daily because of the possibility of existence of tuberculous pneumonia; these 2 drugs were discontinued after all initial cultures for tuberculosis were negative (see "Comment").

Because of refractory hypoxemia, oxygen was administered by ventilator at F_{IO_2} of 0.7. This increased the oxygen tension to 59 and later to 67. Two days later, when attempts were made to reduce the oxygen fraction to 40%, the arterial tension was only 36. After one more day, however, inspired oxygen fractions of 50% provided an arterial tension of 99 and a P_{CO_2} of 35; later an oxygen fraction of 40% produced an oxygen tension of 83 and a P_{CO_2} of 42.

Blood cultures and sputum cultures finally grew numerous colonies of *Streptococcus pneumoniae* on 4 occasions, establishing the cause of the massive pneumonia. When this became known, the use of all antimicrobial agents except penicillin was discontinued.

Two weeks later, while the patient was breathing room air, oxygen tension was 61; P_{CO_2}, 31; and pH, 7.49. A subsequent roentgenogram taken some 5 months after hospital admission still showed some residual pulmonary infiltration, but the patient was clinically well (Fig. 12-12*B*).

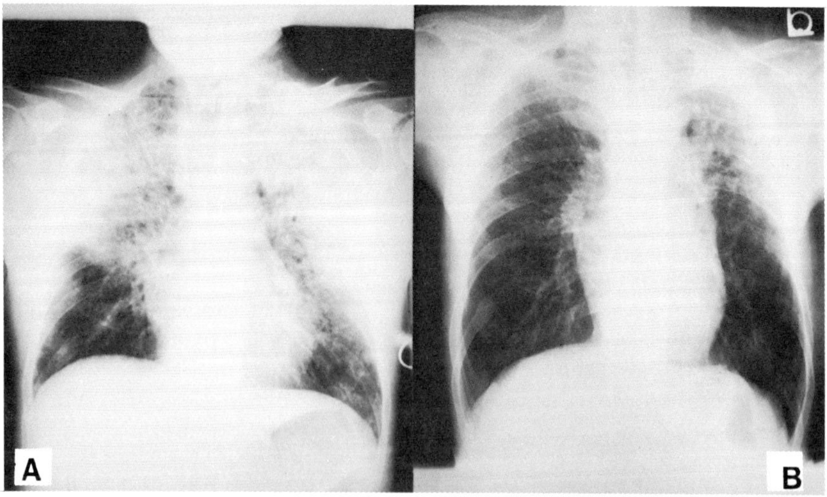

Fig. 12-12. Case 6. Admission film, *A*, shows massive upper lobe infiltrates. Incomplete clearing seen five months later (*B*).

Comment. This was an example of overwhelming pneumonia due to a common organism, *Streptococcus pneumoniae.* Penicillin is the drug of choice and should be given in high dosage in patients with bacteremia. In view of the life-threatening nature of the illness, since the attending physician could not wait for specific cultures, the use of antimicrobial agents directed at additional possibilities was wise. As soon as the etiologic agent became known, chemotherapy could then be more specific.

Interesting is the fact that because of persistent apical infiltrations, repeated cultures for tuberculosis were obtained in the follow-up period. Eight months after the acute bacterial pneumonia, sputum cultures became positive for *M. tuberculosis* for the first time. Organisms were fully sensitive in vitro to INH and ethambutol. These two drugs were instituted along with daily streptomycin for the first three months. The two oral drugs were then continued for a total of two years. Sputum conversion occurred in the third month, and all examinations thereafter failed to grow *M. tuberculosis.* It is likely that the acute bacterial pneumonia activated a quiescent apical focus of tuberculosis in this case.

The development and use of inhalation therapy devices has been an advance in medicine. Nonetheless, these devices may be the source of serious life-threatening nosocomial infection if they are not properly decontaminated.[21,22] An illustrative case follows.

Case 7. B.M., an 18-year-old male college student, was admitted to a hospital because of mild exacerbation of bronchial asthma, first diagnosed 6 months before. He had beeen receiving ephedrine by mouth, and he had had one short course of corticosteroids. Roentgenogram showed a normal chest. He had not been having chills, fever, cough, or expectoration.

In the hospital, IPPB was ordered for 10 minutes, 4 times daily. On the third hospital day, he had an episode of acute chills, fever, cough, purulent expectoration, and hemoptysis. He was given tetracycline. Chest roentgenogram revealed patchy infiltrates in the left upper lung and a thin-walled cavity in the left mid-field of the lung (Fig. 12-13). The patient's condition deteriorated over the next 24 hours, and he was transferred to Colorado General Hospital. On admission, he was desperately ill, evidenced by high fever and prostration. His temperature was 105°F; blood pressure, 80/50; pulse rate 120; and respiration rate, 40. His mucous membranes were injected and dry; the conjunctivae were injected. The left hemithorax was splinted, and loud crackling rales were heard over the left side of the chest. The white cell count was 21,800; some immature leukocytes were present in the smear. Sputum smear demonstrated numerous gram-negative rods and a few gram-positive cocci.

The chest roentgenogram at this time (Fig. 12-14) showed massive infiltration in the left lung with a 4-cm cavity. Arterial blood gas determinations while the patient was receiving nasal oxygen at 2 L/min revealed Po_2 of 55 (normal, 65 to 70); Pco_2, 39; and pH, 7.46.

The diagnosis of necrotizing pneumonia and lung abscess was made. Methicillin (9 g), penicillin (20 million U), and chloramphenicol (4 g) were given daily. On the second hospital day, sputum culture revealed 2 strains of *Pseudomonas aeruginosa,* both of which were susceptible in vitro to colistin and partially susceptible to chloramphenicol, but resistant to other antibiotics. A single colony of *Staphylococcus aureus*—coagulase- and mannitol-positive, resistant to penicillin G, and sensitive to methicillin—was found. Injections of 140 mg colistin intramuscularly were then given every 12 hours along with methicillin; penicillin and chloramphenicol were discontinued. Within 48 hours, marked reduction in fever and tachycardia was observed, and the blood pressure returned to normal. Repeat arterial determinations with the patient breathing room air revealed P_{O_2} of 80; P_{CO_2} of 32; and pH of 7.48, demonstrating normal oxygen transport and mild hyperventilation. The patient then made a

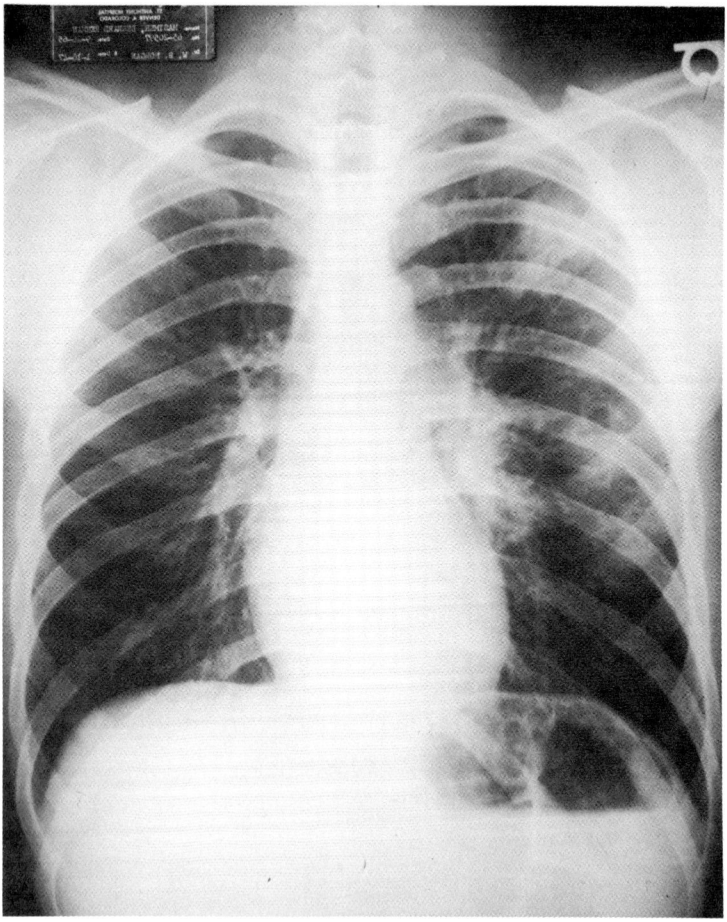

Fig. 12-13. Case 7. X-ray film of chest taken prior to transfer of patient to University Hospital. Patient had chills, fever, and purulent sputum. Note patchy infiltration and the cavity in the left middle lung field. (Reproduced with permission from Med. Clin. North Am., *51*:529, 1967.)

gradual recovery over the next 28 days. Methicillin therapy was continued for a total of 28 days, and colistin for 15 days. Subsequent roentgenograms demonstrated marked clearing; a postinfection thin-walled cyst was the final result over the ensuing 12 months (Fig. 12-15). This case is included to serve as an example of the rare but devastating nature of nosocomial pneumonia that occurred in the past owing to the improper use of respiratory care equipment.

Comment. After careful investigation, it was learned that this patient had received IPPB treatments with a heated mainstream nebulizer that had been passed from patient to patient without sterilization. Since the patient had entered the first hospital with no evidence of pneumonia and in a state of general good health, the nebulizer of the IPPB device was implicated as the most likely source of the necrotizing pneumonia.[21]

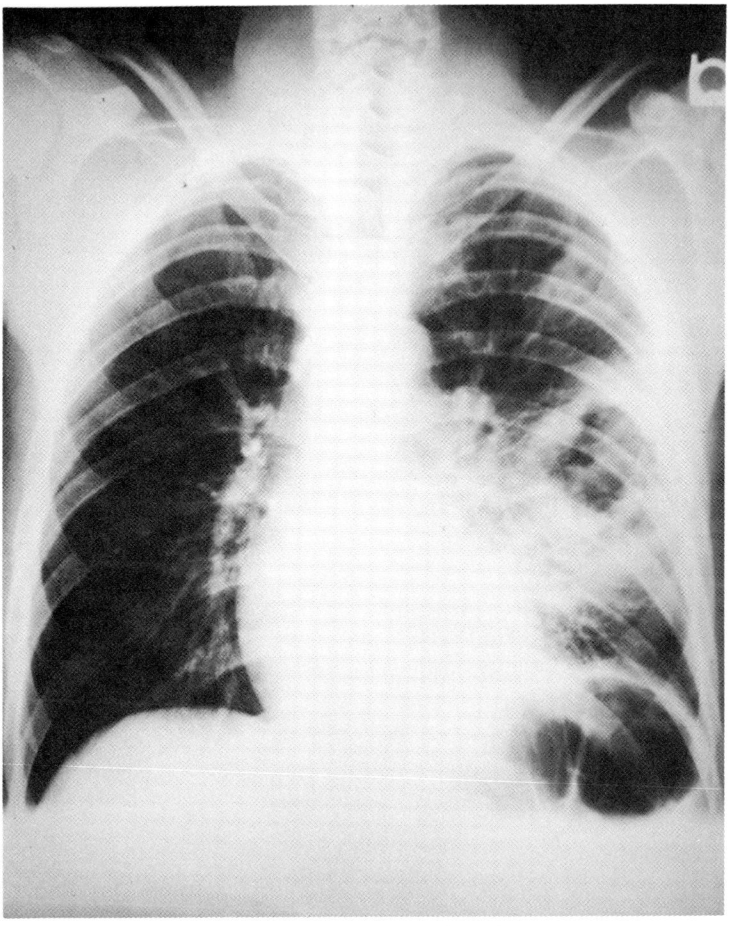

Fig. 12-14. Roentgenogram taken following transfer of patient B.M. to University Hospital. The massive cavity is seen in the left mid-lung field. (Reproduced with permission from Med. Clin. North Am., *51*:529, 1967.)

PNEUMONIAS ASSOCIATED WITH LEUKEMIA

In states of altered immune status due to an underlying disease such as leukemia or lymphoma, or in altered host response due to drugs, previously unusual pneumonia such as that due to *Pneumocystis carinii* may occur and present life-threatening problems.[24,25] The following case illustrates this point.

Case 8. D.W., an 18-year-old female, had acute myelogenous leukemia, diagnosed 8 months before her current hospital admission following a short history of fatigue, back pain, myalgia, and fever. Initially she was given 60 mg prednisone daily, 60 mg mercaptopurine, amethopterin, and vincristine which brought about a hematologic remission. Beginning 2 months later, she was treated with cytosine arabinoside (a potent antimetabolite) administered intramuscularly. Six months later, hematologic relapse occurred, and the frequency and dose of cytosine arabinoside as well as of prednisone were increased. At this time, her

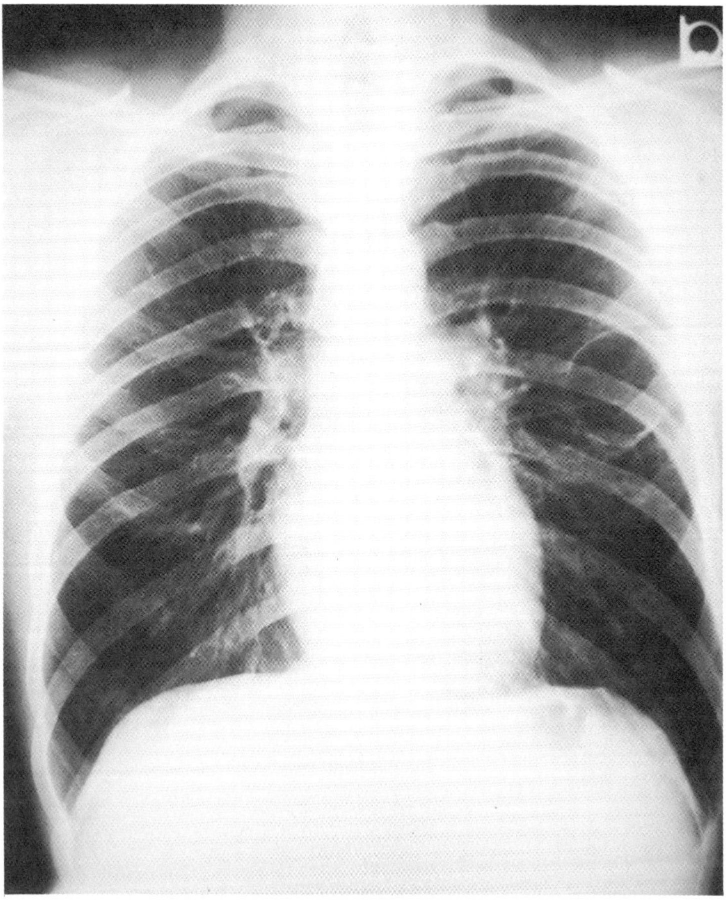

Fig. 12-15. Case 7. Twelve months after recovery. Postinflammatory cysts in the left mid-lung field remain. (Reproduced with permission from Med. Clin. North Am., *51*:529, 1967.) This patient remains well 14 years later.

white count was 1700 with 98% blast forms. Following this, her bone marrow revealed serous atrophy without any organized hematopoietic tissue. Her white count increased from 1400 to 38,000, and she was treated with vincristine and prednisone. The white cell count then dropped to 1400. She received whole blood transfusions for anemia, the hemoglobin determinations averaging 8 g/100 ml.

Five days before she was admitted to the hospital, the patient developed a chill and fever of 101°F. Her white cell count obtained in a physician's office was 350 cells. The patient was admitted to another hospital and was treated with kanamycin twice daily with no improvement. She was then transferred to Colorado General Hospital. Physical examination revealed an oriented, cooperative, but depressed individual who had a fever of 104°F. Her respiration rate was 32; blood pressure, 100/70. No skin lesions were present. Chest examination revealed decreased breath sounds and no rhonchi. Cardiac rhythm was normal, and no extra sounds were heard. No edema was present. Chest roentgenogram (Fig. 12-16*A*) revealed diffuse alveolar infiltrations. Arterial determinations made while the patient was breathing room air revealed Po_2 of 46, Pco_2 of 32, saturation of 85%, and pH of 7.5.

The hectic febrile course continued; on the third hospital day a lung trephine biopsy was performed. Sections of this showed the presence of typical *Pneumocystis carinii*.[25] The patient was given 160 mg pentamidine intramuscularly each day. Beginning on the fifth hospital day, there was defervescence. The patient's temperature was reduced to normal after 10 days of treatment. The patient received pentamidine for 13 days. During this course of treatment marked improvement in the chest condition took place, as shown by roentgenogram (Fig. 12-16*B*), and there was excellent physiologic improvement, the Po_2 being 66 with the patient breathing air; Pco_2, 36; and pH, 7.48.

Comment. The use of immunosuppressive drugs in acute leukemias as well as after transplantation surgery has led to a marked increase in the incidence of unusual pneumonias of a life-threatening nature. When the diagnosis is suspected or proved, antimicrobial agents may bring prompt clinical resolution and may save life.

The advent of a new biopsy or bronchial brushing techniques via fiberoptic bronchoscopy to confirm diagnoses such as this is an important advance in our ability to isolate the etiologic agent in troublesome pneumonias.[26] The advent of use of trimethoprim sulfa has offered a potent oral agent for the effective control of pneumocystis, and today this preparation is considered the drug of choice.[27] This well-tolerated preparation is being used more and more on an empiric basis when pneumocystis is suspected, but not proved. This practice will most likely be lifesaving in many patients.[27]

FUNGAL PNEUMONIAS

A variety of fungi cause pneumonia, usually in compromised hosts. *Candida* pneumonia is particularly perplexing.[28] *Nocardia asteroides* is not a fungus but is rather a true bacterium. *Nocardia* is a genus of the aerobic Actinomycetaceae bacteria but historically has often been lumped together with the fungi.[29] It is an important pathogen because it is readily treated with sulfadiazine or trimethoprim sulfa.[29]

The new oral antifungal agent, ketoconazole (Nizoral), may well change the picture regarding fungal pneumonias; this effective drug is now commercially available.[30]

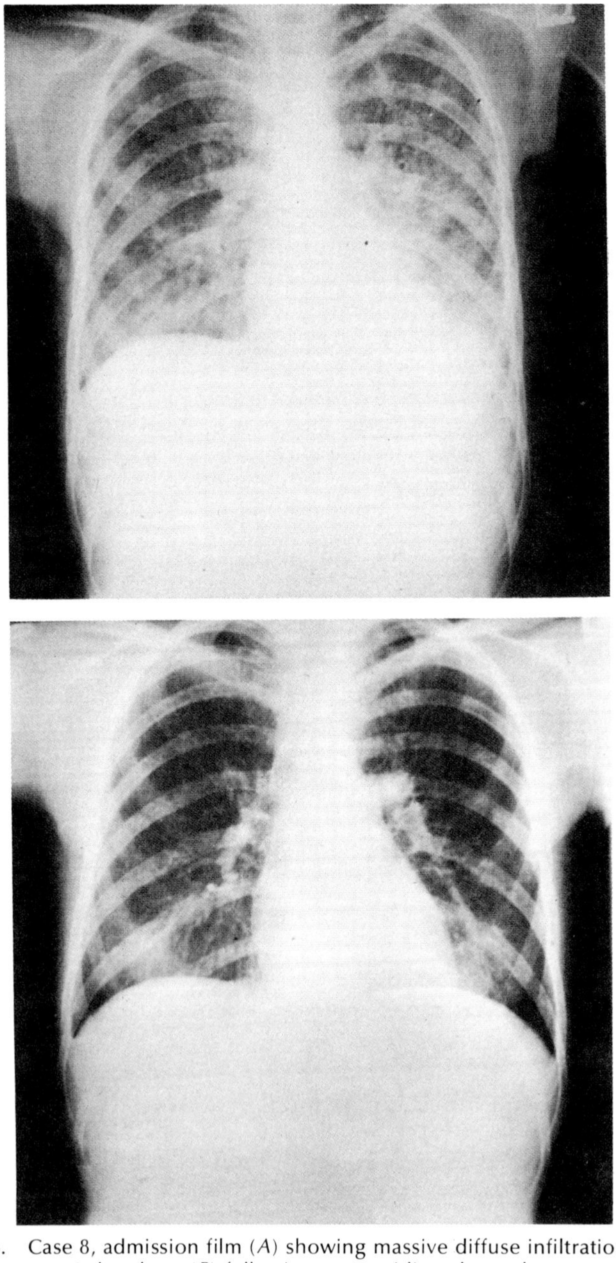

Fig. 12-16. Case 8, admission film (*A*) showing massive diffuse infiltration. Marked clearing is seen 13 days later (*B*) following pentamidine chemotherapy.

PROTOZOAN INFECTIONS

Pneumocystis carinii is the only common protozoan known to cause pneumonia. A case example was presented previously. Rarely, *Trichomonas* and *Giardia* have also been implicated.

HYPERSENSITIVITY AND OTHER NONINFECTIOUS PNEUMONIAS

A variety of drugs can cause acute pulmonary reactions. The classic example is nitrofurantoin.[31] Numerous additional drugs can cause both acute and chronic pulmonary reactions which can contribute to or directly result in respiratory insufficiency.[32] Hypersensitivity reactions and other noninfectious acute infiltrative pulmonary reactions are additional considerations.[33,34]

SUPPORTIVE CARE

Principles of management of overwhelming pneumonias include supportive measures with controlled oxygen therapy, chest physiotherapy (see Chap. 7), upper airway suctioning, and, in certain cases, the judicious application of ventilators to maintain ventilation and oxygen transport (see Chap. 4). Supportive measures gain time, while specific therapeutic measures are directed at the underlying etiologic agent by means of appropriate application of potent antimicrobial agents. This requires identification of the offending agent or the use of broad coverage directed against the most likely to be treatable pathogens. Tracheostomy care, suctioning, and applications of oxygen systems and ventilators useful in the management of pneumonia have been discussed in earlier chapters. During the care of patients with any form of infectious disease, but particularly during intensive respiratory care for the overwhelming pneumonias described in this chapter, the careful practice of appropriate handwashing is mandatory. This regular procedure alone will do more to prevent the spread of pneumonia throughout an intensive care unit than any other single technique.[35]

REFERENCES

1. Rifkind, D., Starzl, T.E., Marchioro, T.L., Waddell, W.R., Rowlands, D.T., and Hill, R.B., Jr.: Transplantation pneumonia. JAMA, *189:*808, 1964.
2. Lattimer, G.L., and Rhodes, L.V., III: Legionnaires' disease (clinical findings and one-year follow-up). JAMA, *240:*1169, 1978.
3. McDade, J.E., Shephard, C.C., Fraser, D.W., Tsai, T.R., Redus, M.A., and Dowdle, R.R.: Legionnaires' disease. (Isolation of a bacterium and demonstration of its role in other respiratory disease.) N. Engl. J. Med., *297:*1197, 1977.
4. Kirby, B.P., Snyder, K.M., Meyer, R.D., and Finegold, S.M.: Legionnaires' disease: Clinical feature of 24 cases. Ann. Intern. Med., *89:*297, 1978.
5. Fay, D., Baird, I.M., Aguirre, A., Haegren, V., Werling, K., and Bell, T.W.: Unrecognized Legionnaires' Disease as a cause of fatal illness. JAMA, *243:*2311, 1980.
6. Everett, E.D., Rahm, A.E., Adaniya, R., Stevens, A.L., and McNitt, T.R.: Haemophilus influenzae pneumonia in adults. JAMA, *238:*319, 1977.
7. Iannine, P.B., Claffey, T., and Quintiliani, R.: Bacteremic pseudomonas pneumonia. JAMA. *230:*558, 1974.

8. Weinstein, L.: The "new" pneumonias: the doctor's dilemma. Ann. Intern. Med., *92:*559, 1980.
9. Broome, C.V., Cherry, W.B., and Winn, W.C.: Rapid diagnosis of Legionnaires' disease by direct immunofluorescent staining. Ann. Intern. Med., *90:*1, 1979.
10. This reference has been deleted.
11. Decuncq, H.G., and Lee, F.A.: Mycoplasma pneumoniae pneumonia (massive pulmonary involvement and pleural effusion). JAMA, *194:*162, 1965.
12. Noriega, E.R., Simberkoff, M.S., Gilroy, F.J., and Rahal, J.J.: Life threatening Mycoplasma pneumoniae pneumonia. JAMA, *229:*1471, 1974.
13. Holmes, K.K., Miller, F.L., Edwards, E.A., and Johnson, D.W.: Etiology of pneumonia in non-recurrent military personnel. Am. J. Med. Sci., *260:*264, 1970.
14. Teutsch, S.M., Martone, W.J., Brink, E.W., Potter, M.E., Eliot, G., Hoxsie, R., Craven, R.B., and Kaufman, A.F.: Pneumonic tularemia on Martha's Vineyard. N. Engl. J. Med., *301:*826, 1979.
15. Lorber, B., and Swenson, R.M.: Bacteriology of aspiration pneumonia. (A prospective study of community- and hospital-acquired cases). Ann. Intern. Med., *81:*329, 1974.
16. Gonzalez-C., C.L., and Calia, F.M.: Bacteriologic flora of aspiration-induced pulmonary infections. Arch. Intern. Med., *135:*711, 1975.
17. Petersdorf, R.G., Fusco, T.J., Harter, D.H., and Albrink, W.S.: Pulmonary infections complicating Asian influenza. Arch. Intern. Med., *103:*262, 1959.
18. Pudding, B.A., Wagner, S.C., Zeller, J.A., Gmelich, S.L., Frencn, G.R., and Top, F.H.: Fatal pneumonia associated with adenovirus type 7 in three military trainees. N. Engl. J. Med., *286:*1289, 1972.
19. Triebwasser, J.H., Harris, R.E., and Bryant, R.E.: Varicella pneumonia in adults. Medicine, *46:*409, 1967.
20. Davidson, M., Tempest, B., and Palmer, D.L.: Bacteriologic diagnosis of acute pneumonia (comparison of sputum, transtracheal aspirates and lung aspirates). JAMA, *235:*158, 1976.
21. Reinarz, J.A., Pierce, A.K., Mays, B.B., and Sanford, J.P.: The potential role of inhalation therapy equipment in nosocomial pulmonary infections. J. Clin. Invest., *44:*831, 1965.
22. Ringrose, R.E., McKown, B., Felton, F.G., Barclay, D.P., Muchmore, H.G., and Rhodes, E.R.: A hospital outbreak of Serratia marcescens associated with ultrasonic nebulizers. Ann. Intern. Med., *69:*719, 1978.
23. Sickles, E.A., Young, V.M., Greene, W.H., and Wiernik, P.H.: Pneumonia in acute leukemia. Ann. Intern. Med., *79:*528, 1973.
24. Ruskin, J., and Remington, J.S.: The compromised host and infection. JAMA, *202:*96, 1967.
25. Vogel, C.L., Cohen, M.H., Powell, R.D., and DeVita, V.T.: Pneumocystis carinii pneumonia. Ann. Intern. Med., *68:*97, 1967.
26. Lauver, G.L., Hasan, F.M., Morgan, R.B., and Campbell, S.C.: The usefulness of fiberoptic bronchoscopy in evaluating new pulmonary lesions in the compromised host. Am. J. Med., *66:*580, 1979.
27. Winston, D.J., Lau, W.K., Gale, R.P., and Young, L.S.: Trimethoprim-sulfamethoxazole for the treatment of Pneumocystis carinii pneumonia. Ann. Intern. Med., *92:*762, 1980.
28. Ramirez, G., Shaster, M., Kozub, W., and Pribor, H.C.: Fatal acute Candida albicans bronchopneumonias. JAMA, *199:*340, 1967.
29. Curry, W.A.: Human nocardiosis. (A clinical review with selected case reports.) Arch. Intern. Med., *140:*818, 1980.
30. Grayhill, J.R., and Drutz, D.J.: Ketoconazole: A major innovation for treatment of fungal disease. Ann. Intern. Med., *93:*921, 1980.
31. Strauss, W.G., and Griffin, L.M.: Nitrofurantoin pneumonia. JAMA, *199:*175, 1967.
32. Rosenow, E.C., III: The spectrum of drug induced pulmonary disease. Ann. Intern. Med., *77:*977, 1972.
33. Lopez, M., and Salvaggio, J.: Hypersensitivity pneumonitis: Current concepts of etiology and pathogenesis. Am. Rev. Med., *27:*453, 1976.
34. Carrington, C.B., Addington, W.W., Goff, A.M., Madoff, I.M., Manks, A., Schwaber, J.R., and Gaensler, E.A.: Chronic eosinophilic pneumonia. N. Engl. J. Med., *780:*287, 1969.
35. Steene, A.C., and Mallison, G.F.: Handwashing practices for the prevention of nosocomial infections. Ann. Intern. Med., *83:*683, 1975.

Chapter 13

NEUROMUSCULAR RESPIRATORY FAILURE AND POISONINGS

By Thomas L. Petty

Several acute neurologic states may cause sudden failure of ventilation due to impaired nerve transmission at the myoneural junction. In acute poisonings, either accidental or self-induced, respiratory center depression results in impaired ventilation. Therefore, it is appropriate to consider these two forms of respiratory failure together because of their common features, which are: (1) the absence of intrinsic pulmonary disease initially, (2) the necessity for ventilatory support for severe cases, and (3) the potential for complete recovery and full rehabilitation. Thus, the purpose of this chapter is to present examples of acute neuromuscular respiratory paralysis and of the poisoned state, and to describe respiratory care of the unconscious patient. Respiratory failure associated with cord trauma is considered in Chapter 14, and chronic progressive respiratory failure due to muscular dystrophies and motor neuron disease is discussed in Chapter 19.

ACUTE NEUROGENIC RESPIRATORY FAILURE

The clinical entities in which neurogenic respiratory failure occurs are listed in Table 13-1. The Guillain-Barré syndrome, myasthenia gravis, and neuromuscular poisonings are the most commonly en-encountered in general hospitals.

The paralytic state, which is the common denominator of these otherwise unrelated conditions, poses special problems in care

TABLE 13-1. Acute Neurologic Respiratory Failure

Clinical Entities
1. Guillain-Barré syndrome
2. Myasthenia gravis
a. Myasthenic crisis
b. Cholinergic crisis
3. Neuromuscular poisons/toxins
a. Parathion and others
b. Aminoglycoside antibiotics
c. Botulism
d. Porphyria
e. Diphtheria
4. Multiple sclerosis
5. Poliomyelitis
6. CNS injury (see "Trauma," Chap. 14)

(Table 13-2). The totally paralyzed patient is helpless, and thus for all body functions he is entirely dependent upon external support from mechanical devices and from medical, nursing, and technical personnel. Patients with no spontaneous ventilatory capacity will die in three to four minutes if disconnected from the respirator. Thus, an alarm system must be used to detect any accidental disruption of airflow between machine and airway.[1]

Either an endotracheal or a tracheostomy tube provides the definitive airway for paralyzed patients. A tracheostomy is preferred in the long-term patient because of its superiority as a route for removal of secretions and because eating normal food may be promoted with use of this airway.

Communication with the patient, maintenance of ventilation, and support of other body functions pose additional problems.

An example of the type of protracted problem one still encounters is that of the acute Guillain-Barré syndrome (Case 1), which is repre-

TABLE 13-2. Special Problems In Care of the Paralytic Patient

1. Total or near-total paralysis
2. Total dependence on respirator
3. Requirements of prolonged care
a. Psyche
b. Nutrition
c. Elimination—ileus, fecal impaction
4. Urinary tract infection
5. Communication

sentative of the reversible forms of neuromuscular paralysis encountered today.

Case 1. N.R., a 56-year-old housewife, was admitted to the hospital with a 3-day history of diarrhea, nausea, myalgias, paresthesias, and weakness of the right leg. The day before admission, progressive weakness of all extremities developed. On admission, the patient was profoundly ill with marked dyspnea and cyanosis. Total respiratory paralysis developed rapidly during the next 6 hours. Oral intubation was followed by tracheostomy and use of a constant-volume ventilator. After stabilization of vital signs, physical examination revealed blood pressure of 210/140, pulse rate of 108, and a flaccid quadriplegia with an insensitivity to pinprick and light touch in the lower extremities. Bilateral facial nerve palsies were present with weakness of the ninth, tenth, and twelfth cranial nerves. No reflexes were present.

Past history included diabetes mellitus requiring 40 to 60 U NPH insulin. There was no history of lead exposure.

Laboratory determinations showed hematocrit level of 54; white blood count of 11,400/mm^2 with 64% polymorphonuclear leukocytes; blood sugar, 537. Urinalysis revealed 3 + proteinuria. Urinary porphyrins were not found. Chest roentgenogram showed no abnormality. Determination of arterial blood gases with controlled ventilation with air revealed oxygen saturation of 94.5%; P_{CO_2} of 39.5 mm Hg; pH, 7.330; base excess, −4.5 mEq/L; and bicarbonate, 20.4 mEq/L. Lumbar puncture revealed an opening pressure of 160 cm H_2O. The cerebrospinal fluid contained 95 mg/100 ml protein; no white blood cells were seen; reaction to tests for syphilis was negative.

Ventilation was maintained with a tidal volume of 600 ml and a rate of 14/min. Corticosteroid therapy was begun one week after admission and failed to produce any significant improvement. *Pseudomonas aeruginosa* was consistently cultured in small numbers from tracheal aspirates but was not associated with evidence of wound sepsis, bronchitis, or pneumonitis.

During the second month, the patient developed thrombophlebitis in the left calf; this was treated with sodium heparin followed by sodium warfarin. One month later, in spite of the anticoagulant therapy, sudden dyspnea, cyanosis, and rales over the left lower lobe appeared; these were thought to be consistent with the signs of a pulmonary embolus, although no ECG or x-ray changes were noted. These conditions subsided during the next 10 days with continued anticoagulation therapy with heparin.

In the fifth month of care, *Pseudomonas aeruginosa* and *Proteus mirabilis* were cultured from the urine. Approximately one month later an episode of gram-negative septicemia due to *Klebsiella* and *Aerobacter* organisms occurred with hypotension and progressive hypoxemia, in spite of adequate ventilatory support. The septicemia was treated with antibiotics. At this time, a right upper quadrant mass was discovered and was thought to be a perinephric abscess. This was believed to be the source of the septicemia. The mass disappeared after antibiotic therapy. Acute tubular necrosis and oliguria also occurred, but recovery followed after 13 days with return of normal renal function.

After 6 months the patient remained totally paralyzed, requiring ventilatory control (Fig. 13-1).

In the seventh month of respiratory paralysis, massive gastrointestinal bleeding occurred, followed one month later by another episode of gram-negative septicemia due to *Pseudomonas aeruginosa,* which was effectively treated with antibiotics.

Beginning recovery of distal arm musculature and the ability to swallow and to move the head took place during the eighth month. Through this entire period, the tidal volume and forced vital capacity were measured daily (vital capacity was 100 to 200 ml and the tidal volume no greater than 50 ml). Normal blood gases could not be maintained without respiratory assistance. One month later, it was noted that a tidal volume had gradually increased to 400 ml and could be maintained by the patient; the forced vital capacity was 750 ml. Beginning on this date, the patient was removed from the respirator several times a day for periods up to 15 minutes. Over a 14-day period, the patient was gradually weaned from the respirator, and after 10 months of ventilatory assistance, the vital capacity was 1.45 liters and normal Po_2 and Pco_2 could be maintained. The patient was then transferred from the intensive care unit to the neurology ward for further care and rehabilitation (Fig. 13-2).

Thereafter, the patient had continued neurologic recovery with increasing strength in the arms, shoulder girdle, and neck area, and total recov-

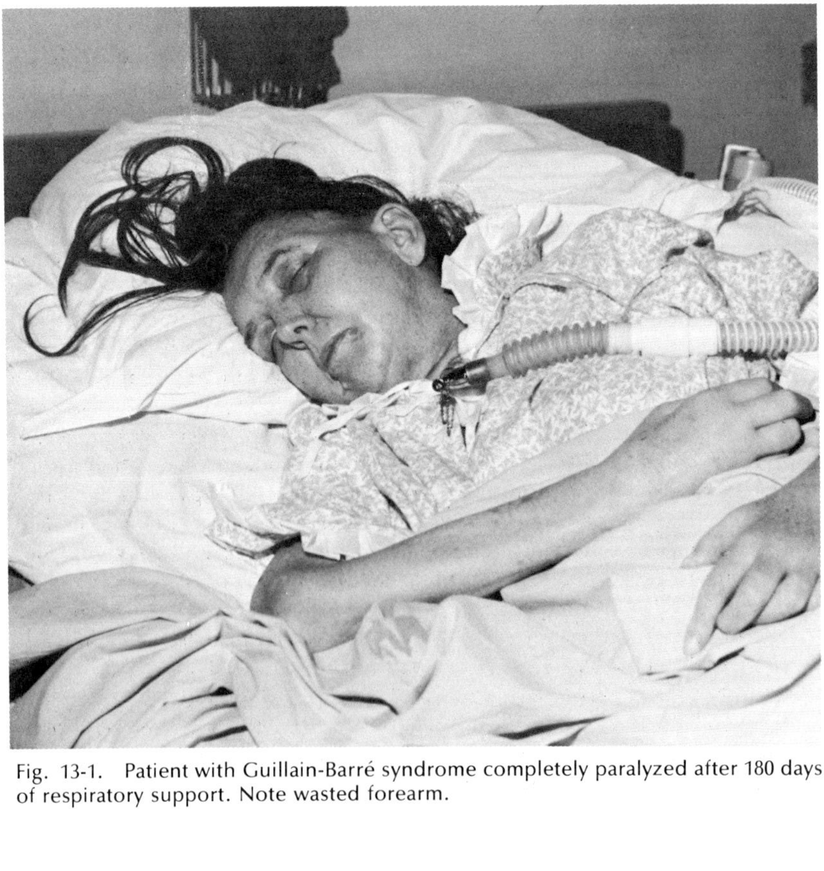

Fig. 13-1. Patient with Guillain-Barré syndrome completely paralyzed after 180 days of respiratory support. Note wasted forearm.

ery of cranial nerve deficits. No residual sensory deficit was observed. The patient was now able to speak well, and bronchoscopy revealed only mild tracheal stenosis in spite of prolonged use of a cuffed tracheostomy tube. The tracheostomy incision healed within 2 months of the removal of the tube. Thirteen months after the onset of her illness, the patient went home to receive further convalescent care. Moderate tracheal stenosis was observed one year after recovery; this responded to tracheal dilation. Six years after hospital discharge, continuing neurologic recovery was observed. (This case has been reported elsewhere.)[2]

Comment. Important features of prolonged respiratory care which are designed to prevent respiratory infection include meticulously aseptic and atraumatic tracheostomy suctioning at least hourly (Chaps. 2 and 7), replacement of the tracheostomy tube frequently, and use of a carefully decontaminated respirator and nebulizer. A second patient has recently required 205 days of respiratory support and has made a full recovery.

A more severe and more dramatically reversible cause of acute neuromuscular respiratory failure is myasthenia gravis. Newer understandings of pathogenesis and management have advanced our

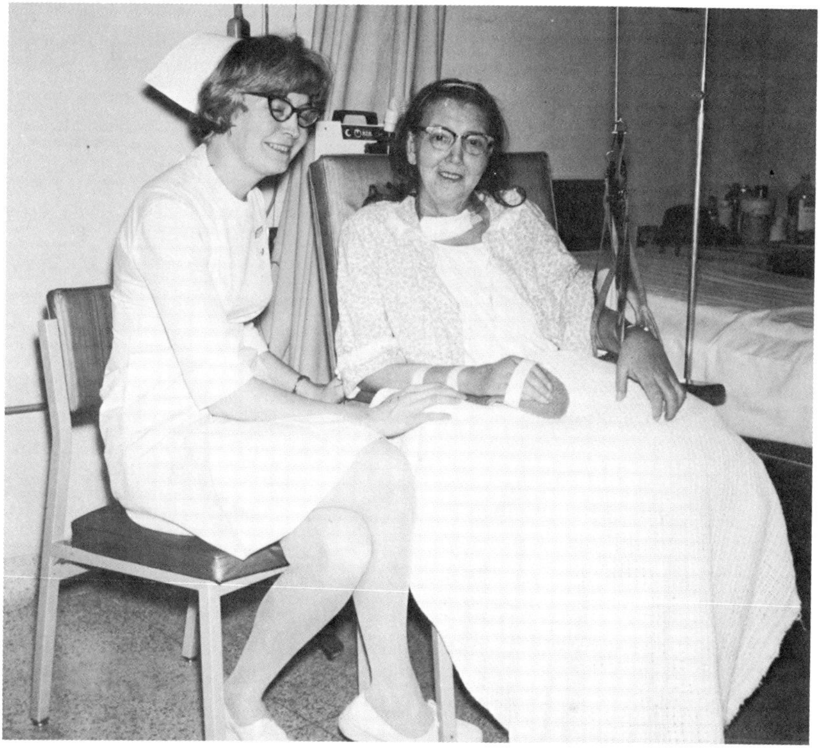

Fig. 13-2. The ability to ventilate and distal muscle strength returned after 266 days of total respiratory support. The tracheostomy wound has now healed. Note the support braces that allow the patient to feed herself.

ability to care for these patients.[3] Principles of management are supportive and are designed to improve neurotransmission by use of cholinergic drugs (anticholinesterase drugs), or to reduce the level of acetylcholine-receptor antibodies by use of corticosteroids, other immunosuppressive drugs such as azathioprine, or plasmapheresis, or following thymectomy. The details and strategies of these therapeutic measures are beyond the scope of this chapter. Recent reviews will augment the reader's knowledge.[3,4]

Another occasionally encountered problem is that of food poisoning due to *Clostridium botulinum*. This type of case is representative of all forms of reversible neuromuscular poisonings.

Case 2. R.S., a 54-year-old housewife on an outing, stopped at a frequently visited bar and grill for a midafternoon snack following a tour of the country. She ate a hamburger on a bun and a small amount of potato salad. Because the potato salad did not "taste right," she left most of it on her plate. Following her return home, approximately 12 hours after eating the potato salad, the patient noted diplopia and weakness of the extremities. She immediately realized that something was amiss and came to the hospital with the help of her husband. On examination she was found to have marked generalized weakness of her muscles, including the external ocular and facial muscles, and muscles of the distal extremities. Over the next 4 hours, her vital capacity measured with a Wright Respirometer dropped from 1500 ml to approximately 350 ml, but at all times normal blood gas values were maintained. Because of the respiratory paralysis, the suspicion of botulism was heightened by the appearance of 2 other individuals who, it was quickly learned, had eaten potato salad in the same restaurant.

A tracheostomy tube was placed immediately, and the patient was ventilated with a volume respirator with a disconnect alarm system.

The patient's course was uncomplicated; however, 17 days of ventilatory assistance were needed before the patient could support her blood gases with her own ventilatory efforts. The tracheostomy tube was then changed to a smaller one, i.e., # 5, which is useful in suctioning and maintaining the tract while allowing the patient to talk, but is not suitable for ventilatory assistance. The patient made a total and complete neurologic recovery.

These features of care, provided in an organized general-purpose respiratory care unit, have produced recovery from reversible neuromuscular paralysis due to a variety of causes, including myasthenia gravis with myasthenic or cholinergic crisis.[5] Probably, nursing care has never been challenged more than it is for the totally paralyzed patient. Almost a 1:1 nurse-to-patient ratio is required for feeding, bathing, personal hygiene, changing of position for comfort, and psychologic support.

As soon as it becomes apparent that prolonged respiratory support will be needed, as with patients in severe paralytic states such as the acute Guillain-Barré syndrome or myasthenia gravis, a feeding tube should be placed and a balanced diet provided three times a day. High-protein diet may cause diarrhea. The tendency toward ileus in patients of this type is great; thus, assistance with elimination by giving laxatives (milk of magnesia) and stool softeners (such as Colace) regularly, and oil retention enemas in the event of fecal impaction are important items of care.

An external catheter should be used in male patients to prevent constant wetness and the likelihood of decubitus ulcer; in females there seems to be no substitute for an indwelling catheter in a totally paralyzed patient. The catheter must be kept as clean as possible and should always be changed at least every other day in an aseptic, atraumatic manner. Water irrigations with antiseptic solution such as neomycin infusions may help prevent heavy colonization of the bladder. As illustrated in Case 1, urinary tract infections and gram-negative sepsis are common life-threatening problems in patients requiring prolonged care with bladder drainage and must be avoided if at all possible. Urine should be cultured frequently to detect the presence of gram-negative rods so that the most likely organism will be known in the event of gram-negative septicemia. At that point, the physician may choose an antibiotic based upon his prior knowledge of the predominant organism present in the bladder. With the urinary catheter in place, almost every patient will become infected within 48 to 72 hours.

In our experience, many cases of the Guillain-Barré syndrome have been complicated by an episode of pulmonary embolism. Therefore, our current practice is to give prophylactic heparin therapy intravenously to all patients with this problem.

One of the greatest problems is the patient's personal comfort. The constant changing of position using pillows for support and the use of a sheepskin will help distribute the pressure and prevent decubiti, which otherwise will inevitably form in patients in bed more than two weeks. This is particularly important when muscle wasting due to poor nutrition occurs.

Communication is an art. One can phrase questions so that they require only a yes or no response to find out if the problem has to do with breathing, stomach, urine, stools, or something external, such as noises made by ventilators. Asking the question, "Is it this or that," giving a simple alternative, will help develop lines of communication. Once facial musculature use returns, many patients can learn to "mouth" words; lip-reading by the nurse will then allow communication. Patience and perseverance are required. For example, in one young college student with the Guillain-Barré syndrome, the patient learned to click her tongue as a signal to nurses. Seizing upon this resource, one of the medical students taught the patient the Morse code so that she could communicate. Later on, as physical strength returns, writing with a pad and pencil becomes possible. Some patients even learn to hold the pencil in their teeth.

As soon as the patient has some strength of the tongue, lips, and pharynx, the tracheal balloon can be slightly deflated. The inflow of air will then regurgitate to the vocal cords and allows the patient to grunt a few words.

Much can be written about psychologic support of such patients. It should always be borne in mind that most paralyzed patients are not mentally clouded or unconscious. A radio, a television set, or a friend's visit can be extremely important. Clergymen should also be welcomed into the unit.

Physical therapy is fundamental in preventing ankylosis of joints, and physical therapists should have at least two sessions each day performing range of motion exercises of all joints. Again it must be remembered that the patient cannot communicate well, but careful scrutiny of the expression will tell whether painful overextension or flexion of the joints is occurring.

The care of patients described herein is immensely frustrating, particularly if the paralysis is protracted. It is important that nurses in the respiratory care unit receive counseling and relief at times of great frustration; conferences with a psychiatric nurse or staff psychiatrist are helpful in aiding the nurses to deal with their frustrations. Certainly, a weekly conference to encourage the nursing personnel is in order in cases such as exemplified by Case 1. The longest duration of respiratory support in our unit was experienced by a unique patient with acute intermittent porphyria coexisting with hyperparathyroidism. She required 14 months of mechanical ventilation before weaning became possible.

Accidental Poisoning

The well recognized association of polymyxin therapy with acute neuromuscular paralysis in patients with underlying chronic renal impairment cautions against the use of polymyxin antibiotics in such patients.[6] An example of acute neuromuscular insufficiency due to polymyxin E is cited in Case 3.

Case 3. E.S., a 66-year-old white housewife, suffered from chronic pyelonephritis and recently had a chronic *Pseudomonas aeruginosa* infection of the urinary tract. She was admitted to the hospital because of fever and flank pain. She had been taking no medications prior to admission.

Physical examination revealed good nutrition; blood pressure, 150/90; pulse rate, 88. Chest and abdominal examinations revealed no abnormality. Bilateral costovertebral angle tenderness was present. Blood urea nitrogen value was 28; serum creatinine, 3.3 ml/100 ml. The white cell count was 15,000 and the hematocrit value, 39%.

Two and one-half hours after admission, 100 mg colistin methanesulphonate were administered intramuscularly. No other medications were given. Three hours later, paresthesias of the hands and pectoral region were noted, but they subsided quickly. Twelve hours after admission, a second dose of 100 mg colistin was administered; 45 minutes later the paresthesia returned. Fatigability, restlessness, and labored respirations followed. One hour and a quarter after the injection, absence of intercostal muscle activity and shallow diaphragmatic breathing were noted. Cyanosis was present. An oral tracheal tube was used until a tracheostomy tube could be placed. Ventilation was supported with a pressure-cycled respirator. External ophthalmoplegia was also present. The patient remained awake and alert with normal vital signs.

Peripheral muscle strength, however, remained good. Four hours after the injection of colistin, blood levels were 3.2/μg %.*

On attempt to remove the patient from the respirator, marked fatigue of the respiratory muscles occurred. Successive measurements of vital capacity gave values of 600 ml, 300 ml, and 50 ml, followed by apnea. Injections of 1.0 mg neostigmine, 10 mg edrophonium, and 10 ml 10% calcium gluconate were given without effect.

While the patient was using the respirator, arterial P_{CO_2} was 33; pH, 7.29; base excess, −11 mEq/L; oxyhemoglobin saturation, 98%. An intravenous injection of 134 mg sodium bicarbonate was given because of the base deficit. This resulted in a pH of 7.39.

On the next morning, with successive forced breaths without use of the respirator, measurements of vital capacity yielded values of 1500 ml, 1100 ml, 900 ml, 500 ml, and 50 ml followed by apnea. On the following day, the patient could maintain her own ventilation for 45 minutes without fatigue. Two days later, use of the respirator was discontinued, and 2 days after that, the tracheostomy tube was removed.

Four months following discharge from the hospital, ventilation tests revealed VC, 2.26 L (2.72); FEV_1, 1.74; MMF, 2.01 L/sec (2.97 ± 0.59); and MVV, 73 L/min (72). Electromyography revealed no abnormalities, and serum enzyme test results were normal.

Comment. Colistin was clearly implicated in this case because no other drugs were administered, and complete recovery occurred after its use was discontinued. Subsequently, 9 additional cases have been encountered in which one of the polymyxin drugs was implicated. In all cases, the respiratory paralysis was completely reversible, usually within 24 to 72 hours.[6] In cases like this, support of respiration can be expected to lead to recovery. In view of the short period of respiratory support required, an endotracheal tube is the preferred definitive airway. Similar acute reversible respiratory paralysis has been occasionally described following other aminoglycoside antibiotic use such as gentamycin.

Case 4. A 47-year-old employee at an insecticide plant developed sudden diplopia, weakness, and excessive salivation and was admitted to the hospital. He had had similar but less striking episodes of weakness

* Determinations were made later.

which he himself thought were due to the fact that he was not using reasonable methods of personal hygiene during his exposure to parathion. Initially he was treated with 2-PAM, but with only temporary effectiveness; thereafter a tracheostomy tube was placed to allow ventilatory support. He was managed with a pressure-cycled respirator for 17 days before respiratory strength again returned; the patient made a complete recovery.

Self-Induced Poisonings

An unconscious flaccid state and respiratory center depression may occur due to a variety of self-induced drug ingestions. Management of these patients is similar to that of patients with other acute neurologic problems, since there must be respiratory support until spontaneous recovery occurs through neutralization or removal of the poison.

Case 5. O.F., a 29-year-old housewife from a rural community 100 miles from Denver, ingested approximately 30 tablets of glutethimide, an unknown amount of meprobamate, a handful of trifluoperazine, a large dose of aspirin, and probably some meperidine. She was found unresponsive by her rancher husband who took her to the local community hospital. At that time, she was unresponsive but was apparently ventilating satisfactorily. Fluid therapy was begun, but she remained unresponsive with deteriorating vital signs over the next 24 hours; she was then transferred to the intensive respiratory care unit. Her pupils were dilated but responded to light; tidal volume was 250 ml; respiration rate, 20. The breath sounds were decreased throughout, and scattered rales were detected in the left base posteriorly. The extremities were flaccid and without reflexes. Chest roentgenogram revealed a left lower lobe infiltrate. Electrocardiogram revealed no abnormality. A gram stain of sputum showed numerous polymorphonuclear leukocytes and gram-positive cocci. The white count was 18,000; hematocrit, 54%.

At the time of admission to the intensive respiratory care unit, an oral endotracheal tube was placed, and ventilation was supported with a self-inflating bag.* The rectal temperature was 38.4°C. Electrolyte determinations revealed sodium, 130; potassium, 3.4; chloride, 104; bicarbonate, 22; and BUN, 5.

Because of the pneumonia, a developing secretion problem, the deteriorating clinical signs, and the predicted long course, a tracheostomy was performed to facilitate the removal of secretions and support ventilation. Penicillin G was given for treatment of pneumonia. The patient became afebrile on the second day but remained unconscious. Two days later she became responsive. The tracheostomy tube was removed after five days. The depressive illness was managed by a psychiatrist. Six months later, the patient was living at home in an apparently happy mental condition.

---

* Hope Resuscitator, Ohio Medical Products, Madison, Wisconsin.

Comment. In most poisonings, an endotracheal tube provides a satisfactory airway because the anticipated period of ventilatory support is short, and the unconscious state precludes feeding. Obviously, comfort is not an immediate consideration in these patients. In the case just described, marked secretions and the profound depression of respiration indicated that a tracheostomy tube was needed from the beginning. Glutethimide and ethchlorvynol produce coma, often persisting for many days; thus, a tracheostomy may be a consideration. For unconscious patients, however, an endotracheal tube is satisfactory, even for long-term use (see Chap. 2). These drugs are also not removed effectively by forced diuresis or hemodialysis. The longest ethchlorvynol coma lasted 17 days with complete recovery (see Chap. 20).

DISCUSSION

The earlier chapters have dealt with principles of management applicable to all forms of acute respiratory failure. In these cases of acute neurologic emergencies and poisonings, the main principles are the support of ventilation, gas exchange, and cardiac output and the maintenance of a normal hydrogen ion concentration. Since patients with these pulmonary insults presumably have no intrinsic pulmonary or cardiac disease and complete recovery is expected, support becomes the major goal of therapy. In addition, the complications of management and the complications of the severe respiratory emergency itself require surveillance. The details of these various complications are discussed in Chapter 15. Special problems of slowly progressive neuromuscular failure are considered in Chapter 19.

REFERENCES

1. Petty, T.L., Nett, L.M., and Schmader, R.D.: A simple ventilator warning device. Inhal. Ther., *14:*67, 1969.
2. Whitehouse, A.C., and Petty, T.L.: Recovery in Landry Guillain-Barré syndrome after prolonged respiratory support. Lancet, *1:*1029, 1969.
3. Smith, L.H.: Myasthenia gravis. West. J. Med., *130:*438, 1979.
4. Martin, D.W., Naughton, J.L., and Smith, L.H.: Myasthenia gravis. West. J. Med., *130:*438, 1979.
5. Petty, T.L., Lakshminarayan, S., Sahn, S.A., Zwillich, C.W., and Nett, L.M.: Intensive Respiratory Care Unit (Review of ten years' experience). JAMA, *233:*34, 1975.
6. Lindensmith, L.A., Baines, R.D., Bigelow, D.B., and Petty, T.L.: Reversible respiratory paralysis associated with polymyxin therapy. Ann. Intern. Med., *68:*318, 1968.

Chapter 14

ACUTE RESPIRATORY FAILURE AFTER SURGERY OR TRAUMA

By Thomas L. Petty

Postoperative respiratory failure, as characterized by a high P_{CO_2} or a low P_{O_2}, is more common than is generally recognized. Fortunately, the insufficiency is usually mild and is well tolerated by a healthy patient undergoing surgery for disease unrelated to the cardiorespiratory system. Severely ill patients, particularly those with respiratory, cardiac, or septic illness, are the most likely to develop respiratory failure that may endanger their lives. Familiarity with both mild and severe forms of this type of respiratory failure can prevent serious morbidity and mortality. Likewise, good respiratory care in the postoperative period can speed recovery and foster a sense of well-being in the patient. In this respect it is far better to err on the side of overtreatment than undertreatment when prescribing measures designed to prevent or treat respiratory failure in the postoperative period. Since postoperative respiratory failure tends to fall into distinct patterns, the groups will be discussed individually.

The Adult Respiratory Distress Syndrome (ARDS), which may occur in the postoperative period, particularly when shock and sepsis are present, is the subject of Chapter 8.

TYPES OF POSTOPERATIVE RESPIRATORY FAILURE

Depression Due to Anesthetic or Narcotic Agents

Etiology. This form of respiratory failure is usually seen after (1) prolonged anesthesia, (2) overdoses of narcotic, and (3) the use of paralytic agents such as curare and pancuronium bromide. Occasionally it occurs after the intraperitoneal injection of neomycin, polymyxin, and other aminoglycoside antibiotics (see Chap. 13) or with high spinal anesthesia.

Physiology. The abnormality seen in these patients is hypoventilation with resultant atelectasis and physiologic shunting.[1] The use of 100% oxygen and hyperventilation at the end of a period of anesthesia just prior to extubation may augment these changes. Since the oxygen may reduce ventilatory drive, its use may lead to atelectasis as the oxygen is absorbed from the alveoli.[2] Blood gas determinations are likely to show a normal or slightly elevated P_{CO_2}, a decreased pH, and a lowered P_{O_2}. If the operative procedure was unusually long or the patient is in shock, metabolic acidosis may also be present. Normal P_{O_2} may coexist with an elevated P_{CO_2} if the patient is receiving oxygen via mask or cannula. This finding should not lull the clinician into discounting the possibility of hypoventilation.

Recognition. The patient is difficult to arouse. Respirations are slow and shallow, and the pulse is usually slow. Blood pressure initially may be elevated, reflecting hypercapnia. The presence or absence of cyanosis is an unreliable sign since peripheral cyanosis can occur despite adequate arterial P_{O_2}; also adequate oxygenation can occur despite hypoventilation when oxygen is being administered via nasal cannula or mask. The administration of narcotics in the immediate postoperative period will further depress respiration.

Treatment. Treatment is directed at restoring adequate ventilation. When hypoxemia exists without hypercapnia, nasal oxygen with flow rates of 1 to 2 L/min will correct hypoxemia. Narcotic overdosage can be treated by naloxone given intravenously; dosage depends on the type and the amount of narcotic given. Ventilation should be assisted in these patients until their own efforts are adequate. Severe respiratory depression caused by anesthetic agents, barbiturates, or paralytic agents is best treated with endotracheal intubation and respiratory assistance with a mechanical respirator. In the absence of underlying pulmonary disease, a pressure cycled ventilator will usually achieve and maintain adequate respiration. Volume-cycled ventilators have nearly replaced all pressure-cycled machines in most units and are preferable because of their capabilities. Ventilation is assisted until the patient is fully awake. Then the use of the respirator is discontinued temporarily while the patient's tidal volume and forced breath are measured. If these are adequate, oxygen is administered through an endotracheal tube with a T-tube assembly (see Fig. 7-7). An arterial blood sample should be taken 15 to 30 minutes after discontinuing use of the respirator. If blood gas levels are normal, the endotracheal tube can be removed. The patient should be carefully observed for several hours in the recovery room or in the intensive care unit in case there should be subsequent relapse.

Postoperative Atelectasis, Hypoventilation, and Hypoxemia

Etiology. This syndrome differs from the syndrome just described in two ways: (1) the patient is usually fully awake, and (2) hypoventilation and hypoxemia persist beyond the immediate recovery phase.

The most common cause is the pain that is associated with upper abdominal or thoracic operations, inhibiting normal ventilation to the extent that atelectasis, hypoventilation, and hypoxemia occur. Abdominal distention, general inanition, debility, and oversedation may also contribute to the respiratory failure.

Physiology. Although rapid shallow respiration may increase minute ventilation, alveolar ventilation is reduced by the increased ratio of dead space to tidal volume. If shallow breathing persists without intermittent deep breaths or coughing, atelectasis may develop in the underventilated portions of the lung, and the ventilation-perfusion ratio is disturbed. When blood flow continues to underventilated areas, physiologic shunting occurs, and the P_{O_2} drops although the P_{CO_2} may remain normal.

Recognition. The patient is usually apprehensive and defensive. He complains of abdominal pain and resists efforts to ambulate or cough. Tachypnea, tachycardia, and moderate fever are commonly found. Breath sounds are decreased at the bases, and the coarse rhonchi of retained secretions are frequently heard on auscultation. Chest roentgenograms may show "plate-like atelectasis." Larger areas of atelectasis may be present, and left lower lobe atelectasis is common following cardiac surgery.

Treatment. Reassurance of the patient, combined with the judicious use of narcotics, physical therapy, and ambulation is usually sufficient in the treatment of this syndrome. The need for deep breaths and frequent coughing is explained to the patient, and he is assured that these exercises will not cause his wound to burst. Narcotics should be administered before sessions of vigorous physical therapy and coughing exercises, but oversedation should be avoided.

The physical therapist interested in pulmonary problems is an invaluable aid to the surgeon and internist in treating the patient having this type of problem. Ideally, the patient should be seen before surgery and taught breathing and coughing techniques. The therapist then visits the patient two or three times daily in the postoperative period to assist him in breathing and coughing. Early ambulation is encouraged, since it relieves muscle stiffness and encourages deep breathing. Frequent postural changes are helpful in improving ventilation-perfusion inequalities.

Intermittent positive-pressure breathing devices may be used in conjunction with other aspects of bronchial hygiene, including steam or mist inhalation and physical therapy. Used alone, an IPPB device is ineffective in preventing pulmonary complications. A controlled study has failed to show that postoperative care with IPPB reduces complications compared with non-IPPB therapy.[3] The patient may receive a nebulized sympathomimetic amine bronchodilator, such as isoetharine, metaproterenol, or isoproterenol for 10 minutes using a pressure-driven small plastic nebulizer (Fig. 14-1). Immediately afterward, he inhales warm mist for 10 to 20 minutes. Following this, vigorous physical therapy, deep breathing, and expulsive coughing are performed. This routine may be repeated 3 to 4 times daily or more if needed.

Blow bottles or the use of an incentive spirometer to give the patient a goal for taking large breaths may be as effective as or even superior to IPPB in combating postoperative atelectasis.[4] The increasing body of evidence favors cough and activity as the best means of increasing mucociliary clearance.[5] Certainly, the use of inhaled bronchodilators with sympathomimetic activity is wise because of the pharmacologic augmentation of mucociliary clearance.[6]

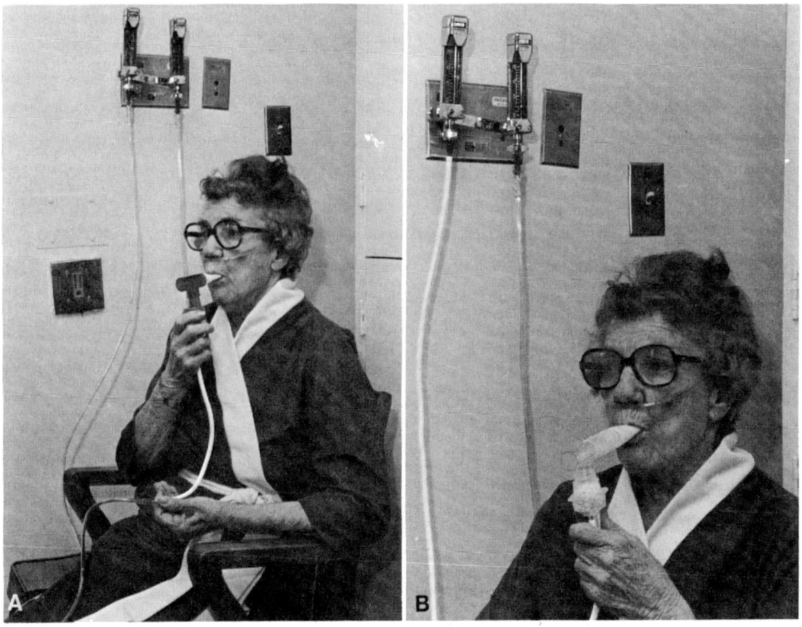

Fig. 14-1. *A*, Postoperative patient receiving inhaled beta agonist drug (Isoetharine) using plastic nebulizer and Y-tube assembly. Patient activates this with her left hand. Nebulizer is powered by a wall oxygen source.

B, Close-up view of powered nebulizer. Patient activates nebulizer during inspiration and inhales slowly to promote deposition of therapeutic aerosol.

"High-Output Respiratory Failure"

The term "high-output respiratory failure" has been historically applied to a particular type of postoperative failure in which high metabolic demands for oxygen are coupled with restriction of ventilation.[7] The prototype is the patient with intra-abdominal sepsis (frequently sub-diaphragmatic), an upper abdominal incision, and high fever. Incipient respiratory failure is often overlooked, since the patient may appear to be breathing adequately. Profound hypoxemia and hypercapnia can occur suddenly in these patients, and preventive treatment is of utmost importance.

Pathophysiology. The high metabolic demands for oxygen imposed by sepsis and fever increase oxygen consumption and cardiac output. Ventilation is increased in response to these demands. The presence of an abdominal incision, abdominal distention, and subdiaphragmatic infection all limit the effectiveness of breathing. The result is rapid, shallow, and mechanically inefficient ventilation, accomplished at great expense of effort by the patient. The oxygen cost of breathing, normally quite small, may become a significant factor in the total oxygen consumption. If treatment is not initiated promptly, the metabolic demands may surpass the ability of the lungs to supply oxygen, or an exhausted patient may be unable to maintain the necessary hyperventilation. Then profound respiratory and circulatory failure rapidly intervene. These mechanisms are operative in ARDS due to sepsis (see Chap.8).

Diagnosis. Any patient with abdominal distention and sepsis should be carefully monitored. An increase in respiratory rate and a decrease in tidal volume are common initial signs of trouble. An increase in respiratory rate to any significant degree is an accurate predictor of emerging acute respiratory failure in most patients.[8] Arterial oxygen tension and saturation are below normal unless additional oxygen is being administered. P_{CO_2} is usually low, reflecting hyperventilation. Although a mild metabolic acidosis may be present, the pH may be alkaline as a result of hyperventilation. Chest roentgenograms show basilar atelectasis and, frequently, elevated diaphragms. These findings may persist relatively unchanged until profound respiratory failure occurs suddenly. At that time, P_{O_2} drops sharply, P_{CO_2} rises, and pH falls.

Treatment. Early therapy, prior to profound respiratory failure, can prevent much of the morbidity and mortality associated with this syndrome. Nasal oxygen should be given to all these patients in an attempt to maintain normal arterial P_{O_2} values. Sepsis must be treated vigorously with antibiotics and drainage of loculated pus from abscesses. Narcotics should be used with extreme caution since any depression of respiration can precipitate severe respiratory failure. Abdominal distention should be relieved if possible. Often, thick secretions and ineffective cough are a problem in these patients. Physical therapy and continuous mist or steam inhalations will aid in mobilizing secretions (see Chap. 7). If improvement does not follow these measures or if the patient worsens, assisted ventilation through an endotracheal tube should be instituted immediately. Respiratory assistance should be continued until the precipitating problems are under control and the patient can maintain normal blood gases without aid. Many patients already septic will develop pneumonia. Frequent monitoring of cultures from the tracheal aspirate will alert the physician to changes in tracheal flora before pneumonia becomes evident. Antibiotics, of course, must be selected according to identification of the predominant organisms by sputum stain or by culture-sensitivity studies.

Surgery with Associated Chronic Lung Disease

Elective operations in patients with chronic bronchitis and emphysema should not be undertaken without preoperative evaluation of the patient and a period of bronchial hygiene in patients with secretion problems. With proper preparation, the incidence of postoperative pulmonary problems will be minimized. In emergency operations without adequate preoperative evaluation, postoperative respiratory management is based on the premise that respiratory failure will occur unless necessary therapeutic measures are undertaken.

Preoperative Evaluation and Care. Careful attention to history and a complete physical examination will lead to the detection of most patients with chronic lung disease. There should be detailed questioning about cough and sputum production. Dyspnea at rest or after minor exertion indicates greatly decreased respiratory reserve. The smoking history is important, since most heavy smokers have some degree of bronchitis. The presence of rales or rhonchi, wheezing, or decreased breath sounds are important clinical signs. Emphysema patients may have an increased anteroposterior diameter of the chest, but this state is not invariably present. A history of decreased exercise tolerance is almost always obtained. Exercise tolerance can be evaluated clinically by having the patient walk briskly and climb stairs along with the observer.

Arterial blood gas analysis of the patient in the resting state should be performed. If limited exercise tolerance has been noted, blood gas studies should be repeated immediately following exercise. A fall in arterial P_{O_2} and a rise in P_{CO_2} indicate a poor respiratory reserve. Ventilation studies, including forced vital capacity (FVC), forced expiratory volume in one second (FEV_1), maximal midexpiratory flow (MMEF), and maximal voluntary ventilation (MVV), are helpful in assessing the respiratory reserve and the degree of impairment.[9]

Preoperative Care. If time allows, a week or more of intensive respiratory care may change a poor-risk patient into a good-risk patient. Bronchial hygiene, antibiotics, exercise, oxygen, and physical therapy play important roles in the welfare of the individual patient (see Chap. 10). Smokers should be encouraged to stop smoking at least two weeks prior to an elective surgical procedure.

ANESTHESIA AND CHRONIC LUNG DISEASE

Local and regional anesthetics are preferred when they can be used without additional sedation. While local anesthesia alone is not dangerous, barbiturate or narcotic premedication can precipitate respiratory failure in patients with chronic lung disease. Spinal anesthetics may paralyze accessory muscles of respiration and precipitate intra-operative respiratory failure. For operations that require adequate sedation or relaxation, the safest procedure is to use a general anesthetic agent and to control ventilation through endotracheal intubation. A competent anesthesiologist is a vital partner in the intraoperative management of these patients.

When a patient with secretion problems must undergo an operation without prior bronchial hygiene or preparation, bronchoscopy and aspiration of secretions at the end of the operative procedure will often prevent serious immediate postoperative problems.

PATHOPHYSIOLOGY OF POSTOPERATIVE RESPIRATORY FAILURE

The presence of an underlying chronic lung disease usually determines the specific abnormalities that occur. Retained secretions, atelectasis, pneumonia, severe hypoxemia, and hypoventilation are commonly encountered in the postoperative period in patients with chronic bronchitis and emphysema. Either restlessness or coma may be present depending on the degree of hypoxemia and the patient's tolerance of it.

Tracheostomy should always be considered in this group of patients, particularly when operations must be performed without adequate preoperative evaluation or preparation. If secretions are a problem or if prolonged ventilatory assistance is anticipated, a tracheostomy should be performed at the end of the operative procedure. The high risk of death from respiratory failure in this group of patients far outweighs the risk of tracheostomy. For anticipated slow recovery, use of a tracheostomy as the definitive airway has many advantages, including comfort, ease of suctioning, and the likelihood that the patient will be able to eat food.

POSTOPERATIVE CARE

Careful monitoring of arterial blood gases is fundamental in the intelligent management of these patients. Blood gas analysis should be performed immediately following termination of the period of anesthesia before the endotracheal tube is removed. Since a good airway is necessary for assisted ventilation, the airway should be removed only when the patient is fully awake and able to maintain ventilation without mechanical assistance (see "Weaning," Chap. 4). Although the need for postoperative ventilatory assistance varies from patient to patient, it has been the custom in this unit in recent years to assist ventilation in patients with chronic lung disease throughout the recovery room period. It is during these first few hours in the postoperative course that acute respiratory failure and cardiac arrest most commonly occur. The endotracheal tube is often left in place until the patient is transferred from the recovery room to the intensive care unit. The patient is then carefully reevaluated by means of physical examination, tidal and forced breath measurements, and blood gas analysis. A trial period of an hour without ventilatory assistance should always be undertaken before extubation. The patient should receive low-flow oxygen to the endotracheal or tracheostomy tube to prevent hypoxemia during this transition period. After extubation, the patient is carefully watched in the intensive care unit for at least an additional 24 hours before transfer out of the unit.

Early ambulation and aggressive physical therapy are important in decreasing postoperative pulmonary morbidity and increasing the patient's morale. This must often be accomplished in the face of great opposition from the patient, his family, and a reluctant nursing staff. It is common in our institution to see a patient ambulating in the hall while a nurse assists ventilation through a tracheostomy tube with a resuscitation bag (see Chap. 7).

ANTIBIOTICS

Antibiotics are frequently used in postoperative therapy of patients with chronic bronchitis. Broad-spectrum antibiotics of the tetracycline group or ampicillin control most of the organisms commonly found in the sputum of patients with chronic lung disease. Frequent cultures of the tracheal aspirates are obtained, and antibiotics are selected on the basis of in vitro sensitivity studies and the patient's general condition.

PULMONARY EDEMA

Pulmonary edema can be a serious cause of respiratory failure in the postoperative period.[9] The use of drugs that depress myocardial contractility, fluid overload, bronchospasm, aspiration, and redistribution of body fluids may participate in the sudden onset of this complication.

Physiology. With the development of pulmonary edema, there is an increase in physiologic shunting. This is in part due to changes in ventilation and in part due to diffusion impairment resulting from increased interstitial and intra-alveolar fluid. Ventilatory changes occur with the obstruction of small airways by foamy edema fluid.[10] The resulting atelectasis and unevenness of ventilation lead to shunting and hypoxemia. Hypoxemia is usually marked and may further depress the myocardium. Hypercapnia is not usually a problem unless the patient is in profound respiratory failure. If aspiration occurs during or after surgery, pulmonary edema is usually secondary to the direct toxic effects of the aspirated material on the alveoli and capillaries, resulting in ARDS (see Chap. 8).

Diagnosis. The classic picture of bubbling rales and frothy, pink-tinged sputum is found only in more severe types of pulmonary edema. Earlier signs are tachypnea, tachycardia, dyspnea, cyanosis, and rales at the bases of the lung. Central venous pressure may increase if the right heart fails; if the right heart remains competent, the central venous pressure may be normal. Monitoring pulmonary artery and wedge pressure via a flow-directed catheter is thus preferable (see Chap. 5). Chest roentgenograms showing perihilar fluffy infiltrates may help confirm the diagnosis. Arterial P_{O_2} is low but usually responds to oxygen administration; P_{CO_2} may range from low to high values depending on the degree of pulmonary edema and on the patient's ability to breathe. Acidemia is common and may be severe when low cardiac output and poor peripheral circulation occur in conjunction with an elevated P_{CO_2}.

Treatment. Administration of supplemental oxygen via mask or nasal cannula is begun immediately. Diuretics and digitalis are given intravenously. Morphine sulfate may be given in small intravenous doses if respiratory distress is not marked. Severe respiratory distress and hypoxemia that do not respond to nasal oxygen indicate the need for assisted ventilation and possibly endotracheal intubation. Intermittent positive-pressure breathing is fairly effective in transiently reducing pulmonary edema and increasing arterial P_{O_2} in this situation. Positive end-expiratory pressure (PEEP) is more effective, however, and in the presence of pulmonary edema does not appear to affect cardiac output seriously (see Chap. 8).

Fluids should be restricted to 1500 ml daily. No cardiac depressant drugs should be given. An intravenous drip of dopamine or dobutamine may be needed to maintain cardiac output, systemic blood pressure, or tissue perfusion.

RESPIRATORY SUPPORT FOLLOWING OPEN-HEART OPERATIONS

The extreme popularity of coronary artery bypass operations has resulted in large numbers of patients receiving mechanical ventilatory support in the immediate postoperative period. Ventilation overnight is almost routine. It presents the advantages of assuring adequate oxygenation and ventilation and provides the work of breathing. Narcotics may be used for pain with confidence so long as hemodynamics are stable. Against the practice of routine postoperative mechanical ventilation, however, are the discomfort of the endotracheal tube, the interference with communication, and the necessity for endotracheal suctioning rather than expulsive coughing to clear secretions. For these reasons, consideration has been given to early extubation.[11-13] Certainly, pharmacologic reversal of muscle relaxants and analgesics would aid in early extubation.[11] Any cardiopulmonary condition resulting in a low mixed venous Po_2 (<35 mm Hg) would make early extubation likely to fail, and these patients should receive continued ventilatory support until hemodynamic stability can be achieved.[12] Prospective studies have shown, however, that the majority of patients requiring coronary artery surgery may be successfully extubated two to five hours after leaving the operating room.[12,13]

RESPIRATORY FAILURE FOLLOWING CRUSHED CHEST INJURIES

Etiology. Crushed chest injuries are due primarily to automobile or industrial accidents.[14] Damage to the rib cage and underlying lung parenchyma can lead to serious respiratory failure in patients with these injuries. Associated injuries, particularly abdominal and neurologic, are commonly seen in conjunction with chest trauma and may contribute to impaired ventilation. Paradoxic motion of unstable segments of the chest wall and the presence of blood or air in the pleural cavities can also impair ventilation and the effective clearance of secretions.

Pathophysiology. It was previously believed that paradoxic rib motion resulting in impaired thoracic mechanics and hypoventilation was the basic reason for respiratory failure in crushed chest injury. Efforts to stabilize the rib cage with sand bags, rib traction in the hospital, and surgical rib repair thus became modes of therapy. It is now recognized that underlying lung contusion is the major reason for impaired oxygenation and, to a lesser degree, CO_2 retention. Thus, the trend in management is away from mechanical ventilation and so-called "internal fixation" unless lung contusion is present. Recent studies have demonstrated the high success rate of nonventilatory management of chest injuries in the absence of severe hypoxemia.[15] Analgesics are used for pain, and surgical rib stabilization is employed in selected patients.[15] Lung contusion is most apt to be associated with major degrees of rib trauma and paradox, however, and thus these two processes occur in parallel, but not as cause and effect. The additional pressure of a hemo- or pneumothorax or both may further seriously interfere with the expansion of the lungs. When air collects under tension in the pleural cavity, complete collapse of the ipsilateral and partial collapse of the contralateral lung may lead to severe respiratory failure. Associated diaphragmatic injuries also interfere with ventilation, both by the loss of the normal bellows action and by displacement of lung by herniated abdominal viscera. Blood gas analysis in post-traumatic injuries of the chest commonly shows a severe hypoxemia and mild to moderate elevations of the P_{CO_2}. Acidemia, which is commonly present, may have a metabolic component as well as a respiratory component.

Diagnosis. Severe restlessness and dyspnea in a patient with chest injury are indications of respiratory failure. Auscultation and percussion will usually reveal a pneumothorax or hemothorax. Tension pneumothorax can be confirmed by aspiration of the chest with a needle and syringe. Flail chest is usually obvious on physical examination. Rib fractures are indicated by the presence of localized tenderness and crepitation. A chest roentgenogram is a valuable diagnostic aid, but it is seldom an emergency procedure and should generally be postponed until immediate problems of resuscitation have been corrected. Pulmonary infiltrates seen immediately following chest trauma are almost always a result of lung contusion.

Treatment.

Rib Fractures. Simple rib fractures in an otherwise healthy patient without known lung disease are best treated with an intercostal nerve block, physical therapy, and good bronchial hygiene. In young patients with good pulmonary reserve, strapping of the chest with adhesive tape may contribute to the patient's comfort, but this procedure should be avoided in patients with limited respiratory reserve. The elderly and those patients with chronic lung disease should be hospitalized so that they may be kept under close observation. Repeated nerve blocks, daily physical therapy, and bronchial hygiene are necessary and valuable adjuncts. Antibiotics are not needed unless there is an underlying pulmonary infection.

Flail Chest. Small segments of unstable chest wall may be tolerated by a young person with good pulmonary reserve. Most patients with flail chest, however, will need hospitalization and respiratory support. The emergency treatment may consist only of stabilization with sand bags or a rolled blanket or towel. This treatment is not satisfactory, however, as definitive care. Prior to the advent of mechanical ventilators, flail chest was usually treated with various methods of traction on the flail segment. This mode of treatment is painful to the patient, is often ineffective in stabilizing the chest, and does not prevent hypoventilation. The current method of therapy used in this institution is internal stabilization of the chest and use of a mechanical ventilator.[15] An endotracheal tube is placed and a volume-type respirator is employed to provide intermittent positive-pressure breathing through the tracheostomy tube. Ventilation should be controlled to the extent that the patient is not initiating respiratory movements on his own. Slight hyperventilation will usually reduce the respiratory drive of most patients in order to allow the respirator to take over the full work of breathing. The flail segment is then stabilized by internal expansion of the lungs. This treatment assures adequate ventilation with the least pain possible. The flail segment will usually stabilize over a period of 12 to 14 days; earlier stability occurs in many patients. At this time, the patient is weaned from the respirator for short periods under close observation. If the flail segment is stable, and if the patient can easily maintain an adequate tidal volume and normal blood gases, the use of the respirator is discontinued, and the tracheostomy is removed.

Hemo- or Pneumothorax. Blood or air in the pleural cavity following chest trauma must be removed through a chest tube. Pneumothorax alone is best relieved by a tube placed in the second or third intercostal space in the midclavicular line. The size of the tube should be sufficient to keep up with any underlying leak in the lung parenchyma. Normally, a 20 to 24 French tube is adequate. In patients with a large air leak from the pulmonary parenchyma, a larger tube may be needed. For hemothorax, the tube should be placed in the sixth intercostal space in the posterior axillary line. A tube of 28 French or larger should be inserted for the removal of blood, and care should be taken that this tube is frequently milked free of blood clots so that it remains open and patent. Hemorrhage that continues in large volumes following insertion of a chest tube is an indication of a major vascular injury that demands prompt exploration of the chest. Likewise, massive continuing air leak is an indication of a torn or ruptured bronchus, which should be surgically corrected. All patients with a simple pneumothorax should have a chest tube inserted prior to the use of positive-pressure assisted ventilation to avoid development of a tension pneumothorax.

A large bronchopleural fistula, whatever the cause, effects a major loss of the tidal volume delivered by the ventilator. Smaller leaks are compensated by an increase in tidal or minute ventilation. Large leaks necessitating the use of positive end-expiratory pressure require more ingenuity. A valving arrangement using Heimlich valves, with placement of the chest tube under water parallel to the ventilator exhalation circuit to balance forces with the chest, has been described and is a useful maneuver in severe cases.[16]

Diaphragmatic Ruptures. Ruptures of the diaphragm are surgical emergencies and are almost always associated with intra-abdominal injury. Diaphragmatic ruptures are usually approached through an abdominal or thoracoabdominal incision, so that the subdiaphragmatic injury may be corrected at the same time that the diaphragm is repaired.

Acute Respiratory Failure following Multiple Trauma. It is now recognized that respiratory failure following multiple trauma is a complex process representing many diverse pathophysiologic processes including lung contusion, fat embolization, impaired thoracic mechanics due to rib fracture, and paradoxic rib motion. Pleural space problems as just described and diaphragmatic injury with associated shock or aspiration produce the full picture of ARDS (see Chap. 8). Because of this final common pathway, mechanical ventilation with PEEP is frequently employed as a routine measure (see Chaps. 5 and 8). The response to PEEP is variable in this setting owing to the different pathologic processes involved.[17] Thus, it is important to monitor gas transfer by serial measurements of Pa_{O_2} on the same FI_{O_2} as PEEP is introduced to identify benefit. PEEP is not a panacea and should not be used unless clear improvement in oxygen transfer across the lungs and augmented tissue oxygen transport does not occur (see Chap. 5).

PULMONARY COMPLICATIONS OF BURNS

Almost all patients who die from severe burns will have some pulmonary complications, and in many patients the pulmonary complications are the direct cause of death.[18]

Early Complications

Thermal damage to the respiratory epithelium is rare, since it is caused by steam or intense heat. This is nearly always fatal, and the victims rarely survive even long enough to receive emergency care. Much more common are complications caused by smoke or chemical inhalation. These patients often have severe bronchospasm, cough, and profuse secretions. Chemical pneumonitis can lead to acute pulmonary edema and to a condition similar to (and probably identical with) the ARDS (see Chap. 8). Hypoxemia is frequently present, but it usually responds to administration of oxygen. Treatment is directed at reducing the irritation, improving the arterial oxygen saturation, and preventing subsequent infection. Adequate moisture is given through a face tent with a heated nebulizer. Corticosteroids are given intravenously until symptoms subside; 100 mg hydrocortisone or the equivalent may be given every 6 to 8 hours. Usually, the use of corticosteroids may be stopped after 3 to 4 days. Oxygen is given via nasal mask or cannula at flows of 1 to 5 L/min, depending on arterial oxygen saturation. A broad-spectrum antibiotic, either ampicillin or tetracycline, is given if the patient has a prior history of bronchitis. Any subsequent antibiotic therapy should be guided by the growth and sensitivity of pathogenic organisms in sputum cultures. Ventilatory assistance may be needed in some instances of severe smoke inhalation, particularly when the patient has major burns or has received other injuries. When assisted ventilation is necessary, a nasotracheal tube is preferred over a tracheostomy tube. The incidence of tracheostomy complications in burned patients is high, and usually a nasotracheal tube can be kept in place for the period of ventilatory assistance that is necessary.[17]

Late Complications

Postburn pulmonary complications are generally related either to fluid overload during the resuscitation period or to sepsis occurring in the post-resuscitation period. Acute pulmonary edema and congestion are largely preventable with careful fluid therapy. Central venous pressure can be misleading and may remain at low values despite pulmonary edema. Pulmonary artery pressure more accurately reflects the status of the pulmonary circulation. Treatment for this condition consists of digitalis, diuretics, and assisted ventilation. Positive end-expiratory pressure breathing has been necessary for most of these patients.

Pneumonias occurring in the postburn period have been divided into hematogenous and airborne pneumonias.[17] The hematogenous pneumonias occur primarily with patients with burn wound sepsis and septicemia. Airborne pneumonias are less common since the advent of topical antibiotics, but both types of pneumonia carry a high morbidity and mortality. Appropriate antibiotics are the most important facet of treatment. Continuous mist or steam inhalation and IPPB therapy will help in the management of secretions. Respiratory failure with pulmonary sepsis in the postburn patient is associated with a high mortality rate despite assisted ventilation, PEEP, and antibiotics. Death, when it occurs, is usually due to a combination of sepsis and respiratory failure. The possible role of oxygen toxicity in this illness, as in other forms of severe respiratory distress, remains unclear. In our experience, all patients with burns over 80% of their bodies have died in spite of excellent supportive therapy. All have had pulmonary complications.

Improvements in burn care have occurred during the past 15 years.[19] These include better approaches to both wound closure and burn-associated sepsis, resulting in improved survival and shortened hospitalization time.[18]

RESPIRATORY FAILURE FOLLOWING CENTRAL NERVOUS SYSTEM TRAUMA

As many as 50% of patients with head or spinal cord injury have significant hypoxemia.[20] Thus, blood gas monitoring is required to detect unsuspected abnormalities. Beyond this are two forms of sudden, devastating central nervous system (CNS) catastrophes that require special mention.

Acute cerebral edema with sudden increase in intracerebral pressure rapidly affects central control of respiration. In advancing cerebral edema, key clinical signs are: (1) level of consciousness, (2) pupillary relexes, (3) ocular reflexes, (4) pattern of respiration, and (5) muscle tone and posture. Progressive signs relative to these occur as damage via increased intracranial pressure following trauma descends from cortex to thalamus, mid-brain, pons, and medulla. Respiration deteriorates from normal, variable, and coordinated (eupnea) to the Cheyne-Stokes pattern—deep and regular to fixed and mechanical. It finally becomes shallow and ataxic as respiration is about to cease through loss of central control. The fixed rhythmic respiration with jaw and laryngeal jerk with each inspiratory effort following trauma or cardiac arrest is a grave clinical sign.

The details of CNS evaluation following head trauma are beyond the intent of this chapter. Briefly, a rapid systematic neurologic examination by a skilled clinician is mandatory, usually followed by a CT scan as preparations for a possible craniotomy are being made by a neurosurgeon. Patients with rapidly deteriorating CNS signs are intubated and ventilated as evaluation proceeds. Forced hyperventilation is traditional and is effective in immediately reducing cerebral edema by reducing cerebral blood flow. Improvement in survival via hyperventilation is probably the result of this ventilating procedure, but clinical studies concerning this technique are necessary.[20] Most experts believe that maintaining Pco_2 at 24 to 28 is appropriate in the short term. Whether or not long-term hyperventilation is useful is not known.

Quadriplegia following Cord Trauma

This is one of the most tragic problems facing the respiratory specialist. Often young, happy, and successful individuals are victims of trauma, usually on the highway or following diving or gymnastics. High cord trauma including cervical fractures or dislocations, or both, in the C_3, C_2, or C_1 region immediately cause mechanical bellows failure because of loss of phrenic nerve innervation in high cord injuries. At times, the sensory level ascends one or two dermatomes following injury, possibly as a result of cord edema following initial trauma. Thus, patients may be brought to emergency rooms with intact diaphragm function (but without intercostals to maintain chest wall stability), only to deteriorate into total respiratory paralysis in 24 to 48 hours.

Few centers are prepared to care for the ventilator-dependent quadriplegic patient. Fortunately, the Craig Rehabilitation Center in Denver has established and pioneered an approach to this form of demanding and heart-rending respiratory care. Their program is briefly described here (with the kind assistance of Allan Wicks, M.D., pulmonologist at Craig Rehabilitation Center).

Initial Care. If death does not occur at the scene of the accident, most patients suffering high cord injury are brought to general hospitals. They may even be accompanied by a friend or family member who is assisting with mouth-to-mouth breathing. They may have been intubated by ambulance personnel. Further manipulation of the neck carries the risk of aggravating the cord injury. Thus, if an endotracheal tube is in place, it should be maintained and changed later. Otherwise, a tracheostomy should be immediately and skillfully performed, because it will be the patient's airway for the remainder of life.

In patients who are still breathing, monitoring of forced vital capacity with a Wright spirometer with face mask is done frequently. Baseline arterial blood gas determinations are performed.

A significant diuresis occurs during the first days or weeks. This is due to muscle atrophy and fat catabolism, and the mobilization of tissue water. All patients develop atelectasis, most have pneumonia, and the majority have pulmonary emboli. Management includes frequent tracheal suction, hyperinflation with IPPB or bag breathing in nonventilated patients, or deep breathing with increasing tidal volumes or "sigh" breaths via ventilators providing these capabilities. A "quad cough" technique employs large breaths and assists a forced expiration by means of rib compression during exhalation. Fiberoptic bronchoscopy will inevitably be tried to help expand atelectatic lobes or segments, but often mucus plugs are not found. Pneumonia is treated empirically or on the basis of sputum-stained smears or cultures. Prophylactic low-dose heparin is used or, in the face of major pulmonary emboli, full-dose heparin.

Weaning requires special skill. Patients are weaned flat in bed when they are alert, cooperative, and willing. No simple rule can be followed. Short T-tube periods off the respirator are best. Use of accessory neck muscle is encouraged. All muscular resources must be mobilized.

Personal hygiene, psychologic support, and management of the family are crucial. Nowhere in medicine are skills in human understanding more necessary.

As soon as possible, an uncuffed metal (silver) Jackson tracheostomy is used. This allows for talking with each inspiration. Lung and thoracic impedance is low, and air fills lungs and larynx readily. Thus, communication is possible. Ability to talk is known as the "great day" in the lives of these patients and their family and friends.

The day of emancipation, however, is discharge home. Preparations for this are immense and parallel a military logistic operation. Now, reliable small and portable volume ventilators are used (see Chap. 19). Two devices, suction equipment, and emergency supplies cost approximately $8000.

This brief description of care only touches on the challenges, frustrations, and despair that surround this form of respiratory care. The rewards in many cases are immense, however. In a recent series, 49 of 98 consecutive patients survived and were discharged home. Many have led productive and reasonably happy lives afterward.

This chapter is one of the most difficult in terms of capturing the drama, details of care, and methods of rehabilitation of a subject applicable to most acute care hospitals. Certainly, the immediate stages of care will be required for all forms of trauma in most community hospitals. Long-term definitive and rehabilitative care will be required in teaching hospitals. This is most likely to be necessary in the case of intra-abdominal sepsis with respiratory failure, major burns, or high cord trauma.

REFERENCES

1. Harman, E., and Lillington, G.: Pulmonary risk factors in surgery. Med. Clin. North Am., *63:*1289, 1979.
2. Dery, R., Pelletier, J., Jacques, A., Clauet, M., and House, J.: Alveolar collapse induced by denitrogenation. Can. Anaesth. Soc. J., *12:*531, 1965.
3. Baxter, W.D., and Levine, R.S.: An evaluation of intermittent positive pressure breathing in the prevention of postoperative pulmonary complications. Arch. Surg. (Chicago), *98:*795, 1969.
4. Van de Water, J.M., Watring, W.G., Linton, L.A., Murphy, M., and Byron, R.L.: Prevention of postoperative pulmonary complications. Surg. Gynecol. Obstet., *135:*229, 1972.
5. Oldenburg, F.A., Dolovich, M.B., Montgomery, J.M., and Newhouse, M.T.: Effects of postural drainage, exercise and cough on mucus clearance in chronic bronchitis. Am. Rev. Resp. Dis., *120:*739, 1979.
6. Pavia, D., Bateman, J.R.B., Sheahan, N.F., and Clark, S.W.: Clearance of lung secretions in patients with chronic bronchitis: Effects of terbutaline and ipatropium bronchial aerosols. Eur. J. Resp. Dis., *61:*245, 1980.
7. Burke, J.F., Pontoppidan, H., and Welch, C.E.: High output respiratory failure—an important cause of death ascribed to peritonitis or ileus. Ann. Surg., *158:*581, 1963.
8. Gravelyn, T.R., and Weg, J.G.: Respiratory rate as an indicator of acute respiratory dysfunction. JAMA, *244:*1123, 1980.
9. Adriani, J., Zepernick, R., Harmon, W., and Hiern, B.: Iatrogenic pulmonary edema in surgical patients. Surgery, *61:*183, 1967.
10. Cook, C.D., Mead, J., Schreiner, G.L., Frank, N.R., and Craig, J.M.: Pulmonary mechanics during induced pulmonary edema in anesthetized dogs. J. Appl. Physiol., *14:*177, 1959.
11. Klineberg, P.J., Geer, R.T., Hirsh, R.A., and Aukburg, S.J.: Early extubation after coronary bypass graft surgery. Crit. Care Med., *5:*272, 1977.
12. Prakash, O., Jonson, B., Meis, S., Bos, E., Hugenholtz, P.G., Nauta, J., and Hekman, W.: Criteria for early extubation after intracardiac surgery in adults. Anesth. Analg., *56:*703, 1977.
13. Quasha, A.L., Noeber, N., Feeley, T.W., Ullyot, D.J., and Roizen, M.F.: Postoperative respiratory care: A controlled trial of early extubation following coronary-artery bypass grafting. Anesthesiology, *52:*135, 1980.
14. Ashbaugh, D.G., Peters, G.N., Halgrimson, C.G., Owens, J.C., and Waddell, W.R.: Chest trauma. Arch. Surg. (Chicago), *95:*546, 1967.
15. Ginsberg, R.J., and Kostin, R.F.: New approaches to the management of flail chest. Can. Med. Assoc. J., *19:*116, 1977.
16. Phillips, Y.Y., Lonigan, R.M., and Joyner, L.R.: A simple technique for managing a bronchopleural fistula while maintaining positive pressure ventilation. Crit. Care Med., *7:*351, 1979.
17. Perel, A., Olshvang, D., Eimerl, D., Katzenelson, R., and Cotev, S.,: The variable effect of PEEP in acute respiratory failure associated with multiple trauma. J. Trauma, *18:*218, 1978.
18. Foley, F.D., Moncrief, J.A., and Mason, A.D.: Pathology of the lung in fatally burned patients. Ann. Surg., *167:*251, 1968.
19. Feller, I., Tholen, D., and Cornell, R.G.: Improvements in burn care, 1965–1979. JAMA, *244:*2074, 1980.
20. Sinha, R.P., Ducker, T.B., and Perot, P.L.: Arterial oxygenation findings and significance in central nervous system trauma patients. JAMA, *224:*1258, 1973.

Chapter 15

COMPLICATIONS AND INTERCURRENT PROBLEMS IN THE MANAGEMENT OF ACUTE RESPIRATORY FAILURE

By Thomas L. Petty

As experience is gained in the management of acute respiratory failure, an awareness of many associated problems develops. When patients survive beyond the acute phase of respiratory failure, a variety of problems involving almost every organ system may develop to delay complete recovery. Complications may arise, of course, in any severely ill patient regardless of the clinical problem; however, the complications associated with acute respiratory failure and its management have been of such magnitude and scope that it is worthwhile to devote a chapter to this subject. A clear delineation between problems that are directly associated with acute respiratory failure (i.e., the clinical manifestations of hypoxia, hypercapnia, and associated acid-base abnormalities) and clinical conditions properly called complications is difficult and frequently a matter of semantics. This chapter presents a review of the important effects of acute respiratory failure and its management on other organ systems and is organized to alert the physician to the major complications that may plague the clinical course of the patient. It has been our experience that treating the precipitating event of the respiratory failure and correcting the hypoxemia and hypercapnia are frequently easy matters compared with dealing with complications. The major complications to be discussed are tabulated in Table 15-1.

TABLE 15-1. Complications Occurring in Respiratory Failure

- I. Cardiovascular complications
  - A. Hypotension
  - B. Hypertension
  - C. Congestive failure
  - D. Low cardiac output during mechanical ventilation
  - E. Cardiac arrhythmias
  - F. Cardiac arrest
  - G. Pulmonary thromboembolism
- II. Gastrointestinal complications
  - A. Ulceration with bleeding and/or obstruction
  - B. Ileus, gastric dilatation
  - C. Fecal impaction
- III. Electrolyte and fluid abnormalities
  - A. Acid-base imbalance
  - B. Alkalemia
  - C. Hypokalemia, hypochloremia
  - D. Water retention
- IV. Neurologic complications
  - A. Mental changes, delirium
  - B. Motor changes
  - C. Local neurologic signs
  - D. Seizures
- V. Pulmonary complications
  - A. Upper airway obstruction
  - B. Tracheal and laryngeal injury
  - C. Pneumothorax, pneumomediastinum
  - D. Super-infections
  - E. Oxygen toxicity
- VI. Other major organ complications
  - A. Hepatic
  - B. Renal
  - C. Hematologic

CARDIOVASCULAR COMPLICATIONS

Cardiovascular complications head the list of problems associated with acute respiratory failure because they may rapidly be fatal. Marked hypercapnia with acidemia can produce extreme vasodilatation by means of local action on blood vessels and thereby create hypotension.

Severe hypoxemia is well known to suppress cardiac output. Hypotension following rapid lowering of the P_{CO_2} has been reported by others, and has been seen on several occasions in our patients.[1,2] When hypotension occurs during respiratory failure, one must consider many possible causes, including myocardial infarction, pulmonary thromboembolism, adrenal insufficiency, sepsis, gastrointestinal hemorrhage, other causes of hypovolemia, severe electrolyte abnormalities, and an adverse reaction to drugs. All these problems have been encountered in our patients at one time or another. Milder forms of hypercapnia can cause a reflex vasoconstriction and hypertension. It is not uncommon to observe systemic hypertension during the time a patient is being "weaned" from a respirator, if moderate degrees of hypercapnia develop.

Cor pulmonale is a well-known complication of chronic lung disease, and the occurrence of repeated episodes of congestive heart failure in patients with chronic bronchitis, chronic hypoxia, and erythrocythemia has been stressed.[3] Both hypoxia and increased hydrogen ion concentration cause pulmonary vasoconstriction and a rise in pulmonary artery pressure.[4] Consequently, correcting reversible features in any form of pulmonary involvement such as infection, bronchospasm, hypoxemia, hypercapnia, and acidemia can often decrease vasoconstriction, lower pulmonary pressure, and thereby improve hemodynamics. Patients who suffer their first episode of acute respiratory failure may also have their first occurrence of congestive heart failure.

Low cardiac output may occur immediately after a patient is placed on a mechanical respirator owing to impairment of venous return by the elevated transpulmonary pressure. Changes in cardiac output are quite variable in patients receiving mechanical respiratory assistance and depend on the underlying lung disease and the type of breathing pattern which is used. Modifications of the pressure-wave form such as inflation hold and the use of positive end-expiratory pressure (see Chaps. 5 and 8) may impair cardiac output, but this is uncommon in the adult respiratory distress syndrome.[5] At times, ideal ventilation must be sacrificed somewhat to allow for adequate cardiac output by shortening inspiration time and by minimizing transpulmonary pressures by employing lower tidal volumes. When a mechanical ventilator produces profound effects on cardiac output, a borderline hypovolemic state may be present. It has been a common observation that placing the patient in the Trendelenburg position or adding fluid volume replacement will frequently correct this problem.

Cardiac arrhythmias have been a very common complication in patients with respiratory failure. Electrocardiographic monitoring during the acute phase of respiratory failure for all patients, especially during mechanical ventilation, is as important as it is in the Coronary Care Unit!

Tables 15-2 and 15-3 review our early experience with cardiac arrhythmias occurring during respiratory failure in patients with chronic airway obstruction in which 848 electrocardiograms were reviewed from a series of 70 consecutive patients. All these patients had had arterial oxygen tensions less than 59 mm Hg at some time during management. Arrhythmias occurred in 61% of patients and in 55% of admissions.[6] Simple sinus tachycardia occurred in 20 patients, 9 of whom expired. Sinus tachycardia with PVC occurred in 25

TABLE 15-2. Prevalence of "Major" Supraventricular and Ventricular Arrhythmias Associated with Acute Respiratory Failure of CAO

Arrhythmia	*By Patient*	*By Admission*
"Major" supraventricular	23/70	38/148
Ventricular	20/70	24/148
"Major" supraventricular and/or ventricular	33/70	54/148

patients, 12 of whom expired. Atrial or ventricular tachyarrhythmias occurred in 20, 14 of whom expired. All 20 were receiving digitalis.

One cannot help being impressed by the implication that digitalis can be deleterious in this clinical setting. It is worth reiterating that in the patient with chronic airway obstruction, cor pulmonale, hypoxemia, and acidemia, the likelihood of digitalis intoxication is enhanced. These data are included in this edition for background. Today all critically ill patients receive continuous electrocardiographic monitoring in modern intensive care units.

Ventricular fibrillation is known to occur after a rapid lowering of the P_{CO_2}.[7,8] Several episodes of unexplained ventricular fibrillation and sudden death were likely to be associated with a too-rapid lowering of P_{CO_2} in our series. As improvement occurs during mechani-

TABLE 15-3. Prevalence of Arrhythmias Associated with Acute Respiratory Failure of CAO

	By Patient (Total = 70)	*By Admission (Total = 148)*
Normal sinus rhythm	49	82
Sinus tachycardia	43	79
Sinus bradycardia	2	2
Sinus arrhythmia	3	3
Ectopic atrial pacemaker	9	13
Wandering atrial pacemaker	5	5
Atrial tachycardia	11	19
Atrial flutter	7	8
Atrial fibrillation	6	6
Multifocal atrial tachycardia	12	17
AV junctional arrhythmia	5	5
Ventricular bigeminy	5	7
AV dissociation	4	5
Idioventricular rhythm	4	4
Ventricular tachycardia	4	4
Cardiac arrest	15	15

cal ventilation, the increased physiologic dead space associated with disease may rapidly diminish, leading to alveolar hyperventilation. When pressure-cycled ventilators are used, cycling pressure settings that were originally required to maintain an adequate P_{CO_2} may now become excessive, and there may be a sudden, rapid fall in the arterial P_{CO_2}. Prevention of this emphasizes the need for frequent monitoring. Use of volume-cycled ventilators minimizes this problem.

The management of cardiac arrhythmias lies predominantly in the correction of blood gas abnormalities and the discontinuation of use of cardiac stimulants such as sympathomimetic amines and aminophylline.[8] Intravenous injection of lidocaine (50 to 100 mg) followed by continuous infusion is useful in managing premature ventricular contractions, which may be the precursor of potentially fatal tachyarrhythmias or cardiac arrest. Electrolyte replacement is also required (see Chap. 6).

In the digitalized patient with a predilection for hypoxemia and potassium depletion, digitalis intoxication is always a threat.

The high incidence of pulmonary thrombosis or embolism found at autopsy in patients with advanced chronic airway obstruction has been reported from this institution.[9] Pulmonary thromboembolism has also been found in a significant number of patients dying during respiratory failure and has been evident on clinical grounds in a number of patients who have survived an episode of acute respiratory failure.[10] Diagnosing pulmonary thromboembolism during life is difficult since the classic clinical signs and symptoms of pulmonary infarction are rarely present. Electrocardiograms, chest roentgenograms, lung scans, and enzyme studies often show poor correlation with the extent of pulmonary thromboembolism found at autopsy. Clinical-pathologic correlations in deaths occurring during respiratory failure have indicated that unexplained tachycardia, dyspnea, or mild fever is often the only clue to thromboembolism during life. Such evidence is an indication for intravenous heparin therapy in patients suspected of having pulmonary thromboembolism. However, this is not without significant hazard because a substantial number of patients develop spontaneous retroperitoneal and cerebral hemorrhage during well-controlled heparin therapy. The diagnosis and management of pulmonary thromboembolism during respiratory insufficiency and failure remains one of our most difficult and frustrating problems. Ventilation and perfusion scans are helpful, but they may be abnormal owing to the presenting pulmonary problem, such as COPD, pneumonia, or chest trauma. Angiography remains the "gold standard" of diagnosis.

Figure 15-1 shows an extensive flank ecchymosis in a patient with respiratory failure who had evidence of pulmonary thromboembolism. Heparin therapy was well controlled, and no trauma oc-

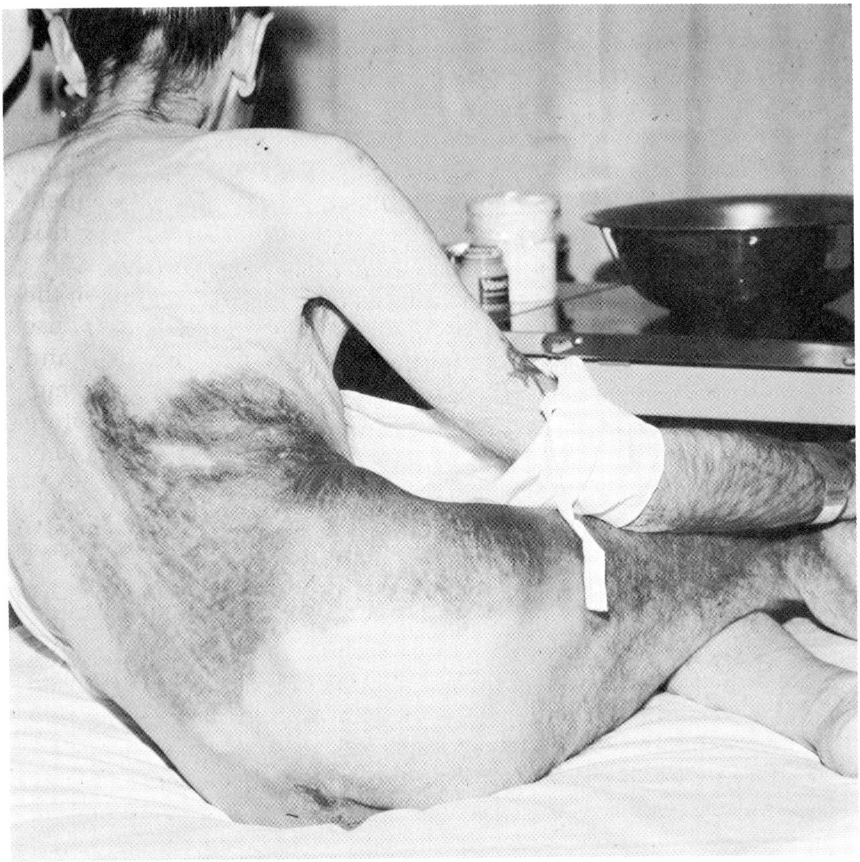

Fig. 15-1. Extensive flank ecchymosis after a spontaneous retroperitoneal hemorrhage in a patient receiving heparin. See text for explanation.

curred. The patient suddenly developed signs of retroperitoneal hemorrhage and hypovolemia. With reversal of heparin activity with protamine and blood replacement, his condition stabilized. Several days later, the ecchymosis appeared in the flank.

Acute myocardial infarction during acute respiratory failure management has occurred on occasion, as it does in any clinical situation. Heart failure and associated arrhythmias present additional problems.

GASTROINTESTINAL COMPLICATIONS

The association of peptic ulcer in patients with chronic airway obstruction is well known. During the stress of respiratory failure, peptic ulceration complicated by hemorrhage or obstruction, or both, is common. Profound hemorrhage which requires massive blood replacement, may develop in patients with no prior history of peptic disease.

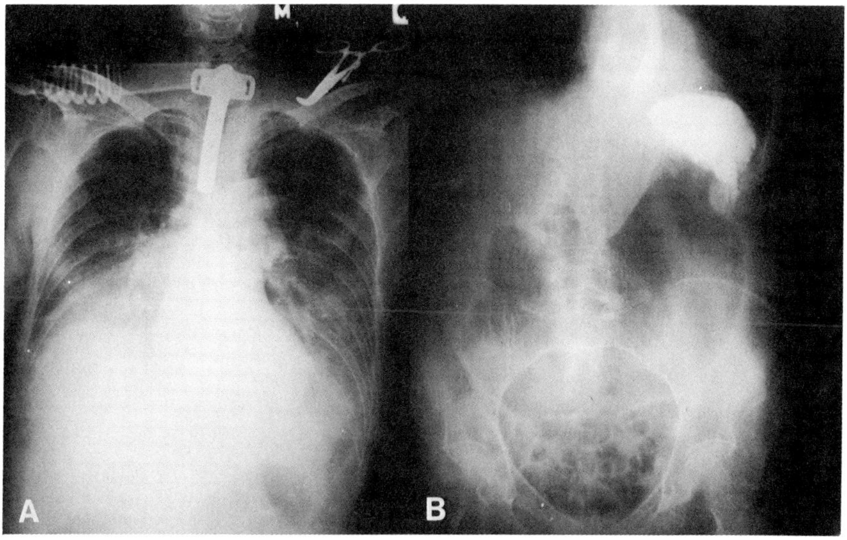

Fig. 15-2. Chest and abdominal x-ray films of patient with respiratory failure receiving mechanical ventilation. Note dilated stomach.

Adynamic ileus is frequently encountered with or without associated hypokalemia. Gastric dilatation also occurs in patients who are receiving mechanical ventilation, possibly due to esophageal peristalsis due to the inflated balloon in the adjacent trachea. Figure 15-2 shows the roentgenogram of a patient suffering respiratory failure and receiving mechanical ventilation. This patient developed extreme gastric dilatation suddenly. She also had the additional complication of gastrointestinal hemorrhage and outlet obstruction. Gastric dilatation is best managed by means of a nasogastric tube and intermittent suction. Care must be exercised to avoid hypokalemia and hypochloremia caused by excessive gastric suctioning.

Fecal impaction of the most severe form, extending retrograde to the right colon, has occurred in two patients suffering respiratory failure as a consequence of the Guillain-Barré syndrome (see Chap. 13). As a result, great care is taken to avoid this problem in paralyzed patients; dioctyl sodium sulfosuccinate (Colace), a stool softener, is useful in preventing this problem.

ELECTROLYTE AND FLUID ABNORMALITIES

Any combination of acid-base imbalance may occur either acutely or chronically during the recovery phase of respiratory failure (see Chap. 6). It is worth stressing that severe alkalemia associated with potassium and chloride losses may occur after assisted ventilation and can precipitate serious cardiovascular and neurologic complications.

Fluid retention *without* evidence of cardiac failure in patients managed with prolonged mechanical ventilation has been the subject of considerable interest.[11] This problem has been associated with radiologic evidence of pulmonary edema, significant weight gain, reduction in pulmonary compliance, and impaired oxygen transport. It has been speculated that the causes for this are relative water overload, an increase in antidiuretic hormone activity, or subclinical cardiac failure.[11] Other investigators have shown a precapillary arteriolar leak of fluid thought to be due to a variety of insults to the lungs.[12] We have seen similar problems in patients with respiratory failure and mechanical ventilation. A review of the details of fluid administration often reveals that intravenous therapy has been *excessive*. Our policy for patients receiving mechanical ventilation is to maintain a state of *slight* underhydration by watching intake and output closely and following daily weights whenever possible. The use of intravenous saline solution is kept to the barest minimum because there is evidence of sodium retention during mechanical ventilation.[13] When volume replacement is needed, colloid preparations or whole blood were once preferred, since it was believed that pulmonary edema could be diminished. No convincing study has shown that this is true. This crystalloid fluid replacement is usually employed unless the basic problem is blood loss. It should be remembered that the humidification systems used on some mechanical respirators can add a significant amount of water by absorption through the lungs. Intake and output values must be judged with this in mind.

NEUROLOGIC COMPLICATIONS

A variety of neurologic abnormalities occurring during respiratory failure have been discussed by a number of authors.[15–19] Changes in mentation such as restlessness, lassitude, drowsiness, forgetfulness, personality changes, confusion, disorientation, delirium, or coma have all been described. A close correlation between the state of consciousness and the arterial P_{O_2} and P_{CO_2} has been reported.[19] Motor changes with generalized or localized weakness, tremors, twitching, asterixis, myoclonic jerks, gross clonic movements, generalized convulsions, and flaccid immobility may occur in any combination. Localized and focal neurologic signs may develop, such as muscle palsies and abnormal pupillary reflexes.[17,18] Differentiating the neurologic complications of respiratory failure from a space-occupying lesion or intracerebral bleeding can be difficult, but is important in management. Subjecting patients to unnecessary diagnostic neurologic studies can increase morbidity and mortality by interfering with the proper treatment of respiratory failure. Consequently, the physician managing respiratory failure, as well as his neurologic consultant, must be aware of the spectrum of neurologic complications which can occur in this setting. Watchful waiting and control of the blood gas abnormalities are often the approach that must be taken in such patients, even those with profound neurologic findings. Clinical judgment must dictate whether vigorous diagnostic neurologic studies need to be performed. In our experience, intracranial catastrophes during respiratory failure are rare, except in patients receiving anticoagulant drugs, although profound neurologic abnormalities are frequent, particularly early in management.

Several experiences in our series are worth relating. We have observed a few patients who tolerate profound hypoxemia and severe hypercapnia well during the acute state with little change in mentation and few neurologic signs. Many hours after the blood gas abnormalities have been corrected, the patient may deteriorate with almost continuous seizure activity and focal neurologic findings. This cerebral catastrophe is usually followed by death. Careful postmortem brain examination has recorded nothing more than mild to moderate cerebral edema with no focal lesions or vascular changes.[10]

Serious neurologic signs and seizure activity can result from mechanical hyperventilation.[20] Figure 15-3 presents such a situation with pH and P_{CO_2} changes outlined.

RENAL FAILURE

The development of coexisting renal failure from any cause greatly compromises chances of survival.[14] In a large series, 80% of patients with coexisting respiratory and renal failure died.[14] Predisposing factors were gastrointestinal bleeding, sepsis with associated shock, drug-induced nephrotoxicity (aminoglycosides), and hypotension from any cause.[14] Urinary output should be maintained with adequate fluid and potent diuretics, but not at the cost of aggravating pulmonary edema. Tradeoffs occur. The respiratory-renal-circulatory interrelationships are complex. Hemodynamic, fluid, and urinary flow parameters are mandatory in the most complex situations (see Chap. 5).

Case History. A patient with severe chronic airway obstruction was admitted to the hospital with respiratory insufficiency and hypoxemia, but with the P_{CO_2} only slightly above normal. During the first day, she appeared to improve with conservative management. On the second day her respiratory efforts fatigued, and she lapsed into a coma. Before coma, the arterial blood gases showed a rising P_{CO_2} and falling pH. At the moment coma developed, physicians were too busy with resuscitation to draw an arterial blood sample. However, it is estimated, from earlier determinations, that her P_{CO_2} was 90 mm Hg. (She had been receiving supplemental oxygen.) The patient was placed on a mechanical ventilator,

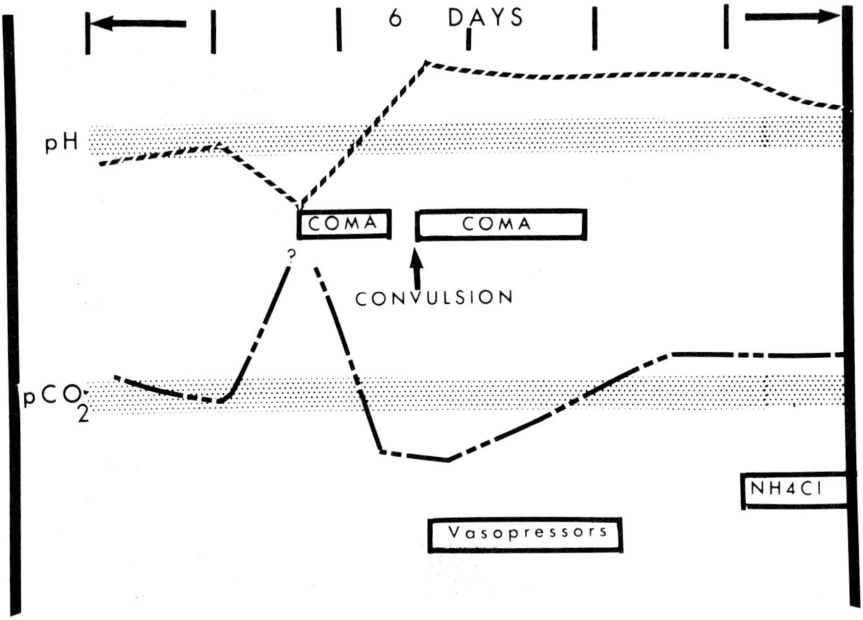

Fig. 15-3. Sudden drop in Pco_2 and rising pH after institution of mechanical ventilation with resultant respiratory alkalemia. Stippled areas denote normal pH and Pco_2 level. See text for explanation.

resulting in rapid fall of the Pco_2 and rise of the pH, at which time she awoke from her coma. A short time later, she began to have convulsions, then lapsed back into a coma with complete flaccid immobility. It can be seen in Figure 15-3 that the Pco_2 had been reduced below normal levels (Pco_2, 29) and the pH had risen to alkalemic levels (pH, 7.53). This occurred because of unanticipated ease of mechanical ventilation so that hyperventilation was produced. (The goal is to strive for normal pH and not necessarily normal Pco_2.) At the time the patient lapsed into coma, she also became hypotensive and required vasopressors for a short period. The minute ventilation with the mechanical ventilator was decreased, and the Pco_2 was allowed to elevate slightly above normal. By this time the patient had developed potassium and chloride deficits and remained alkalemic. Potassium chloride and ammonium chloride were infused intravenously. Figure 15-3 shows that the pH returned to near normal values after NH_4Cl was added. Mental status improved rapidly, and the patient awoke.

Comment. This case represents several problems: overventilation with neurologic as well as cardiovascular consequences, respiratory alkalosis with alkalemia, and the need for potassium chloride replacement and occasionally the correction of hydrogen ion deficit with ammonium chloride, which is rarely used today. Hydrogen ion replacement with dilute HCl infused into central venous lines is more commonly applied to this kind of clinical situation.

PULMONARY COMPLICATIONS

In addition to the respiratory failure itself, complications involving the pulmonary system may occur.

Early in our experience, we used tracheostomy tubes with latex balloons that slipped over the tracheostomy tube like a sleeve. Upper airway obstruction produced by herniation of the cuff over the lumen of the tube accounted for three deaths early in our experience. Figure 15-4 shows one of these tracheostomy tubes after it was removed from a patient. The balloon is overinflated, distorted, and herniated in such a manner that it occludes the orifice of the tube. The patient from whom this was removed suddenly developed respiratory distress and could not be ventilated. Before the cause of obstruction was realized the patient became hypoxemic, and cardiac arrest occurred. Mucus plugs can also occlude the tracheostomy or endotracheal tube and prevent ventilation. It is important that all medical and nursing personnel be aware of these possibilities; if the slightest indication of upper airway obstruction occurs, the cuff should be deflated immediately, and the tracheostomy or endotracheal tube should be replaced. Tracheostomies and care of the airway are discussed in Chapter 2, including the indications, management, and complications. The most common complications of tracheostomy we have experienced have been fatal hemorrhage from erosion of the tracheostomy tube into the innominate artery, tracheal stenosis, and erosion into the mediastinum.[21,22] Fortunately, these complications have been few, even though our use of the tracheostomy is extensive. Complications are minimized by the frequent changing of the tube (approximately every 48 hours) and use of minimal amounts of air for balloon inflation.

A great deal has been written about the problems of prolonged endotracheal intubation.[23-27] Complications of endotracheal intubation include laryngeal edema, ulceration, granulomas, membrane formation, and fibrosis (see Chap. 2). Special problems can occur from tissue reaction due to the use of tubes composed of polyvinyl chloride.[28,29] Endotracheal tube design has improved in the past few years. Further advances are likely. Our contemporary experience with both endotracheal tubes and tracheostomies has recently been published.[30] Much of this experience is cited in Chapter 2.

When using mechanical respirators, there is always the risk that the rupture of a bleb on the surface of the lung may lead to pneumothorax with rapidly developing tension which may become life-threatening. Diagnosis must be made quickly and the tension immediately released by placement of chest tubes (see Chap. 14). Occasionally, tension pneumothorax may be bilateral; unless there is immediate release of pressure by the placement of chest tubes or

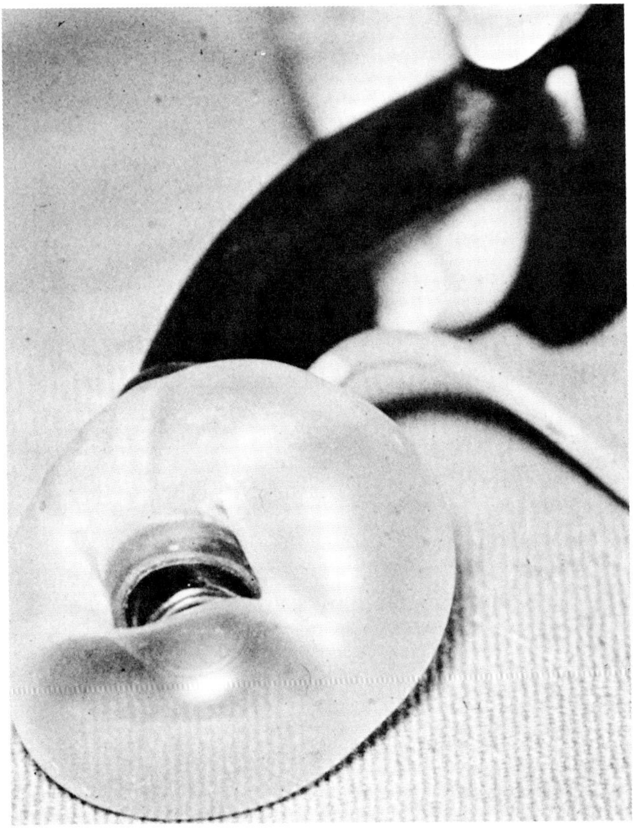

Fig. 15-4. Tracheostomy tube removed from a patient who developed sudden upper airway obstruction. Note that latex balloon includes lumen. This type of tube is no longer used, and many of these problems have been obviated. See Chapter 2 for complete discussion of tracheostomy and endotracheal tube complications.

multiple needles, the result will be fatal. Once the chest tubes have been placed and the tension reduced, mechanical ventilation can be continued even at high pressures, if necessary. We have successfully ventilated patients for prolonged periods after they have developed large bronchopleural fistulas secondary to rupture of a bleb. We have had certain patients in whom a large portion of the tidal volume was lost through a bronchopleural fistula, but ventilator adjustments and increasing tidal volumes could still allow adequate ventilation and oxygen transport. Therefore, the development of a pneumothorax which can be successfully managed with the placement of chest tubes, connected to underwater seal or suction, is not a reason to cease ventilation.

The hazard of superinfection with gram-negative necrotizing pneumonias arising from contamination by respirators which employ mainstream nebulizers has gained much interest in recent years (see Chap. 14).[31] The organism most commonly encountered is *Pseudomonas aeruginosa*; however, a wide spectrum of gram-negative organisms has been involved. A statement regarding the significance of superinfection is important. Patients with endotracheal or tracheostomy tubes frequently develop *colonization* of the airways with a wide variety of gram-negative organisms. This is especially true of any patient who is receiving antibiotics. It is our belief that routine cultures during antibiotic therapy are important in surveillance, but small growths of pathogenic organisms do not require the institution of an antibiotic unless there is clear-cut clinical evidence of secondary infection such as fever, leukocytosis, or new pulmonary infiltrates. Most generally, low growths of organisms indicate colonization but not necessarily tissue invasion.

The technique of obtaining bacteriologic specimens from patients who have developed evidence of secondary infection is of great importance. Collecting sputum samples by suctioning the lower respiratory tract and catching the sample in a sputum trap is one technique (see Chap. 7). However, we have found it necessary to perform a needle aspiration of the infiltrate on certain occasions to identify correctly the organism invading the lung parenchyma.

Oxygen toxicity has become a popular subject (see Chaps. 3 and 8). The lung has a limited response to insult or injury. The pathologic findings associated with oxygen toxicity are, in our opinion, similar to those found after other insults to the lung. Extensive aspiration, contused lung, fat emboli, massive fluid overload, or oxygen toxicity can all have similar pathologic features. Rapidly developing interstitial fibrosis has been thought to be an indication of oxygen toxicity. However, we have seen interstitial fibrosis develop in 10 to 14 days in association with nonspecific inflammation in patients who have not received high oxygen concentrations.[10] Consequently, interpreting pathologic changes of the lung noted at autopsy as resulting from toxicity, simply because a patient has received oxygen, ignores the fact that a variety of insults can give the same pathologic picture. Our policy, however, is to use respirators with precise oxygen control in order to deliver the lowest possible inspired oxygen concentration that will provide arterial oxygen tensions in the 65 to 75 mm Hg range (see Chap. 4). At no time are patients given more oxygen than is absolutely necessary. However, if a patient requires 100% oxygen to maintain arterial blood gases compatible with life, it is provided for as long a period as needed. At the present time, it is fair to say that all the factors involved in oxygen toxicity and its precise recognition have not been delineated.

The popular and necessary use of flow-directed pulmonary artery catheters has been associated with expected complications. Infection resulting in bacteremia and septicemia and fatal pulmonary hemorrhage have been described.[32,33] All medical advances have associated complications. Judgment in the selection of each invasive technique is the best method of minimizing this problem.

OTHER COMPLICATIONS

In an older review of the complications of acute respiratory failure, Asmundsson and Kilburn commented on their experience with hepatic and renal abnormalities.[34] Refsum has reported that patients with pulmonary insufficiency and profound arterial hypoxemia had elevated SGOT, SGPT, and LDH levels and central lobular liver cell necrosis.[35] We have seen transient and mild elevations of liver enzymes during acute respiratory failure, but extensive liver cell necrosis has not been a problem in our series.[10]

An association between poor survival and anemia in chronic obstructive pulmonary disease has been reported, but we have not been able to associate anemia with acute respiratory failure unless hemorrhage occurs.[33]

Another report from this institution has indicated a poor prognosis in patients with chronic airway obstructive pulmonary disease who had secondary erythrocytosis.[36] Phlebotomy was frequently employed in patients with secondary erythrocytosis and hematocrits above 60%. Furthermore, patients with chronic airway obstruction and erythrocythemia may have a higher incidence of pulmonary thromboembolism.[36] However, precise correlations between hematocrit levels per se and thromboembolism are not evident in our series.

THE "RESPIRATOR-BOUND" PATIENT

Not exactly a complication of management, but a feared outcome of care, is the patient who survives the initial episode of acute respiratory failure but who remains dependent on the respirator to provide adequate maintenance of oxygenation and ventilation. Fortunately, this problem is uncommon; our data indicate that for more than 18 years, approximately 75% of patients have survived and have returned to their home environment. Those who do not survive usually succumb in a short time to acute respiratory failure, complications, or intercurrent problems such as infection. In 18 years' experience, only 3 patients became totally dependent on respirators. One, a 55-year-old woman with CAO, lived on a respirator for 8 months in a nursing home, but with relative comfort once nurses became acquainted with her care and needs. The second, a 26-year-old man with congenital hypogammaglobulinemia and repeated chest infections, lived at home with a respirator providing ventilation through a tracheostomy tube for 6 months with care provided by his mother. The third case is described in Chapter 20. The success in weaning patients with minimized respiratory reserve is a tribute to the nurses and therapists of the respiratory care unit.

SUMMARY

Complications and intercurrent problems occurring during the management of acute respiratory failure are important; the prevention, early identification, and management of the compounding problem are essential for a successful outcome.

REFERENCES

1. Miller, F.A., Brown, E.B., Buckley, J.J., Van Bergen, F.H., and Varco, R.L.: Respiratory acidosis: its relationship to cardiac function and other physiologic mechanisms. Surgery, *32:*171, 1952.
2. Young, W.G., Jr., Sealy, W.C., and Harris, J.S.: The role of intracellular and extracellular electrolytes in cardiac arrhythmias produced by prolonged hypercapnia. Surgery, *36:*636, 1954.
3. Mitchell, R.S., Vincent, T.N., Ryan, S., and Filley, G.F.: Chronic obstructive bronchopulmonary disease: IV. The clinical and physiological differentiation of chronic bronchitis and emphysema. Am. J. Med. Sci., *247:*513, 1964.
4. Harvey, R.M.: The influence of hydrogen ion in the control of pulmonary artery pressures in patients with obstructive diseases of the lungs. Med. Thorac., *22:*108, 1965.
5. Lutch, J.S., and Murray, J.F.: Continuous positive-pressure ventilation: effects on systemic oxygen transport and tissue oxygenation. Ann. Intern. Med., *76:*193, 1972.
6. Hudson, L.D., Kurt, T.L., Petty, T.L., and Genton, E.: Arrhythmias associated with acute respiratory failure with chronic airway obstruction. Chest, *63:*661, 1973.
7. Brown, E.B., Jr., and Miller, F.: Ventricular fibrillation following a rapid fall in alveolar carbon dioxide concentration. Am. J. Physiol., *169:*56, 1952.
8. Sealy, W.C., Young, W.G., Jr., and Harris, J.S.: Studies on cardiac arrest: The relationship of hypercapnia to ventricular fibrillation. J. Thorac. Cardiov. Surg., *28:*447, 1954.
9. Ryan, S.F.: Pulmonary embolism and thrombosis in chronic obstructive emphysema. Am. J. Pathol., *43:*767, 1963.
10. Petty, T.L., and Bigelow, D.B.: Unpublished data.
11. Sladen, A., Laver, M.D., and Pontoppidan, H.: Pulmonary complications and water retention in prolonged mechanical ventilation. N. Engl. J. Med., *279:*448, 1968.
12. Martin, A.M., Jr., Simmons, R.L., and Heisterkamp, C.A., III: Respiratory insufficiency in combat casualties: I. Pathologic changes in the lungs of patients dying of wounds. Ann. Surg., *170:*30, 1969.
13. Gett, P.M., Jones, E.S., and Shephard, G.F.: Pulmonary oedema associated with sodium retention during ventilator treatment. Br. J. Anaesth., *43:*460, 1971.
14. Kraman, S., Khan, F., Putel, S., and Seriff, N.: Renal failure in the respiratory intensive care unit. Crit. Care Med., *7:*263, 1979.
15. Sieker, H.O., and Hickam, J.B.: Carbon dioxide intoxication: the clinical syndrome, its etiology and management with particular reference to the use of mechanical respirators. Medicine, *35:*389, 1956.
16. Hamilton, J.C., and Gross, N.J.: Unusual neurological and cardiovascular complications of respiratory failure. Br. Med. J., *2:*1092, 1963.
17. Miller, A., Bader, R.A., and Bader, M.E.: The neurologic syndrome due to marked hypercapnia with papilledema. Am. J. Med., *33:*309, 1962.
18. Pitt, B., Alkaloy, I., Sweet, R., and Stein, M.: Respiratory failure with focal neurological signs. Arch. Intern. Med., *115:*714, 1965.
19. Refsum, H.E.: Relationship between state of consciousness and arterial hypoxemia and hypercapnia in patients with respiratory insufficiency breathing air. Clin. Sci., *25:*361, 1963.
20. Rotheram, E.B., Safar, P., and Robin, E.D.: Central nervous system disorder during mechanical ventilation in chronic pulmonary disease. JAMA, *189:*993, 1964.

21. Ivankovic, A.D., Thomasen, S., and Rattenberg, C.C.: Fatal hemorrhage from the innominate artery after tracheostomy. Br. J. Anaesth., *41:*450, 1969.
22. Sara, C.: Histological changes in the trachea and bronchi with tracheostomy. Med. J. Aust., *12:*1174, 1967.
23. Donnelly, W.H.: Histopathology of endotracheal intubation. Arch. Pathol. (Chicago), *88:*511, 1969.
24. Schlorf, R.A., and Duvall, A.J., III: Post-intubation granuloma of the larynx. Minn. Med., *52:*717, 1969.
25. Harrison, G.A., and Toukin, J.P.: Prolonged (therapeutic) endotracheal intubation. Br. J. Anaesth., *40:*241, 1968.
26. Hedden, M., Ersoz, C.J., Donnelly, W.H., and Safar, P.: Laryngotracheal damage after prolonged use of orotracheal tubes in adults. JAMA, *207:*703, 1969.
27. Dixon, T.C., Sando, M.J.W., Bolton, J.M., and Gilligan, J.E.: A report of 342 cases of prolonged endotracheal intubation. Med. J. Aust., *2:*529, 1968.
28. Guess, W.L., and Stetson, J.B.: Tissue reactions to organotin-stabilized polyvinyl chloride (PVC) catheters. JAMA, *204:*624, 1968.
29. Rendell-Baker, L.: Hazards of prolonged intubation and tracheostomy equipment. JAMA, *204:*624, 1968.
30. Stauffer, J., Olson, D.E., and Petty, T.L.: Complications and consequences of endotracheal intubation and tracheostomy. (A prospective study of 150 critically ill adults.) Am. J. Med., *70:*65, 1981.
31. Reinarz, J.A., Pierce, A.K., Mays, B.B., and Sanford, J.P.: The potential role of inhalation therapy equipment in nosocomial pulmonary infection. J. Clin. Invest., *44:*831, 1965.
32. Michel, L., Marsh, M., McMichan, J.C., Southorn, P.A., and Brewer, N.S.: Infection of pulmonary artery catheters in critically ill patients. JAMA, *245:*1032, 1981.
33. Pape, L.A., Haffajee, C.I., Markis, J.E., Ockene, I.B., Paraskos, J.A., Dalen, J.E., and Alpert, J.S.: Fatal pulmonary hemorrhage after use of the flow-directed balloon tipped catheter. Ann. Intern. Med., *90:*344, 1979.
34. Asmundsson, T., and Kilburn, K.H.: Complications of acute respiratory failure. Ann. Intern. Med., *70:*487, 1969.
35. Refsum, H.E.: Arterial hypoxemia, serum activities of GO-T, GP-T and LDH and centrilobular liver cell necrosis in pulmonary insufficiency. Clin. Sci., *25:*369, 1963.
36. Mitchell, R.S., Webb, W.C., and Filley, G.F.: Chronic obstructive bronchopulmonary disease. III. Factors influencing prognosis. Am. Rev. Resp. Dis., *89:*878, 1964.

Section C

Special Problems of Respiratory Failure and the Young and Old

Chapter 16

PEDIATRIC PROBLEMS

By Ernest K. Cotton and Margo A. Pinney

In children, as well as in adults, respiratory care depends upon basic principles of physiology and pathology. Mature physiologic responses are established at birth, with differences residing in the anatomy of the airway. These differences in anatomy are essentially confined to three areas of the airway: support, size, and smooth muscle mass. These anatomic alterations account for the abruptness and severity of diseases involving the lung of infants and children. An example would be the response to hypoxia, which physiologically is identical in infants and adults. Because of the relative increase in smooth muscle mass in the pulmonary vascular bed of the infant, the resultant pulmonary hypertension is more pronounced.

In the treatment section, techniques that are unique for children are discussed, but treatments discussed elsewhere in this book are to be considered appropriate for children as well as adults.

ANATOMIC DIFFERENCES IN INFANTS AND CHILDREN

Until the age of three months, little smooth muscle is present in the airways, although an abundance of smooth muscle exists in the pulmonary vascular bed. This relationship results in a different timing of reactions than in the adult. Adults generally react with some airway signs while the infant reacts with abrupt respiratory and cardiac failure. The support of the airways is dependent upon surrounding structures. Cartilage is poorly developed before adolescence, resulting in a functional "airway malacia." Because of this airway instability, positioning of the head becomes important in premature infants or in infants with endotracheal or tracheostomy tubes. For example, if the head is positioned to one side, the stiff tube can obstruct with a resultant "ball-valve" effect. This "flabby airway" can modify well-established signs of obstruction in the airway, such as stridor and wheezing (Fig. 16-1).

Newborns are nasal breathers, and significant airway obstruction can occur with only nasal obstruction. The most obvious anatomic difference between children and adults is the airway size. The airway is smaller, but the number of conducting airways is the same as in the adult.

Peripheral airways are disproportionately narrow in the early years of life. A decrease in size of the small airways will have a greater effect on increasing the resistance to flow in the young infant than in the adult. Damage of small airways will have greater clinical consequence in the infant than in the adult, causing the infant to develop severe aspects of bronchiolitis. Moreover, the infant will develop more atelectasis than the adult because of lack of collateral ventilation.

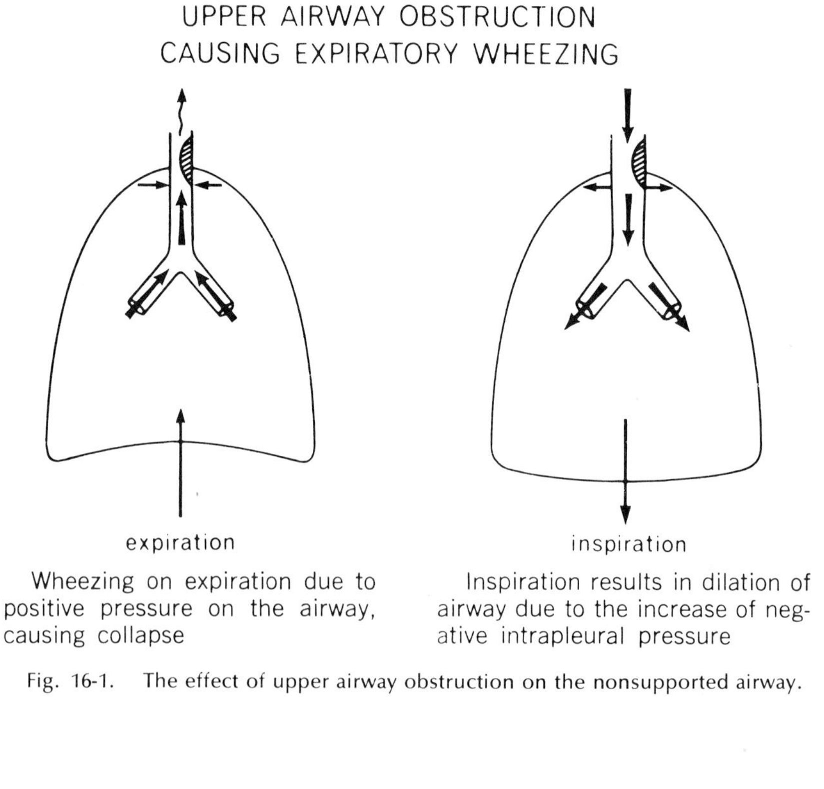

Fig. 16-1. The effect of upper airway obstruction on the nonsupported airway.

SPECIFIC RESPIRATORY PROBLEMS COMMON TO INFANTS AND CHILDREN

Hyaline Membrane Disease

General Considerations. Hyaline membrane disease (HMD) occurs mainly in infants born prematurely and is the expression of an immature lung whose small respiratory units inflate with difficulty and collapse between respiratory efforts.[1,2] HMD is characterized by increased pulmonary vascular resistance and decreased or absent surface-active substances, resulting in stiff lungs (loss of compliance). Widespread atelectasis of the lung and injury to the pulmonary parenchyma result. Vascular engorgement and hemorrhage are frequent. Hyaline membranes form from plasma clots composed of fibrin, other blood products, and cellular debris. Babies with severe disease who die within the first few hours of life may not show evidence of the membrane, although the rest of the pathologic process is consistent with the disease.

Clinical Findings: Symptoms and Signs. Retractions and expiratory grunting begin shortly after birth and become progressively more severe.[1] Decreased air exchange, cyanosis, and increased respiratory rate occur as the disease progresses. Symptoms increase in severity until about 36 to 72 hours of age, when the disease process reaches its peak. The respiratory rate will rise to 70 to 80/min. Inspiratory retraction of the sternum and lower costal margin is often associated with abdominal distention. Poor air entry is the main auscultatory finding; rales are not heard in the early state of the disease. Edema is common, especially in the hands and feet. The limbs are flaccid, and bowel sounds are poor or absent. Progressive ventilatory insufficiency may cause death by 3 days of age.

When recovery ensues, reparative processes result in progressive ventilatory improvement. With supportive care only, babies with the respiratory distress syndrome will have about a 30 to 60% mortality rate. However, when given optimal metabolic and respiratory support, the mortality rate drops to 10% or less.

Laboratory Findings. Blood gas values show the effects of ventilatory insufficiency: acidemia, CO_2 retention, and diminished oxygen tension.[3] In severely affected infants, the arterial oxygen tension is low, with a low arterial blood pH due to metabolic products. P_{CO_2} elevation is a poor prognostic sign. Continued low arterial oxygen tension despite oxygen administration is an unfavorable sign that indicates an increase in right-to-left shunting. Lactate, the main metabolic product causing metabolic acidosis, reflects tissue hypoxia. Serum potassium levels rise as the disease progresses.

X-ray Findings. Roentgenograms of the chest frequently demonstrate the characteristic "ground glass" appearance and an air bronchogram.[4] Their main use, however, is to rule out some other causes of respiratory distress that need specific therapy.

Special Examinations. Pulmonary function studies show small lungs with a reduced effective pulmonary blood flow.[1]

Differential Diagnosis. Respiratory distress syndrome must be differentiated from cold stress, pneumonia, pneumothorax, pneumomediastinum, lobar emphysema, pulmonary hemorrhage, diaphragmatic hernia, CNS hemorrhage, and congenital heart disease.[1,2]

Complications. If the disease is mild, recovery is usually evident by 72 hours of age. Elevation of the arterial CO_2 tension is an unfavorable prognostic sign that indicates the that baby will die unless he receives assisted ventilation.[2] Pulmonary fibrosis and an increased incidence of pulmonary infection are being reported more often in patients receiving certain types of ventilatory assistance. Bronchopulmonary dysplasia (BPD) has become one of the major chronic lung disease problems in pediatrics. BPD is a result of loss of alveolar lining, alterations of lung water, and damage secondary to treatment. Since the alveoli are mainly damaged, growth will completely repair even the most severe case of BPD if secondary infections do not occur. The iatrogenic factors that add to the damage are oxygen and pressure. The macrophage system seems to be altered with high inspired oxygen administration and will result in fibrotic changes. High inspiratory pressures (greater than 20 cm H_2O) may also prevent lung clearance of water and debris. Treatment of BPD rests on provision of calories, adequate oxygen, adequate pulmonary toilet, and prevention and treatment of infections. With an increased survival rate and with more immature infants now being treated, an increase in intracranial bleedings has occurred. The CNS bleed is probably due to a combination of immaturity and iatrogenic causes. Even with the severe pulmonary and CNS complications, the outlook for an infant to recover completely without residual sequelae is good.

Prevention. Prematurity is one factor that is clearly involved in the development of this disease. Therefore, every effort should be made to prevent preterm births. The mothers at risk (those with diabetes, toxemia, and histories of other premature birth or respiratory distress syndrome in other babies) should receive meticulous prenatal care. Transfer to a center where advanced techniques are available for caring for the mother and infant should be considered.

Prediction of Respiratory Distress Syndrome. The use of amniocentesis to predict lung maturity by means of the lecithin:sphingomyelin ratio appears promising.[6] As the infant matures, the amount of lecithin increases in relation to the sphingomyelin. A mature lung is associated with a lecithin:sphingomyelin ratio of 2:1 or greater. Severe respiratory distress syndrome can be expected when the ratio is 1:1 or less. Intermediate disease occurs when the ratio is between 1:1 and 2:1. Fetal heart rate monitoring is also prognostic, with bradycardia being a poor sign. Caesarean section is commonly done for fetal distress.

Treatment of Mild Respiratory Distress Syndrome. Early recognition is important so that the baby can be evaluated and treatment begun as soon as possible.[2] Since prematurely born infants with asphyxia are at highest risk of developing HMD, they should be resuscitated vigorously at birth. The lungs should be expanded with positive pressure, since the infant's spontaneous breaths do not completely expand the lung. If progressive atelectasis or failure to maintain an arterial oxygen tension of 50 mm Hg in an oxygen environment of 60 to 80% exists, continuous distending pressure to the lung will usually augment inspiration and impede expiration by opposing the high surface tension. If continuous ventilation and continuous distending pressure cannot be maintained at the primary hospital, then the infant should be transported together with an airway and continuous positive pressure. This early intervention has been responsible for lower mortality and reduced morbidity. Transport of the high-risk mother prior to premature delivery is ideal. Optimal care can therefore be given to both mother and infant by an experienced team.

Maintenance of normal body temperature (37°C) during all procedures is essential. (For specifics on ventilatory procedures, see Treatment section.) Intravenous administration of water, glucose, and electrolytes appears to be beneficial: water to maintain adequate hydration and renal output, glucose to provide calories, and electrolytes for maintenance requirements and for specific correction of metabolic derangements. A satisfactory solution is the following: 250 ml 10% dextrose in distilled water plus 50 ml concentrated $NaHCO_3$ solution (giving a solution containing 8.3% dextrose and 150 mEq HCO_3/L), administered at a rate of 65 ml/kg/day by continuous drip. In the sicker infant hypovolemia may be present, and the infant will be in shock. Therefore, therapy for the severely affected infant is directed at correcting hypoxemia and acidosis, improving pulmonary blood flow and expansion of the lung, and correcting blood volume.[2] To this end, inspired oxygen, arterial P_{O_2}, P_{CO_2}, pH, and systemic blood pressure must be monitored. If possible, central venous pressure is also monitored.

Intravenous fluids may be given via a peripheral vein or the umbilical vein. The latter presents some danger to the infant because of the possibility of portal vein thrombosis. Arterial blood is necessary for monitoring oxygen tension, pH, P_{CO_2}, and systemic blood pressure. A satisfactory route for monitoring blood gases and administering fluids is the umbilical artery when fluids are introduced at a constant rate with an infusion pump.

The need for massive amounts of bicarbonate has decreased since the advent of early vigorous resuscitation and maintenance of alveolar stability. However, if the pH remains below 7.20, respiratory and metabolic corrections should be instituted. Assisted ventilation (see "Treatment") should be improved so that the arterial CO_2 can be maintained between 30 and 40 mm Hg. Metabolic acidosis should be corrected using a standard sodium bicarbonate (0.89 mEq/ml) diluted with 5 or 10% glucose water and infused at a rate of 1 mEq/kg min. The amount required to correct the metabolic acidosis is calculated from the following formula:

$$\text{mEq of bicarbonate} = \text{body weight in kg} \times \text{the base deficit (negative base excess)} \times 0.3$$

Oxygen Therapy. Guidelines from the American Academy of Pediatrics stress the importance of monitoring inspired oxygen concentration as well as arterial oxygen tension.[7] Hypoxemia must be corrected, but too high an arterial oxygen tension may lead to the development of retrolental fibroplasia or pulmonary oxygen toxicity. Therefore, the physician must maintain a balance between the inspired oxygen concentration and the arterial oxygen tension so that hypoxemia is corrected with as little inspired oxygen as possible. The goal is to maintain the arterial oxygen tension between 50 and 70 mm Hg. The oxygen may be given in the incubator up to a concentration of 40%, after which a clear plastic hood is preferred. The oxygen should be warmed and humidified. Flow through the hood should be at least 5 L/min to prevent CO_2 rebreathing.

Hypovolemia. This condition may be assumed whenever the central venous pressure is less than 2 mm Hg or the mean arterial pressure is less than 25 mm Hg.[1,2] Volume may be replaced by whole blood or salt-poor albumin (4 g/100 ml).

Temperature. The oxygen requirement is reduced if the infant remains in a "thermal neutral" state. Moreover, pulmonary blood flow is reduced if the infant is cool. Therefore, the body temperature should be maintained at 37° ± 0.5°C (98.6° ± 1°F) by means of an incubator or a radiant heater.

Fluid and Electrolytes. Intravascular fluids are infused at a rate of 60 to 80 ml/kg body weight/24 hr.[2] Dextrose, 10% in water, should be used, with added maintenance electrolytes or those electrolytes required to treat specific needs.

Prognosis. The prognosis depends upon the ability of the nursery staff to give intensive care. The prognosis is good if the infant survives 72 hours.

Croup

Croup is a term applied to a symptom complex consisting of a resonant "barking" cough, inspiratory stridor, and variable respiratory distress related to the degree of laryngeal obstruction. Three separate clinical entities of separate etiology are recognized: laryngotracheobronchitis, epiglottitis, and spasmodic laryngotracheitis.

Differential Diagnosis. Diphtheria must be ruled out by an immunization history. Aspiration of a foreign body must also be considered. Angioneurotic edema may present as acute respiratory obstruction but is rare in infants and children; epinephrine and antihistamines give prompt relief.

Laryngotracheobronchitis (Viral Croup, Subglottic Croup)

General Considerations. This is the most common form of croup; it usually occurs in children between six months and three years of age. It is thought to be a viral disease most commonly due to infection with parainfluenza virus, adenovirus, and respiratory syncytial virus. Measles and influenza viruses have been isolated and have been associated with a prolonged course of croup. The viruses involve mainly the subglottic area (larynx, trachea, and bronchi). Symptoms may vary depending upon which anatomic area is more heavily infected.

Clinical Findings: Symptoms and Signs. The onset is usually gradual, with a history of upper respiratory tract symptoms for several days prior to the onset of barking cough and stridor. Fever is generally mild, and the child does not appear "sick." If the lower respiratory tract is involved early, wheezing may be present. As the laryngeal obstruction progresses, stridor becomes associated with sternal, intercostal, and abdominal retractions, and the expiratory phase of respiration is also prolonged. Auscultation reveals decreased breath sounds. The child becomes anxious and restless as hyperoxemia ensues. Cyanosis is a late sign and may herald complete obstruction.

Laboratory Findings. Leukocyte count is less than 15,000/ml.

Complications. The principal complication of viral croup is asphyxia secondary to laryngeal obstruction. Other complications are related to misadventures in attempting to supply an airway in an emergency situation or are associated with management of a tracheostomy or endotracheal tube after an airway has been provided.

Treatment: Medical Measures. Mist is effective in reducing laryngeal edema and relieving respiratory distress. This may be administered in the hospital as cool mist in a "croup tent" or fog room, or at home by means of a cold-mist humidifier or by steaming up the bathroom by running hot water in the bath or shower. Steam vaporizers carry the risk of scalding the child and should not be recommended to parents. Subemetic doses (105 ml) of syrup of ipecac (not fluid extract) have also been thought to be effective. The dose may be repeated in one hour if respiratory symptoms persist. Vomiting often gives remarkable relief from symptoms. Antibiotics are not indicated except in the case of bacterial superinfection. Sedation is contraindicated since it may depress the respiratory center, promoting hypoventilation and hypoxemia, and since it may mask the anxiety and restlessness which are important signs of hypoxemia.

Oxygen must be used with caution. Administration of oxygen in high concentrations (per mask) may delay the signs of complete airway obstruction (increasing restlessness). If oxygen is used, experienced personnel should be at the bedside. If intubation becomes necessary, oxygen in high doses is mandatory. The use of corticosteroids is controversial, and recent well-controlled studies indicate that they are of no value.[8] Still, many clinicians claim good results with dexamethasone (Decadron), 2 to 4 mg given intramuscularly every 6 hours.[9] Racemic epinephrine in dilutions of 1:4 or 1:8 given by positive pressure has been reported to relieve this condition. This therapy should be used only in an environment where proper observation and intubation can be done.[10] The duration of observation should be 6 to 8 hours, since airway obstruction can occur within this time period. If the treatment leads to an increase in anxiety, it should be discontinued. A crying child may accept the treatment effectively if it is administered in a patient, calm manner.

Artificial Airways. If these measures are not successful in relieving respiratory distress and the patient remains restless and agitated, an airway must be provided. Blood gas analyses are of little value since the invasive technique cannot evaluate the steady state of the patient.

Patients requiring an artificial airway to relieve airway obstruction need either prolonged nasotracheal intubation or tracheostomy. The important feature of either is to avoid a "crash" intubation or tracheostomy; it is preferred to perform a controlled intubation or tracheostomy under optimum conditions. Once the decision to provide an artificial airway has been made, the child should be given high concentrations of oxygen while arrangements are made. If a nasotracheal tube is employed, it should be small enough to provide a small leak of air around it in order to reduce trauma to the glottis and subglottic area. Tracheostomy should be performed in the operating room over an endotracheal tube or bronchoscopy tube. Postoperative care includes careful suctioning, postural drainage, and pulmonary toilet, including administration of humidified air to the nasotracheal or tracheostomy tube. The patient usually may be extubated or decannulated in three to five days.

Prognosis. Most children do not progress beyond the stage of cough, stridor, and mild retractions, and the disease runs its course in three to seven days, with gradual improvement leading to complete recovery.

Epiglottitis (Bacterial Croup, Supraglottic Croup)

This form of croup generally affects children between the ages of three and seven years. It has a rapidly progressive, fulminant course. It is most commonly caused by *Haemophilus influenzae* type B, although beta-hemolytic streptococci and pneumococci have been implicated in rare cases.

Clinical Findings: Symptoms and Signs. The onset of the illness is abrupt.[11,12] Younger children present with high fever and respiratory distress; older children complain of difficulty in swallowing and severe sore throat. Because of the dysphagia, pooling of secretions in the pharynx and drooling are prominent. Since the site of the pathologic process is the epiglottis, the larynx is not involved, and the patient may not be hoarse. Phonation is muffled, but voice quality is normal. Fever is usually high (38.5°C), and the patient appears "sick" or even shock-like. Blood cultures are frequently positive for *H. influenzae* type B. Within hours after onset, the child may be in marked respiratory distress, with stridor and retractions. The pharynx is inflamed, and excessive secretions may be noted. The diagnosis can be made by visualizing the large, swollen, cherry-red epiglottis with a tongue blade. However, this maneuver must be undertaken with great caution because stimulation of the epiglottis has produced abrupt laryngospasm and death.

Laboratory Findings. Leukocytosis greater than 15,000/ml is usually present.

X-Ray Findings. Lateral roentgenograms of the pharynx may be of value in confirming enlargement of the epiglottis without resorting to direct visualization. The roentgenogram should be taken when resuscitation equipment is readily accessible. The film should be taken with the patient in the sitting and most comfortable positions.

Treatment. When the diagnosis of epiglottitis is confirmed, the only approach is to provide an artificial airway. Preparations should be made for controlled intubation. In the operating room, direct visualization of the epiglottis can be performed by the anesthesiologist or someone competent in intubation.[11] If the diagnosis is confirmed, an airway can be immediately provided. Nasotracheal intubation is now considered the airway of choice, and tracheostomy for this short period of time (24 to 72 hours) is no longer appropriate. Corticosteroids are of no value. Parenteral antibiotics, preferably given intravenously, are indicated. Chloromycetin is the drug of choice in a dose of 100 to 150 mg/kg/day.

Prognosis. The disease process usually responds rapidly to antibiotics, and the patient may be extubated in 48 to 72 hours. If an airway is not provided promptly, the mortality rate may be as high as 50%.

Spasmodic Croup (Allergic Croup)

This form of croup may affect any age group. There is often a past history or family history of croup. The cause is not known, but the disease may be allergic in nature. The onset is abrupt (usually at night) with a barking cough and, in some cases, moderate stridor. There is usually no fever or other symptoms.

Treatment. This disease rarely progresses to airway obstruction, and almost any treatment is effective: change in environmental temperature, enemas, emetics, mist, weather fronts moving through, bronchodilators, or antihistamines. The attack may abate as suddenly as it presented and may not recur. More frequently, the symptoms will lessen during the daytime for a few days, only to increase at night.

Pneumonia

General Considerations. Pneumonia in children can be produced by bacterial organisms as well as by viral agents. Beyond infancy, bacteria account for only a minority of cases, the vast majority being viral. Early recognition and treatment of pneumonia can well make the difference between relatively simple home treatment and hospitalization with an increased incidence of complications.

Clinical Findings. The pattern of clinical illness varies with the age of the patient and the etiologic agent. Bacterial pneumonias are usually preceded by an upper respiratory tract infection. Typically, the child with a mild rhinitis suddenly becomes anorexic, listless, and febrile. The loss of desire for food or liquid in a small child with a cold is a danger signal. The cough, previously loose because of postnasal drip, now becomes dry and painful. The pain may be referred to the abdomen and can simulate appendicitis.

Older children (5 years and older) may complain of headache and chills. Small children (0 to 2 years) often have vomiting or mild diarrhea initially. In infants, convulsions occur frequently at the onset. The temperature is elevated, usually to 38.5° to 40°C (103° or 104°F). The respiratory rate increases to 50 to 80 per minute. Respirations are rapid and shallow and are frequently accompanied by an expiratory grunt. The pulse rate is often doubled.

By the second day of illness, cough, dyspnea, and diminished breath sounds and rales over the involved area of the lungs usually enable the physician to diagnose pneumonia correctly. A chest roentgenogram is helpful to confirm the diagnosis. The child begins to improve about 24 hours after appropriate antibiotics are initiated. There are no foolproof laboratory tests to prove or disprove bacterial pneumonia, so one's clinical acumen is of utmost importance. In addition to antibiotics, treatment should include increased fluids, bed rest while febrile, and postural drainage. There is no evidence to support the use of nebulized mist or cough medicines in the treatment of bacterial pneumonia. A "home brew" dose consisting of equal parts (1/4 to 1/2 oz) of whiskey, honey, and fresh lemon juice is inexpensive and soothing, and giving it satisfies the parents' urge to do something for the child with pneumonia, especially when antibiotics are not required.[13]

Viral or atypical pneumonias and mycoplasma pneumonias are in general less striking. The older child with viral pneumonia does not appear as ill as his fever might indicate. Cough may be absent or infrequent initially, later becoming dry and irritating. Paroxysmal cough, simulating pertussis, is common in small children. The pulse is slower than expected: A fever of 40°C may be accompanied by a pulse rate of 100 R. Petechiae on the soft palate and conjunctivitis occur frequently.[14] Rales are usually heard at the posterior of both lungs.

There is frequently a discrepancy between the physical examination and radiologic findings. Rales may be present with minimal x-ray changes at the onset. Later, the x-ray film may demonstrate extensive pulmonary infiltration, while physical findings are minimal or absent.

Influenza viruses, adenoviruses, rubeola, varicella, and human cytomegalovirus have been associated with primary pneumonias in children. The morbidity and mortality rates from viral pneumonias vary with the age and physical condition of the patient as well as with the agent involved. Viral respiratory infection is the second leading cause of death in infants and young children and may contribute to the sudden infant death syndrome as well.[13] Severe viral pneumonias, especially in children less than 1 year of age, may require hospitalization.

Treatment. Acute treatment is symptomatic with antipyretics given for fever and discomfort. If the dry, irritating cough interferes with sleep, codeine can be used to suppress it. Antibiotics are of no use in viral pneumonia except with mycoplasmal, rickettsial, or chlamydial species or when a bacterial infection is superimposed.

Mycoplasma pneumonia is the most common single etiologic agent of primary atypical pneumonia in older children (5 to 30 years), but it can also be seen in the young child. The onset is usually insidious. Fever, cough, and malaise are seen in most patients. Sore throat and headache reportedly occur in about half the patients. Erythromycin or tetracycline, 250 mg qid (50 mg/kg, up to 1 g) given for 5 to 7 days is effective for this agent. The other, more rare, atypical pneumonias are not discussed in this chapter.

Complications. The sequelae from acute respiratory viral infections may include chronic interstitial pneumonia, obliterative bronchitis and bronchiolitis, bronchiectasis, and chronic segmental or lobar atelectasis. These pulmonary sequelae cause acute and chronic ill health, significant discomfort, inability to participate in physical education and recreational activities, social deprivation, and interference with learning.[15] Outpatient follow-up is important until the chest roentgenogram is clear. There is evidence that even a simple upper respiratory infection (URI), let alone viral pneumonia, can cause airway damage in children.[16] Postural drainage preceded by use of an inhaled bronchodilator is helpful in clearing the lung. We recommend that parents do postural drainage two to three times per day until the child's chest is clear. In some cases, this can take months.

It has been reported that adults with lung disease had less reversibility if they had significant respiratory infection before 16 years of age.[17] It is important for children who have had viral disease involving the airways never to smoke, to avoid pollution, and always to receive influenza vaccine when available.

Prevention. Prevention of pneumonia is limited to avoiding exposure to children who are obviously ill, being aware of epidemic influences and avoiding large crowds during that time, and receiving proper immunizations and flu vaccine when available. For those children with chronic illnesses such as cystic fibrosis and asthma, it is crucial to avoid viral infections. When pneumonia does occur, prompt action by the parent and physician will help prevent sequelae.

Summary. Pneumonia may be classified as typical (bacterial), or atypical (viral). After infancy, viral pneumonia is more common. Bacterial pneumonia has the more toxic symptoms, with a rapid onset, and is treated with penicillin, whereas viral has a more gradual onset, is less toxic, and cannot be treated with antibiotics unless the eitologic agent is mycoplasmal. The viral pneumonias cause a more diffuse lung involvement and can cause airway damage and possibly chronic lung disease in adults. Therapy consists of symptomatic treatment in the acute phase and postural drainage in the recovery state, to be carried out until the chest roentgenogram clears. Prevention consists of avoidance of affected individuals and immunizations.

Severe Asthma in Childhood

Childhood asthma is usually triggered by a respiratory viral disease, which can lead the patient to the intensive care ward when the arterial carbon dioxide level starts to increase. In previous years, the number of children admitted to the intensive care ward was 40 to 60 per year. However, these numbers have decreased with better outpatient management resulting from laboratory determination of serum theophylline levels and the use of high-dose steroids for short periods of time (burst techniques).

Our therapy does not differ greatly from the treatment of adult asthma, except that we do use isoproterenol intravenously in children; this mode of therapy is contraindicated for adolescents and adults.

The decision if and when to ventilate becomes critical because delay may result in death or the necessity for emergency resuscitation. The advantages of early use of a ventilator must be weighed against the difficulties and complications of the procedure.

Useful clinical and biochemical guidelines for the institution of assisted ventilation in severe asthma are as follows:[18]

1. Severe inspiratory retractions
2. The so-called "silent chest" (decreased wheezing and breath sounds)
3. $Paco_2$ that is increasing.

The most important criterion for intubation is an increasing $Paco_2$ in the presence of full medical therapy. The rise in $Paco_2$ need not reach 65 mm Hg but may merely go from 40 to 45. This criterion of the rising $Paco_2$ will give a greater margin of safety for the intubation procedure.

Treatment. There are six factors in the treatment of asthma. (1) Preoxygenation is essential to successful intubation prior to ventilation. (2) One should correct acidosis, if possible, and maintain acid-base balance while the ventilator is being used. (3) Aminophylline therapy (4 mg/kg every 4 to 6 hours) should be continued. (4) Intravenous isoproterenol, starting at 0.1 μg/kg/minute, should be given. (5) Corticosteroid therapy should be maintained while on intravenous isoproterenol or the respirator. (6) A ventilator capable of producing high pressures (up to 100 cm H_2O) is required in conditions of high airway resistance.

Severe asthma in childhood is a medical emergency which causes appreciable mortality.[18] Death can occur during a severe attack. The use of assisted ventilation and intravenous isoproterenol has undoubtedly reduced the mortality.

In most cases, therapy has been started before admission to the intensive care ward, and it should be continued. Serial arterial blood gases enable the respiratory status of the patient to be followed closely. Indwelling radial artery lines are often used for this purpose. When tolerated, postural drainage may effectively clear plugs, which could prevent further progression of the disease.

Drug therapy during assisted ventilation consists of aminophylline and corticosteroids. Epinephrine is discontinued. If the patient is difficult to ventilate because of agitation, and hypoxia has been excluded as a cause, morphine, curare, or flaxedil alone or in combination can be used. The average time on a ventilator is about 36 hours. Discontinuance of ventilation depends on the ability of the patient to cycle the ventilator. We no longer place a patient in the pediatric age range on a T-piece for 6 to 12 hours as a guide to extubation. Patients are maintained on self-cycling models with a 2- to 4-cm H_2O end-expiratory pressure. If blood gases remain satisfactory, the nasotracheal tube is removed, and the clinical status and blood gases are monitored. A percutaneously placed arterial line (radial artery) greatly facilitates management.

Many patients have received intravenous isoproterenol.[18,19] Isoproterenol is started in patients for whom ventilation is being considered. It is given intravenously through a separate vein starting at a dose of 0.2 μg/kg/minute, and it is increased based on the results of blood gas analysis and heart rate. The usual effect occurs within 15 to 20 minutes. If PCO_2 has not dropped or heart rate of 200 per minute has not occurred within this time, then the dose is increased in increments of 0.1 μg/kg/minute. A heart rate of 200/minute cannot be exceeded, but our experience indicates that patients who favorably responded to this drug had a heart rate of 190 to 200/minute at the time their $PaCO_2$ dropped. If a heart rate of 200 has occurred without a lowering of the $PaCO_2$, the patient is intubated and ventilated.

From the experience in the adult and adolescent age range, the use of intravenous Isuprel is contraindicated because of the increased incidence of arrhythmias.

Cystic Fibrosis

Cystic fibrosis is a genetically transmitted autosomal-recessive disease characterized by widespread involvement of the exocrine glands. Approximately 5% of the Caucasian population are carriers of the recessive gene, and one in 2000 births is affected by the disease. Multiple organ systems are involved as well as the lungs, including the gastrointestinal tract, the biliary tree, the sweat glands, and the testes.[20]

The basic pathophysiology in the lungs resides mainly in the small airways of 2 mm in diameter or less. There is a derangement in the mucous glands which results in an end-product which is thick and tenacious.[21] The respiratory cilia, which beat at a faster rate, are unable to move the thick mucus layer of the mucociliary escalator system owing to the loss of the sol component of this system. This leads to complete or partial obstruction of the bronchioles and eventually results in air trapping or atelectasis. Bronchospasm has recently been shown to be a component of airway narrowing in this disease. Secondarily acquired infection occurs and may result in destruction of the respiratory epithelium and bronchioles, resulting in bronchiectasis. The disease is progressive and leads to respiratory failure and death. There is wide clinical variability, with some patients severely affected as infants while others remain asymptomatic until adolescence. Any patient with malabsorption problems or repeated pulmonary infections should be suspected of having cystic fibrosis. An elevated sweat chloride (>70 mEq/L) is diagnostic.

Clinical Findings: Symptoms and Signs. Typical symptoms consist of foul-smelling fatty stools, failure to thrive, and repeated pulmonary infections with chronic productive cough.[21,22] Symptoms resemble asthma. Newborns may present with intestinal obstruction secondary to inspissated stool (meconium ileus).

Physical findings range from normal to severe signs of pulmonary involvement, including hyperexpansion of the thoracic cage, rales and rhonchi, cyanosis, and clubbing.

Laboratory Findings. Laboratory test results are normal except for elevated sweat sodium and chloride levels and increased stool fat.

Pulmonary function tests reveal obstructive lung disease with increased total lung capacity and residual volumes.[22] Vital capacity is decreased. Airway conductance and flow rate are reduced.

X-Ray Findings. Chest roentgenograms reveal hyperexpansion with flattening of the diaphragm early in the disease. Later there are diffuse infiltrates, peribronchial cuffing, and areas of atelectasis.

Differential Diagnosis. Cystic fibrosis must be differentiated from allergic diseases, immunologic deficiency diseases, chronic recurrent pneumonia, and alpha-1-antitrypsin deficiency disease.

Complications. Complications include pneumothorax, hemoptysis, empyema, cor pulmonale, and respiratory failure.[23]

Treatment. Treatment of the pulmonary component of cystic fibrosis is aimed at relieving the obstruction of the bronchioles by mobilizing the tenacious secretions. Postural drainage and percussion are the mainstays of treatment. Bronchodilators systemically used as aerosols prior to postural drainage have been found effective in maintaining the patency of the airway so that mucus can be effectively coughed out. Antibiotics are indicated for infection and are usually used intermittently in the less involved patient, but on a continued basis with severe disease. Cor pulmonale is treated with oxygen therapy.[24] Tolazoline can effectively relieve pulmonary vascular spasm, but it has been used less with the more liberal use of oxygen. Constant low-flow oxygen therapy in severely cyanotic patients may add immeasurably to their comfort and productivity at home.

Prognosis. Although recent advances in treatment have prolonged the lives and usefulness of patients with cystic fibrosis, the prognosis remains poor, with the median life expectancy being 18 to 20 years.

Foreign Body Aspiration and Aspiration Pneumonia

Diagnostic accuracy in these conditions depends upon maintaining a high index of suspicion and proper radiologic examination. Children aged six months to three years are particularly susceptible. The cardinal manifestations are coughing interspersed with symptom-free periods and recurrent pneumonitis in a specific area of the lung. Vomiting when the cough reflex is absent (e.g., unconsciousness) leads to aspiration of vomitus. Physical examination discloses absence of air entry in the involved area.

The clinical pattern will vary from immediate death when the trachea is obstructed to unexplained recurrent pneumonia in a peripheral area of the lung. A detailed history must be taken, questioning the parents about coughing episodes when material such as a peanut or sunflower seed could have been aspirated. Aspiration pneumonia will also occur with ingestion of gasoline, kerosene, or other hydrocarbons. In the infant and small child, wheezing can be an immediate and persistent finding. Hyperexpansion occurs early, followed by atelectasis. Inflammation occurs if obstruction has been incomplete and airway damage has occurred.

Properly performed inspiratory and expiratory roentgenograms will show air trapping.[25] An excellent expiratory roentgenogram can be obtained by using the "gloved fist technique." The technician will push in the epigastrium of the child, allowing an optimal expiration. If cooperation is still not obtained, cinefluoroscopy is warranted.[26]

Treatment consists of removal by either endoscopy or postural drainage.[26] Obstruction of a large airway such as the trachea is an immediate indication for endoscopy; however, urgency in removal of the segmental foreign body is not necessary, and an increased morbidity and mortality are seen when proper facilities are not available.[26]

Postural drainage preceded by a bronchodilator aerosol has been successful in the removal of a variety of foreign matter, especially when the latter is located in a segmental area of the lung.[26]

Antibiotics are of limited value and, if used, should be as specific as possible. Corticosteroids have not been shown to be effective in reducing morbidity or mortality.

Prognosis. The prognosis is excellent after removal. Continued postural drainage treatment is necessary until the chest roentgenogram is normal.

DIAGNOSTIC AND TREATMENT METHODS

When the first edition of this book was originally written, the diagnostic and treatment procedures for infants and children were modifications of the invasive procedures used on adults. Noninvasive techniques for both blood gas determinations and pulmonary function testing are now being developed for pediatric use. The obvious value of such techniques will be not only the comfort and safety of the patient but also the potential for evaluation of the patient in a natural or steady state. Data from these noninvasive methods are leading to a reevaluation of treatment procedures used on the critically ill patient. For example, postural drainage and tipping of the premature infant recovering from severe hyaline membrane disease was thought to be a benign procedure until recently. Today, continual arterial oxygen monitoring has shown that tipping alone can result in a low Pa_{O_2} (30 to 40 mm Hg), from which the patient takes hours to recover. It is hoped that the future will bring objective and noninvasive pulmonary function testing for the age range of three months through five years. The remainder of this chapter deals with diagnostic and treatment procedures that relate specifically to pediatric problems.

Specific Diagnostic Procedures

Radiographic Procedures

1. "Gloved-fist technique." To achieve maximum expiration in a noncooperative infant or child, the technician firmly places his lead-gloved fist on the child's epigastrium. This procedure is most beneficial in diagnosis of an aspirated foreign body. The foreign body is easily recognized because of differential inflation of the lung; the obstructed lung will remain expanded on forced expiration, and upon comparison with the inspiratory film, one can see unilateral air trapping.[27]
2. Barium swallow. Barium can be given to an infant by nipple and to the older child by glass. This test is used in conjunction with a milk scan to diagnose chronic aspiration, which is a cause of chronic lung disease in children. The upper lobes are the main target for involvement. Swallowing coordination and function should be noted as well as retention of barium in the pharynx after swallowing has been completed.
3. Milk scan. A radiolabeled liquid (milk with technetium) will be given the patient prior to sleep. The lungs are scanned eight to ten hours later. Chronic regurgitation occurring during sleep can thus be diagnosed.

In conjunction with the barium swallow and milk scan, a nonradiographic test for analysis of esophageal acidity is often performed. A pH probe is passed into the mid or upper third of the esophagus, and continual pH recordings are made during the various sleep and awake states.

Arterial Blood Gases

The basic arterial gas analysis is identical to the technique explained in Chapter 1 except that volumes of 0.5 to 0.6 ml are obtained. A 25-gauge needle is used with a heparinized tuberculin syringe. A complete gas analysis can be done with 0.5 ml of blood. If multiple sampling will be required, percutaneous arterial lines can be placed, or the umbilical artery can be catheterized in newborns.

Since arterial pressure cannot be used as an indicator for the success of puncture, the radial artery is the preferred site because there is no associated vein. Other potential sites are the temporal, brachial, and femoral arteries. There is little or no place for using "arterialized" capillary blood. The radial artery can be used just as easily in newborns as in older children. All commonly used blood gas analyzers can be adapted for low volumes.

Umbilical Artery Technique. The use of an indwelling catheter in an umbilical artery or vein has become a common procedure in hospital nurseries. Catheterization of the artery generally provides a more useful source of diagnostic information and is safer than catheterization of the more frequently used umbilical vein.

Diagnostic Uses:

1. To obtain blood samples for analysis (particularly blood gas and pH analysis).
2. To measure intravascular pressures (arterial and venous).
3. For cardiac catheterization and angiocardiography.

Therapeutic Uses:

1. In exchange transfusion.
2. In administration of fluids, blood, antibiotics, electrolytes, alkali (sodium bicarbonate, tromethamine), and so forth.

Procedure. The catheter should be made of flexible, nontoxic radiopaque material that will not kink when advanced through a vessel and that will not collapse during blood withdrawal. Nonwettable material and a single, smooth-surfaced end hole reduce clot formation. A # 3.5 (Aloe Medical Corporation) catheter is used for infants weighing less than 1500 g, and a # 5 for larger infants. Dead space of the catheter system should be determined prior to catheterization.

The infant is loosely restrained and is warmed (preferably under an overhead radiant heater), and the procedure is carried out under sterile conditions. In normal infants, arterial constriction may prevent catheterization after the first 15 to 30 minutes of life. (In the presence of hypoxia and acidosis, arterial constriction is usually diminished.) A standard cut-down tray is opened, and the wide end of the umbilical artery catheter is cut off so that the blunt needle adapter fits snugly into the catheter. The catheter capacity is reduced by discarding the wide end and utilizing the needle adapter. A sterile syringe is filled with flushing fluid (e.g., heparinized saline solution) and attached to a 3-way stopcock and, in turn, to the umbilical catheter. The entire system is filled with flushing fluid. An assistant may elevate the umbilical cord by the cord clamp while the operator prepares the cord and adjacent skin with an iodine solution, which should then be removed with alcohol to prevent an iodine burn of the skin. The area is then draped. A purse-string suture (taking care not to puncture the umbilical vessels) or a loop of umbilical tape is placed at the base of the umbilical cord and tied loosely in order to control bleeding if necessary. The cord is then cut 1 to 1.5 cm above the skin with scissors or a scalpel blade.

The two thick-walled, cord arteries and the single thin-walled vein are identified. The rim of the cut vessel is grasped with a pointed forceps or mosquito clamp. The lumen of the vessel is then dilated with the tips of the forceps. Initially, the lumen may allow only one tip to enter. Both tips may then be inserted and allowed to spread, further dilating the vessel. The fluid-filled catheter is inserted into the lumen of the artery or vein and is advanced. Any obstruction to advancement usually can be overcome with steady, gentle pressure. Forceful probing may lead to increased arteriospasm or perforation of the vein or artery. If the obstruction in one of the arteries cannot be overcome, the catheter should be removed and an attempt made to catheterize the other umbilical artery. If a similar obstruction occurs, the catheter should be removed and filled (0.1 to 0.2 ml) with 1 to 2% lidocaine (Xylocaine) in epinephrine. The catheter should be reinserted up to the obstruction and the lidocaine injected. This usually relaxes the arteriospasm after one or two minutes and allows the catheter to advance.

Frequent aspiration will demonstrate blood return. In arterial catheterization, the tip should be positioned at the bifurcation of the aorta (approximately at the level of the third lumbar vertebra on x-ray examination).

The catheter is tied in place by means of a purse-string suture at the base of the cord, securing the ends of the suture to the catheter, and the catheter is taped to the infant's abdomen. An antibiotic ointment is applied to the stump, which is examined frequently for signs of infection. Routine systemic antibiotics are not indicated.

Complications. The principal complications of this procedure are infection ("prophylactic" systemic antibiotics do not reduce the incidence of infection), hemorrhage, vasospasm and thrombosis, and embolism. Thrombosis is rare in arterial catheterization, but is common (3 to 33%) in venous catheterization. Embolization occurs when air or clots are introduced. This complication is seen more often in the shocked and debilitated infant in whom the clotting factors are altered or absent. Vascular perforation is a rare complication of portal vein catheterization. Vascular and tissue damage may occur secondary to the rapid infusion of hypertonic solutions.

Transcutaneous Oxygen and Carbon Dioxide Monitoring

The amount of oxygen in the arterial circulation can be determined by analysis of oxygen diffusing from the skin heated to 44°C.[27] Similar electrodes are also available for the analysis of carbon dioxide. These electrodes analyze the partial pressure of the gases and in addition can determine the blood flow to the area by measuring the energy required to obtain a skin temperature of 44°C. In the small infant or stressed child, the analysis is usually carried out by placing the electrode on the abdominal or thoracic area (See Fig. 16-2). Stress will often cause peripheral vasoconstriction, resulting in an artificially low Po_2. In the unstressed older child or adult, the medial surface of the forearm can be used.

This technique gives the ability to measure Pao_2 continually. In the past, continual measurements could be obtained only by using an indwelling oxygen electrode (3 to 5 mm in diameter). This method often resulted in complications and was invasive. Continuous transcutaneous monitoring of oxygen (Tco_2) has given data that have altered some treatment routines previously considered nonstressful for the patient. Experience with the electrode has given us the following findings.

1. Handling (turning, chest physiotherapy, feeding) of the stressed infant will cause the Tco_2 to drop to low levels (10 to 40 mm Hg), requiring several hours to recover.

2. Abrupt elevations of Tco_2 can occur with oxygen therapy given with brief stress. The levels are potentially damaging to immature retinal arterioles (Retrolental Fibroplasia—RLF). Even with frequent intermittent analysis of blood gases with the invasive techniques, the abrupt Po_2 elevations were missed. The amount of inhaled oxy-

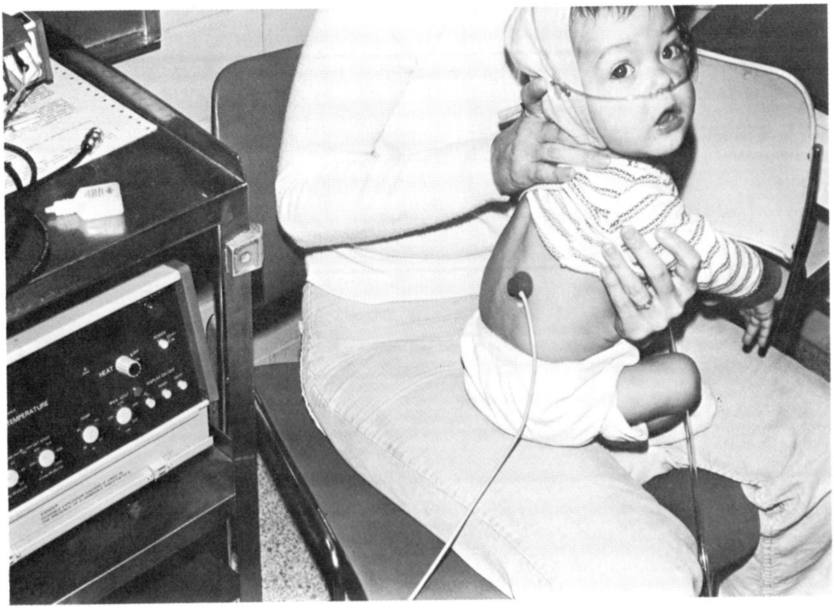

Fig. 16-2. Transcutaneous oxygen monitor attached to boy with lung disease (bronchopulmonary dysplasia).

gen needed for recovery from stress is best determined by the transcutaneous technique.

3. The effects of sleep and feeding on the arterial oxygen tension have been best analyzed with this noninvasive technique. In patients with chronic lung disease or central nervous system abnormalities, the arterial oxygen will often drop with certain stages of sleep.

Although this technique was originally developed for the newborn, recent data indicate its usefulness in the infant, child, and adult.[27,28]

Pulmonary Functions

When a child reaches the age of six years or is able to cooperate, complete pulmonary function values can be obtained. Because coop-

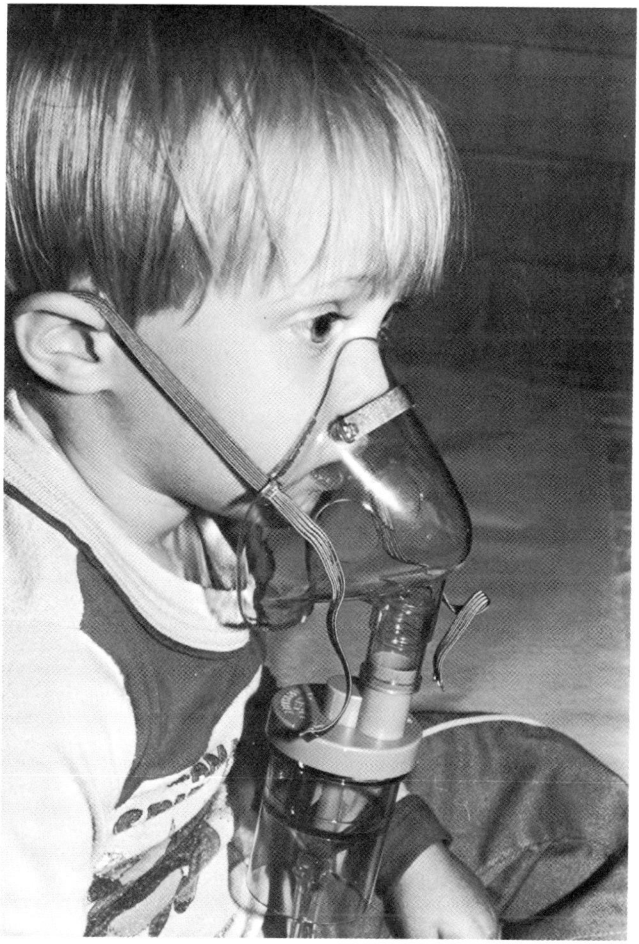

Fig. 16-3. Mist delivery system for hospitalized patients.

eration and attention span are limited in the child, techniques of analysis that are quick and noninvasive should be used. Determinations of thoracic gas volume (TGV) using a body box will be more accurate than functional residual capacity (FRC), which requires 5- to 7-minute washout by nitrogen or helium equilibration techniques. Complete cardiopulmonary function studies can be obtained for the newborn (birth to three months) with noninvasive techniques, but for the age range of three months to six years, techniques are not available unless the patient is sedated.[29]

Other Invasive and Specialized Procedures

1. Bronchoscopy. This procedure is most commonly used for the removal of an aspirated foreign object, for upper airway evaluation, and as a check on endotracheal tube position. As with adults, we do not find it effective in the treatment of atelectasis.

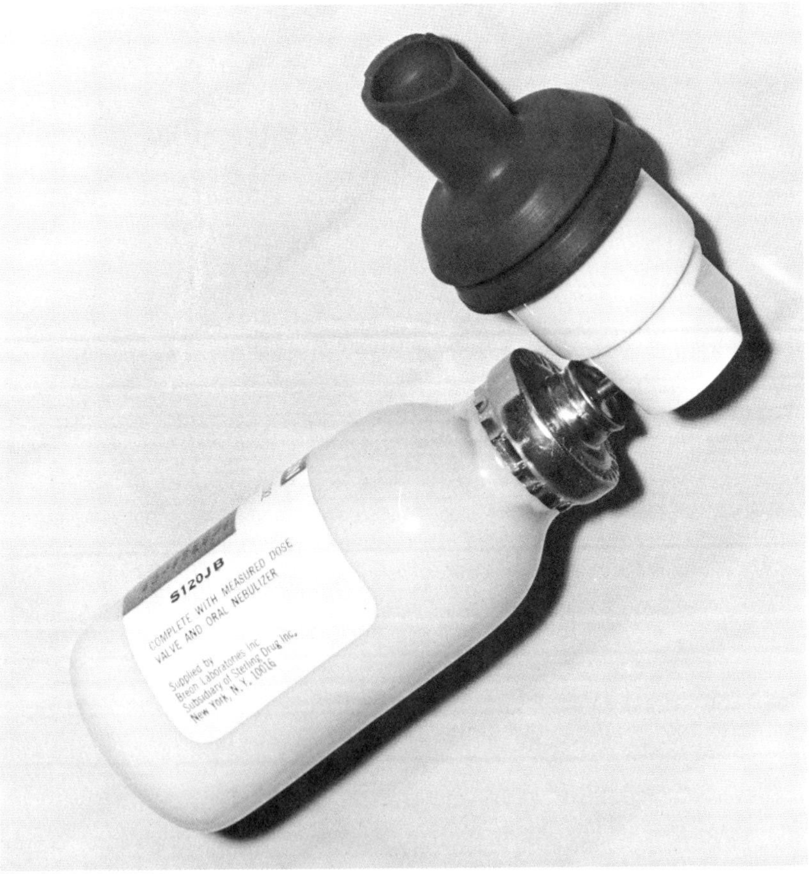

Fig. 16-4. Bronkometer with cut-off nipple applied, used to deliver bronchodilator to infant.

2. Open lung biopsy. This procedure is used for lesions requiring complete tissue, pathologic, and immunologic evaluation. Common lesions needing formal lung biopsy are viral disease that has progressed to a chronic state and hemosiderosis-like lesions. Lung aspiration or tap is done only when an unusual bacterial infection may be present.

3. Sputum analysis. Deep tracheal suction is needed to obtain culture material that would indicate the cause of an inflammatory lesion. A coughed-up sample is not usually diagnostic unless a pure culture is obtained. With thick sputum, such as from patients with cystic fibrosis, the material must be homogenized under sterile conditions. The technique will obtain bacteria from the center of the specimen that will correlate more with the cause of a lower airway inflammation.

GENERAL PRINCIPLES OF RESPIRATORY CARE FOR INFANTS AND CHILDREN

1. Children have developmental needs that must be met in addition to the care their particular illness demands. This requires knowledge of normal child development. The nurse caring for children must also have an appreciation of the need a child has for his parents and must allow for their participation in care. Any institution caring for infants and children should have nursing personnel that are experienced in that role.

2. Personnel working in small hospitals can usually be trained in a short period of time at a university center. There, they can be taught commonly used treatment and diagnostic techniques and also stabilization methods needed to enable adequate patient transport to a more specialized center.

3. Centers specializing in respiratory care for the newborn and child should be used for the following problems:

a. Premature intensive care
b. Long-term assisted ventilation
c. Cardiopulmonary surgical problems
d. Severe trauma requiring specialized equipment and ventilation
e. Bronchoscopy—treatment and diagnosis
f. Specialized care for the child with asthma and cystic fibrosis
g. Patient needing formal lung biopsy

Treatment is similar to that for the adult, but techniques have been modified for several age ranges depending on either size or cooperative ability, or both.

Airway Maintenance. In infants with an artificial airway, the head should be sandbagged to maintain a neutral position. Suctioning and irrigation of tubes must be carried out diligently, since only a little mucus can obstruct a small airway. Pressures used with a self-inflating bag should be monitored, since slow high pressure—40 cm—could cause alveolar ruptures.[30,31]

Bronchodilators. The normal airway is in part supported by smooth muscle, which can be relaxed with bronchodilators. The dilated airway allows for better exchange of air and easier expulsion of mucus. The most efficient mode of administration is via an air- or oxygen-driven nebulizer (Fig. 16-3). A bronchodilator can also be given with a freon-propelled unit as shown in Figure 16-4. The nipple adaptation is useful when treating infants. The goal of treatment is for the child to take slow deep inhalations of the medication. The small child and infant are not likely to cooperate so the nose is held, causing mouth breathing and crying, and therefore deep breathing. Inhaled bronchodilators precede postural drainage. Isoproterenol can cause granulation formation in rats when given in extremely high doses, but this side effect has not been reported in the low doses used in humans (two to three breaths of a 1:400 solution prior to postural drainage).

Humidity Therapy. The only place humidity has in the treatment of pediatric lung disease is in croup and with the use of artificial airways.

Postural Drainage. Postural drainage and percussion is a technique readily used in pediatric patients to aid resolution of atelectasis as well as removal of aspirated foreign bodies and mucus from the lung. The duration of therapy and which segments are drained are dependent upon the lesion and the infant or child's condition. The size of the patient will determine whether the procedure is done in the bed or on the therapist's lap. Vibration is often utilized in the premature infant because percussion may be too stressing. The therapist must monitor the infant's or child's color throughout the procedure. If the procedure causes hypoxia, then oxygen should be given. Generally, the maximum duration for postural drainage at one setting is a half hour, which allows for coughing and changing positions. Premature or sick infants may only tolerate five minutes at a time. As in any treatment, the results must be evaluated and the procedure modified as necessary. Nursing care of children and infants is a specialty. There must be an appreciation of the sudden changes in condition that can take place and of how to respond appropriately.

Coughing and Deep Breathing. Methods used to achieve deep breathing and coughing in the infant or uncooperative child are:

1. Postural drainage and percussion
2. Balloon blowing
3. Incentive spirometers

Emphasis must be put on inspiration for best results.

Exercise. Children as well as adults with lung disease need activity; therefore, bedrest is contraindicated. Infants can be placed in infant seats, strollers, or a playpen for periods of time. Older children should be encouraged to be up and about. Play therapists are key people on a pediatric ward.

Oxygen. Enough oxygen should be given via nasal cannula, mask, or hood to maintain an arterial gas tension between 65 and 85 mm Hg.

Oxygen tents have no place in pediatrics, since O_2 concentration cannot be maintained owing to necessary nursing care.

Nasal prongs are available for children; for infants, a nasal cannula can be constructed from soft rubber or polyvinyl tubing and taped just under the nares (Fig. 16-5). With nasal prongs or a catheter, up to a 30% concentration of oxygen can be achieved. When nasal obstruction is present or a higher concentration of oxygen is necessary, a face mask or hood is necessary. The flow through a nasal catheter or prongs should not exceed 3 L/min.

High concentrations of oxygen should be avoided. Arterial blood gases at a tension of 80 mm Hg or more can cause eye damage in

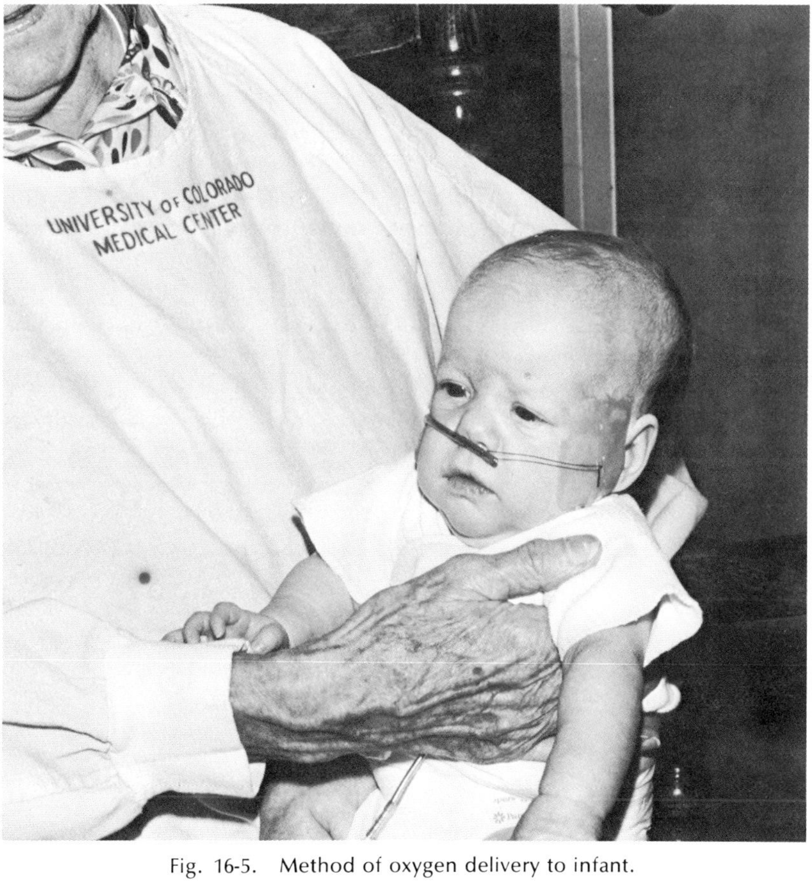

Fig. 16-5. Method of oxygen delivery to infant.

immature infants. Inspired oxygen concentrations greater than 240 mm Hg (40%) administered for prolonged periods can cause alveolar damage and interstitial fibrosis of the lung. Inspired O_2 concentrations should be monitored with arterial oxygen tension measurement or transcutaneous monitors, which should be maintained between 65 and 85 mm Hg.

Endotracheal Tubes. Endotracheal tubes are classified on the basis of the internal diameter of the tube in millimeters.[30] The range of size is 3.5 to 9.5 mm. The correct tube size is that which comfortably passes through the vocal cords. In general, a tube that will pass through the external nares will pass through the cords. For an approximate guide to the endotracheal tube size appropriate for infants and children, see Table 16-1.

Continuous Positive Airway Pressure (CPAP). CPAP (Fig. 16-6) was first used by Gregory in babies with severe hyaline membrane disease.[32] Since loss of surfactant results in loss of alveolar stability, continuous airway pressure can prevent alveolar collapse and can maintain the functional residual capacity. The stability of the alveoli will result in normalizing of the arterial oxygen tension. CPAP is now often used in other conditions such as pulmonary edema in which the arterial oxygen is low. Adequate CPAP will not only increase the pulmonary capillary uptake of oxygen, but also will decrease the amount of oxygen to be given. The decrease in the inspired oxygen will eliminate one of the factors that may lead to alveolar damage. When alveoli are stabilized at a correct FRC, the pulmonary compliance will improve and the work of breathing will decrease.

CPAP is contraindicated in the hyperexpanded and the normal lung. If used in patients who are hyperexpanded, barotrauma

TABLE 16-1. Guide to Appropriate Size of Endotracheal Tubes

Age	*Weight (kg)*	*Internal Diameter (mm)*	*Length (cm)*
Newborn	2.0–2.5	3.5	10
Newborn	2.5–3.0	4.0	12
1 month	3–4	4.5	13
6 months	6	4.5	14
1 year	10	5.0	15
2 years	12	5.5	16
3 years	14	5.5	16
4 years	16	6.0	17
5 years	18	6.0	17
6 years	22	6.5	18
8 years	30	6.5	18
10 years	36	7.0	20
12 years	45	7.0	20
14 years	50	7.5	24

(pneumomediastinum, pneumothorax) can occur. If used in normal lungs or if used with too great a pressure, the effective pulmonary blood flow will be decreased, resulting in drops in arterial oxygen and cardiac output.

Because of possible complications, CPAP should be used only when a widespread loss of FRC (pulmonary edema, RDS, bronchiolitis), airway closure, or both, may occur.

CPAP is available on most modern ventilators but can be set up without assisted ventilation (Fig. 16-6).

The procedure recommended is taken from Gregory's recommendations[32]: CPAP should be initiated when a Pa_{O_2} of less than 50 mm Hg breathing 40 to 60% occurs or when the infant is apneic. Noninvasive (such as nasal) means can be applied early, but if CPAP has increased to 15 cm H_2O and O_2 requirement has increased to 80%, then an endotracheal tube is inserted and CPAP applied. If further deterioration occurs, mechanical ventilation is begun. Distending pressure should be kept low, starting at 4 to 6 cm H_2O and increasing by 2 cm H_2O until the Pa_{O_2} goes to 50 mm Hg. When the Pa_{O_2} reaches 70 mm Hg, the inspired O_2 should be dropped. When the inspired oxygen reaches 40%, then CPAP is reduced in 2-cm H_2O decrements every 2 to 4 hours, being aware that the Pa_{O_2} must remain between 50

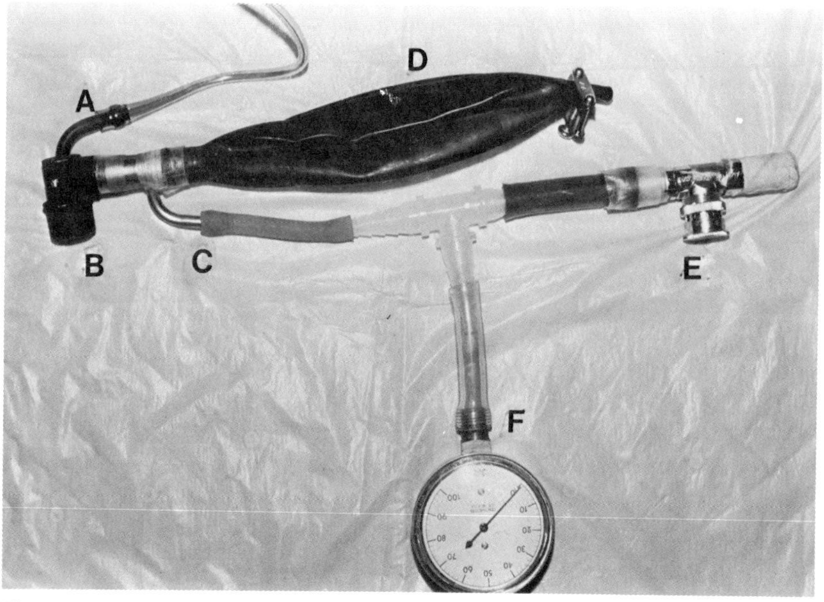

Fig. 16-6. Constant positive airway pressure (CPAP) equipment. Equipment is used when added assisted ventilation is not needed. *A* = inlet for oxygen-enriched mixture; *B* = Norman Elbow, allowing low resistance from airway to bag (*D*) relief valve (*E*); *C* = relief valve and pressure recording vent; *D* = 1.5 L reservoir bag with reduction clamp; *E* = relief valve, which now replaces the water seal; *F* = pressure gauge measuring pressure in cm of H_2O.

and 70 mm Hg. One should not go to zero CPAP but should extubate when CPAP reaches 2 to 4 cm H_2O.

CPAP has increased survival in disease states for which the mortality rate was 80% or more. Now 90% or more of these infants will survive.

For short-term resuscitation (e.g., resuscitation of the newborn), oral tubes are generally used. If the tube is to be left inside more than a few hours, a nasal tube is indicated, since they are more comfortable for the patient and more easily fixed in place.

Endotracheal tubes are obtainable with cuffs from size 5.0 mm on up. The purpose of using a cuffed tube is to provide an airtight seal in the patient-ventilator circuit (which may be essential if high inflation pressures are used) and to isolate the respiratory tract from the gastrointestinal tract, thus preventing aspiration. If an endotracheal tube is cuffed, the volume of air placed in the cuff should be just enough to produce an airtight seal (a small leak is permissible), since excess pressure in the cuff may produce tracheal necrosis and stenosis. The cuff should be deflated for five minutes each hour to prevent persistent ischemia of the tracheal mucosa.

All patients in respiratory distress should be intubated by a person experienced in the technique, since the intubation is usually done with the patient awake and breathing spontaneously. Preoxygenation is an essential prerequisite of intubation, but in many cases, the arterial oxygen tension will not be markedly elevated despite preoxygenation, thus providing only a short time to intubate the patient.

Tracheostomy. Tracheostomy should always be performed as an elective procedure, preferably in the operating room. All tracheostomies should be done over a previously placed endotracheal tube under controlled conditions. Tracheostomy is occasionally required as an urgent lifesaving procedure.

Manual Resuscitating Devices. Manual resuscitation can be performed with a self-inflating bag (Ambu, Hope, and so forth), but these bags can only deliver a maximum of approximately 50% oxygen no matter how great the supplementary oxygen inflow is; this is due to the entrainment of room air as the bag fills, and it limits their usefulness.[31] A simple anesthetic T-piece and bag can also be used. A high flow of oxygen, 5 to 7 L/min, is used to prevent rebreathing. This apparatus should be used whenever 100% oxygen is indicated.

REFERENCES

1. Hodson, W.A.: Lung Biology in Health and Disease. Development of the Lung. Vol. 6. New York, Marcel Dekker, 1977.
2. Thibeault, D.W., and Gregory, G.A.: Neonatal Pulmonary Care. Menlo Park, California, Addison-Wesley, 1979.
3. Behrman, R.E.: The use of acid-base measurements in the clinical evaluation and treatment of the sick neonate. J. Pediatr., *74:*632, 1969.
4. Capitanis, M.A., and Kirkpatrick, J.A., Jr.: Roentgen examination in the evaluation of the newborn infant with respiratory distress. J. Pediatr., *75:*896, 1969.

5. Hallman, M., Kulovich, M.V., Kirkpatrick, E., et al.: Phosphatidylinositol and phosphatidylglycerol in amniotic fluid: indices of lung maturity. Am. J. Obstet. Gynecol., *125:*613, 1976.
6. Nelson, N.M.: On the etiology of hyaline membrane disease. Pediatr. Clin. N. Am., *17:*943, 1970.
7. Tunnessen, W.M., and Feinstein, A.R.: The steroid-croup controversy: An analytic review of methodologic problems. J. Pediatr., *96:*751, 1980.
8. James, J.A.: Dexamethasone in croup. Am. J. Dis. Child., *117:*511, 1969.
9. Westley, C.R., Cotton, E.K., and Brooks, J.G.: Nebulized racemic epinephrine by IPPB for croup: A double blind study. Am. J. Dis. Child., *132:*484, 1978.
10. Battaglia, J.D., and Lockhart, C.H.: Management of acute epiglottitis by nasotracheal intubation. Am. J. Dis. Child., *129:*334, 1975.
11. Moltini, R.A.: Epiglottitis; incidence of extraglottic infection; report of 72 cases and review of literature. Pediatrics, *58:*526, 1976.
12. Todd, J.K.: Pneumonia in children. Postgrad. Med., *61:*254, 1977.
13. Green, M., and Haggerty, R.J.: Ambulatory Pediatrics. Philadelphia, W.B. Saunders Co., 1968.
14. Laraya-Caasay, L.R.: Pulmonary sequelae of acute respiratory viral infection. Pediatr. Ann., *7:*42, 1978.
15. Taussig, L.M., Loughlin, G.M., and Cota, K.A.: Longitudinal assessment of the effects of upper respiratory illness on lung function. Pediatr. Res., *12:*570, 1978.
16. Burrows, B., Knudson, R.J., and Lebowitz, M.D.: The relationship of childhood respiratory illness to adult obstructive airway disease. Am. Rev. Resp. Dis., *115:*751, 1977.
17. Downes, J.J., Wood, D.W., Striker, T.W., et al.: Advances in the management of status asthmaticus. Pediatrics, *38:*286, 1966.
18. Wood, D.W., Downs, J.J., Scheinkopf, H., and Leceks, H.I.: Intravenous isoproterenol in the management of respiratory failure in childhood status asthmaticus. J. Aller. Clin. Immunol., *59:*75, 1972.
19. Cotton, E.K., and Parry, W.: Treatment of status asthmaticus and respiratory failure. Ped. Clin. North Am., *22:*163, 1975.
20. Wood, R.E., Boat, T.F., and Doershuk, C.F.: State of the Art: Cystic Fibrosis. Am. Rev. Resp. Dis., *113:*833, 1976.
21. Mellins, R.B.: Site of airway obstruction in cystic fibrosis. Pediatrics, *44:*315, 1970.
22. Zapletal, A., Motoyama, E.K., Gibson, L.E., et al.: Pulmonary mechanics in asthma and cystic fibrosis. Pediatrics, *48:*64, 1971.
23. Monset-Couchard, M., Mason, C.V., and Moss, A.J.: Cor pulmonale in children. Curr. Prob. Pediatr., *5:*3, 1975.
24. Petty, T.L., et al.: Outpatient oxygen therapy in chronic obstructive pulmonary disease. Arch. Intern. Med., *139:*28, 1979.
25. Blumhagen, J.D., Wesenberg, R.L., Brooks, J.G., and Cotton, E.K.: Endotracheal foreign bodies: Difficulties in diagnosis. Clin. Pediatr., *7:*480, 1980.
26. Cotton, E.K., Abrams, G., Van Houtte, J., and Burrington, J.: Removal of aspirated foreign bodies by inhalation and postural drainage. Clin. Pediatr., *12:*270, 1973.
27. Huch, R., Lubbers, D.W., and Huch, A.: Reliability of transcutaneous monitoring of arterial Po_2 in newborn infants. Arch. Dis. Child., *49:*213, 1974.
28. Tremper, K.K., et al: Continuous transcutaneous oxygen monitoring during respiratory failure, cardiac decompensation, cardiac arrest, and CPR. Crit. Care Med., *8:*377, 1980.
29. Accurso, F., et al.: Comparison of magnetometry and body plethysmography for determination of respiratory timing and amplitude in infants. Am. Rev. Resp. Dis., *121:*283, 1980.
30. Smith, R.M.: Anesthesia for Infants and Children. St. Louis, C.V. Mosby, 1968.
31. Carden, E.B., Chir, B., and Bernstein, M.: Investigation of the nine most commonly used resuscitator bags. JAMA, *212:*589, 1970.
32. Gregory, G.A., Kitterman, J.A., Phibbs, R.N., Tooley, W.H., and Hamilton, W.K.: The treatment of the idiopathic respiratory distress syndrome with continuous positive airway pressure. N. Engl. J. Med., *284:*1333, 1971.

Chapter 17

RESPIRATORY CARE OF THE ELDERLY

By David J. Pierson

The effectiveness of modern respiratory intensive care has now been well established for the management of acute respiratory failure in a wide variety of clinical settings.[1] Improved survival of patients in all diagnostic groups, as shown in Table 17-2, may be achieved in any hospital providing comprehensive care for its patients. Paradoxically, however, in hospitals capable of such life-saving care, it is sometimes withheld from a significant number of patients solely on the basis of advanced age. A considerable number of physicians and at least one geriatrics textbook continue to maintain that "such extreme measures" as tracheal intubation and mechanical ventilation "could seldom be justified" in elderly patients.[2]

Data justifying statements and policies such as withholding aggressive respiratory care from patients older than 70 or some other arbitrary age have not been published, although it is widely observed that patients withstand severe illnesses of all types less well with advancing age. Because of the increasing numbers of old people in our population and in our hospitals, knowledge of the problems to which the elderly are prone and the appropriate use of current methods of management are of prime importance in providing them the best possible care.

The purpose of this chapter is to review the special problems of older patients with acute respiratory illness and to examine the usefulness of intensive respiratory care in the elderly.

THE AGING LUNG

The effects of aging on the respiratory system are summarized in Table 17-1. Significant alterations occur in all aspects of respiratory function with advancing age, some of which are difficult to separate from the effects of disease.[3,4] For example, progressive enlargement of the respiratory bronchioles, alveolar ducts, and alveoli with age makes the distinction between "normal" and "emphysema" difficult, and using strict pathologic criteria, most individuals have changes consistent with emphysema by age 90.[5]

The lungs become progressively more distensible with age as elastic recoil decreases. The total amount of elastic tissue does not change, but its distribution within the lung is altered, and overall surfactant function declines, probably owing to loss of total alveolar surface area. Vital capacity declines progressively by age 70 to about 75% of the value at age 20. At the same time, the loss of lung recoil results in a steady increase in residual volume (by about 50% at age 70) and functional residual capacity. Total lung capacity does not

TABLE 17-1. Effects of Aging on the Respiratory System

Function	*Process*	*Clinical Effect*
Mechanics	↓ Lung elastic recoil ↑ Chest wall stiffness	↓ Vital capacity ↑ Residual volume and functional residual capacity No change in total lung capacity ↓ Flow rates
Gas Exchange	↑ Airway closure in dependent portions of lung ↑ Ventilation/perfusion mismatching	↓ Pa_{O_2} (~4 mm Hg/decade) No change in Pa_{CO_2} or pH
Pulmonary Circulation	↓ Alveolar-capillary surface area	↓ Diffusing capacity
Ventilatory Control	↓ Sensitivity of peripheral chemoreceptors ? ↓ Function of central chemoreceptor	↓ Ventilatory response to hypoxia and hypercapnia
Bellows Function	↓ Strength of respiratory muscles ↑ Chest wall stiffness	↓ Maximum voluntary ventilation ↓ Exercise capacity
Defense Mechanisms	↓ Airway clearance mechanisms ↓ Humoral immunity ↓ Cellular immunity	↑ Susceptibility to infection

change significantly with normal aging; the increases in lung compliance and chest wall stiffness roughly balance one another.

Tests of mechanics such as FEV_1 and FEF_{25-75} show progressive decline with age; FEV_1 falls about 30 ml per year in normal individuals and the FEV_1/VC ratio decreases slightly.

As an individual ages, there is a progressive increase in the number of airways closed in dependent portions of the lung during tidal breathing. Progressive mismatching of ventilation and perfusion results, with widening of the normal alveolar-to-arterial oxygen partial-pressure difference. Arterial Po_2 falls about 4 mm Hg per decade, so that at sea level a healthy individual with Po_2 of 95 at age 20 would have an expected Po_2 of about 80 at age 60, and a value approaching 70 by age 80.[6] At an altitude of 5280 feet, these values would be approximately 75, 62, and 55 mm Hg, respectively. Predictable changes in the pulmonary circulation with age result in progressive loss of alveolar-capillary surface area and a parallel decline in measured diffusing capacity, although this change is of little clinical significance. Pulmonary capillary blood volume stays about the same as age increases, and overall perfusion as assessed by lung scanning remains normal.[7]

Ventilatory control, as indicated by the responses of the peripheral and central chemoreceptors to hypoxia and hypercapnia, becomes blunted with age, as does the heart rate response to these stimuli.[8] Mechanical ability to ventilate deteriorates with age as reflected by the bellows apparatus: Chest wall stiffness increases and the strength of both respiratory and nonrespiratory muscles falls. Thus, there is a progressive decline in maximum voluntary ventilation and in exercise capacity with age.

Finally, pulmonary defense mechanisms weaken with age. Upper airway reflexes become less vigorous, and mucociliary clearance probably deteriorates. There is a gradual decline in the ability both to synthesize antibody in response to antigen and to manifest cellular immunity. This finding is consistent with the high frequency of active tuberculosis in the elderly and with the observed general decrease in resistance to all types of infection.

SPECIAL CONSIDERATIONS FOR ELDERLY PATIENTS IN THE INTENSIVE CARE UNIT

Along with the impaired respiratory and immunologic functioning which accompany normal aging, elderly patients are likely to have coexisting chronic disease in other systems that can increase morbidity and mortality in acute respiratory failure. Elderly patients are less able to withstand insults to the cardiovascular system and are particularly vulnerable to dehydration, fluid overload, and electrolyte imbalance, disorders that frequently occur in the management of acute respiratory failure (Table 17-2). They are more prone than

TABLE 17-2. Special Hazards to the Elderly Patient in the Intensive Care Unit

1. Disorders of medical management
   a. Fluid depletion
   b. Fluid overload
   c. Electrolyte imbalance
2. Masked infection
   a. Respiratory
   b. Urinary
3. Masked acute respiratory failure
4. Intensive care psychosis

younger patients to aspiration of food or gastric contents and to the development of pulmonary emboli in the face of poor peripheral circulation and sudden immobilization, particularly when congestive heart failure is present. Because of the potentially serious nature of the latter complication, prophylactic anticoagulation with low-dose heparin should be part of routine management in high-risk patients.

Acute respiratory failure is associated with a high incidence of cardiac arrhythmias, especially in chronic airway obstruction, which is common in the elderly.[9] These patients should therefore be observed with continuous electrocardiographic monitoring in the respiratory intensive care unit.

Frequent monitoring of respiratory secretions, by tracheal suction when necessary, is important in the elderly because of their impaired ability to manifest infection by usual signs such as fever and leukocytosis. The routine use of prophylactic antibiotics, however, is to be discouraged, since it increases the risk of hospital-acquired resistant superinfection. Specific antimicrobial drugs should be given when indicated on the basis of bacteriologic data or clinical evidence of infection.

TABLE 17-3. Practical Points for the Elderly Patient in the Intensive Care Unit

Things to monitor routinely:
- EKG
- Respiratory secretions
- Sensorium

Things to avoid:
- Excessive sedation
- Urinary catheters
- Indwelling intravenous catheters
- Restraints
- Fecal impaction

The avoidance of procedures or devices that carry a high risk of infection—such as indwelling urinary or intravenous catheters—is of prime importance in the elderly (Table 17-3). External catheters can often be used in male patients, and less hazardous scalp-vein needles should be tried before plastic catheters are inserted.

The clinical manifestations of acute respiratory failure (Table 1-2) are nonspecific and seldom point directly to the lung; in the elderly they may be especially subtle. The most frequent signs—restlessness, confusion, and tachycardia—may be interpreted in the elderly patient as "sundowning," "senility," or just "cantankerousness," and may not arouse concern until respiratory arrest or other serious complication occurs. The physician and nurse must think of acute respiratory failure whenever a change in behavior, mental status, or vital signs occurs, and must pursue this diagnosis with arterial blood gas determination and clinical reassessment of the patient.

Whenever possible, physical restraints should be avoided in the elderly. When necessary, they must be carefully positioned so as not to restrict chest movement and thus promote hypoventilation. Likewise, because of the sensitivity of older patients to the respiratory-depressant effects of sedatives, anesthetics, and most analgesics, these should be used with caution. This is particularly true when renal insufficiency, liver disease, or chronic airway obstruction is present.

Elderly patients are especially prone to intensive care unit psychosis and to less severe mental disturbances resulting from severe illness and unfamiliar surroundings.[10] Frequent family visits and constant efforts to maintain orientation—an easily visible clock, having patients' beds close to the window, and frequent reminders by the staff to patients of where they are and why—will help to minimize these complications.

Pulmonary complications represent the most frequent and most serious of postoperative problems, and it has long been established that these are most common in elderly patients.[11,12] Since the increased incidence of complications parallels the increased incidence of chronic airway obstruction in older individuals, identification of high-risk patients through preoperative pulmonary function tests and arterial blood gas determinations is imperative when the presence of chest disease is suggested by history or physical examination.

Such high-risk patients, once identified, must have preoperative instruction in bronchial hygiene, and rigorous postoperative care.[13] The latter should include the use of a mechanical ventilator whenever spontaneous ventilation is inadequate, and frequent nasotracheal suctioning, chest physiotherapy, and postural drainage if excessive secretions or atelectasis are evident.

Finally, application of the principles of rehabilitation (Chap. 18) is especially important in the elderly, who are susceptible to rapid weight loss, skeletal demineralization, and the development of decubitus ulcers whenever they are placed at total bed rest. The encouragement of adequate nutrition—often by selecting favorite foods on the recommendations of family or friends—and avoidance of fecal impaction through the use of stool softeners, along with early and vigorous ambulation, may make the difference between recovery and continued morbidity or death.

ILLUSTRATIVE CASES

The following case examples illustrate how the principles and methods of intensive respiratory care may be applied effectively to elderly patients, sometimes with surprisingly favorable results in what appear to be irreversible clinical situations.

Case 1. V.C., an 84-year-old woman who did not speak English, was admitted with productive cough and dyspnea. Physical examination showed respiratory distress and signs of consolidation of the left lower lobe. Initial laboratory data revealed gram-positive diplococci in her sputum and a left basilar infiltrate on chest roentgenogram. In the absence of prior medical information, the patient was thought to have pneumococcal pneumonia exacerbating chronic obstructive pulmonary disease, and was treated with penicillin, bronchodilators, and corticosteroids. Sputum cultures revealed no pathogens, however, and over the first four days in the hospital the patient deteriorated despite vigorous routine treatment for pneumonia. On the fifth day acute respiratory failure developed, manifested by progressive fatigue, decreased responsiveness, and fall in arterial pH from 7.49 to 7.27 with rise in P_{CO_2} from 28 to 52 mm Hg.

Despite reluctance on the part of some of the physicians participating in her care to proceed with "heroic" measures in what seemed to be a chronic and perhaps irreversible situation, the patient was intubated and placed on a volume-cycled ventilator. At this point a positive cold-agglutinin titer of 1:2038 was reported in a blood specimen from the third hospital day, and tetracycline was begun for presumed *Mycoplasma* pneumonia. The patient improved dramatically during assisted ventilation and was extubated after 24 hours. Thereafter, she recovered uneventfully and was discharged on the tenth hospital day. At initial follow-up 3 months later the patient had no respiratory symptoms whatever and had resumed her previous active life.

Comment. This patient appeared at first to have "end-stage" chronic airway obstruction with irreversible respiratory failure. A fatal outcome was avoided through the use of tracheal intubation and assisted ventilation. This case illustrates the hazards of withholding available therapy from a patient whose history is not thoroughly known to the managing physician; the decision to "let him go" cannot be made without a complete familiarity with the patient and the certainty that the acute episode is irreversible, information which is seldom available in the acute "crash" situation.

Case 2. S.I., a 70-year-old man, was admitted during an influenza epidemic with an acute febrile illness and increasing shortness of breath. His history included chronic airway obstruction, manifested by dyspnea, productive cough, and mild arterial oxygen desaturation. Three days prior to admission he noted malaise, fever, sore throat, and a change from white to greenish yellow sputum. Because of continued symptoms after a trial of broad-spectrum antibiotic he was admitted to the medical ward.

The patient was afebrile on admission, with physical findings of chronic airway obstruction. Laboratory data included mild leukopenia, moderate arterial oxygen desaturation, and bilateral basilar infiltrates on chest roentgenogram. After cultures were obtained, treatment was begun with bronchodilators, humidification, supplemental nasal oxygen, and broad-spectrum antibiotics.

Over the first 4 hospital days the patient deteriorated: he remained dyspneic with daily fevers to 39°C, and chest roentgenograms showed increasing lower lobe infiltrates. All cultures were negative for pathogens, and corticosteroids were added to the treatment regimen. Because of increasing respiratory distress and progressive hypoxemia on increasing flows of nasal oxygen, the patient was transferred to the respiratory intensive care unit, intubated with a nasotracheal tube, and placed on a volume-cycled respirator.

Initial ventilator settings using 100% O_2 (F_{IO_2} = 1.0) failed to raise the patient's P_{O_2} to acceptable levels, and positive end-expiratory pressure (PEEP) was added. After initial further deterioration, during which he required 10 cm PEEP and F_{IO_2} = 1.0 for 36 hours, the patient gradually improved. His extensive bilateral pulmonary infiltrates gradually cleared, and PEEP was reduced and finally discontinued once an acceptable reduction in F_{IO_2} to 0.45 had been achieved.

The patient was successfully weaned from the respirator and was extubated on the sixteenth hospital day. Supplemental nasal oxygen was dis-

TABLE 17-4. Diagnoses of Patients over Age 70 Ventilated Between January 1, 1971, and December 31, 1972

I.	Acute respiratory failure in patients with chronic airway obstruction
II.	Acute respiratory failure in patients with other pulmonary diseases (overwhelming pneumonia, status asthmaticus, kyphoscoliotic lung disease)
III.	Acute respiratory failure in surgical patients (those requiring ventilation for more than 12 hours postoperatively; acute respiratory failure occurring within 6 days postoperatively; massive trauma, extensive burns)
IV.	Short-term postoperative ventilation (12 hours or less)
V.	Miscellaneous cases of acute respiratory failure (cerebrovascular accidents, coma of other causes, poisonings, cardiorespiratory arrest of a variety of causes)

continued after another three days, after which time the patient's Po_2 remained within the acceptable range breathing room air.

The patient was discharged after 20 days in the hospital, and soon thereafter returned to his usual activity. He was well when seen 6 months after his initial episode of respiratory failure.

Comment. This patient entered with a flu-like illness which progressed despite treatment to the adult respiratory distress syndrome. Aggressive management, including mechanical ventilation with PEEP, resulted in a gradual but complete recovery. Although culture confirmation is lacking, he is presumed to have had bilateral viral pneumonia, with the adult respiratory distress syndrome occurring as a recognized complication of this illness.

Case 3. W.T., a 76-year-old man, first noted dyspnea on exertion 15 years prior to admission. For 5 years he had had productive cough, episodes of wheezing, and increasingly incapacitating dyspnea. In the year prior to admission he had been treated continuously with bronchodilators, corticosteroids, and intermittent nasal oxygen, and he had been hospitalized on one occasion for shortness of breath.

The patient entered the hospital with a severe episode of wheezing, which had not responded to aggressive outpatient therapy, and within hours of admission developed acute respiratory failure. His arterial pH fell from 7.44 to 7.22 over 2 hours, with a rise in Pco_2 from 39 to 79, at which time a nasotracheal tube was inserted and the patient placed on a volume-cycled respirator. He improved with high-dose corticosteroids, antibiotics, and bronchodilators, was extubated after 24 hours of assisted ventilation, and went home on the sixth hospital day.

The patient received continuous low-flow nasal oxygen at home and returned to an active life for 3 months following his initial episode of respiratory failure. At that time he again required hospitalization for increasing shortness of breath. Shortly after admission he suffered a cardiorespiratory arrest, was successfully resuscitated, and underwent mechanical ventilation for 18 hours. He again improved and was discharged on the fifth hospital day.

TABLE 17-5. Overall Survival—Assisted Ventilation in Patients over Age 70

Result	*Number*	*Percentage*
Lived—went home	33	29
Lived—transferred to other hospitals	5	4
Lived—transferred to nursing homes or rehabilitative facilities	20	18
Died while on ventilator	29	26
Died in hospital after discontinuation of assisted ventilation	26	23

The patient suffered a third exacerbation 5 months after discharge, which was successfully managed without mechanical ventilation. He has since done well and was self-sufficient at home on continuous oxygen therapy 22 months after his first episode of acute respiratory failure.

Comment. This patient was managed aggressively despite a previous history of long-standing, disabling chronic airway obstruction requiring continuous supplemental oxygen, a prior episode of acute respiratory failure, and the development of cardiorespiratory arrest. His acute respiratory failure proved to be readily reversible on three separate occasions, although in each instance this might not have been predicted at the outset. On each occasion the patient was able to resume a reasonably productive life despite his age and the seriousness of his illness.

ASSISTED VENTILATION IN THE ELDERLY

Because of several anecdotal cases similar to those just described, in which mechanical ventilation and other aspects of current respiratory intensive care were used successfully in elderly patients, a retrospective analysis of a series of such patients was recently undertaken at our institution to examine the efficacy of this treatment.[14]

All patients 70 years of age or older who underwent mechanical ventilation for any reason at either Colorado General Hospital or Denver General Hospital during the 24 months ending December 31, 1972, were included in the study. These two hospitals together serve a large and varied patient population representative of the greater Denver area, as well as patients referred from nearby cities and adjacent states. All acute respiratory care in these hospitals, including the use of mechanical ventilators, is provided by the members of the Division of Pulmonary Medicine of the University of Colorado Medical Center.

The patients were classified into the diagnostic groups shown in Table 17-4. Information was sought regarding the presence of chronic lung disease prior to hospitalization, as defined by symptoms, physical examination, chest roentgenograms, and pulmonary function testing when available. Smoking history, when available, was noted.

TABLE 17-6. Relationship of Age to Survival among Patients Treated with Assisted Ventilation

Age	*Number*	*Survived*	*Percentage of Survival*
70–74	49	28	57
75–79	36	19	53
80–95	28	11	39

Complications occurring during assisted ventilation were recorded, as was the outcome of each hospitalization. Chi-square analysis was used to assess statistical significance.

During the 24-month study period, 61,196 patients were admitted to the two hospitals. Out of this number, 1178 adults underwent continuous assisted ventilation, of whom 113, or 9.6%, were from 70 to 95 years of age. Forty-nine patients were between 70 and 74, and 85 were under age 80. There were 69 men and 44 women; 95 were white and 18, nonwhite.

Fifteen patients required ventilatory assistance more than once during a given admission. Volume-cycled machines accounted for two-thirds of all ventilator usages. The total duration of assisted ventilation in these patients ranged from one hour to 71 days; 71 were ventilated for 3 days or less. Total hospital stay averaged 20 days.

The overall survival of the patients studied is shown in Table 17-5. Fifty-eight patients (51%) survived acute respiratory failure and were discharged from the hospital. Of these, 57% went home, 9% were transferred to other hospitals for acute care, and 34% were transferred to rehabilitation centers or nursing homes. Of the 55 patients (49%) who died in the hospital, 53% succumbed while on the ventilator and 47%, from 6 hours to 31 days after respiratory support was discontinued.

Survival decreased as age increased in these patients as shown in Table 17-6, although the differences were not statistically significant. Similarly, survival following assisted ventilation was not significantly related to duration of ventilatory support (Table 17-7). Indeed, of the five patients alive at the end of two weeks on the respirator, four survived.

Table 17-7 shows survival among the patients in the different diagnostic groups. Included in Group I (acute respiratory failure in chronic airway obstruction) are two patients who survived this and a subsequent episode requiring assisted ventilation during another hospital admission; four had had previous episodes of acute respiratory failure not requiring a respirator, and seven were receiving sup-

TABLE 17-7. Relationship of Duration of Assisted Ventilation to Survival in Acute Respiratory Failure

Duration	*Number*	*Survived*	*Percentage of Survival*
24 hours or less	49	29	59
1–2 days	22	11	50
3–6 days	17	6	35
7 days or longer	25	12	48

plemental oxygen at home prior to admission. Of the latter group, six left the hospital alive.

Among the surgical patients, 29 were ventilated following emergency procedures and 15 after elective operations. Survival in these 2 groups was identical. Respiratory failure occurred in the 8 other surgical patients after the surgical procedure (Table 17-8).

Neither the availability of prior historic information nor laboratory data nor the presence of pre-existing chronic lung diseases, as defined, had a significant correlation with patient survival. Likewise, among these patients, cigarette smoking had no effect on prognosis; those who smoked and those who did not had the same rate of survival.

Table 17-9 shows the associations between severe specific complications occurring during assisted ventilation and patient survival. Pneumonia developing after the patient had been placed on the ventilator was associated with a decrease in survival that was significant ($P < .02$) when compared with patients who did not develop this complication. However, the occurrence of congestive heart failure, as diagnosed by chest roentgenogram, and the development of pneumothorax, both considered grave events in patients with acute respiratory failure, carried no statistically significant increase in mortality in this series.

Patients who were resuscitated from cardiorespiratory arrest and then placed on assisted ventilation survived as often as those ventilated without a previous arrest. However, cardiac arrest occurring while the patient was on the respirator was fatal in all but 2 of 15 patients. Simultaneous occurrence of two or more of these complications in a patient receiving assisted ventilation was not associated

TABLE 17-8. Survival in Assisted Ventilation among Different Diagnostic Groups

Group	*Diagnosis*	*Number*	*Survived*	*Percentage of Survival*
I	Acute respiratory failure in chronic airway obstruction	19	14	74
II	Acute respiratory failure in other pulmonary diseases	10	4	40
III	Acute respiratory failure in surgical patients	38	17	45
IV	Short-term postoperative ventilation	14	11	79
V	Miscellaneous cases of acute respiratory failure	35	12	34

with increased mortality. Gram-negative sepsis and massive pulmonary embolism were fatal in every instance.

Although the overall survival in this group of elderly patients was poorer than that observed in all patients placed on ventilators at this institution, it is clear from the data presented that vigorous resuscitation in the elderly patient with acute respiratory failure can often be successful. Indeed, in the group of patients with acute respiratory failure complicating chronic airway obstruction, the overall survival rate of 74% is well within the range reported in most series for all patients with this disease. This study refutes the assumptions that assisted ventilation is less applicable to elderly patients than to others and that an unfavorable outcome can be predicted from history, seriousness of presentation, or development of complications.

SUMMARY

This chapter has reviewed aspects of pulmonary function and acute respiratory illness in the elderly and has presented data on the effectiveness of current methods in treating respiratory failure in these patients. Although nothing in the care of older patients is qualitatively different from the treatment of younger individuals, several

TABLE 17-9. Effect of Specific Complications during Assisted Ventilation on Survival of Patients over Age 70

Complication	*Number*	*Survived*	*Percentage of Survival*
Pneumonia	47	18	38
Did not develop pneumonia	66	40	61
Heart failure by x-ray examination	30	12	40
Did not develop heart failure	83	46	55
Pneumothorax	10	5	50
Did not develop pneumothorax	103	53	51
Cardiorespiratory arrest prior to being placed on ventilator	26	13	50
Ventilated without prior arrest	87	45	52
Cardiac arrest while on ventilator*	13	2	15
Did not arrest on ventilator	100	56	56
Any combination of 2 or more of the above 5 complications	32	16	50
Sepsis (positive blood culture while on ventilator)	6	0	0
Pulmonary embolism (diagnosed during life)	2	0	0

* For which resuscitation was attempted.

aspects of respiratory intensive care in the elderly deserve special attention. These include meticulous attention to fluid and electrolyte balance, the cautious use of respiratory depressant drugs, careful treatment and prevention of infection, measures to prevent mental disturbances, the provision of adequate nutrition, and efforts toward earliest possible ambulation and physical rehabilitation.

The physician caring for the elderly patient with acute respiratory failure should not hesitate to use all the means at his disposal to treat it. There may be pressure from fellow physicians, nurses, family members, and occasionally even the patient, to avoid "heroics" and aggressive measures. While occasionally this may be appropriate, the decision to withhold current respiratory intensive care must not be made without a thorough familiarity with the patient, and cannot be urged on the presumption that this treatment is likely to fail. Indeed, acute respiratory failure may be as reversible in the elderly as in any patient, and the physician must be as aggressive as with the young in all aspects of its treatment.

REFERENCES

1. Petty, T.L., Lakshminarayan, S., Sahn, S.A., Zwillich, C.W., and Nett, L.M.: Intensive respiratory care unit: Review of ten years' experience. JAMA, *233:*34, 1975.
2. Agate, J.: The Practice of Geriatrics. 2nd Ed. London, William Heinemann Medical Books, 1970, p. 174.
3. Murray, J.F.: The Normal Lung. Philadelphia, W.B. Saunders Co., 1976, pp. 307–324.
4. Campbell, E.J., and Lefrak, S.S.: How aging affects the structure and function of the respiratory system. Geriatrics, *33:*68, 1978.
5. Liebow, A.A.: Biochemical and structural changes in the aging lung: Summary. In Aging of the Lung. Edited by L. Cander, and J.G. Moyer. New York, Grune & Stratton, 1964, pp. 97–104.
6. Sorbini, C.A., Grassi, V., Solinas, E., and Muiesan, G.: Arterial oxygen tension in relation to age in healthy subjects. Respiration, *25:*3, 1968.
7. Kronenberg, R.S., L'Heureux, P., Ponto, R.A., Drage, C.W., and Loken, K.M.: The effect of aging on lung perfusion. Ann. Intern. Med., *76:*413, 1972.
8. Kronenberg, R.S., and Drage, C.W.: Attenuation of the ventilatory and heart rate responses to hypoxia and hypercapnia with aging in normal men. J. Clin. Invest., *52:*1812, 1973.
9. Hudson, L.D., Kurt, T.L., Petty, T.L., and Genton, E.: Arrhythmias associated with acute respiratory failure in patients with chronic airway obstruction. Chest, *63:*661, 1973.
10. Wilson, L.M.: Intensive care delirium. Arch. Intern. Med., *130:*225, 1972.
11. Dripps, R.D., and Deming, M.V.N.: Postoperative atelectasis and pneumonia: diagnosis, etiology, and management based upon 1240 cases of upper abdominal surgery. Ann. Surg., *124:*94, 1946.
12. Zeffren, S.E., and Hartford, C.E.: Comparative mortality for various surgical operations in older versus younger age groups. J. Am. Geriatr. Soc., *20:*485, 1972.
13. Lorhan, P.H.: Anesthesia for the Aged. Springfield, IL, Charles C Thomas, 1971, pp. 125–138.
14. Pierson, D.J., Neff, T.A., and Petty, T.L.: Ventilatory management of the elderly. Geriatrics, *28:*86, 1973.

Section D

Extended Care

The development of a comprehensive respiratory care program demands the establishment of effective outpatient and home care for selected patients. The use of home oxygen—including portable oxygen systems and oxygen concentrators, and simple techniques of bronchial hygiene—is now established. Many patients with severe respiratory insufficiency can be effectively maintained at home with a great economic saving and with enhanced comfort. Home ventilation is possible in patients with advanced muscular dystrophy. This section deals with pulmonary rehabilitation and home care in COPD and new methods of care for the neuromuscular patient.

Chapter 18

PULMONARY REHABILITATION FOR COPD

By Thomas L. Petty

Patients with chronic obstructive pulmonary disease (COPD)—also called chronic airflow obstruction or limitation—and other chronic respiratory diseases who recover through intensive efforts to reverse acute respiratory failure often require an organized extended care period designed for functional improvement and further physical rehabilitation. In addition, patients with chronic airway obstruction who are less severely ill benefit from sytematic outpatient care.[1] It must be remembered that COPD represents this country's most rapidly growing health problem in the adult population.[2] For example, it has been estimated that 8 million Americans suffer from emphysema and chronic bronchitis; 500,000 are receiving social security benefits for disability.[3]

It has now been determined that the systematic application of certain forms of well-established therapy may lead to improved functional ability and increased work efficiency in spite of the fact that severe expiratory airflow obstruction persists.[1,4,5]

In order to provide extended care for patients recovering from chronic airflow obstruction and to provide for comprehensive clinic and home care for patients with chronic respiratory insufficiency, an organized multidisciplinary approach is needed. The major methods include patient education, bronchial hygiene, breathing retraining, physical reconditioning, and, in some cases, continuous oxygen therapy in the home. Oxygen is discussed later in the chapter.

Education is the cornerstone of management of all chronic diseases. This has long been true for diabetic individuals, who are taught sophisticated self-care including concepts of insulin dosage, methods of hypodermic needle administration, and principles of controlled diet, activity, and total care. So it is with the COPD patient. The enlightened patient must become a member of his own health team and must provide for his own day-to-day self-care. We have found that individual instruction or small group instruction is most helpful (Fig. 18-1). At least three initial sessions, two individual and one group, should be held. Patients are taught a fairly complete review of pulmonary anatomy and physiology, as well as the pathology of emphysema, chronic bronchitis, and associated disorders. Simple drawings and illustrations in booklets supplement the instructions given by trained nurses.[6] Clinic instruction is reinforced by visits from the public health nurse when this is possible.

Prevention is a fundamental concept in COPD management. All efforts to stop smoking should be made; although no set formula exists that will insure that patients can stop smoking, the straightforward intellectual approach is probably the best. This must be supported by the physician's belief in the continued harm of smoking and the demonstration that the physician himself will not tolerate smoking in his office. Avoiding air pollution is desirable when possible; effective air-conditioning systems in the patient's home and place of work may help in urban areas having severe air pollution.

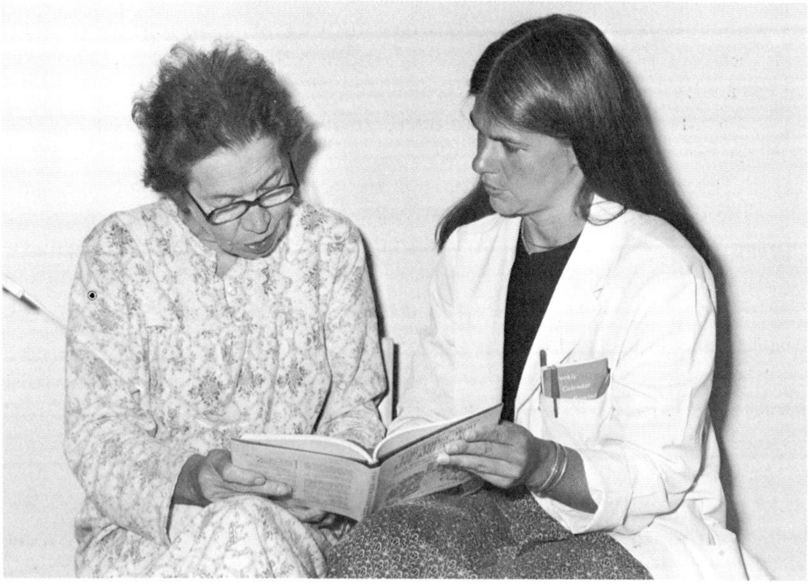

Fig. 18-1. Respiratory care nurse instructing patient using patient care manual. Hand-made scrapbooks are also used.

Influenza vaccine should be administered each fall for whatever protection it will afford. Patients should avoid individuals with communicable respiratory diseases whenever possible. They should have a home supply of tetracycline, ampicillin, or trimethoprim-sulfa for self-administration when they develop deep chest infections with obvious purulence or fever, or both. Generally, an initial dose of 2 g tetracycline daily or 2 to 4 g ampicillin is followed in 48 hours with half this dose. Trimethaprim-sulfa is given in a convenient fixed combination morning and night for 7 to 10 days in exacerbations of chronic bronchitis. It is an important addition to our antimicrobial arsenal.

Each patient needs to learn a method of home bronchial hygiene that is applicable to his own situation. Bronchial hygiene—the protection and cleansing of the airways—involves inhalation of bronchodilator drugs, followed by inhalation of moisture, followed in turn by expulsive coughing or postural drainage, or both (see Chap. 7).[5,7] It is now appreciated that bronchodilators, particularly beta agonists such as isoetharine, stimulate mucociliary clearance.[8] Thus, this pharmacologic effect may be useful even in patients who do not demonstrate an improvement in airflow on laboratory testing. Theophylline also improves mucociliary clearance in man.[9]

A variety of bronchodilator drugs is available. Those in most common use are isoetharine (Bronchosol), metaproterenol (Alupent, Metaprel), and albuterol (Proventil, Ventolin) or isoproterenol (Isuprel) by metered dose device. Isoetharine, metaproterenol, and isoproterenol are used as inhalant solutions. Albuterol is not currently available as a solution. The duration of effectiveness ranges from half an hour to 6 hours, depending on dose and choice of drug. Isoproterenol lasts 60 to 90 minutes, isoetharine and metaproterenol 3 to 4 hours and occasionally longer, and albuterol 5 to 6 hours. With all these beta-agonist bronchodilators, longer activity periods occur in patients with the greatest degree of reversibility. Side effects vary.

Generally, 0.2 or 0.3 ml or 5 to 10 drops of a bronchodilator drug are diluted with an equal amount of water and consumed over a 5- to 10-minute period in a hand-powered or pump-driven nebulizer. It must be stressed that this is simply a starting dose; in the event of palpitations, the drug should be diluted more or used for shorter periods of time, or both. If, by contrast, no clinical benefit is observed, longer periods of nebulization and increasing dosages may be tried. Some patients tolerate undiluted bronchodilator drugs. Although ventilatory function tests are helpful as guides to the therapeutic effectiveness of a drug, they have insufficient sensitivity to small changes in airway resistance; thus, the physician should be partly guided by the patient's own judgment of relief of symptoms.

Bronchodilator drugs may be administered by a variety of means, such as a hand bulb nebulizer (Fig. 18-2), a pump-driven nebulizer, or a pressure breathing machine. A hand-held IPPB device has also been effective in both the hospital and home administration of bronchodilator drugs.[10] The popularity of IPPB for bronchodilator administration has been waning greatly in recent years. Currently, a controlled multicenter clinical trial is underway comparing the effectiveness of bronchodilator administration by IPPB with that provided by a powered nebulizer. This study promises to answer many questions about IPPB.

Thus far, no controlled study has shown that delivering a bronchodilating drug via an IPPB machine is any more effective than delivering it by a hand nebulizer or a pump-driven nebulizer.[11,12] Tidal volume and alveolar ventilation can be increased transiently in severe COPD by use of IPPB, but on discontinuance of this technique, the previous level of tidal volume and alveolar ventilation returns (unless bronchospasm is improved with drugs or clearance of secretions is accomplished).[12] Clinical experience, however, dictates that certain patients either subjectively or objectively benefit from bronchodilators delivered via IPPB. These are generally individuals with very severe obstruction, meaning an FEV_1 of considerably less than 1 liter per second. It should be remembered that the devices already mentioned are effective and are easy and safe to use in the home. If, therefore, following a trial, IPPB appears to be useful in the overall therapeutic plan, there should be no hesitation to use it.

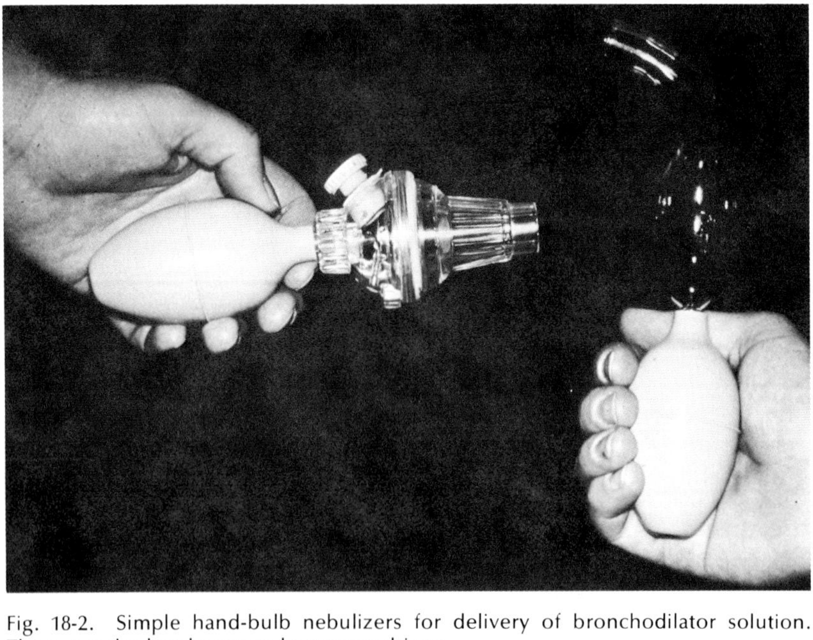

Fig. 18-2. Simple hand-bulb nebulizers for delivery of bronchodilator solution. These may be hand powered or pump driven.

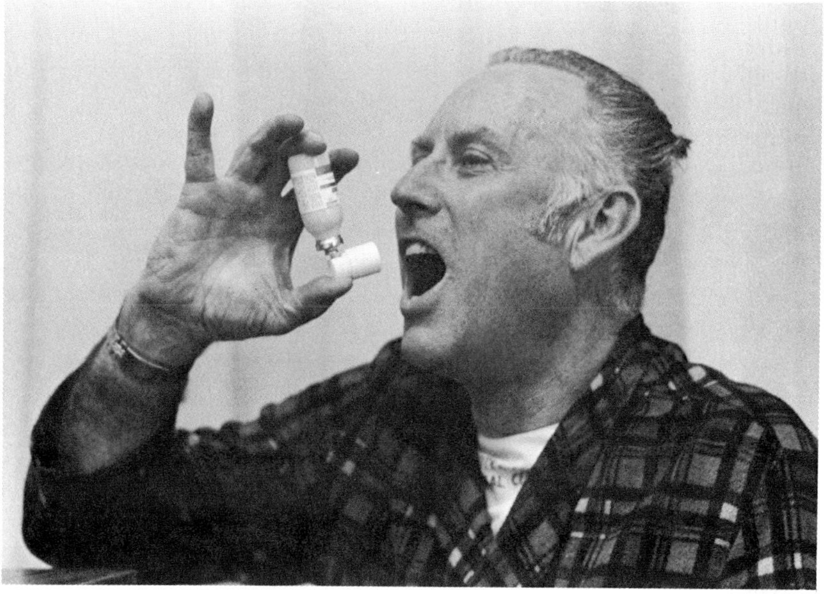

Fig. 18-3. Bronkometer device being properly used. Notice nozzle is held in front of teeth to allow large particles to precipitate out. Patient inhales slowly from mid-lung volume following actuation of device, and pauses and exhales against pursed lips to promote deposition. Other metered-dose devices such as Alupent, Metaprel, Ventolin, and Proventil are used in similar manner.

It should be emphatically stated, however, that if a patient benefits from IPPB, he should have his own device and should not be dependent upon trips to the physician's office or the "puffing parlor" of an outpatient inhalation department, with its attendant costs and risks of cross-infection. Each patient should be taught to use and clear his own machine at home for convenience and safety.

Moreover, a simple, inexpensive pump-driven nebulizer* is useful as a means of delivering therapeutic aerosols. Today, however, the metered-dose aerosol is the most common method of administration of inhaled bronchodilator (Fig. 18-3). Previous questions about particle size must be re-evaluated in view of new knowledge about the fate and deposition of inhaled drugs in general. Fears of overuse can be overcome by instruction and by the patient's understanding of pharmacologic principles and objectives of therapy. The patient is taught to inhale from midlung volume, to activate the device into the open mouth while inhaling, and to pause at the end of inspiration to encourage deposition of drug. Exhalation slowly against pursed lips is also taught. This sequence can be repeated one to four times depending upon side effects.

* Maxi-Myst, Meade Johnson, Evansville, Indiana.

Immediately after bronchodilator administration, there should be a period of moisture inhalation. Simple devices—nursery humidifiers and steaming devices—are capable of providing sufficient moisture (Fig. 18-4). Simple devices are preferred. Although a high-density mist can be delivered by newer ultrasonic nebulizers, clinical experience with these devices fails to indicate their superiority, and ultrasonic mist may have an adverse effect on pulmonary mechanics in patients with asthma and chronic bronchitis.[14] Following moisture inhalation, expulsive coughing will generally clear the airways of the retained secretions.

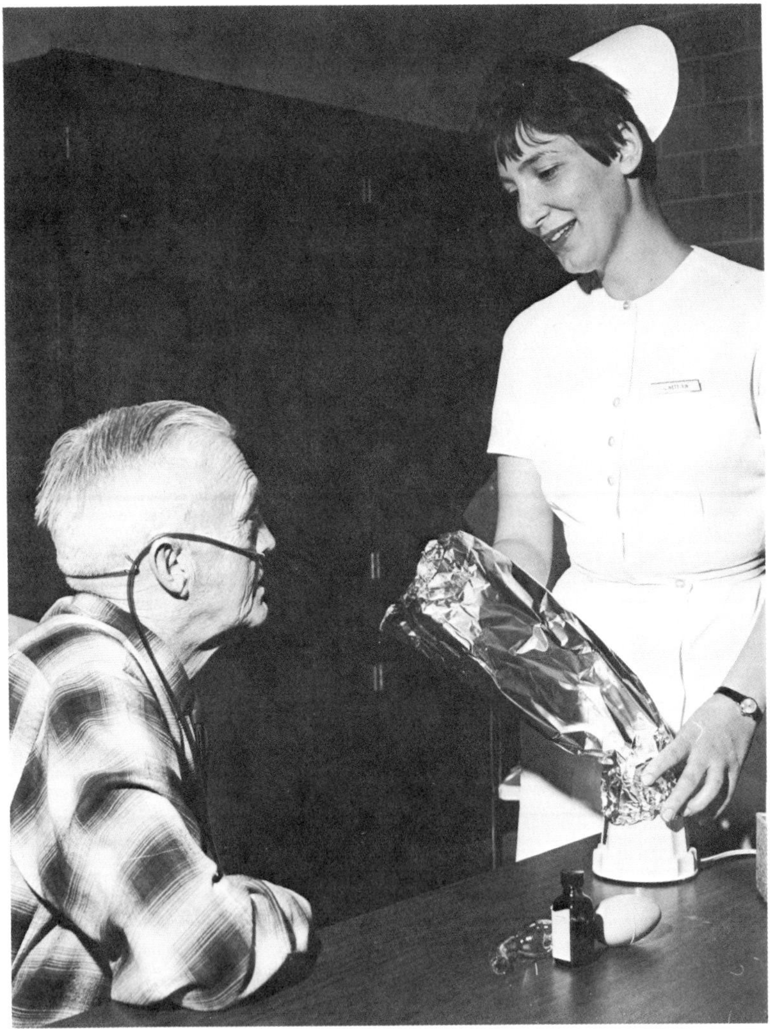

Fig. 18-4. Nursery-type humidifier, which is an adapted baby bottle warmer used with metal foil for steaming.

Many expectorant drugs are in common use today. Although the iodides will provide a serous bronchorrhea, their long-term use may cause bronchial irritation. Saturated solution of potassium iodide (10 drops in water three times daily) may be used for one or two days in patients in whom this is clinically effective. Glyceryl guaiacolate is widely used today. Whereas this drug probably does no harm, there is little objective evidence that it is effective in producing bronchorrhea. In a controlled trial, the drug has been found ineffective both in vitro and in vivo.[15]

It should be stressed that moisture inhalation is the most important means of thinning secretions. Also, in the absence of congestive heart failure, liberal intake of fluids, up to three quarts daily, is desirable and will help thin secretions.

Special mention should be made of the high degree of effectiveness of steroid drugs in exacerbations of bronchitis and bronchiolitis that are marked by sudden worsening dyspnea with reduced sputum production and profound hypoxemia. Corticosteroid therapy in doses of 30 mg prednisone daily given for approximately 3 days is effective in most cases. At times, low maintenance doses of corticosteroids (5 to 10 mg) have been associated with objective functional improvement in patients with chronic bronchitis.[16] The overall effectiveness of corticosteroids is a matter of a current study, but at the present time a trial of corticosteroids in the treatment of a bronchitic

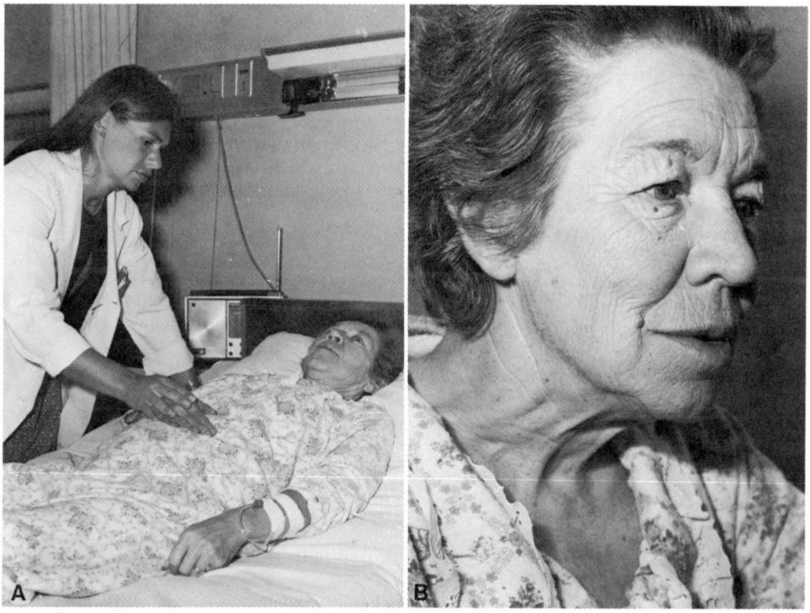

Fig. 18-5. Respiratory care nurse stressing abdominal-diaphragmatic breathing with exhalation against pursed lips with patient in recumbent position. Similar techniques are used with patients sitting and leaning forward.

patient with wheezing attacks seems warranted. It is now recognized that symptomatic benefit is often supported by objective evidence of improvement in forced vital capacity (FVC) and forced expiratory volume in one second (FEV_1).[17] When corticosteroids bring benefit, they may be continued in a low morning dose or on alternate days. Inhaled beclomethasone (Vanceril, Beclovent) may also maintain the benefit. If not, the physician and the patient will have to decide whether or not the benefit achieved by oral corticosteroids is worth the risks of long-term side effects, such as osteoporosis and cataract formation. In most cases, men tolerate long-term systemic corticosteroids better than women. Additional "baseline" pharmacology often includes oral theophylline in addition to an inhaled beta agonist and corticosteroids, if they are found beneficial. Controlled

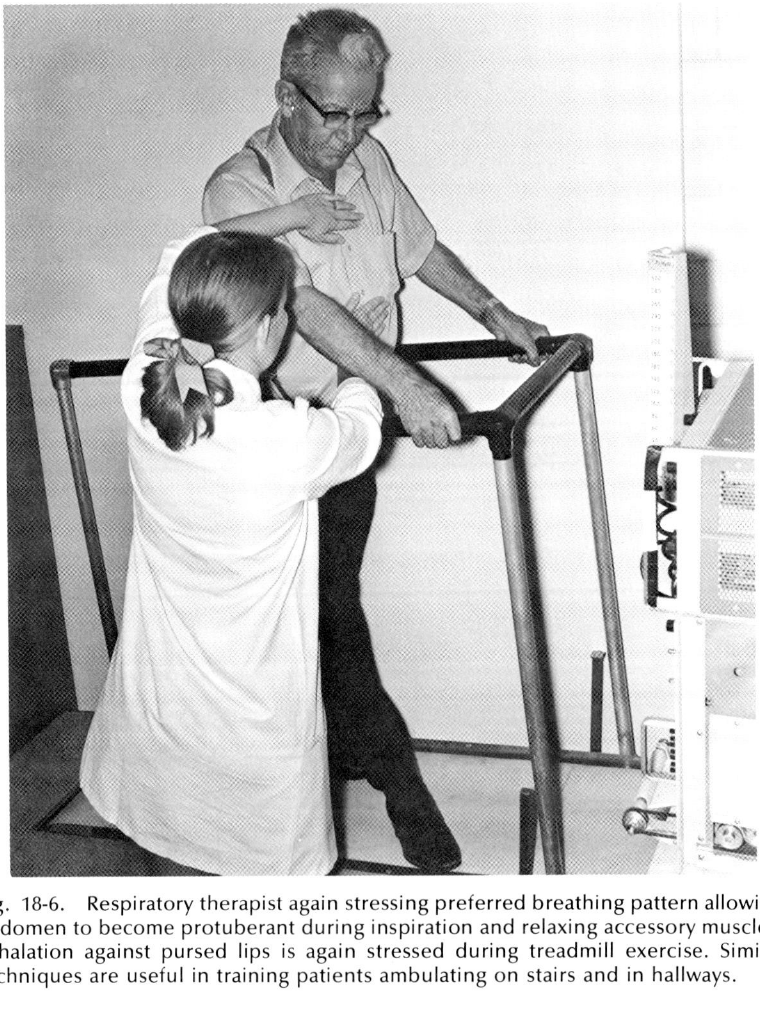

Fig. 18-6. Respiratory therapist again stressing preferred breathing pattern allowing abdomen to become protuberant during inspiration and relaxing accessory muscles. Exhalation against pursed lips is again stressed during treadmill exercise. Similar techniques are useful in training patients ambulating on stairs and in hallways.

clinical trials do not support the use of theophylline in all patients. Most "responders" could be predicted on the basis of improved flow rates following inhalation of a beta agonist.[18] The long-used combination tablets with theophylline and ephedrine are rapidly being replaced by separate use of theophylline and, at times, an additional oral beta agonist such as metaproterenol (Alupent, Metaprel) or terbutaline (Brethine, Bricanyl). Tremor may be a problem with oral beta agonists, but generally this subsides or is simply tolerated in favor of symptomatic and objective benefit.

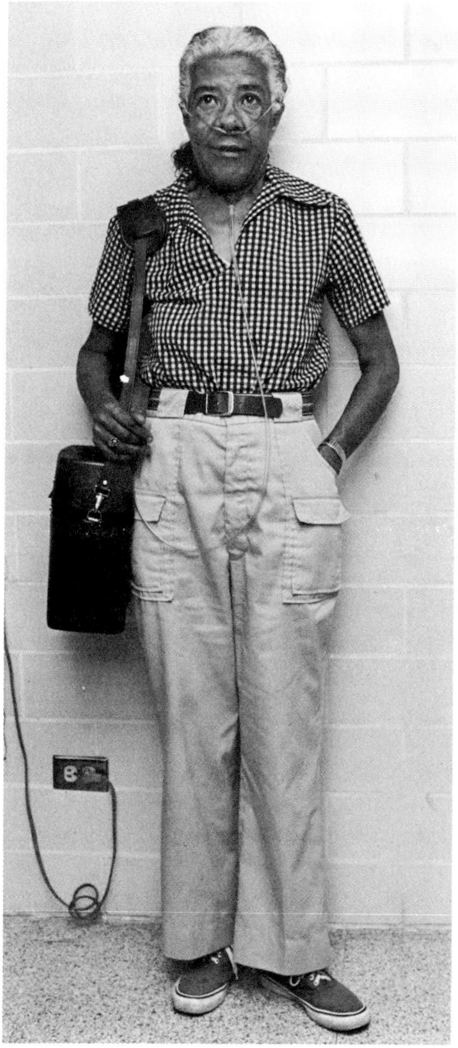

Fig. 18-7. Patient using new lightweight Linde walker, which weighs 6.5 lb and gives approximately 4-½-hrs oxygen supply.

Breathing retraining is the next step in extended ambulatory care. The efficacy of breathing training has been appreciated by patients for several years.[19–21] Patients with CAO usually breathe in a rapid, shallow, inefficient manner. They must be taught slowed breathing and abdominal-diaphragmatic breathing with exhalation against pursed lips at rest (Fig. 18-5) and during exercise (Fig. 18-6). Measurements have shown that pursed-lip breathing decreases minute ventilation without reducing alveolar ventilation, enhances oxygen transport, promotes carbon dioxide elimination, and thus, in short, is more efficient.[20]

Physical reconditioning with graded exercise decreases the exercise impairment of patients with COPD, and often they can then perform more physical activity with lower oxygen consumption.[21–23] The greatest benefit of physical training is that the patient becomes more efficient in his delivery of oxygen to the tissues. Exercise devices can be used at home in cold weather when outdoor exercise may cause bronchospasm; the best exercise is, however, walking outdoors at a pace that causes only mild dyspnea. In spite of the fact that pulmonary function may not change during extended care and rehabilitation, experience has shown that graded exercises allow patients to function at a higher level of activity with greater comfort.

Continuous ambulatory oxygen therapy is valuable for hypoxemic patients with marked disability. The development of portable liquid oxygen systems has made continuous ambulatory therapy more convenient, since as much as a nine-hour supply is available.[24] Figure 18-7 shows a newer lightweight model, a fourth-generation Linde oxygen walker. These types of devices are now widely used throughout the United States (see discussion of oxygen later in this chapter). Use of this system allows a patient to engage in various activities away from the oxygen source.

RESULTS OF A PULMONARY REHABILITATION PROGRAM FOR ADVANCED COPD

In our original series—a demonstration project designed to evaluate the methods, logistics, costs, and effectiveness of pulmonary rehabilitation—we chose to evaluate a large number of patients with all degrees of COPD. A consecutive series of patients was chosen so that the selection would reflect no bias based upon preconceived notions or upon presumed favorable background factors such as youth, high motivation, or mildness of the illness. The aim was to study the overall effectiveness of programs for ambulatory outpatient and home respiratory care treatment.[5] This program began to enroll patients in August, 1966—all patients were finally enrolled by May, 1968.

Patients were selected consecutively on request if they (1) had a well-established diagnosis of COPD (emphysema and chronic bron-

TABLE 18-1. Background Features of 182 Patients in Care-Study Program

	Average	*Standard Deviation*	*Range*
Age	61	9	33 to 81
Sex	87.3% male		
Weight	142 lb	29	88 to 265
Height	67.9 in.	3.0	58.5 to 75
VC	2.58	.79	1.22 to 5.17
FEV_1	.94	.38	.26 to 2.21
MMF	.41	.22	.11 to 1.77
MVV	35.5	15.1	6.4 to 80.9

chitis), and (2) were free from other confusing respiratory or cardiac disorders, and other serious disease which would alter the natural course or prognosis of individuals participating in this care-study program. Patients selected had a demonstrable loss of pulmonary function (usually loss of FEV_1 or MVV of 50% or more), a definable functional impairment of daily activity (by personal definition), and professed ability or apparent willingness to participate in an outpatient program. Patients were not excluded on the basis of age, sex, or national origin. Patients may have recently been ill with acute respiratory failure or may have required continuous oxygen before entry into the study.

Following the initial physician and nurse evaluation to establish suitability for participation, the care-study patients were instructed in the details of therapy just discussed.

Background factors in the 182 patients admitted to this study, summarized in Table 18-1, indicate marked severity of disease. Predominantly an elderly male sample was selected.

The early effectiveness of this program has been reported.[25] In brief, the majority of patients appreciated symptomatic relief and had significantly improved exercise tolerance. When studied, most patients could perform the same amount of exercise at a lower oxygen

TABLE 18-2. Four-Year Observations of 47 Patients from the Comprehensive Care Program

	Preliminary (Mean)	*Four-Year (Mean)*	*"P" Value**
VC (L)	2.79	2.44	<.005
FEV_1 (L)	1.09	0.89	>.001
MMEF (L/sec)	0.49	0.38	<.01
MVV (L/min)	44.4	37.6	<.005

* Single-tailed Student's T Test.

consumption. We were also initially pleased that the expected rate of pulmonary function deterioration did not occur early in the study. As the program progressed, however, pulmonary function did decline, but only at a rate of 50 ml/year over a 4-year period (Table 18-2).[25]

No claim was made that survival was altered by the therapy, enthusiastically designated "Pulmonary Rehabilitation" by the author and his associates.

Late Follow-Up of the Pulmonary Rehabilitation Program

The 10-year survival curve using the life-table method is presented in Figure 18-8, compared with survival of white men of age 61 in 1968 (actuarial data). The 10-year survival of the COPD patients participating in our rehabilitation program was only 17% compared with 69% in the general male population (Fig. 18-8).[26]

One hundred forty-three patients died during the 10-year follow-up. Three-fourths of these deaths (110) were due to pulmonary causes, with progressive COPD being the most common cause. The most frequent nonpulmonary causes of death were myocardial infarction (in 8) and suicide (in 5) (Table 18-3).

We found several factors present on initial examination that were associated with decreased survival (Table 18-4). On physical examination, these were a resting tachycardia and the presence of right

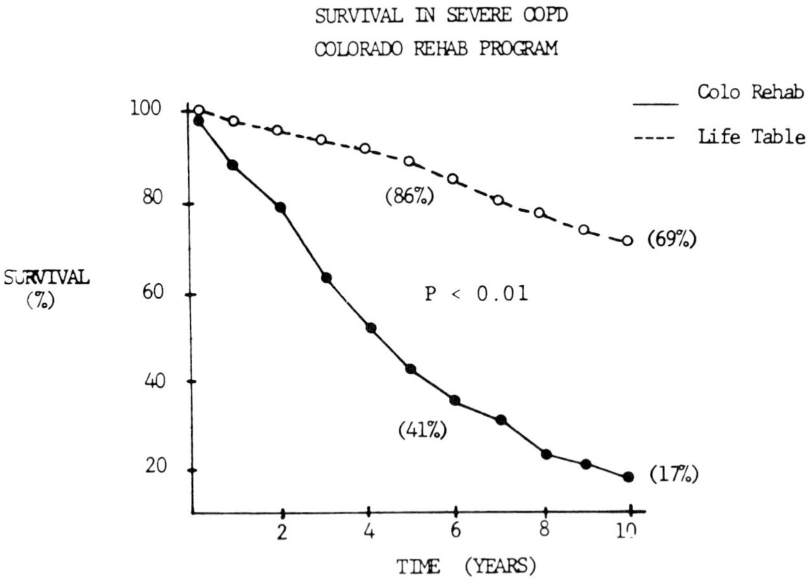

Fig. 18-8. Survival in patients with COPD in the Colorado rehabilitation program compared with the survival of white men, age 61 years in 1968. The 10-year survival curve in the COPD patients (*solid line*) was only 17%, vs 69% in the general population from actuarial data. The difference in survival curves is excess mortality due to COPD in spite of the benefits of a rehabilitation program.

TABLE 18-3. Causes of Death at 10 Years—Colorado Rehabilitation Program (n = 143)

Pulmonary		*Nonpulmonary*	
Progressive COPD	58	Myocardial infarction	8
Progressive COPD with RHF	35	Suicide	5
Pneumonia	12	Other cardiovascular	3
Pulmonary embolus	1	GI bleeding	3
Lung cancer	1	Other known	9
Other pulmonary	3	Unknown	5
	110		33

heart failure (both $P < 0.05$). Abnormal gas exchange was also associated with decreased survival. Patients with a Pa_{O_2} of less than 60 mm Hg, hypercapnia greater than 46 mm Hg, and hypocapnia less than 32 mm Hg had a decreased survival as compared with those who did not have those abnormalities (all $P < 0.05$). Other laboratory data associated with decreased survival were anemia (hematocrit less than 38 vol/100 ml) and polycythemia (hematocrit greater than 51 vol/100 ml), and the electrocardiographic abnormalities of right axis deviation, right atrial hypertrophy, and right ventricular hypertrophy (all $P < 0.05$). In general, those patients with the worst pulmonary function had the worst prognosis. A forced vital capacity of less than 2.5 L, an FEV_1 of less than 1.0 L, and MMEF of less than 0.5 L/sec, and an MVV of less than 40 L/min were markers of a poor prognosis.

There were 28 10-year survivors. The 10-year survivors had significantly better gas exchange, lower hematocrit levels, and fewer hospital days in the year prior to entry than those who did not survive 10 years (all $P < 0.05$). In addition, they had significantly better

TABLE 18-4. Factors Present on Admission Associated with a Decreased Survival (All $P < 0.05$)

Physical Examination	*Gas Exchange*
Resting tachycardia	Pa_{O_2} (<60 mm Hg)
Right heart failure	Pa_{CO_2} (<32 or >46 mm Hg)
Pulmonary Function	*Other Laboratory*
FVC (<2.5 L)	Hematocrit (<38 or >51 vol/100 ml)
FEV_1 (<1.0 L)	ECG abnormalities
MMEF (<0.50 L/sec)	Right axis
MVV (<40 L/min)	Right ventricular hypertrophy

pulmonary function. The percentage bronchodilator response in the 28 survivors (percentage of change in MMEF) was 70 ± 17% (mean ± SEM) vs 47 ± 5% in the nonsurvivors ($P < 0.05$) (Table 18-5).

Over the 10-year period, the forced vital capacity decreased at an average of 117 ml/year, while the FEV_1 decrement per year was 46 ml. In the 28 survivors, however, the FEV_1 decrement per year was only 9 ml. There was a 0.77 mm Hg fall in Po_2 per year. Over the 10 years, there was a 1.6 lb weight loss per year.

There was a significant reduction in hospitalization due to pulmonary causes. In both a group of 54 of the patients who survived 5 years and a group of 44 who survived 6 years, pulmonary hospital days were reduced ($P < 0.05$).

The last 30 patients admitted to the program received psychologic testing for evaluation of their symptom complex on admission to the study and again after one year. Significant improvement was found in the patients' symptom trend and in the physicians' evaluation of the patients' symptom trend ($P < 0.05$). In addition, patients had a significant reduction in affective distress, i.e., anxiety, depression, and somatic concern ($P < 0.05$). These patients also demonstrated a 2-½ fold increase in their ability to walk ($P < 0.05$).[27]

In summary, a systematic outpatient care program for patients with severe COPD was established using existing hospital personnel. Survival was 41% at 5 years and 17% at 10 years. These survival data are similar to those of others obtained at sea level.[28–30] However, our patients resided at high altitude, a factor known to increase the incidence of cor pulmonale and death in patients with COPD.[29] When our 2-½ year data were compared with those of the only other study of COPD patients residing at high altitude, we found a significantly better survival over that of those in the VA Cooperative Study (67% vs 50%, $P < 0.05$, Fig. 18-2).[29] The FEV_1 decreased at the rate of

TABLE 18-5. Ten-Year vs Non-Ten-Year Survivors in the Colorado Rehabilitation Program

	10-Year Survivors (n = 28)	*Nonsurvivors (n = 143)*
Pao_2*	63 ± 1**	57 ± 1
$Paco_2$*	38 ± 1	42 ± 1
Hematocrit*	47 ± 1	50 ± 0
Pulm. hospital days*	7 ± 3	14 ± 2
FEV_1*	1.28 ± .08	0.87 ± .03
Bronchodilator response (%)*	70 ± 17	47 ± 5

* $P < 0.05$. One patient lost to follow-up.
** Mean ± SEM.

46 ml/yr over the 10 years. This figure is at the lower end of the spectrum of FEV_1 decrements per year, but it may be affected by variables such as the length of follow-up and the initial FEV_1.[28,31,32] The longer the follow-up, the lower a decrement one tends to find in the FEV_1, since the end-stage patients who have more rapid deterioration die earlier while the patients with more stable pulmonary function live longer.

The Colorado Rehabilitation Program was able to show a significant reduction in "pulmonary" hospital days and in some patients an improvement in symptom complex and life style. A detailed cost analysis was not performed. However, because of the reduction in hospital days and the ability of some patients to maintain or regain employment in the setting of an outpatient program using existing hospital personnel—and returning the majority of patients to the care of their primary physician—the cost/benefit ratio was low.

Whether or not pulmonary rehabilitation improves survival is sometimes debated. Although no adequately controlled trial has been reported, one attempt from our program has been to compare the survival rate among patients in a rehabilitation program with that among similar patients living in the Denver metropolitan area who received their medical care primarily from private physicians within the community. This latter group served as a "control" group, but it must be emphatically stated that this was not a randomized control group, nor was it even a contemporary control group, because many of the patients had been studied and followed before the popularization of pulmonary rehabilitation techniques—the fundamental basis of comprehensive care for advanced COPD. Thus, at best, the control group can be viewed only as a "historic control" group with obvious limitations. The matching of the groups by age, height, forced expiratory volume in one second, and O_2 saturation while breathing room air was excellent (Table 18-6). All patients were men. The comparison of survival at 8 years is shown in Figure 18-9; there was little difference in the cumulative mortality, and the difference in survival between the 2 groups ($n = 72$) at 8 years was of borderline significance ($p = 0.08$).

TABLE 18-6. Rehabilitation Versus Emphysema Registry Cases*

	Rehabilitation	*Emphysema Registry*	*2 Tailed t-Test*
Age, yr	58.5	57.9	NS
Height, cm	175	175	NS
FEV_1, L	1.08	1.15	NS
SaO_2, 0/0	89	88	NS

* Data are given as the mean values for the matched groups. Definitions of abbreviations: FEV_1 = forced expiratory volume in one second; SaO_2 = arterial O_2 saturation.

Comment

The past decade has seen the establishment of pulmonary rehabilitation as an established method of care for advanced stages of COPD.[33–35] The goals of pulmonary rehabilitation are well stated and laudable. The methods of care are all based on a reasonable scientific rationale, and the value of rehabilitation in reducing the impact of symptoms on the patient, improving exercise tolerance, and reducing hospital needs is reasonably well established. The question of improved survival has not yet been answered, but the possibility is there. How best to provide these services has not been critically evaluated, but a simple pragmatic outpatient approach is suggested, because hospitalization per se appears to offer no clear-cut advantages. Moreover, no hospital-based program has reported an outcome superior to those of programs not using a period of hospitalization.

It is the opinion of the author that most patients with advanced COPD can be effectively cared for by experienced physicians assisted by a nurse or a therapist, and that this simple "team" can provide most or all of the benefits associated with more elaborate rehabilitation programs. If this proves to be true, the benefit from pulmonary

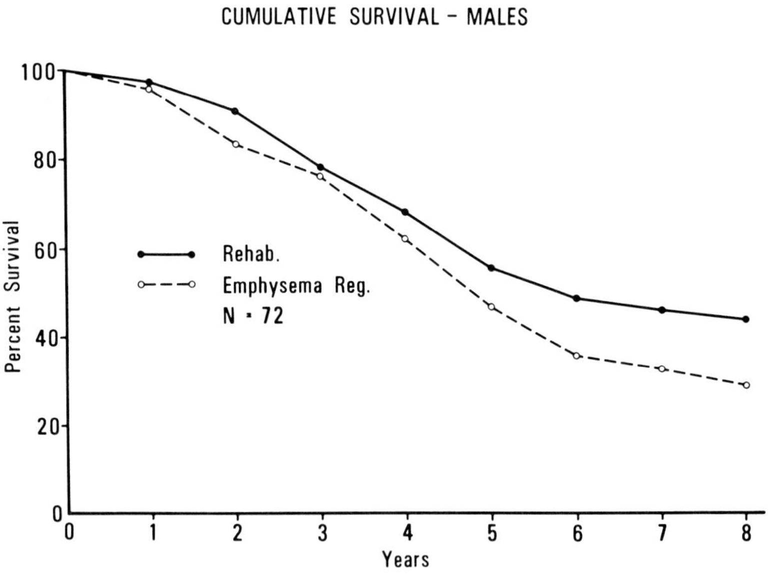

Fig. 18-9. Comparison of cumulative survival between a group of men in the rehabilitation program and a "historical control group" (data presented in Table 18-6) followed eight years. Equal groups of patients were cared for, but the Emphysema Registry patients were not part of a rehabilitation program but rather received care from their personal physicians. They resided in the same environment. At eight years, the difference between the groups was of borderline significance ($p = 0.08$).

rehabilitation will be within reach of most patients via their own personal physicians.

LONG-TERM HOME OXYGEN IN ADVANCED COPD AND HYPOXEMIA

Numerous reports have suggested that continuous oxygen is useful in reducing the impact of hypoxemia in selected patients with advanced COPD.[24,36,37] Suggestions that similar benefit might be possible using less than so-called "continuous" oxygen formed the basis of the now-famous nocturnal oxygen therapy trial (NOTT).[38,39] Briefly, this trial enrolled 203 stable patients with Po_2 of 55 or less into either nocturnal oxygen therapy (NOT), including the hours of sleep, or continuous oxygen therapy (COT), which was intended to be as close to 24-hour oxygen administration each day as possible.[39]

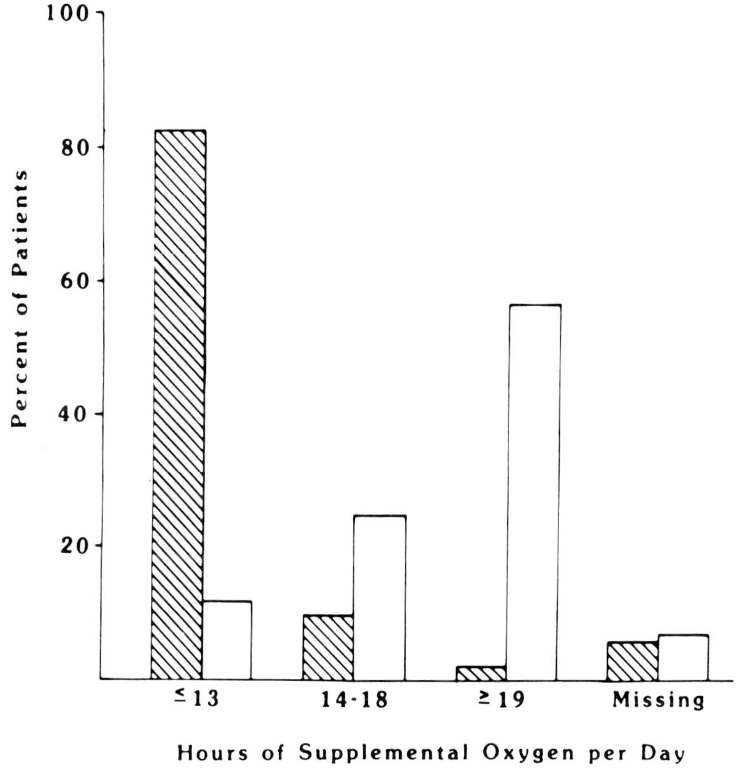

Fig. 18-10. Compliance with treatment regimens as assessed by patient diaries, expressed as a frequency distribution of the daily oxygen use. Hash bars represent patients on nocturnal oxygen therapy, open bars those on continuous oxygen therapy. Missing bars indicate patients in whom data are missing. A statistically significant difference in the amount of oxygen used between continuous (COT) and nocturnal (NOT) was present. (From Nocturnal Oxygen Therapy Trial Group: Continuous or nocturnal oxygen therapy in hypoxemic chronic obstructive lung disease. Ann. Intern. Med., *93*:391, 1980.

Supplementary criteria for the study included patients with a Po_2 as high as 59 if they also revealed ECG evidence of "P pulmonale" with P waves > 3mm in standard leads II, III, and AVF, a hematocrit of ≤ 55%, or leg and ankle edema suggesting congestive right heart failure.[39] Fortunately, background factors including age, sex, ethnic background, years of formal education, and baseline physiologic parameters matched almost identically in both the NOT (N = 102) and COT (N = 101) groups.[39] Of equal importance to the successful outcome of this study was the good adherence to the NOT vs COT duration of oxygen therapy (Fig. 18-10). A simple view of outcome, of course, is survival. Figure 18-11 compares the survival of COT with that of NOT and reveals a significant difference in mortality at 1 and 2 years ($P < 0.01$). COT was also better than NOT in terms of hospital requirements.[39] The NOT survival curve was almost identical to the survival curve of patients receiving 15 hours of oxygen participating in the British Medical Research Council clinical trial. This study compared oxygen given for 15 hours with no oxygen. The survival curve for those receiving no oxygen proved to be significantly worse than the North American NOT (12 hr) patients and the British MRC 15-hr oxygen groups.[40] Thus, some oxygen is better than

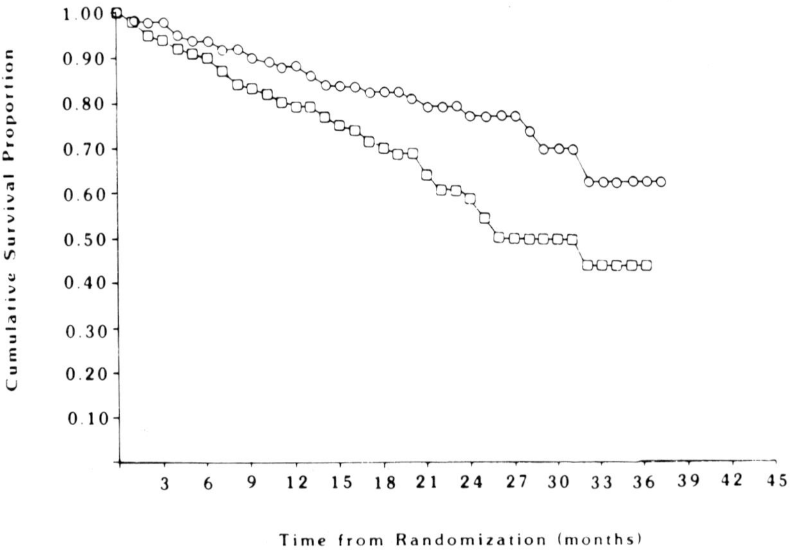

Fig. 18-11. Overall mortality. Ordinate is fraction of patients surviving; abscissa is time for randomization or duration of treatment. Open circles represent continuous oxygen therapy group; squares represent nocturnal oxygen therapy group. Of the total group, 80 nocturnal O_2 and 87 continuous O_2 therapy patients were followed 12 months, and 29 nocturnal O_2 and 37 continuous O_2 patients were followed 24 months. (From Nocturnal Oxygen Therapy Trial Group: Continuous nocturnal oxygen therapy in hypoxemic chronic obstructive lung disease. Ann. Intern. Med., *93*:391, 1980.)

none, and nearly continuous oxygen is better than lesser amounts in these two related studies.

Today, a variety of oxygen systems is available including oxygen in high-pressure cylinders, liquid systems, or home oxygen concentrators. The relative advantages and disadvantages of each system are briefly considered.

Systems of Oxygen Administration

Compressed Gas

This type has been used longer than liquid or concentrator systems. Oxygen tanks of varying sizes are available in most communities. They can be stored and safely transported but have the disadvantages of being heavy, of providing a short supply (even the large cylinders), and of posing a torpedo hazard should inadvertent damage result in the opening of the control valve.

Small tanks can be conveniently transfilled from large tanks, and at least 2 systems—the Mada and Erie (Table 18-7)—are in widespread use. These compressed-gas systems contain approximately a 3.5-hour supply at a flow of 2 L/min. Although fears of accidents during transfilling have been publicized, mishaps have been essentially nonexistent. The major precaution in transfilling is to avoid use at the transfilling connections of any lubricant derived from a pe-

TABLE 18-7. Features of Commonly Used Compressed Gas and Liquid Oxygen Systems for Home Use

Manufacturer	*Name or Model*	*Capacity of Transfillable Device (L)*	*Continuous Oxygen at 2 L/min (hr)*	*Weight (lb)*
Compressed gas systems				
Mada Medical Products	Mada cylinder	240	2	5.5
Carlstadt, NJ 07072	No. 1415	400	3.3	6.5
		682	5.7	8
Erie Controls, Division	Traveler	247	2	6.5
of Erie Mfg. Co.	Traveler	406	3.3	9.5
Milwaukee, WI 53221				
*Liquid systems**				
Union Carbide Corp.	Linde oxygen walker	1030	8–9	9.5
Linde Division	Linde oxygen walker II	500	4	6.5
Indianapolis, IN 46224				
Cryogenic Associates	Stroller	1000	8–9	9.5
Indianapolis, IN 46268	Stroller 2	500	4	6.5
Cryomed Corp.	Travelair	1200	10	13
Elletsville, IN 47429				

* All liquid systems have 13,800-L reservoir canister for transfilling portable device.

troleum product. New Erie aluminum cylinders that can be transfilled are available in 2 sizes (Table 18-7). Both are equipped with a convenient carrying case and shoulder strap.

Liquid

When oxygen is required 24 hr/day, the most convenient system for achieving portability with the greatest range is the liquid transfilling type. The newest designs (Table 18-7) include large reservoir canisters and transfillable portable devices that offer an 8- to 10-hour range of continuous oxygen at 2 L/min. Also available are new, small, lightweight systems offering about a 4-hour supply at 2 L/min.

Most patients can be easily taught to transfill from liquid systems. The oxygen supply available in this type of system reduces the number of deliveries required and thus offers convenience. Cost, however, is high, currently averaging $380/mo in the Denver area (based on 2 L/min for 24 hr/day).

Concentrator

The latest technology for home oxygen uses a separation principle—either a molecular sieve or a semipermeable membrane—to concentrate oxygen from room air. Most of these so-called "oxygen concentrator systems" employ an aluminum silicate sieve that separates oxygen from nitrogen on the basis of the difference in molecular size. Many devices are now available from different manufacturers. Features of the most frequently used models are summarized in Table 18-8.

TABLE 18-8. Features of Commonly Used Oxygen Concentrators for Home Use

Manufacturer	*Name or Model*	*Output Range (L/min)*	*% O_2 at 2 L/min*	*Weight (lb)*	*Unit Size (H×W×D, to nearest inch)*
Bendix	4000	1–4	93	112	30×17×17
Briox	2100A	1–6	>90	125	30×24×16
Bunn	Boras 290+	1–4	92	70	18×17×10
Cryogenics	Roommate	1–4	>92	75	32×17×16
DeVilbiss	955 DVO_2	1–4	94	88	27×19×17
Linde	Loc II	1–3.5	>92	95	36×16×15
Marx	850	1–10	94	90	26×17×14
Mountain Medical	Econ-O_2	1–5	>92	115	27×18×16
OECO*	OECO	1–6	40	110	30×14×16

* Uses semipermeable membrane to concentrate oxygen from room air. Other devices use molecular sieve.

A flow of 2 L/min is adequate for most patients with advanced COPD. In fact, most require only 1 to 2 L/min while awake. Slightly greater oxygen flows may be required during sleep or exercise. In the NOTT study, 1 L/min more was used during sleep and exercise than during rest while awake.

The concentrator system is convenient for providing a continuous oxygen supply. Patients can be active and ambulatory around the home while using the concentrator with a 50-ft tube. The system is, of course, dependent upon electricity and would not be suitable in areas where electrical outrages occur often.

Small tanks cannot be filled from the concentrator. Thus, if continuous oxygen is required, a separate portable system, such as compressed gas, will be needed. Alternatively, the portable device could be filled from a large K cylinder which would also be a useful backup

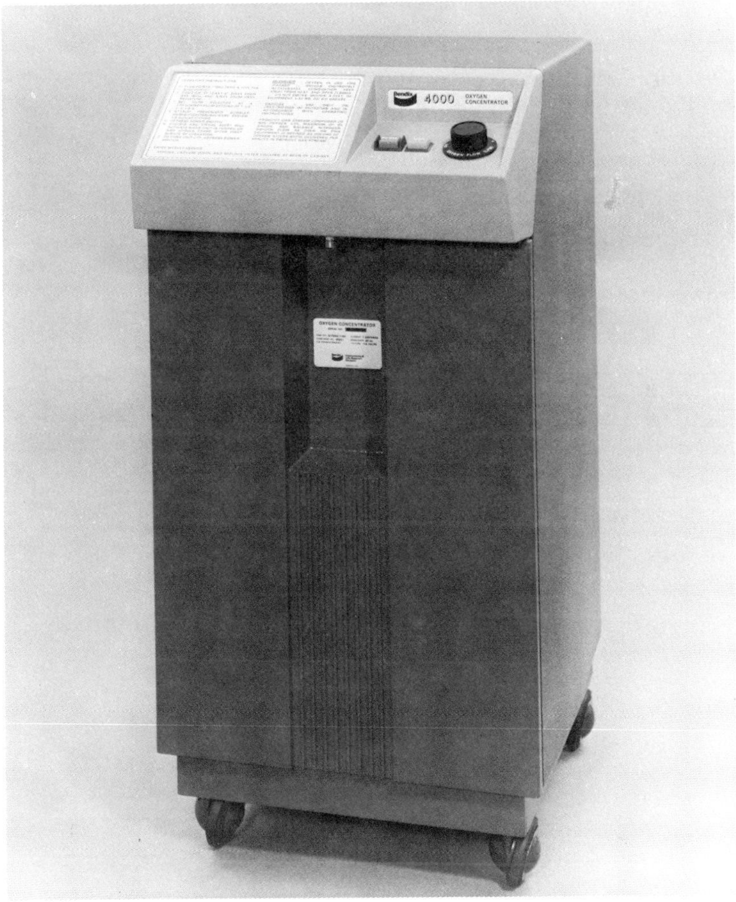

Fig. 18-12. Bendix 400 oxygen concentrator for home use.

cylinder, convenient during a power outage. Three of the most popular concentrator models are shown in Figures 18-12 to 18-14.

An isolated abnormal arterial blood gas measurement should not be the sole criterion for instituting home oxygen therapy. In the NOTT study, in which the criterion for inclusion was a Po_2 of 55 mm Hg or less, a large number of patients "washed out" because during a 3-week stabilization period, their arterial oxygenation improved with therapy directed at secretions, bronchospasm, and infection. Thus, the prescribing physician should be certain that the presence of hypoxemia is well documented and, further, that the hypoxemia cannot be corrected by more conventional means directed at the underlying pathophysiologic feature.

Patients with less severe degrees of hypoxemia but evidence of the ravages of oxygen lack, such as cor pulmonale, should also be strongly considered as candidates for home oxygen therapy. On the basis of large prospective studies, such patients have the poorest prognosis of any group with COPD.[29]

The presence of secondary polycythemia alone should not be considered an indication for long-term oxygen therapy. In most patients with advanced COPD, the RBC mass increases slightly as an adaptive

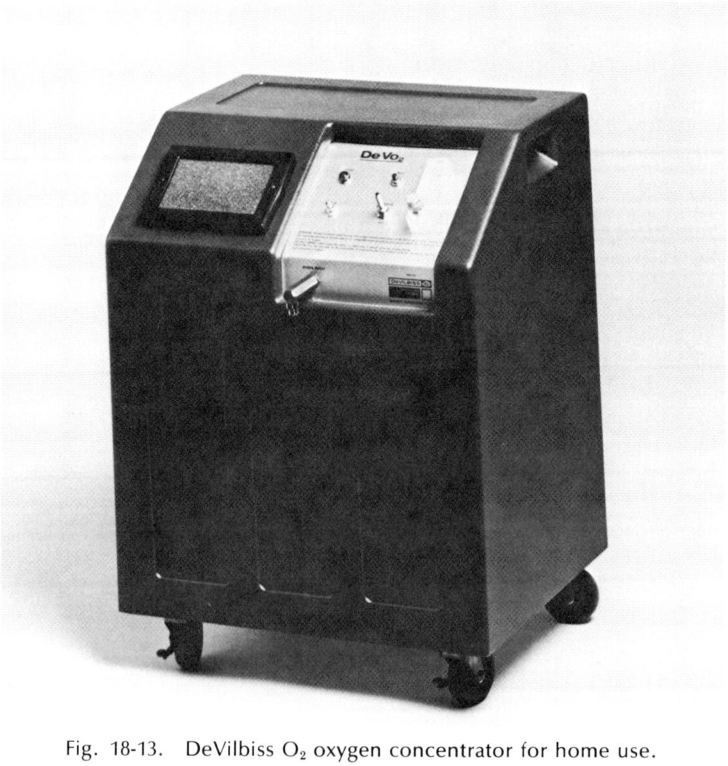

Fig. 18-13. DeVilbiss O_2 oxygen concentrator for home use.

response to hypoxemia. Many patients with a hematocrit value in the 52% to 58% range are not troubled by symptoms of polycythemia. Phlebotomy is required only in symptomatic patients.

Thus, clear indications for home oxygen therapy are emerging, although all the clinical situations in which such therapy may be useful in COPD have not yet been clearly defined. In short, it now appears that home oxygen therapy should be reserved for patients who fail to respond to an otherwise comprehensive program for COPD, including rehabilitation techniques designed to minimize the degree of physiologic and psychosocial impairment.

Management of Patients

Certainly, home oxygen therapy should not be considered a panacea. It does not solve all the problems of the patient with advanced COPD, who requires a comprehensive care program consistent with the goals and principles of pulmonary rehabilitation (see later). Each patient and family should be well indoctrinated regarding total care. Oxygen therapy techniques should receive special emphasis, and careful instructions are required for use of liquid and compressed gas systems. Troubleshooting in the event of device failure must also be taught so that patient and family thoroughly comprehend the procedures.

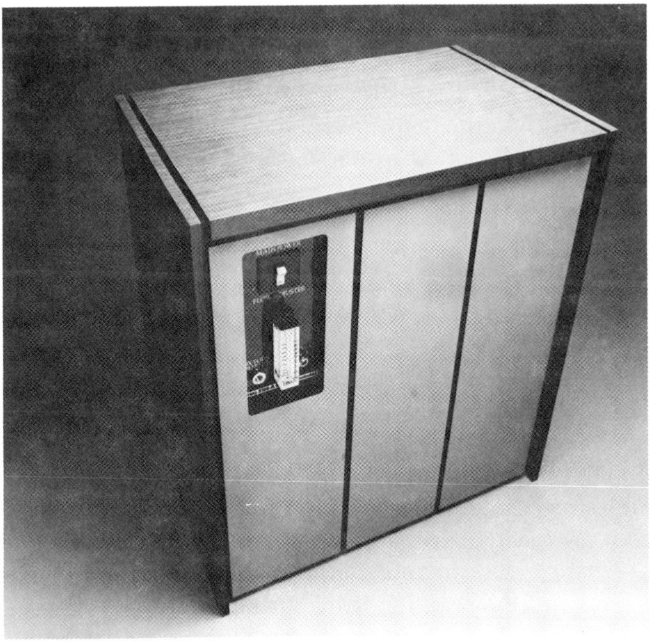

Fig. 18-14. Briox oxygen concentrator for home use.

Oxygen does not replace all other therapy known to be useful in advanced COPD; these therapies are described earlier in this chapter.

Economic Considerations

The cost of oxygen therapy is considerable. The NOTT study, which clearly shows that continuous oxygen therapy is associated with better survival than 12 hr/day therapy, also raised important issues. Reasonable estimates indicate that this form of therapy "purchases" 2 additional years of life in selected patients. The cost difference between continuous and nocturnal oxygen therapy is estimated conservatively at $580 a year. If only 500,000 of the 9 to 10 million persons with advanced COPD in this country today were to receive continuous oxygen, the cost would be $290 million more than if only nocturnal oxygen is used.

Naturally, the decision to use oxygen at home and the choice of number of hours per day must be made in the context of the patient's and the family's life style, with consideration of what life means to the patient. These costs, of course, are far lower than those of other high-technology forms of "maintenance management," such as hemodialysis. On the other hand, the indiscriminate, premature, or unnecessary use of oxygen could perhaps be disastrous in terms of available resources for such care. Thus, the disciplined clinician should make the decision on behalf of the patient, with serious consideration of costs and burdens to the patient and society.

Personal Concerns and Problems

Many patients fear the use of oxygen. Some concerns, such as fears of fire or explosion, can be quickly dispelled. That oxygen will not explode or burn must be emphasized. Oxygen, of course, supports combustion, and direct ignition of oxygen tubing or nasal cannulas causes flash fires. I have cared for two patients who received serious facial burns after igniting oxygen tubing when trying to light a cigarette while intoxicated. A few patients have skin reactions to the tubing.

Nasal dryness and stuffiness may occur during oxygen therapy. This problem can be minimized by occluding one of the nasal prongs or by using a single nasal prong, which is just as effective as double prongs in controlling hypoxemia. It is then possible to use alternate nostrils for oxygen administration.

Probably the most vexing problem is the fantasy believed by many patients—that oxygen therapy signifies the end of life, or at least the end of useful and independent existence. Many fear oxygen "addiction" and for this reason reject or forestall the use of oxygen. These attitudes usually respond to patient counseling.

That oxygen is truly palliative, well tolerated, nonaddicting in the pharmacologic sense, and safe must be emphasized. It is often useful to have another patient who is receiving oxygen therapy visit and help counsel the oxygen therapy candidate. Sometimes this is effectively accomplished through emphysema clubs.

It can be honestly stressed that many patients have been able to work during continuous oxygen therapy. Most restaurants gladly accommodate patients receiving continuous oxygen via a portable system, as do planes, buses, and trains if advance arrangement is made with the medical director of the carrier. These passengers naturally are assigned to the nonsmoking section. Finally, most motor vehicle departments issue driver's licenses to oxygen therapy patients. This group has had an almost perfect safety record for more than 15 years in Colorado.

Future Directions

The foregoing discussion has naturally focused on patients with advanced, severe hypoxemia because of the scientific data establishing the value of oxygen therapy in this group. Is oxygen useful in less severe forms of disease? Could oxygen forestall or prevent the development of cor pulmonale and other ravages of hypoxemia resulting from COPD? These two questions are just beginning to be investigated.

It is now established that in some patients with COPD who are normoxic while awake, hypoxemia develops during sleep.[41] Transient nocturnal pulmonary hypertension has been documented under these conditions.[41] Could it be that the presence of nocturnal hypoxemia plays an important early role in the prognosis of COPD and its complications? The development of reactive pulmonary hypertension, the increased platelet consumption during hypoxemia, the possibility of microemboli reaching the lungs in this setting, and the possibility of platelet-mediated pulmonary hypertension allow the hypothesis that nocturnal hypoxemia plays such a role.[42] If this were the case, the use of oxygen at night to correct nocturnal hypoxemia would be entirely rational. Oxygen does correct the increased platelet consumption that accompanies hypoxemia in COPD.[42]

It is not possible on the basis of today's scientific knowledge to recommend oxygen therapy at night in these patients, but the suggestion that it would be beneficial exists. It is likely that clinical trials will someday answer these important questions concerning the possible efficacy of nocturnal oxygen therapy in early stages of disease.

Finally, some patients have hypoxemia, often profound, only while exercising as part of normal daily activity but return to relative normoxia when resting. These patients may benefit from oxygen therapy during exercise only. In these instances, use of small aluminum cylinders transfilled from large tanks seems most appropriate and least costly.

Logistic and economic considerations will determine the most feasible and appropriate method of home oxygen use, but the principles of home oxygen therapy appear to be established, and no question concerning safety or efficacy should remain.

PULMONARY REHABILITATION IN PERSPECTIVE

The definition of pulmonary rehabilitation as expressed by the committee on pulmonary rehabilitation of the American College of Chest Physicians is as follows:

> Pulmonary rehabilitation may be defined as an art of medical practice wherein an individually tailored, multidisciplinary program is formulated which through accurate diagnosis, therapy, emotional support, and education, stabilizes or reverses both the physio- and psychopathology of pulmonary diseases and attempts to return the patient to the highest possible functional capacity allowed by his pulmonary handicap and overall life situation.

The objectives of pulmonary rehabilitation in advanced COPD must be realistic and consistent with our current knowledge of the

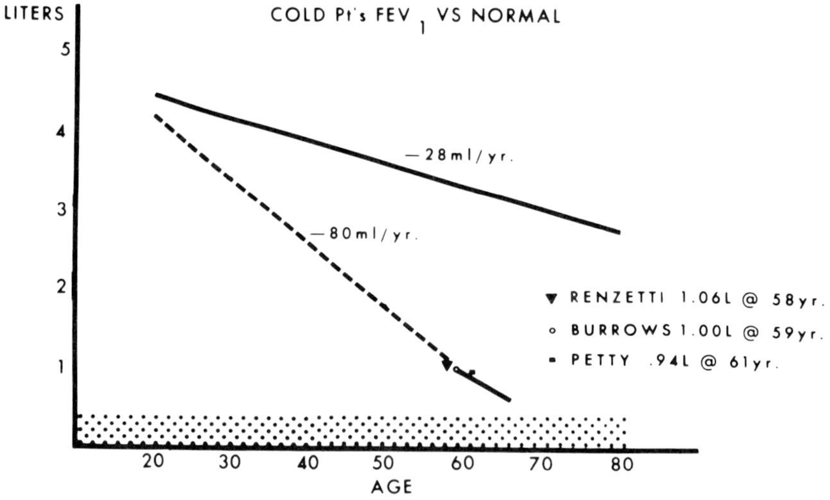

Fig. 18-15. Normal loss of pulmonary function by age is 28 ml per year (*solid line*). The 3 points are representative of age and FEV_1 of 3 large series that dealt with the course and prognosis of COPD. It is projected that an average loss of 80 ml per year has occurred (*dotted line*) since the patients from these 3 series were first evaluated. Solid extension of line (*arrow*) is data from Burrows study on the course and prognosis of chronic airway obstruction.[28] (From Petty, T.L., Neff, T.A., and Hudson, L.D.: Methods of ambulatory care. Med. Clin. North Am., *57:*751, 1973.)

natural history of the disease spectrum. This is a disease process that covers 20 to 35 years. Recent studies indicate that the progress of pulmonary function deterioration continues in almost a predictable way.[28,43] Pulmonary function losses may occur in a linear or even exponential manner.[43] Figure 18-15 depicts the linear loss of pulmonary function averaging approximately 28 ml/yr in FEV_1, using the data of Kory in normal men.[44] Three points are added to this figure from studies of Renzetti, Burrows, and ourselves (87% of our series were men).[5,28,29] The age and FEV_1 on entry to these long-term studies agree remarkably. Thus, in three large series, the average age was near 60 and the FEV_1 nearly 1.0 L. If one assumes that these patients were normal at age 20 and if one makes a simple back calculation, it is apparent that the average pulmonary function loss in FEV_1 has been 80 ml/yr. It really makes no difference whether the progressive loss of pulmonary function is exponential or linear. It is likely that the slope of the dashed line in Figure 18-15 is reasonably correct, because the prospective study of Burrows continues to show nearly the same rate of pulmonary function loss per year over a 5-yr period in spite of systematic therapy.[28]

The challenge for the future focuses on early or at least earlier identification and treatment. It has been established that simple spirometric parameters, e.g., FEV_1 and FEV_1/FVC percentage, along with symptoms of dyspnea, cough, and expectoration identify a population at increased risk of developing progressive disease or of dying from respiratory as well as all causes.[45] Further, the cessation of smoking in patients with only mild to moderate airflow abnormalities retards the rate of deterioration of lung function. Thus, by simple office spirometry, behavior modification, and meticulous management of chest infections as well as the judicious use of bronchodilating drugs, it is likely that the course and prognosis of advancing COPD could be altered.[46]

Today we need a truly comprehensive approach to the multiplicity of problems inherent in the COPD situation. This approach to care is within reach of all practitioners of medicine and has been nicely chronicled in a brief monograph published and distributed by the American College of Chest Physicians.*[47] The problems of COPD are amenable to solution, but only in primary care physicians' offices, in much the same way that the solution, or at least the partial solution, to hypertension has been fashioned.

REFERENCES

1. Miller, W.F.: Rehabilitation of patients with chronic obstructive lung disease. Med. Clin. North Am., *51*:349, 1967.

---

* Available from the American College of Chest Physicians, 911 Busse Highway, Park Ridge, IL 60068.

2. Stone, R.W.: Magnitude of the problem. Arch. Environ. Health, *6:*306, 1963.
3. Facts about Selected Respiratory Conditions in the U.S. [Publication AL-63]. New York, American Lung Association, 1978.
4. Nett, L.M., and Petty, T.L.: Effective treatment for emphysema and chronic bronchitis. J. Rehab., *33:*10, 1967.
5. Petty, T.L., Nett, L.M., Finigan, M.M., Brink, G.A., and Corsello, P.R.: A comprehensive care program for chronic airway obstruction. Ann. Intern. Med., *70:*1109, 1969.
6. Petty, T.L., and Nett, L.M.: For Those Who Live and Breathe. A Manual for Patients with Emphysema and Chronic Bronchitis. 2nd Ed. Springfield, IL, Charles C Thomas, 1975.
7. Petty, T.L., and Nett, L.M.: Patient education and emphysema care. Med. Times, *97:*117, 1969.
8. Foster, W.M., Lagenback, E., and Bergofsky, E.H.: Measurement of tracheal and bronchial mucus velocities in man: relation to lung clearance. J. Appl. Physiol., *48:*465, 1980.
9. Matthys, H., and Kohler, D.: Effect of theophylline on mucociliary clearance in man. Eur. J. Resp. Dis., *61*[Suppl. 109]:98, 1980.
10. Petty, T.L., and Broughton, J.O.: A new simple IPPB device for hospital and home care. JAMA, *203:*871, 1968.
11. Goldberg, I.L., and Cherniack, R.M.: The effect of nebulized bronchodilator delivered with and without IPPB on ventilatory function in chronic obstructive emphysema. Am. Rev. Resp. Dis., *91:*13, 1965.
12. Chester, E.H., Racz, I., Barlow, P.B., and Baum, G.L.: Bronchodilator therapy: comparison of acute response to these methods of administration. Chest, *62:*394, 1972.
13. Petty, T.L., and Guthrie, A.G.: The effects of augmented breathing maneuvers on ventilation in severe chronic airway obstruction. Resp. Care, *16:*104, 1971.
14. Pflug, A.E., Cheney, F.W., Jr., and Butler, J.: The effects on an ultrasonic aerosol on pulmonary mechanics and arterial blood gases in patients with chronic bronchitis. Am. Rev. Resp. Dis., *101:*710, 1970.
15. Hirsch, S.R., Viernes, P.F., and Kory, R.C.: The expectorant effect of glyceryl guaiacolate in patients with chronic bronchitis. Chest, *63:*9, 1973.
16. Petty, T.L., Brink, G.A., Miller, M.W., and Corsello, P.R.: Objective functional improvement in chronic airway obstruction. Chest, *57:*216, 1970.
17. Williams, I.P., and McGavin, C.R.: Corticosteroids in chronic airways obstruction: Can the patient's assessment be ignored? Br. J. Dis. Chest, *74:*142, 1980.
18. Alexander, M.R., Dull, W.L., and Kasik, J.E.: Treatment of chronic obstructive pulmonary disease with orally administered theophylline (A double-blind controlled study). JAMA, *244:*2286, 1980.
19. Miller, W.F.: A physiologic evaluation of the effects of diaphragmatic breathing training in patients with chronic pulmonary emphysema. Am. J. Med., *17:*471, 1954.
20. Mueller, R.M., Petty, T.L., and Filley, G.F.: Ventilation and arterial blood gas changes induced by pursed lips breathing. J. Appl. Physiol., *28:*784, 1970.
21. Miller, W.F.: Physical therapeutic measures in the treatment of chronic bronchopulmonary disorders. Am. J. Med., *24:*929, 1958.
22. Pierce, A.K., Taylor, H.F., Archer, R.K., and Miller, W.F.: Responses to exercise training in patients with emphysema. Arch. Intern. Med. (Chicago), *113:*28, 1964.
23. Guthrie, A.G., and Petty, T.L.: Improved exercise tolerance in patients with chronic airway obstruction. Phys. Ther., *50:*1333, 1970.
24. Petty, T.L., and Finigan, M.M.: The clinical evaluation of prolonged ambulatory oxygen therapy in patients with chronic airway obstruction. Am. J. Med., *45:*242, 1968.
25. Petty, T.L., Hudson, L.D., and Neff, T.A.: Methods of ambulatory care. Med. Clin. North Am., *57:*751, 1973.
26. Sahn, S.A., Nett, L.M., and Petty, T.L.: Ten year follow-up of a comprehensive rehabilitation program for severe COPD. Chest, *77*[Suppl.]:311, 1980.
27. Fishman, D.B., and Petty, T.L.: Physical, symptomatic and psychological improvement in patients receiving comprehensive care for chronic airway obstruction. J. Chronic Dis., *24:*775, 1971.

28. Burrows, B., and Earle, R.H.: Course and prognosis of chronic obstructive lung disease. N. Engl. J. Med., *280:*397, 1969.
29. Renzetti, A.D., McClement, J.H., and Bertram, D.L.: The Veterans Administration Cooperative Study of pulmonary function. III. Mortality in relation to respiratory function in chronic obstructive pulmonary disease. Am. J. Med., *41:*115, 1966.
30. Davis, A.L., and McClement, J.H.: The course and prognosis of chronic obstructive pulmonary disease. *In* Current Research in Chronic Respiratory Disease. Proceedings of the Eleventh Aspen Emphysema Conference. Arlington, U.S. Department of Health, Education and Welfare, 1968, p. 219.
31. Jones, N.L., Burrows, B., and Fletcher, C.M.: Serial studies of 100 patients with chronic airways obstruction in London and Chicago. Thorax, *22:*327, 1967.
32. Emirgil, C., and Sobol, B.J.: Long-term course of chronic obstructive pulmonary disease. Am. J. Med., *51:*504, 1971.
33. Pulmonary Rehabilitation Study Group: Community resources for rehabilitation of patients with chronic obstructive pulmonary diseases and cor pulmonale. Circulation, *49*[Suppl. A1], 1974.
34. Lertzman, M.M., and Cherniack, R.M.: Rehabilitation of patients with chronic obstructive pulmonary disease: state of the art. Am. Rev. Resp. Dis., *114:*1145, 1976.
35. Moser, K.M., Bokinsky, G.E., Savage, R.T., Archibald, C.J., and Hansen, P.R.: Results of a comprehensive rehabilitation program. Physiologic and functional effects on patients with chronic obstructive pulmonary disease. Arch. Intern. Med., *140:*1596, 1980.
36. Levine, B.E., Bigelow, E.B., Hamstra, R.D., Beckwitt, J.H., Mitchell, R.S., Nett, L.M., Stephen , T.A., and Petty, T.L.: The role of long-term continuous oxygen administration in patients with chronic airway obstruction with hypoxemia. Ann. Intern. Med., *66:*639, 1967.
37. Neff, T.A., and Petty, T.L.: Long-term continuous oxygen therapy in chronic airway obstruction. (Mortality in relationship to cor pulmonale, hypoxia and hypercapnia.) Ann. Intern. Med., *72:*621, 1970.
38. Stark, R.D., Finnegan, P., and Bishop, J.M.: Daily requirement of oxygen to reverse pulmonary hypertension in patients with chronic bronchitis. Br. Med. J., *3:*724, 1972.
39. Nocturnal Oxygen Therapy Trial Group: Continuous or nocturnal oxygen therapy in hypoxemic chronic obstructive lung disease (a clinical trial). Ann. Intern. Med., *93:*391, 1980.
40. Stuart-Harris, C., et al.: Long-term domiciliary oxygen therapy in chronic hypoxic cor pulmonale complicating chronic bronchitis and emphysema. Lancet, *1:*681, 1981.
41. Boysen, A.G., Block, A.J., Wyme, J.W., Hunt, L.A., and Flick, M.R.: Nocturnal pulmonary hypertension in patients with chronic obstructive pulmonary disease. Chest, *76:*536, 1979.
42. Johnson, T.S., Ellis, J.H., Jr., and Steele, P.P.: Improvement in platelet survival time with oxygen in patients with chronic obstructive airway disease. Am. Rev. Resp. Dis., *117:*255, 1978.
43. Emigril, G., and Sobol, B.J.: Long-term course of chronic obstructive pulmonary disease. (A new view of the mode of functional deterioration.) Am. J. Med., *51:*504, 1971.
44. Kory, R.C., Callahan, R., Borne, H.G., and Syner, J.C.: Veterans Administration airway cooperative study of pulmonary function. I. Clinical spirometry in normal men. Am. J. Med., *30:*243, 1961.
45. Petty, T.L., Pierson, D.J., Dick, N.P., Hudson, L.D., and Walker, S.H.: Follow-up evaluation of a prevalence study for chronic bronchitis and chronic airway obstruction. Am. Rev. Resp. Dis., *114:*881, 1976.
46. Fletcher, C., and Peto, R.: The natural history of chronic airflow obstruction. Br. Med. J., *1:*2645, 1977.
47. Hodgkin, J.E., (Ed.): Chronic Obstructive Pulmonary Disease (Current Concepts in Diagnosis and Comprehensive Care). Park Ridge, IL, American College of Chest Physicians, 1979.

Chapter 19

HOSPITAL AND HOME CARE FOR CHRONIC NEUROMUSCULAR PATIENTS

By Thomas L. Petty

Polio, the classic chronic neuromuscular disease with respiratory muscle involvement, presented the major challenge to physicians, nurses, and therapists in a past era. Fortunately, in advanced countries at least, this medical tragedy has yielded to modern preventive vaccines. Slowly progressive motor neuron disease with late-onset respiratory failure, however, still occurs in some of the veterans of this disease. This shares certain features with amyotrophic lateral sclerosis, a much more rapid motor neuron disease that is considered briefly at the end of this chapter.[1,2]

The challenge today focuses on the potential for care of potentially large numbers of patients with chronic progressive muscular dystrophies or motor neuron diseases. This chapter discusses certain aspects of hospital and home care for selected patients with these respiratory problems.

MUSCULAR DYSTROPHIES

A simple classification of the muscular dystrophies is presented in Table 19-1. The largest group of patients who will develop inevitable involvement of the respiratory muscles has Duchenne's muscular dystrophy. Because of recent concern about this problem and the possibilities for long-term home care, as well as the seeming enigma that surrounds these considerations, a major emphasis of this chapter is Duchenne's muscular dystrophy as a progressive form of neuromuscular respiratory failure affecting the young.

Clinical Vignettes

Probably the most accurate and dramatic way to summarize the possibilities for care of Duchenne's muscular dystrophy is illustrated by the four consecutive cases from my experience seen in the Colorado University Hospital between March 1977 and April 1980. Each case is presented as a clinical vignette with no attempt to capture all the clinical details.

Case 1. L.B., a 23-year-old man with long-standing Duchenne's muscular dystrophy, had been followed closely in the Muscle Clinic of the Colorado University Hospital. He had been deteriorating slowly with marked weight loss, poor appetite, and depression. His mother was advised that there was "no hope" for the problem. Nonetheless, he was brought to the emergency room early one Sunday morning by his mother, who accosted me just before morning rounds, demanding to know, "Why does my son have to die?" Summarizing a series of rapidly developing events, I went to the emergency room, intubated the patient, and provided the mechanical ventilatory assistance which the mother knew was available and insisted upon. The patient immediately awoke from the coma of respiratory failure. He was cachectic but within 24 hours became awake and alert. Feeding by means of a nasal gastric tube was commenced immediately. The patient's best measured forced breath via a Wright respirometer was 50 to 75 ml. During the following 35 days the patient gained weight and strength, but forced vital capacity was no more than 150 to 200 ml, and fatigue occurred rapidly. Tracheostomy was performed, and limited oral feeding became possible during the end of this hospitalization. Plans were made to transfer the patient home under the care of his mother, who was instructed in necessary respiratory care procedures, including tracheostomy suction, the use of a mechanical ventilator (Emerson postoperative ventilator), and all the "nitty gritty" required to support such patients.

Amazingly, the patient gradually gained strength and weight. Forced vital capacity gradually improved to be 400 to 800 ml over the next year. In fact, a degree of ventilatory weaning became possible, and the patient could be off the respirator as long as 4 to 6 hours, and at times even longer. He enrolled in Opportunity School, counseled other patients with muscular dystrophy, provided advice and counsel to respiratory therapy

TABLE 19-1. Major Types of Muscular Dystrophy

1. Pseudohypertrophic (Duchenne)
2. Facio-Scapulo-Hummeral (Landouzy-Dejerine)
3. Limb-Girdle (Erb)
4. Distal dystrophy (Gower)—late onset
5. Myotonic dystrophy (Steizhert's disease)

personnel and residents and fellows in training, and participated in national conferences on respiratory care. He made contributions to the muscular dystrophy campaign by making local television appearances and remained an active member of the family unit. At this writing, almost exactly 5 years after initiation of ventilatory assistance, the patient is a productive citizen living at home, requiring partial mechanical ventilatory support including the hours of sleep. He is clinically stable and enjoying life. Figure 19-1 is a picture of the patient seated in a chair at home. An inventory of his home respiratory care equipment is presented in Table 19-2.

Case 2. R.L., a 22-year-old male with Duchenne's muscular dystrophy diagnosed at age 6, was admitted to the hospital in October 1978. He had been evaluated at another hospital, and the parents were advised that there was nothing more that could be accomplished. Immediately prior to admission, the patient had retained secretions and suffered progressive weight loss and weakness. He was admitted to another community hospital and immediately suffered cardiorespiratory arrest in the emergency room. He was successfully resuscitated, and a bronchoscopic examination was performed to evaluate secretions. He was placed on mechanical ventilation and transferred to the University Hospital four weeks later. Unfortunately, no feeding was done. On admission he was cachectic, but awake and alert. Immediate nasogastric feeding was instituted, which was followed by an improvement in strength. The patient's forced vital capacity was 150 ml. Quickly he was able to tolerate oral feedings and gained further strength. Vital capacity gradually increased to 850 ml over the subsequent 2 weeks, and there was an accompanying weight gain. It was

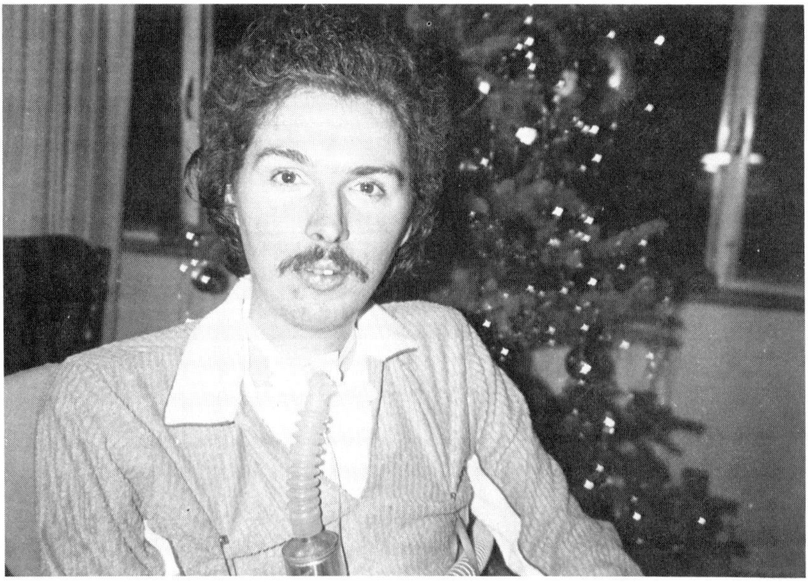

Fig. 19-1. Patient 1, living at home five years after initiation of ventilatory support.

a rather simple matter to extubate the patient, and he was discharged to home breathing without assistance. He has been comfortable at home is assisted by his parents in mobilizing secretions via nasotracheal suctioning. Careful emphasis has been placed on nutrition. He remains in a stable condition nearly 3-½ years following discharge.

Case 3. K.K., a 21-year-old man with long-standing Duchenne's muscular dystrophy, was admitted to the Colorado University Hospital in June 1979. His condition had been slowly deteriorating. Recently, an acute respiratory illness had occurred when he was living in a neighboring state. His nutritional status was deteriorating, and he was having numerous palpitations. He was treated with propranolol by his personal physician. He was referred to the muscular dystrophy clinic for further evaluation and treatment. While seated in a wheelchair, apparent respiratory arrest occurred. He was intubated and transferred to the intensive care unit. Evidence of aspiration pneumonia was present, and mechanical ventilation was continued for the next 14 days. Weaning was begun, but because of "chest tightness," a bronchoscopic examination was performed. Granulation tissue was seen at the tracheostomy site. Radiation therapy to reduce the granulation tissue was initiated. Three days later, an episode of "bronchospasm" occurred following suctioning. We attempted to place a new tracheostomy tube because of the difficulty in using a self-inflating bag. Immediately after replacing the tracheostomy, good breath sounds were heard bilaterally. A sudden cardiac arrest

TABLE 19-2. Home Respiratory Care Equipment, Supplies, Medications (Case 1—Patient with Duchenne's Muscular Dystrophy)

Durable Equipment	*Disposable Supplies*	*Medications*
A. 2 LP_2 Life Products volume ventilators: 1 attached to wheelchair 1 at bedside B. 2 cascade humidifying units C. 2 ventilator circuits D. 1 resuscitation bag E. 3 suction units: 1 in bedroom 1 in family room 1 portable unit F. 1 hospital bed G. 1 patient lift H. 1 bedside table I. 1 Wright Respirometer J. B.P. measureometer K. 1 powered nebulizer	A. Suction catheters B. Gloves C. Shiley trach tubes and fenestrations (change as often as every 2 months, for balloon malfunction; as infrequently as every 6 months without evidence of infection).	A. Isoetharine for nebulizer use B. Anhydrous theophylline C. Tetracycline (rarely used)

followed, however, and resuscitation was unsuccessful, with numerous intractable ventricular arrhythmias present on the monitoring scope. It is likely that the reintubation procedure precipitated an intractable cardiac arrhythmia.

Case 4. S.C., a 23-year-old man with Duchenne's muscular dystrophy for many years, was admitted to the hospital in April 1980. Two brothers had previously died of muscular dystrophy. The patient was first seen 7 years earlier when he was wheelchair bound. At that time, the forced vital capacity was 1.55 L, and FEV_1 was 1.43 L/sec. The mother was taught several bronchial hygiene techniques. The patient was next seen in 1975 and was doing well, with good appetite. He was followed regularly in the muscle clinic. Over the subsequent 5 years, however, he had suffered progressive weakness and weight loss. Secretion problems were becoming a concern. He was evaluated for elective tracheostomy, which was performed immediately following admission. His postoperative course was complicated by left-upper-lobe atelectasis, and mechanical ventilation was required because of profound secretions and emerging weakness. Numerous complications occurred including major airway plugging, cardiac arrhythmias, and a massive pneumothorax requiring chest-tube placement. The patient's condition finally stabilized, and he could be supported with mechanical ventilation. He was awake, alert, and cooperative. Total duration of hospitalization was 43 days. The patient was finally discharged home, with his parents receiving instructions re-

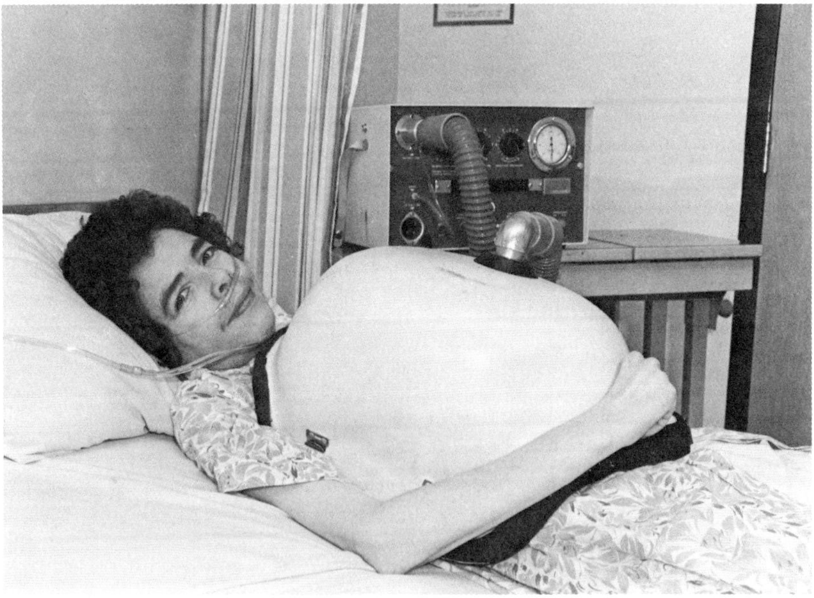

Fig. 19-2. Patient with long-standing and progressive weakness as a residual of poliomyelitis receiving ventilatory assistance with an external curias (shell) respiratory device. Shell connects to pump by large-bone tubing. Rate and inflation pressure as well as inspiratory and expiratory ratio are adjustable.

garding all aspects of respiratory care including tracheostomy suctioning, monitoring, and the use of a mechanical ventilator. During the subsequent year, the patient gained strength and at this writing is able to be without ventilatory assistance as long as an hour. He remains interested in life, enjoying sporting events on television and participating in hobbies, two years following discharge.

Comment. These four cases from my experience raise many questions. Why is it that the patient described as case 1 has improved so dramatically? What will the ultimate outcome of the three survivors be? What burdens to society have been created by the care briefly described in these case histories? How many patients with Duchenne's muscular dystrophy and related disorders are candidates for mechanical ventilation? Is it right and moral to keep these patients alive under the conditions of a progressive and ultimately fatal disease?

These are but a few of the questions and challenges that have been presented to me and my colleagues. Certainly, all answers are not available. The cases are presented as examples of what can be accomplished under certain circumstances.

It is fascinating that the three survivors have gained strength. One must conclude that a degree of weakness must have been due to factors other than the muscular dystrophy. Poor nutrition had likely contributed to muscular weakness, and the patients were thus failing far before they would have failed as a consequence of their muscular

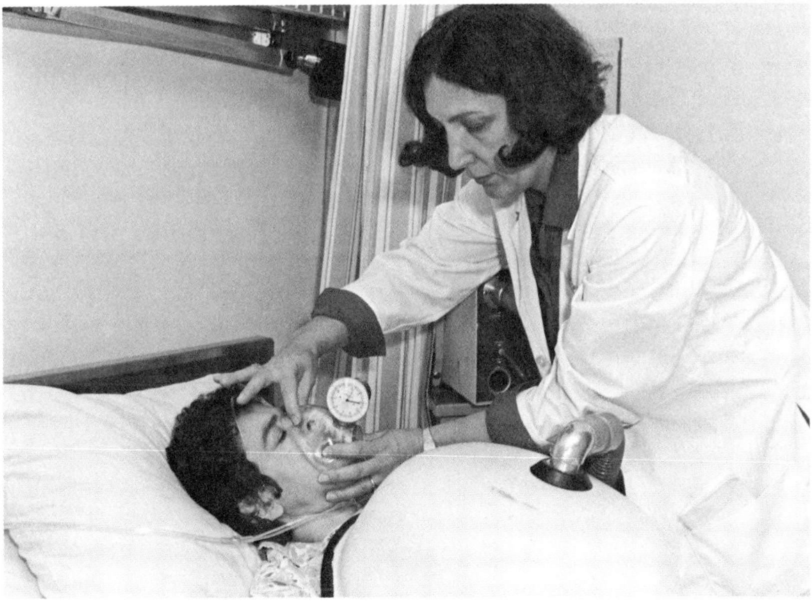

Fig. 19-3. Method of measuring tidal volume and minute ventilation with tight-fitting face mask attached to hand spirometer.

dystrophy. Certainly none of our therapy could be expected to change the course of the muscular dystrophy.

The practicality of home care for these patients is exemplified by cases 1 and 4. The return to pleasant and a partially productive life must be considered. The burdens of the family must also be considered. It is certain that both mothers have been kept from other pleasurable pursuits such as vacations, travel, and so forth because of the responsibilities of caring for their sons. On the other hand, numerous discussions, conversations, and observations have clearly indicated that both families are happy with the outcome.

The care of patient 2 was much simpler, without the requirement of mechanical ventilatory assistance. The fatal outcome in patient 3 was most likely due to cardiomyopathy, sometimes associated with Duchenne's muscular dystrophy, but the possibility of hypoxia-induced cardiac arrhythmia must also be recognized.

The ultimate solution to the heart-rending problems just outlined briefly must rest with a biologic solution to the problem. An immense amount of research is currently ongoing. Until the basic problem of the muscular dystrophy is solved, however, supportive therapy is all that remains. Whether or not this should be offered and the questions of the logistics of care and of available resources loom as major challenges.

MOTOR NEURON DISEASE

Similar problems with motor neuron disease, also called "amyotrophic lateral sclerosis," are frequently encountered. In this situation, the progressive disease leading to paralysis and, ultimately, respiratory failure occurs in much older individuals. Few of these patients are considered candidates for mechanical ventilatory assistance, since the progress of the disease is inexorable. A few patients requiring mechanical ventilators have been successfully weaned from mechanical support.[3] Nonetheless, it is likely that respiratory care specialists will be called upon to provide mechanical ventilatory assistance in the advanced stages of this disease. Certainly, this would be appropriate for external precipitating illnesses such as pneumonia in patients with otherwise adequate respiratory muscles. Whether or not long-term mechanical ventilation would be reasonable for advanced cases in the absence of a remedial cause of respiratory failure remains debatable, and the final decision for or against supportive therapy must be made on an individual basis.

The subject of chronic respiratory insufficiency associated with the residual effects of poliomyelitis was cited earlier in this chapter, including the interesting phenomenon of slowly progressive motor neuron disease.[1,2] Several patients in our area are managed with curias-type ventilators, as illustrated in Figure 19-2. Supplemental oxygen may be used as illustrated. A tracheostomy is not necessary with this type of long-term respiratory support, although some patients find tracheostomy suctioning an advantage. Patients with "old polio" often have impaired respiratory drives which worsen during sleep. Thus, both impaired respiratory muscle function and central hypoventilation are managed with this form of ventilatory support. (Figure 19-3 shows the method of measuring tidal volume with a well-fitting face mask attached to a hand spirometer.)

COMMENT

This chapter is presented as a brief discussion of what can be done in muscular dystrophy, citing anecdotes from my experience. Others have had similar experiences.[4] The future will tell much more about the advisability of this form of therapy for both muscular dystrophy and motor neuron diseases.

REFERENCES

1. Lane, D.J., Hazleman, B., and Nicholas, P.J.R.: Late onset of respiratory failure in patients with previous poliomyelitis. Q. J. Med., *43:*551, 1974.
2. Scott, J.H., Anderson, C.L., and Shankar, P.S.: Late-onset respiratory failure in previous poliomyelitis: Two cases. Resp. Care, *25:*755, 1980.
3. O'Donohue, W.J., Baker, J.P., Bell, G.M., Muren, O., Parker, C., and Paterson, J.L.: Respiratory failure in neuromuscular disease. (Management in a respiratory intensive care unit.) JAMA, *235:*733, 1976.
4. Alexander, M.A., Johnson, E.W., Petty, J., and Stauch, D.: Mechanical ventilation of patients with late stage Duchenne's muscular dystrophy: management in the home. Arch. Phys. Med. Rehabil., *60:*1979.

Section E

Ethical Considerations in Respiratory Failure

Chapter 20

MANAGING DEATH AND OTHER DIFFICULT SITUATIONS

The importance of healing the whole and not the parts is insisted on.—Sir William Osler

By Thomas L. Petty

High-technology medicine, some of which is emphasized in this book, has created its own problems. It has spawned the mechanical doctor, nurse, and therapist. Warmth, compassion, sympathy and concern for the individual, and personal dignity are replaced by "code blue," "cor zero," or a frantic call to the "911" ambulance system. To be sure, many have survived "sudden death," but we are somehow driven to resuscitate, intubate, ventilate, monitor, and drive the human spirit into a black hole rather than allow life's planned transition into death.* We have not learned how to deal with one of nature's most fundamental processes.

This last chapter might well have been written first. Why is it not the first chapter? After all, what we are really doing in respiratory care, indeed in all of medicine, is forestalling premature morbidity and mortality. People are living longer, but the age of death of the oldest is not increasing. It is exactly the same as at the turn of the century. There are no more 80-, 90-, or 100-year-old persons living per 100,000 births than a century ago.[1] Thus, we have a final biologic clock, preset by fundamental biologic processes, controlled and bequeathed by genetics, but modified (or perhaps shortened) by en-

* All death is sudden in one sense and gradual in another. In reality, we begin to die at the moment of conception.

vironmental factors. ("The days of our years are three score years and ten; and if by reason of strength they may be four score years . . ., Psalms 90:10) It has been wisely said that how long and in fact how we live beyond age 10 is determined in large degree by what we smoke, eat, and drink, and by how we drive our car. Thus, we must be careful to pick our parents well and our adventures in life with this caveat. This chapter is intended to give a perspective about managing death as it relates to the problem of acute and chronic respiratory failure described in this book.

CARDIAC ARREST

The following expresses my thoughts regarding the event of acute cessation of circulation and respiration. It is reprinted with permission from an editorial, "Don't Just Do Something, Stand There!"[2]

> The apparent transposition of the phrase that titles this editorial is not a mistake. It is intended to make the point that, at times, what appears at first to be a medical emergency is, in fact, nature's blessing that should be allowed to remove the suffering patient from hopeless and intolerable agony. Certainly our skills at respiratory and cardiac resuscitation should be deftly applied to individuals whose vital functions have suddenly failed by accident, disease, or trauma, to gain time for the resolution of acute reversible life-threatening processes affecting the circulatory and respiratory systems. By contrast, there are individuals for whom these resuscitation techniques only prolong the dying process and impose unnecessary suffering before the inevitable death occurs.
>
> Faced with a patient with sudden cessation of respiratory and cardiac function, how does one decide whether intubation, mechanical ventilatory support, and reestablishment of cardiac function with closed chest massage and/or pharmacologic agents should be instituted? The systematic review of four basic questions provides major assistance in this important decision. These questions are as follows: (1) Do I know the patient's underlying disease process and its course and prognosis? (2) Do I know the patient's quality of life in the context of his disease process? (3) Do I have anything more to offer the patient by resuscitative efforts designed to gain more time? (4) Do I wish to gain more time through resuscitative efforts to resolve these other questions?
>
> The physician and nurse should be able quickly to answer these questions in order to determine if the patient is best served by initiating respiratory and cardiac support. If one is unable to answer the first two questions in the affirmative, it is still highly likely that support should be offered until the answers become clear. One should not fear making a mistake in the direction of vigorous support, for certain patients will be saved to lead meaningful lives once again. If "yes" is the clear answer to the first two questions, and the third and fourth are clearly "no," then the physician, nurse, or allied health worker should simply stand by and offer whatever comfort and assistance they can to the patient or the family, or both. When the patient's life is known to be miserable at best, and when the patient has indicated no wish to have his suffering extended by technological means—in short, when there is nothing to be gained by the

additional hours, days, or weeks one might achieve by supporting respiration and circulation—then intervention such as tracheal intubation, mechanical assistance, and cardiopulmonary support should be set aside on behalf of the patient. Classic examples of these situations might include patients with advanced disabling emphysema with no hopes for recovery from respiratory failure or patients with uncontrolled metastatic carcinoma in whom respiratory failure develops. There are many other similar clinical situations, of course.

It should be clear by now that all patients do not have to die while being assisted by ventilators or in intensive care units with their circulation supported artificially. After all, our job as physicians and health workers is to serve the patient, and not one or another of their failing organ systems, in a desperate attempt to extend physiological life. Withholding of supportive measures in certain highly selected instances will prevent tragedies in which patients hover for extended periods between life and death, with all of the attendant social, economic, legal, and psychological implications that such cases raise. Fortunately, the legal profession and the clergy alike realize that the decision to support life or not requires skillful medical judgment, and the final analysis, should be a contract between the physician and the patient he or she serves.

MECHANICAL VENTILATION OF THE HOSPITALIZED DYING PATIENT

It is recognized that this commentary on cardiac or respiratory arrest, seriously written, does not deal with all the complexities of medicine as it is practiced today. Too often, medicine is practicied by committee. It is hard to tell who is in charge. Consider the patient with a disseminated malignant tumor. Who is finally responsible for the patient in room 1313? Is it the internist, the surgeon, the radiotherapist or the hematologist-oncologist? The oncologist will kill cancer. He will kill every cancer cell in the body. "She's just about to go into remission again," he will say. You know, however, that this is the fifth "remission" in a devastating downhill course. The surgeon may say, "We're going back to the O.R. again to stop the bleeding. Keep her on the respirator." You know, however, that after 88 U blood, ARDS, and super PEEP/IMV, and with an F_{IO_2} of 1.0 for 2 weeks, septic shock, no platelets, and hemodialysis, the likelihood of success is less than 50%. On the other hand, the radiotherapist may insist, "3000 more rads may control the pleural effusion and bone pain." However, you know that after years of a losing battle with metastatic breast cancer, this 82-year-old grandmother with total endocrine ablation, the ravages of previous radiotherapy, recurrent pneumonia, sepsis, and a recent operation for bowel obstruction is only seeking a little peace and quiet.

These problems can best be managed by the personal physician. Here is where all decisions must be made on behalf of the patient. What does one do, however, when the "onk," the "knife" and the "ray"—the "body mechanics"—attack in force? The body mechanics are aggressive, often evangelistic, and certainly supersalesmen of their trade. They will not promise a remission, but the nagging suggestion is there. They call for action and often suggest to the patient or family that everything that could be is not being done (by you). One way to buffer their endless striving for the supremacy of "chemosurgiotherapy" over cancer is a "second opinion." If one hunts enough, he can find support in any medical specialty. Another way is a "summit conference" during which a consensus may be reached, but the final decision must be made by the personal physician. This may include a decision *not* to ventilate a dying patient if respiratory failure intervenes.

Managing the Patient

Above all, the patient must be informed of the decisions the personal physician is making on his behalf. The fact that the physician is in charge and that he will continue to care for the patient no matter what happens must be stressed. Many times, it is good to say, "I don't believe using a respirator would be appropriate at this time," or "I have decided that putting a tube in your windpipe or operating on your throat so that we can breathe for you would not be the best thing." This usually leads to a meaningful interchange between patient and physician, and many times the patient is relieved to know that unnecessary prolongation of life and extension of death via a respirator is not planned. The personal physician can be positive about what will be done in terms of relieving dyspnea, pain, and suffering. Frequent visits for counseling and the liberal use of sedatives and analgesics are stressed. It is best to make more than the usual number of visits to the dying patient. When does a patient need a caring physician more than when he is dying? We have specialties that preside over the moment of birth, but few that look after the dying from a management point of view. The amount of good that the pleasant, cheerful, patient, thoughtful physician can do for the dying patient has been fantastically underestimated. The patient may respond with cheerfulness, humor, pathos, or any combination of these. Almost never is anger expressed, but if it is, it can always be dealt with by the experienced physician. Handholding, sitting on the bed, aiding with feeding, and holding the patient in one's arms are entirely appropriate for the dying patient, even though this may break certain rules and rituals. One should remember that medical care is supposed to serve the patient—not the medical hierarchy, nursing supervisor, or hospital administrator.

Managing the Family

This is almost as important as managing the patient. The family should be told that a decision has been made whether or not to intervene with a respirator. Some of the same comments are appropriate: "I have decided that your father will not benefit from a respirator," or "In these cases the respirator cannot be expected to save life, but only to promote suffering," or "I don't think it's in the best interest of your mother to go on any further." This type of statement on behalf of the suffering patient takes the decision-making out of the hands of the family. True, they may oppose this judgment, but usually with counseling regarding the likelihood of the outcome, they handle the situation nicely. People are much more reasonable than many believe and often are relieved when the physician sits down and explains that no further intervention is appropriate or will be followed. It is unusual for a family to oppose these decisions, to threaten, or to sue. As a matter of fact, it almost never happens and essentially will not happen if honesty, sincerity, and patience on behalf of the family are exercised.

Many times, the family themselves have decided that nothing more should be done. Occasionally, they have decided this prematurely, which is something that can usually be handled effectively if the physician points out that intervention *is* appropriate, that the patient still has a reasonable chance to recover, and that the pathway to ultimate recovery will not be a devastating, painful, or threatening experience. This is particularly important in older patients in whom reversible features are still present. The physician can say, "I believe we have a chance to make your mother comfortable and have a real chance for recovery," or "I'm not ready to give up yet, are you?," or, "I think we should have one more shot at it." These comments are good lead-ins to more detailed discussions about future plans for management. Another good policy is to have a daily conference with the family by promising to be available at a given time for at least 20 minutes to answer all questions. This is a particularly good time for the managing physician to emphasize that he will be making all the decisions, with the family's consent, and to remind the family that no matter what they hear from some well-meaning person, nothing is true until they hear it from *the physician in charge*. Therefore, if students, interns, residents, fellows, or other specialists become involved inappropriately, little harm will be done, since they know that the *primary physician* is making all the final decisions on behalf of the patient. It is recognized that this brief commentary regarding patient and family management is an oversimplification of a complex matter, but the principles and approach are valid.

REQUEST TO VENTILATE A DYING PATIENT

All too often, physicians are unwilling to accept the inevitability of death in a hopelessly ill and suffering patient. Thus, specialists in respiratory care are frequently asked to take over the ventilatory management of patients who have absolutely no chance for recovery. This is particularly the case in patients with disseminated malignant disease or even in patients who are judged by the primary care physician to be "no code." It has always seemed incredible that a decision is made that should cardiac arrest occur, no intervention will take place, *but* if the patient stops breathing, there will be an immediate clamor for intubation and ventilation. The paradox of this practice is obvious. The primacy of responsibility of the managing physician, however, must be maintained. If a surgeon, oncologist, or radiotherapist is in charge, the respiratory care team has no alternative but to provide the requested service. The only thing that makes this practice tolerable to most pulmonologists, respiratory care nurses, and respiratory therapists is the hope that *perhaps* the respiratory team does not know all the information available, the dynamics of disease, and the contract the managing physician has made with the patient or family. This is really not the major problem. The *real* problem occurs when patient care deteriorates to committee medicine and no one is really in charge. Again, we are told, "Another remission is possible," or "I think he's just about to stop bleeding," or "There's no question that we can fix it this time," and on and on. In the quiet of a conference room with no family present and only the specialists in attendance, it is perfectly appropriate for the knowledgeable respiratory care physician to disagree with his colleagues. Why is it that so many physicians delude both themselves and the patient, to say nothing of the family, when the outcome is certain? The problem is lack of experience, lack of intellectual honesty, lack of courage, and combinations of these common failings. The outcome for patients receiving mechanical ventilation with hopeless malignant disease is dismal.[3] The hopeless patient is best allowed to die before resuscitation, according to most experienced physicians.[4]

DISCONNECTING THE RESPIRATOR FROM DEAD PATIENTS

Although this should never be a problem, unfortunately it is. Here again, medicine has failed the dying or dead patient and the family and has timidly turned to law for a solution. It is so simple. When brain death is clearly present, the respirator should be discontinued. Well-publicized tragedies, endless rhetoric, and unnecessary and at times irresponsible jurisprudence could well have been avoided had physicians been trained to be realistic about the fact of death. *The only problem is, how does one define death?* Clearly, our profession and society in general does not demand the historical and traditional definition based upon cessation of all organ function. Brain death criteria have been accepted, and in the absence of pharmacologic agents such as long-lasting sedatives and certain other poisons, there should be no question about recovery with the presence of fixed and dilated pupils, the absence of oculocephalic reflex, so-called "doll's eyes" (made more certain with instillation of cold water into ear canals to augment this reflex), and no respiratory activity. After all, these are signs of deep midbrain and brainstem damage. A "flat line" EEG and no angiographic evidence of brain perfusion are also excellent criteria for irreversible brain death. Complete suppression of cortical activity with long-duration sedation is possible, however, and I have had the experience of ventilating a 72-year-old woman with self-induced ethchlorvynol (Placidyl) poisoning for 17 days with recovery, during which absolutely no electroencephalographic activity was present. This was an unusual situation, and knowledge of the peculiar pharmacokinetics of this drug (fat-bound and extremely slow clearance) plus certain hopeful neurologic reflexes suggested that a hopeful outcome was possible. Thus, again, medical decisions must be made on behalf of the individual patient and the family.

In cases of post-cardiac-arrest coma, if no drugs are present, failure to recover brainstem function and lack of any integrative recovery after 24 hours of resuscitation always identify irreversible brain damage. The ventilator can simply be disconnected in these cases. If respiratory center activity, no matter how primitive, supports respiration, the body will continue to survive for a time. At least this allows discharge from the intensive care unit. If the underlying problem is head trauma or drugs, or if any hopeful signs of recovery are present, the ventilator should be continued. After all, the purpose of the ventilator is to gain time so that Nature, with a little help, can heal the patient. Thus, the decision to continue or discontinue a ventilator is not difficult in cases in which there is no cortical activity.

I might end the discussion at this point, but I would never get away with it. What about the awake, alert, thinking, fearful, anxious, determined, loving person who, for reasons of hopelessly impaired ventilatory mechanics, has life and a conscious state and is maintained solely by mechanical ventilation? As I write this, we have two such individuals in the ICU. The family of one with end-stage COPD could not face death (nor could she), demanding a second episode of mechanical ventilation after the patient had been weaned from mechanical ventilation with great difficulty on transfer from another hospital only three months before. In this case, the patient had not accepted the transition to death which had been discussed with her earlier. The other patient, an elderly man, is slowly recovering from overwhelming bacteremic pneumococcal pneumonia, even though he is still receiving mechanical ventilation after three months, he is eating, walking, and talking, and predictably will go home soon. The woman will too, but with a mechanical ventilator to be used for the remainder of her life. Thus, she will become the third patient who was not able to be weaned in our more than 16 years of experience. Her family is being trained in respiratory care in a fashion similar to the approach used for the neurologic cripple with muscular dystrophy (see Chaps. 14 and 19).

On occasion, following discussions with the patient and the family, I have provided a sedative or narcotic, and I have removed the respirator from a suffering patient with a hopeless malignant tumor. This followed periods of deep thought and a final visit with family, friends and the clergy; a beautiful moment to say good-bye. We simply must not abandon our responsibility to serve our patients and to help them with unnecessary suffering at the time of approaching death.

". . . . and then the spirit takes wings and
flies away". . . (Psalms 90:10)

PREPARING THE AMBULATORY PATIENT FOR DEATH

In chronic lung disease, advanced stages of respiratory insufficiency may be reached, and patients can survive an unbelievably long period of time in spite of extreme physiologic derangements. These patients may be admitted to intensive care units repeatedly for intervention, but there comes a time when this is just as inappropriate as the ventilation of a patient with metastatic carcinoma or overwhelming multiple organ system failure. When the managing physician determines—on the basis of his knowledge, the patient's course, the quality of life, and the dynamics of the disease process—that death may occur at any time or that return to the hospital is inappropriate (see "Home Care of the Dying Patient"), it is time for this knowledge to be shared with the patient. Although this is difficult for many physicians to do, it is critically important for the patient and is the first step in the skillful management of a dying patient.

It is difficult to specify when it is best to have what the author calls "THE TALK." This is the talk about how it will be when death begins to supervene. As a matter of fact, it is important to realize that all patients with advanced chronic obstructive pulmonary disease or other devastating and advancing disease characterized by respiratory insufficiency know well that they are going to die. They do not even care too much that this eventuality is certain but they are panicked about *how* they will die. It is a fact, they are often panicked about some of the scenes described above where a committee or a body mechanic will not exercise proper judgment. They are well aware that at some moment a trained or untrained person may run into the hospital room or be called into the patient's home, break every rib in their body, put a tube down the esophagus, hook the patient to some kind of respirator and come screaming into the hospital emergency room. Our public is sophisticated about medical knowledge, and these tragedies are all too well known. However, these patients often have fantasies about climbing the wall, floating around the room, and gasping for every last breath. That this does not occur in slowly progressive respiratory failure, such as in COPD, offers great peace of mind to many patients and their families. Death is likened to a long sleep. The peaceful and restful nature of sleep is stressed. The patient and family are told that we are all attuned and accustomed to a short sleep, awakening refreshed. The concept of the long sleep is not really intolerable. Death is considered a transition. Religion may play a role at this point in the discussion or it may not, depending upon the beliefs of the patient. The transition, however, is an honest notion. After all, the human spirit came from somewhere and probably will go somewhere else even though uncontrovertible evidence for this fact is not accepted by everyone. But the transition is a nice thought. It can almost be put in terms of an adventure. After all why *isn't* it adventure? All of the rest of life is.

In any case, it is possible in a nonthreatening way to put forward an account that is acceptable to patients and family and has immense therapeutic value. Often the patient or family weeps; it is good if they do and is particularly good if the physician weeps too. I am an uncontrolled sentimentalist and have had this moving and meaningful experience with my patients many times. Why has it been suppressed? It is salutary for all concerned. After the patient and family work through their feelings, an amazing thing happens. There is a *détente with death:* a period of peace and often survival for months or years. One patient, a physician with advanced COPD, returned on many occasions for "THE TALK." The first return was a little more than one year following the first; the second was abouh six months later; and the third three months after that. Further talks were less beneficial as the therapeutic effect became exhausted. Death finally came at home quietly and calmly, as it does in more than 50% of my patients with chronic obstructive lung disease.

HOME CARE OF THE DYING PATIENT

I reported previously that the majority of my private patients with advanced COPD die at home.[5] After all, what better place to be than in the comfort and love of the family or with friends? Most patients are receiving oxygen and have slowly compensated CO_2 retention. Most simply fall asleep and enter the transition comfortably and quietly. It does no harm to offer sedation in the extremely dyspneic patient, and in fact the skillful use of diazepam in patients driven to breathe is being accepted. One must be cautious never to admit to students, interns, or residents that this art of medicine is being practiced, lest it be inappropriately used with disastrous consequences. There is no doubt that death is hastened at home by patients or even by the family in some cases. This does absolutely no harm. Unfortunately, our society has too little compassion for the dying patient. Excessive consumption of alcohol, the overuse of sedative or tranquilizing drugs, or the discontinuance of oxygen is in no way immoral, unethical, or inappropriate in selected patients, in my opinion. No author would ever admit that this has been overtly condoned or encouraged, but it is likely that this has happened a time or two in the past.

SUMMARY

In our society, death and dying are difficult. We are not prepared for it by any segment of society including most religions. The medical profession in its entirety fails badly in this responsibility. We must do better, and we can.

"And thus this man died, leaving his death for an example of noble courage and a memorial of virtue." (2 Maccabees 6:31)

REFERENCES

1. Fries, J.F.: Aging, natural death and the compression of morbidity. N. Engl. J. Med., *303:*130, 1980.
2. Petty, T.L.: Don't just do something, stand there! Arch. Intern. Med., *139:*920, 1979.
3. Snow, R.M., Meller, W.C., Rice, D.L., and Ali, K.: Respiratory failure in cancer patients. JAMA, *241:*2039, 1979.
4. Arena, F.P., Perlin, M., and Turnbull, A.D.: Initial experience with a "code-no code" resuscitation system in cancer patients. Crit. Care Med., *8:*733, 1980.
5. Petty, T.L.: Managing the COPD Patient and Family at Home. *In* Chronic Obstructive Pulmonary Disease. Chap. 9. Edited by T.L. Petty. New York, Marcel Dekker, 1978.

SUGGESTED ADDITIONAL READING

1. Sampson, W.I.: Dying at home. JAMA, *238:*2405, 1977.
2. Clouser, K.D.: Allowing or causing: Another look. Ann. Intern. Med., *87:*622, 1977.
3. Veith, F.J., Fein, J.M., Tendler, M.D., Veatch, R.M., Kleiman, M.A., and Kalkines, G.: Brain death. 1. A status report of medical and ethical considerations. JAMA, *238:*1651, 1977.
4. Veith, F.J., Fein, J.M., Tendler, M.D., Veatch, R.M., Kleiman, M.A., and Kalkines, G.: Brain death. II. A status report of legal considerations. JAMA, *238:*1744, 1977.
5. Downer, D.J., Snyder, J.V., and Grenvik, A.: Brain death certification (a review). Crit. Care Med., *5:*230, 1977.
6. Cohen, C.B.: Ethical problems of intensive care. Anesthesiology, *47:*217, 1977.
7. Lynch, E.C., Young, J.B., Wickemeyer, W.J., Engelhardt, H.T., and Jackson, D.: To treat or not to treat—the dilemma. Heart Lung, *7:*499, 1978.
8. Vanderpool, H.Y.: The ethics of terminal care. JAMA, *239:*850, 1978.
9. Curran, W.J.: The brain death concept: Judicial acceptance in Massachusetts. N. Engl. J. Med., *298:*1008, 1978.
10. Schoenfeld, M.R.: Terror in the ICU. Forum in Medicine. Philadelphia, American College of Physicians, Sept., 1978.
11. Robin, E.D.: Determinism and humanism in modern medicine. JAMA, *240:*2273, 1978.
12. Lo, B, and Jonsen, A.R.: Clinical decisions to limit treatment. Ann. Intern. Med., *93:*764, 1980.
13. Kass, L.R.: Ethical dilemmas in the case of the ill. 1. What is the physician's service? JAMA, *244:*1811, 1980.
14. Callan, J.P.: Therapeutic talk. JAMA, *244:*2202, 1980.
15. McCormick, R.A.: The Fox case. JAMA, *244:*2165, 1980.

Appendices

These appendices are included as a possible special interest section for the reader. Appendix A is a brief synopsis of clinical pulmonary phsysiology and is offered as a succinct review and reference.

Appendix B was kindly prepared by N. Balfour Slonim, M.D., Ph.D. of Denver. It presents a convenient means of estimating alveolar oxygen tension from inspired oxygen concentration and pressure. If the alveolar-arterial oxygen tension difference is known, this nomogram will allow estimates of arterial oxygen tension from changes in inspired oxygen concentration or pressure. Alveolar-arterial tension differences increase with increasing oxygen concentration, so direct arterial oxygen tension measurements will still be required in many patients.

Appendix C gives a brief discussion of my views on the future of respiratory care.

Appendix A

SYNOPSIS OF CLINICAL PULMONARY PHYSIOLOGY

By Giles F. Filley

A. PRESSURE-VOLUME CONCEPTS IN NORMAL AND ABNORMAL LUNGS

1. Pulmonary Compliance

Cough and dyspnea are closely related to disturbances of pulmonary mechanics; clinical measurements of these disturbances, thoughtfully considered, can illuminate these two major symptoms of pulmonary insufficiency. The vital capacity (VC) is a simple measurement of volume—the largest volume that can be expired from the lungs after a full inspiration—but it is also, if interpreted with care, an estimate of pulmonary compliance, a complex concept with important implications.

The tissues of the lung must be stretched (deformed) during inspiration. An easily deformed lung is compliant; a stiff lung is noncompliant. The ease of deformation is measured by the pulmonary compliance. This is the ratio of two laboratory determinations: the volume change (ΔV) resulting from an intrathoracic (intraesophageal) change (ΔP) developed by the respiratory muscles (Fig. A-1). The vital capacity is a useful clinical estimate of the compliance because it is the maximum (and easily measured) volume change resulting when the patient makes a maximum (and easily reproducible) effort to stretch his lungs.

To use the vital capacity thoughtfully as an estimate of compliance requires (a) the exclusion of conditions that change the vital capacity other than stiffness and (b) the full realization of the significance of a compliance change.

a. A low vital capacity can result from causes obviously not related to lung stiffness, e.g., failure to make a maximum effort, chest deformity, small stature, muscular paralysis. Less obvious causes, such as old age, obesity, or pleural thickening, should also be excluded before concluding that a low vital capacity indicates low compliance of the lung.

b. Even when it has been correctly concluded that a low vital capacity resulted from a change within the lung itself, it must not be assumed that the lung parenchyma is therefore necessarily stiff. Mucous plugging of airways can, for example, simply by preventing part of the lung from being ventilated, produce a low vital capacity.

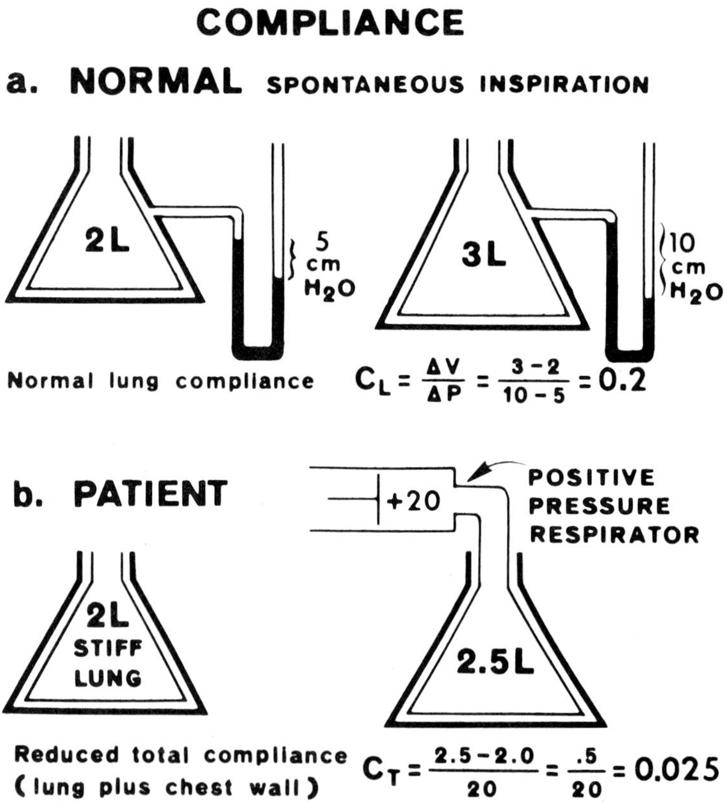

Fig. A-1. The pressure needed to keep the normal lung distended is about 5 cm H_2O; to distend the lung further by taking a breath of 1 L normally requires another 5 cm H_2O. In patients needing respiratory assistance, the lung and chest wall compliances are usually considered together; an airway pressure of 20 mm H_2O may produce a breath of only ½ L because a stiff lung reduces C_T, the total compliance.

In this case, since the unobstructed portions would have to be stretched more to achieve the same volume change, a compliance measurement would decrease even if no actual stiffening of lung tissue had occurred.

2. *Causes and Consequences of Lung Stiffness*

Lung stiffening in pure form occurs when alveolar walls and other parenchymal structures, e.g., perivascular areas, septa, and so forth, are replaced by collagen. Such chronic restrictive lung disease is properly called "pulmonary fibrosis" although this term is loosely used to designate other diseases causing low compliance such as pulmonary granulomas, chronic inflammatory conditions, and the pneumoconioses (see Chap. 11). Acute reduction of pulmonary compliance is caused by atelectasis in many forms, by loss of surfactant, and by pulmonary edema. The underlying conditions may be pulmonary embolism, pneumonia, or congestive heart failure.

The extra work required of the respiratory muscles to stretch uncompliant lungs leads to dyspnea and to rapid shallow breathing. Such breathing may be inefficient since the proportion of dead space breathing is high when the tidal volume is low. Cyanosis from hypoxemia of arterial blood is often severe. It results not only from an inefficient breathing pattern but also from complex disturbances of ventilation-perfusion relationships which cause much of the right ventricular output to leave the lungs unsaturated with oxygen.

The energy needed to ventilate the lungs can be temporarily supplied by mechanical respirators. The implications of compliance changes are therefore of practical importance.

B. PRESSURE-VOLUME-FLOW CONCEPTS

1. *Airway Resistance*

In addition to the work needed to stretch the lung, even greater energy may be required to drive air through bronchi which are narrowed by disease (see Chaps. 9 and 10). The physiologic measure of the severity of such narrowing is the airway resistance, i.e., the ratio of airflow to the pressure drop between alveolus and mouth.

In clinical work, this latter measurement is virtually impossible to obtain by usual methods. It is therefore customary to interpret a *slowing* of airflow under standard conditions to indicate the presence of airway narrowing. This slowing is almost always most marked during expiration. The forced expiratory volume (FEV) that patients can voluntarily expire in one second (FEV_1) when expressed as a percent of normal or of the vital capacity has become the standard practical means of evaluating changes in airway function in clinical medicine. As shown in Figure A-2, the maximum mid-expiratory flow (MMF) is a particularly sensitive index for estimating *changes* of airway resistance.

2. *Chronic Airway Obstruction (Chap. 10)*

This term stands for the "diseases" chronic bronchitis or emphysema, or both. It is chosen because (a) these two conditions often occur together, (b) when occurring separately they are difficult to distinguish, and (c) their outstanding measurable characteristic is an increased airway resistance, whether produced by partial or complete obstruction of bronchi or bronchioles.

The nature of this obstruction has not been conclusively proven. In severe or terminal asthma, plugging of the small airways with viscous mucus is clearly the mechanism. In most patients with emphysema, obvious collapse of the larger bronchi (3 to 5 mm in diameter) can be demonstrated during forced expiration and during cough. Whether this collapse occurs at "flow-limiting segments" of the tracheobronchial tree is questionable; it is known, however, that the bronchial wall in these segments is histologically thin and atrophic in appearance. Increased tone of bronchial muscle, mucosal edema, and submucosal thickening, as caused by hyperplasia of mucous glands, are obstructing mechanisms of potential but unknown importance.

The major symptom of airway obstruction is dyspnea. Major clinical consequences are disability for exercise, derangement of blood

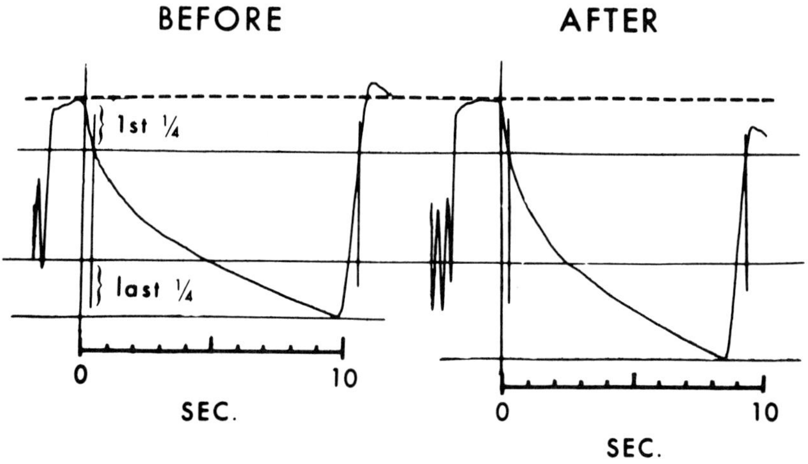

Fig. A-2. Reproduction of an actual spirogram used to measure the change in a patient's expiratory flow rate after use of a "bronchodilator." Before the mean flow rate at which the middle half of the forced expiratory volume is expired is the MMF. *After bronchodilator*, the same volume measured *at the same distance* from the top of the spirogram is used to calculate the flow rate. The first 25% of any spirogram is effort-dependent because initially the airways are held open so widely by the forces generated by a full inspiration that flow is only slightly limited by bronchial caliber and depends mainly on the force and rapidity with which the expiratory muscles contract. The last 25% of the spirogram discriminates poorly between normal and obstructed airways because even normal airways become narrow toward the end of expiration. By comparing the spirograms at similar levels of lung inflation, the effects of drugs on the bronchial tree can be separated from the effects of the lung volume change.

gases, and eventual respiratory failure. These consequences do result directly from mechanical interference with airway function. For example, CO_2 is retained in chronic bronchitis not simply as a direct result of narrowed bronchi, but because the increased work of breathing forces the body to compensate by allowing the alveolar CO_2 concentration to increase. This makes possible a normal CO_2 output at a lower ventilation and thus conserves energy. In the process, a normal arterial P_{CO_2} is sacrificed. Direct and compensatory effects are difficult to distinguish in chronic airway obstruction.

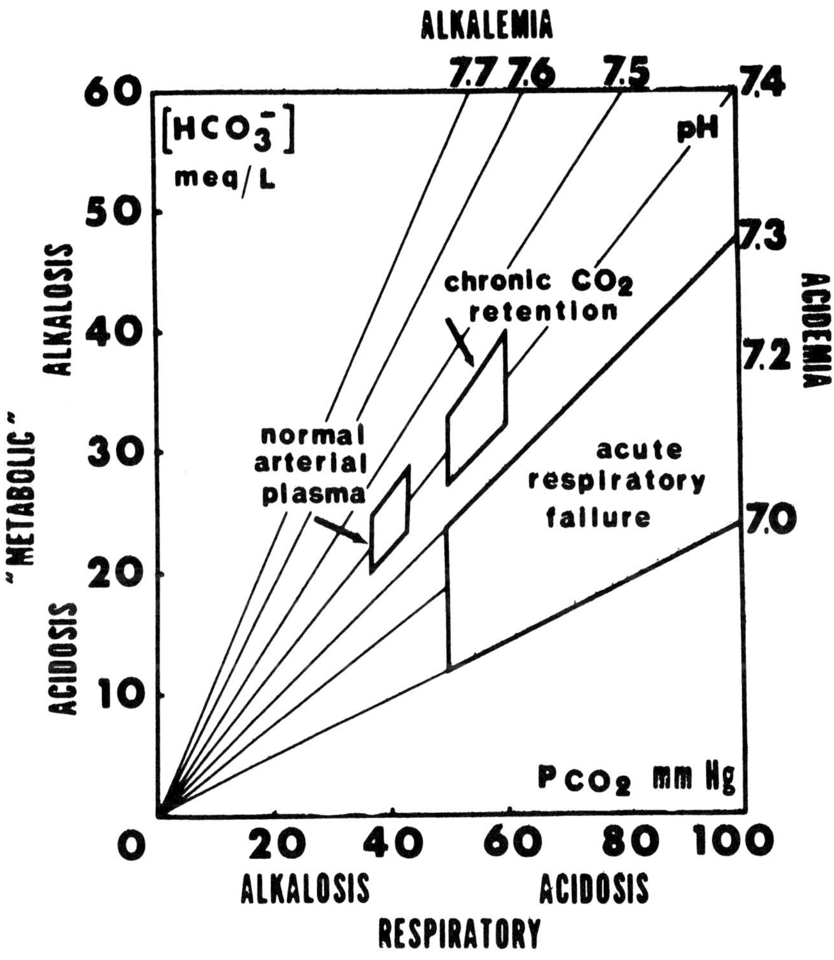

Fig. A-3. The acid-base diagram on which CO_2 dissociation curves can be plotted. The range of values of bicarbonate concentration, CO_2 pressure, and pH encountered in acute and chronic respiratory acidosis is indicated. The diagram is both a graphic presentation of the Henderson-Hasselbalch equation and a means of correctly associating clinical terms with chemical measurements.

RESPIRATORY GAS EXCHANGE
A. CARBON DIOXIDE TRANSPORT

1. Ventilation and Acid-Base Balance

The elimination of CO_2 is ventilation dependent in contrast to the uptake of oxygen, which depends as much on circulatory as on ventilatory factors. The effectiveness with which CO_2 is eliminated is best measured by the level of the arterial P_{CO_2} because this is proportional to the ratio of CO_2 production to the alveolar ventilation. When CO_2 production exceeds the rate of its removal from the lungs, the P_{CO_2} rises.

The P_{CO_2} of blood is also a key variable among those determining the acid-base balance of the body. Acute rises of P_{CO_2} as a result of inadequate ventilation rapidly cause the blood pH to fall.

$$\text{pH}\downarrow \; = 6.1 + \log \frac{[HCO_3^-]}{0.03\ P_{CO_2}\uparrow}$$

Such acidemia normally stimulates central chemoreceptors, and ventilatory efforts are increased. With patent airways, such efforts are usually effective in blowing off CO_2, and a fall in P_{CO_2} occurs, returning the pH toward normal. In chronic airway obstruction,

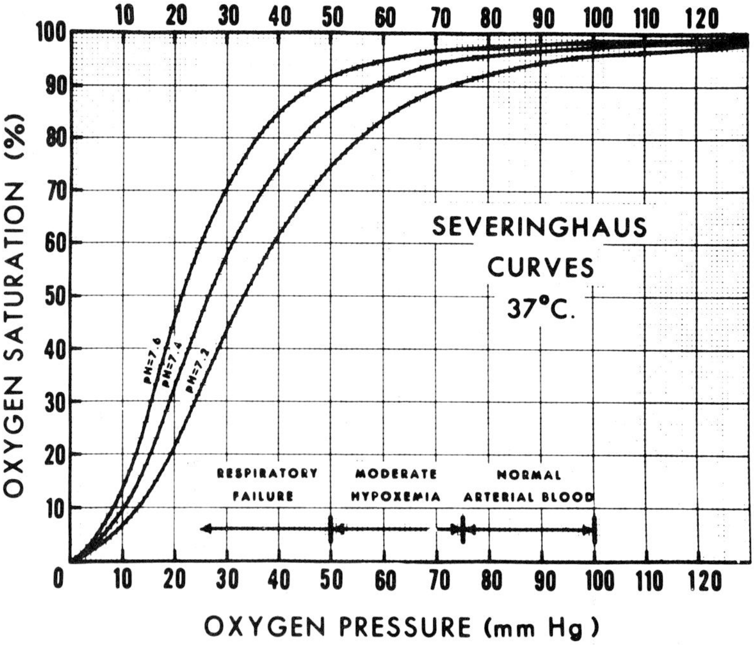

Fig. A-4. Oxyhemoglobin dissociation curves, based on the data of Severinghaus (1966). The range of arterial oxygen pressure values encountered in respiratory failure is indicated.

however, not only is the work of breathing (and hence CO_2 production) greatly increased, but also the effectiveness of ventilation is impaired. The result is usually a permanent elevation of P_{CO_2}, or chronic CO_2 retention. (See Chapter 10.)

Patients with a chronically elevated arterial P_{CO_2} often have a normal pH. This results from the renal generation of bicarbonate, which restores the ratio of HCO_3^- to 0.03 and P_{CO_2} to its normal value of 20:1. In "fully compensated" respiratory acidosis, therefore, the pH is normal. These relationships are determined by the Henderson-Hasselbalch equation above and are illustrated in Figure A-3, which is simply a graphic representation of this equation.

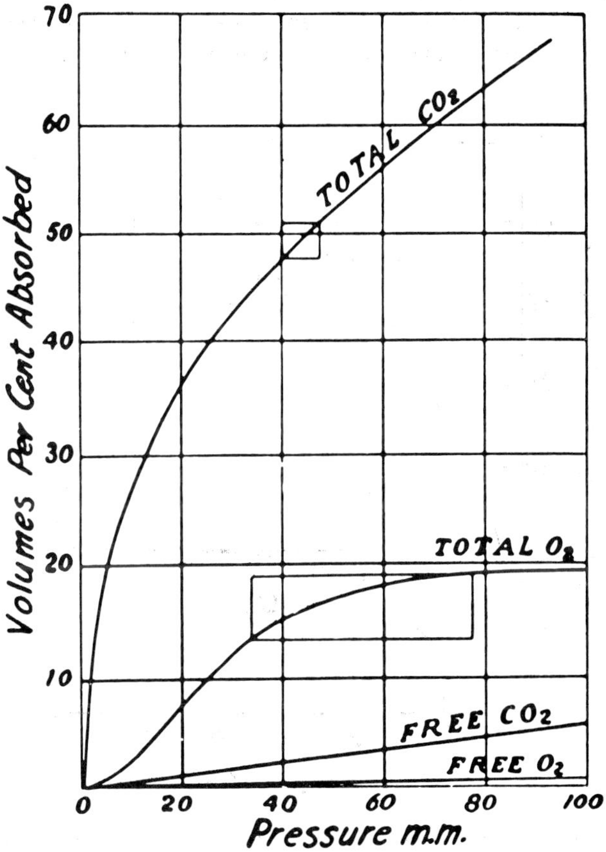

Fig. A-5. Normal CO_2 and O_2 dissociation curves plotted on the same scale. The rectangles indicate the range of values between arterial and mixed venous blood CO_2 and O_2 concentrations and partial pressure. (From Henderson, L.J.: Blood: A Study in General Physiology. New Haven: Yale University Press, 1928.)

2. *Acute Respiratory Acidemia*

It is not known that a high P_{CO_2} per se is toxic to vital organs; more likely, disturbances of cell function are caused by pH changes which almost always accompany rapid P_{CO_2} changes. Local H^+) disturbances occur because local buffering mechanisms and local means of adjusting bicarbonate levels cannot keep pace with the rapid movement of molecular CO_2 from one body compartment to another. These considerations are becoming important to physicians who, with efficient modern respirators and rapidly acting buffer solutions, can bring about pH changes in the brain and other tissues which are not necessarily reflected in the blood.

Patients in acute respiratory acidemia are subject to a large number of complications—cardiovascular, gastrointestinal, renal, and cerebral. There are five complications that should be emphasized because they can be the direct result of mismanagement.

a. Oversedation. It must be remembered that restlessness and sleeplessness in patients with CO_2 retention may be signs of increas-

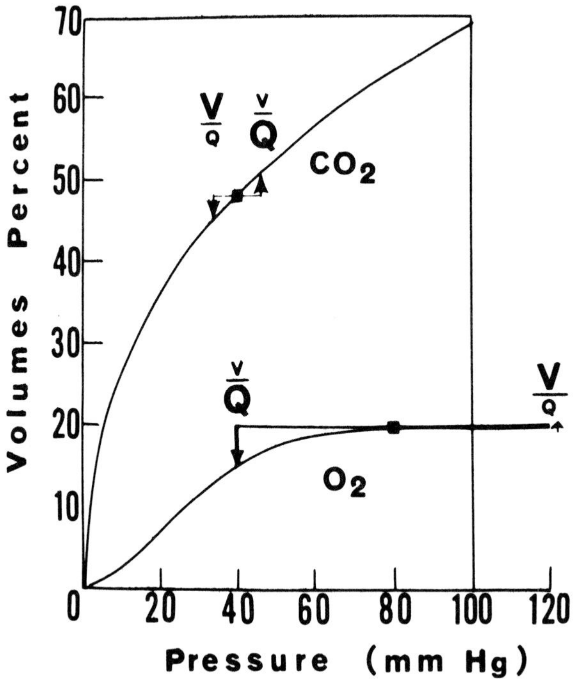

Fig. A-6. The ventilation-perfusion theory explanation for arterial hypoxemia in pulmonary disease illustrated on L.J. Henderson's diagram. Blood leaving normal portions of lung has a P_{CO_2} of 40 and a P_{O_2} of 80 mm Hg (solid squares). Hypoventilated portions yield blood higher in CO_2 but much lower in O_2 content (larger downward-pointing arrow). The hyperventilated portions lower the CO_2 but do not increase the O_2 content appreciably (smaller upward-pointing arrow).

ing hypoxemia. Sedation without respiratory assistance or adequately controlled oxygen therapy can be fatal.

b. Misapplied mechanical ventilatory "assistance." In patients who "fight" the respirator or in cases in which machine pressures, tidal volumes, respiratory rates, or total flows are ill suited to a patient's needs, acidemia may become worse, not better. The only sure way of knowing that mechanical ventilatory assistance designed to wash out CO_2 is in fact doing so is to perform frequent measurements of P_{CO_2} in the arterial blood.

c. A third complication, arterial *hypocapnia* and pH *increases* in the blood, may result from too rapid a loss of CO_2 by mechanical ventilation. Such transient alkalosis and alkalemia may or may not be important depending on whether or not the brain and other tissues undergo similar sudden fluctuations. It is known that the blood can be alkalemic and the cerebral spinal fluid acidic in patients under vigorous treatment for respiratory failure.

d. Potassium tends to move from tissue cells to plasma in acute respiratory acidemia. Such mobilization and the use of diuretics and corticosteroids may cause potassium deficiency in respiratory failure. Since chloruresis also tends to occur, a hypokalemic hypochloremic alkalosis may be a complication of respiratory failure, and replacement of both potassium and chloride is often needed (see Chap. 6).

e. High concentrations of oxygen may, by removing the hypoxic stimulus in respiratory failure, so depress respiration that CO_2 ten-

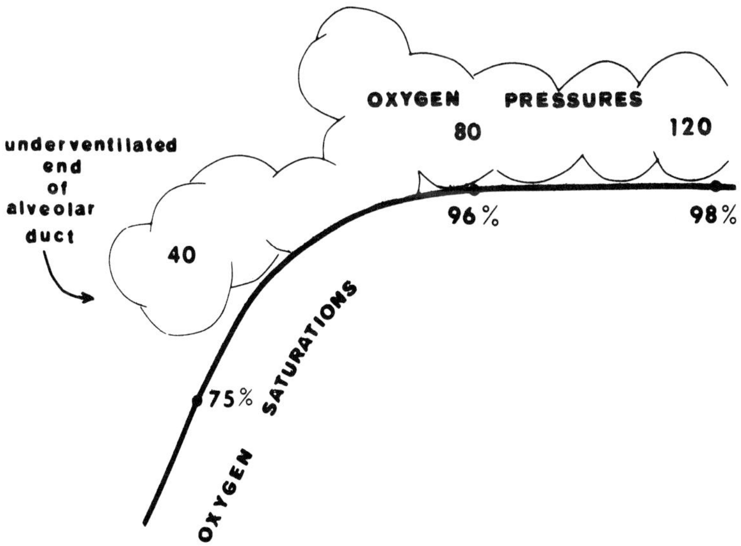

Fig. A-7. The effect on oxygen saturation of underventilating the terminal portions of the alveolar duct system.

sion may rise rapidly to 150 mm Hg or higher and the pH may drop precipitously. Such a danger should not lead to the withholding of oxygen, since all patients with severe CO_2 retention are always hypoxemic on air and *must* receive controlled oxygen. Intermittent use of oxygen is, however, contraindicated. The solution to the problem lies in (a) the controlled use of oxygen at low flows, and (b) frequent monitoring of the arterial blood P_{O_2} and P_{CO_2} (see Chap. 3).

B. OXYGEN TRANSPORT

1. Ventilation-Perfusion Relationships

Exactly how arterial unsaturation results from disturbed lung function is a challenge to both the physiologist and the clinician. Intrapulmonary shunts and diffusion impediments are obvious possible causes of low arterial oxygen content, but pure shunts and pure diffusion blocks are uncommon in pulmonary disease. What is common is a distribution disturbance such that some portions of the lungs are underventilated in proportion to their blood flow (local hypoventilation). These ventilation-perfusion (V/Q) abnormalities cause hypoxemia without CO_2 retention and hence imitate shunting and diffusion effects.

The key to understanding these effects is the shape of the particular hemoglobin dissociation curve relating oxygen saturation to oxygen pressure (Fig. A-4). Not only does this shape explain physiologically how V/Q disturbances cause hypoxemia, but also its graphic representation provides a means of visualizing the abnormalities of oxygenation encountered in clinical medicine.

If for any reason (e.g., a plugged bronchus) a portion of the lungs fails to receive oxygen from the atmosphere at an adequate rate, the alveolar O_2 pressure in that portion will fall. Therefore, the blood perfusing that portion will have a low oxygen pressure. If some other portion of lung is hyperventilated, the blood leaving it will have a high oxygen pressure. But the two blood samples will not have proportionally low and high oxygen contents because of the nonlinear relationship between the content and the pressure of oxygen in blood: if these samples are mixed in equal proportions in the left ventricle, the resulting arterial blood will be low in oxygen although it may be normal with respect to CO_2.

Figure A-5 is a reproduction of the illuminating relationships first grasped by L.J. Henderson. It contrasts the oxygen curve with the physiologically linear CO_2 dissociation curve and reveals the basis for the V/Q theory or respiratory gas exchange. In Figure A-6 the concepts of the previous paragraph are indicated in two ways. It may be seen how local hyperventilation cannot compensate for the lowering of oxygen content caused by a low V/Q in one portion of lung, since a high V/Q elsewhere increases P_{O_2} but hardly increases content along the horizontal portion of the curve; in the case of CO_2, however, hyperventilation can blow off CO_2 to compensate for a locally low V/Q. In Figure A-7 is depicted one of many anatomic visualizations of the type of distribution disturbance that leads to hypoxemia.

2. *Hypoxemia and Hypoxia*

Hypoxemia means deficient oxygen in the blood; hypoxia can mean low oxygen content or pressure anywhere in the body and can imply a much more serious deficiency—an inadequate rate of oxygen delivery. We must distinguish between a low oxygen level and a low oxygen supply to understand how the body adjusts to such stresses as high altitude, exercise, and diseases of the heart and lung.

Since cyanosis may reflect stagnation of flow rather than arterial hypoxemia, and in any case is an insensitive guide, the recognition of arterial hypoxemia requires arterial blood sampling and analysis for oxygen pressure (PO_2) or percentage of saturation (SAO_2). There is no satisfactory substitute for arterial puncture either in the physiologic study of oxygen transport or in the clinical management of respiratory failure. In fact, the practical criteria for the presence of respiratory failure are an *arterial* PO_2 of less than or a PCO_2 of more than 50 mm Hg. The ease and safety of repeated arterial puncture have been established. New technologies may soon make this statement obsolete, however (see "The Future," Appendix C).

The recognition of tissue hypoxia is far more difficult though probably more important. Adjustments in ventilation, in hematocrit level, in cardiac output, and particularly in the distribution of the cardiac output continually operate to insure an adequate supply of oxygen to vital organs whether this supply is threatened by the stress of exertion or cardiopulmonary disease. These adjustments may be costly: The effort of breathing, the viscosity of blood, the work of the heart, and the temporary ischemia of certain tissues need to be considered in evaluating the appropriateness of the body's response.

The oxygen tension in the blood of the great veins (central venous PO_2) is a useful index of the adequacy of the overall tissue oxygen supply since it is proportional to the cardiac output. The physiologist and clinician should, in addition, attempt to estimate how the available oxygen is being distributed to respiratory and heart muscles, to the kidneys, and to the brain. Such estimates are important in evaluating dyspnea, oliguria, and cerebral function in health and disease.

The mechanism of the pulmonary hypertension in all cases of reactive pulmonary hypertension due to hypoxemia or acidemia, or both, is well established. Acute exacerbations of chronic bronchitis lead to alveolar hypoxia and arterial hypoxemia, to acidemia in both venous and arterial blood, and to acidity in the cerebrospinal fluid and probably the brain. Obstruction to pulmonary blood flow is associated with some or all of these changes: muscular contraction of precapillary pulmonary arterioles probably occurs causing pulmonary hypertension and increased right ventricular work. Cor pulmonale with or without congestive heart failure is intimately related to the chemical changes by which respiratory failure is recognized and by which its management must be largely guided.

Appendix B

NOMOGRAM FOR ESTIMATING ALVEOLAR OXYGEN TENSION FROM INSPIRED OXYGEN CONCENTRATION OR PRESSURE (TENSION)

By N. Balfour Slonim

ALVEOLAR OXYGEN PRESSURE AS A FUNCTION OF INSPIRED OXYGEN CONCENTRATION AND PRESSURE

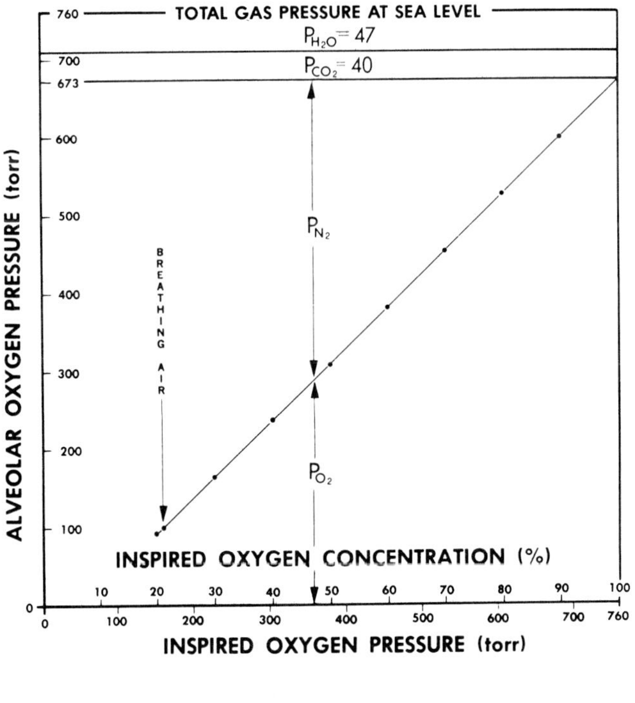

Appendix C

THE FUTURE

By Thomas L. Petty

As with any era, the future promises exciting developments in the field of respiratory care. In the past decade, scientists and care deliverers were fascinated by the possibilities of extracorporeal membrane oxygenation (ECMO). Certainly, this advance in technology has not added greatly to our ability to support many patients. A major controlled multicenter clinical trial did not result in better survival of severely injured patients with use of ECMO compared with use of mechanical ventilation and PEEP.[1] The value of ECMO in selected patients, particularly the young, still remains a potential, and further developments will be required to learn more about the possibilities for ECMO in critical-care situations.[2]

Today, the unending fascination for new support systems focuses on high-frequency jet ventilation (HFJV).[3–5] Certainly, it is possible to support life by breathing at high frequency at a tidal volume much less than the dead space volume. Exactly how this is accomplished is somewhat conjectural. Probably, gas concentration gradients are developed which augment diffusion respiration. Co-axial flow of inspired and expired gas may occur. In any case, oxygenation and carbon dioxide elimination may be maintained by HFJV, which may minimize barotrauma, the hemodynamic effects of conventional ventilation, and massive leaks through bronchopleural fistulae. It is fascinating that the patient's spontaneous ventilatory efforts cease during HFJV. Certainly, careful clinical trials are warranted in selected patients in order to determine what impact this technologic advance will offer to our field.

Currently, an immense amount of research focuses on markers and mechanisms of the adult respiratory distress syndrome (ARDS). A basic biologic approach to lung injury and repair is needed. Can we find a common denominator resulting in ARDS which occurs in so many diverse situations?[6] Supportive measures, although they save many lives, have not improved survival much since their introduction to medicine 16 years ago.[7,8] Preventive therapy based upon early identification of the emerging syndrome; the development of pharmacologic blockers; methods to enhance oxygen tolerance; and a protection of the lung from dreaded sepsis are essential steps for future progress. Already, one marker possibly involved in the basic pathogenesis has been identified by members of our group.[9] Future progress is promised which will ultimately provide a basic cellular and pathologic approach to the problem.

Certainly, we must focus on nutritional problems associated with respiratory failure. Nutritional deficits are likely present in stages of chronic neuromuscular deterioration such as the muscular dystrophies and in cystic fibrosis, and they become intertwined in emerging respiratory failure. Children and young adults with muscular dystrophy and cystic fibrosis probably become weak and develop respiratory failure before their time. Similar problems may occur in patients with COPD. A ventilator patient may be difficult to wean because of poor nutrition. Thus, we must learn more about feeding patients and must employ the wisdom of the body in its selection of nutrients by feeding food into the gastrointestinal tract. We must also learn more about the respiratory muscles, the most vital pump.[10]

The rehabilitation of patients with chronic obstructive pulmonary disease has been an exciting chapter of respiratory care. Pragmatic approaches based upon patient education and involvement of the family, the use of oxygen systems which are more practical and less expensive, and physical conditioning techniques will continue to serve millions. We must learn more about sleep-disordered breathing in COPD.[11] Perhaps nocturnal events play a role in the early pathogenesis of this disease spectrum.

The high cost of modern critical care is of great concern.[12] Resources are soon to be limited. We will need better means of predicting recovery of brain function, and more realistic use of intensive care facilities.[13,14] The continual problem of shortages of trained nurses and of their retention needs a solution at all levels of medicine and nursing.[14] Bedside research in noninvasive and on-line monitoring is needed; costs are an almost overwhelming limitation today.[15] Cost considerations and solutions for the growing number of patients requiring home oxygen need attention.[16]

We must now place our priorities for research on prevention. Many of the problems described in this book are due to behavioral problems and are thus to an extent self-induced. Smoking, what we eat and drink, and how we drive our car or travel, and how we choose recreation determine the length and happiness of life for many people. Certainly, we must adventure, and not be constrained by unnecessary prohibition, and live a free and uninhibited life as much as possible. Mature and appropriate adventure, abandonment of certain imposed conventions, and taking chances here and there add zest and special meaning to life. The reverse is boredom, depression, and its attendant disasters. Living and breathing are intertwined, and it is with extreme gratification that we can accomplish this ourselves as we serve our patients today and beyond.

REFERENCES

1. Zapol, W.M., Snider, M.T., Hill, J.D., Fallat, R.J., Bartlett, R.H., Edmonds, L.H., Morris, A.H., Pierce, E., Converse, I.I., Thomas, A.N., Proctor, H.J., Drinker, P.A., Pratt, P.C., Bagniewski, A., and Miller, R.G.: Extracorporeal membrane oxygenation in severe acute respiratory failure (A randomized prospective study). JAMA, *242:*2193, 1979.
2. Kolobow, T., Stool, E.W., Sacks, K.L., and Vurek, G.G.: Acute respiratory failure (survival following ten days' support with a membrane lung). J. Thorac. Cardiovasc. Surg., *69:*9471, 1975.
3. Sjöstrand, U.H., and Eriksson, I.A.,: High rates and low volumes in mechanical ventilation—not just a matter of ventilatory frequency. Anesth. Analg., *59:*567, 1980.
4. Carlon, G.C., Kahn, R.C., Howland, W.S., Ray, C., and Turnbull, A.D.: Clinical experience with high frequency jet ventilation. Crit. Care Med., *9:*1, 1981.
5. Curlon, G.C., Miodownik, S., Ray, C., and Kahn, R.C.: Technical aspects and clinical implications of high frequency jet ventilation with a solenoid valve. Crit. Care Med., *9:*47, 1981.
6. Sanders, A.P., and Baylin, G.J.: A common denominator in the etiology of adult respiratory distress syndrome. Med. Hypothesis, *6:*951, 1980.
7. Ashbaugh, D.G., Bigelow, D.B., Petty, T.L., and Levine, B.E.: Acute respiratory distress in adults. Lancet, *2:*319, 1967.
8. Petty, T.L., and Ashbaugh, D.G.: The adult respiratory distress syndrome. Clinical features, factors influencing prognosis and principles of management. Chest, *60:*233, 1971.
9. Haynes, J.B., Hyers, T.M., Giclas, P.C., Franks, J.S., and Petty, T.L.: Elevated fibrin(ogen) degradation products in the adult respiratory distress syndrome. Am. Rev. Resp. Dis., *122:*841, 1980.
10. Rochester, D.F.: Respiratory disease: Attention turns to the air pump. Am. J. Med., *68:*803, 1980.
11. Block, A.J.: Respiratory disorders during sleep. Part I. Heart Lung, *9:*1011, 1980.
12. Zook, C.J., and Moore, F.D.: High-cost users of medical care. N. Engl. J. Med., *302:*996, 1980.
13. Wagner, I., and Greenbaum, D.M.: Central function monitoring in deeply comatose patients. Crit. Care Med., *9:*305, 1981.
14. Cullen, D.J.: Surgical intensive care: current perceptions and problems. Crit. Care Med., *9:*295, 1981.
15. Gothand, J.W.W., Basst, C.M., Branwaith, M.A., Davies, N.J.H., and Denison, D.M.: Applications of respiratory mass spectrometry and intensive care. Anesthaesia, *35:*890, 1980.
16. Roberts, S.D.: Cost-effective oxygen therapy. Ann. Intern. Med., *93:*499, 1980.

INDEX

Page numbers in *italics* refer to figures; page numbers followed by t refer to tables.